McNabb's Practical Guide to Joint and Soft Tissue Injection

Fifth Edition

James W. McNabb, MD
Private Practice—Family Medicine
Full Circle Family Medicine of Piedmont HealthCare
Mooresville, North Carolina

Francis G. O'Connor, MD, MPH
Professor
Department of Military and Emergency Medicine
Uniformed Services University of the Health Sciences
Bethesda, Maryland

Chad D. Hulsopple, DO
Director, Sports Medicine Fellowship
Associate Professor
Department of Military and Emergency Medicine
Uniformed Services University of the Health Sciences
Bethesda, Maryland

Wolters Kluwer
Philadelphia • Baltimore • New York • London
Buenos Aires • Hong Kong • Sydney • Tokyo

Acquisitions Editor: Joe Cho
Development Editor: Cindy Yoo
Editorial Coordinator: Anthony Gonzalez
Editorial Assistant: Kristen Kardoley
Marketing Manager: Janet Feeney
Senior Production Specialist: Bridgett Dougherty
Manager, Graphic Arts & Design: Stephen Druding
Manufacturing Coordinator: Lisa Bowling
Prepress Vendor: Straive

Fifth Edition

9 8 7 6 5 4 3 2 1

Printed in United States of America

Cataloging-in-Publication Data available on request from the Publisher

ISBN: 978-1-9752-6012-5

---

shop.lww.com

DEDICATION

This book is dedicated to those who make our work possible. We especially want to thank and recognize the understanding and support given by our wives, families, colleagues, staff, and patients.

Foreword

"Primary care providers trained to provide in-office procedures for their patients offer expertise, affordability, and convenience in a familiar, comfortable, and trusted setting."

—Thomas White, MD
Past president NCAFP and rural direct primary care family physician

Congratulations on the fifth edition of *McNabb's Practical Guide to Joint and Soft Tissue Injection*. If there is one medical text you choose to purchase and read this year, this should be it. I have known Dr. Jim McNabb for over 30 years, having taught with him at Cabarrus Family Medicine Residency Program and practiced with him as well. I can attest to his passion and competence in patient care. He is dedicated to medical education as well as providing to his patients the full breath of Family Medicine. Not only is he an expert in providing the care outlined in this book, but he also understands the need for additional training and resources in this area for primary care providers. He has made it his mission to advance this knowledge to the primary care community through this work and having taught hundreds of courses to colleagues around the country. The passion for the skills outlined in this book is evident in this latest release by Dr. McNabb and his coauthors. This is a text that should be on every primary care physician, PA or FNP's bookshelf and referred to regularly. If you have not had experience with these procedures, this book serves as a step-by-step educational resource to show you how. It is well illustrated with practical tips, evidence-based references, consent forms, patient instructions, and billing and coding procedures. The included point of view injection and ultrasound videos deliver the final layer of clarity—translating theory into sharp, practical focus.

The fifth edition's major enhancement is Dr. Chad Hulsopple's considerable contribution of ultrasound-guided injections in almost all the clinical injection chapters. This builds on Dr. Francis O'Connor's work in the fourth edition. This new fifth edition includes links to videos and will walk you through how to use ultrasound to enhance your ability to perform these procedures. The availability and affordability of ultrasound in the primary care setting opens up additional opportunities for service to our patients. It also improves the ability of primary care clinicians to confidently and effectively provide all the procedures and services outlined in this text.

Why are these skills important for primary care?

Musculoskeletal, soft tissue, and skin complaints are some of the most frequent conditions encountered in primary care practice. Given adequate training, the majority of these conditions can be competently treated by primary care providers. Patients referred for common conditions that we could easily treat must take another day off from work and sometimes travel to another location or city to see another physician. This is particularly a problem for those who practice in small or rural communities. If you are elderly or poor, the option for referral becomes even more problematic for many of the conditions easily treated by primary care.

Having managed Medicaid in North Carolina and having worked for decades on access to primary care for patients, I can speak directly to the fact that improving the access to comprehensive primary care for patients not only improves the health of the population but saves money. Community Care of NC was a 20-year experiment that proved this fact in the Medicaid population.

Congratulations again on the fifth edition of *McNabb's Practical Guide to Joint and Soft Tissue Injection!*

L. Allen Dobson Jr, MD
Family Physician 40 years (retired)
Editor-in-Chief, Medical Economics
President and CEO Community Care of North Carolina (retired)
Former President and Residency Director—Cabarrus Family Medicine and Cabarrus Family Medicine Residency Program
Emeritus Clinical Professor of Family Medicine—UNC School of Medicine
Former Assistant Secretary and Medicaid Director—NC DHHS

Preface

"The ability to perform procedures in the office setting allows family physicians to treat the whole person, not just the symptoms. This continuity not only improves outcomes, but ensures patients feel seen, heard and cared for at every stage of life."

—Jen Brull, MD,
Past president, American Academy of Family Physicians

Mercy! Have times changed. The last edition of this text was written at the onset of the COVID-19 coronavirus pandemic. At that time, we, as medical providers, were fighting an unseen monster without the benefit of diagnostic tests, treatment, or immunizations. Patients and colleagues died. Just going to work was seen as a near-heroic action. Wearing full PPE, masking, and keeping 6 ft apart were drilled into each of us. Care in the early phases at my small family practice office shifted to parking lot car visits and telemedicine. For quite some time, close contact was just not possible. But as caring primary care providers and emotional human beings, we crave that nearness. That of course extends into our relationships with our patients. Performing a careful physical examination, assessing causality, and administering treatment are all intimate actions that require close contact. Fortunately, we made it through the difficult times and are probably stronger and more resilient because of it. Telemedicine has its role, but in-person office visits remain the gold standard. This is the setting where we have the greatest impact. The primary potential disruptor now is the introduction of artificial intelligence. At this early point, it is being used beneficially to data mine opportunities to aid diagnosis of difficult medical cases, reduce administrative burden with care authorizations, improve the care of individual patients and populations, and significantly streamline patient visit documentation. Time will tell its impact, but only we as compassionate beings can lay our warm hands on the patient and provide immediate treatment as indicated, possibly by administering a therapeutic injection. Care by a human will always be better than a machine-derived algorithm.

In writing this new, completely updated, fifth edition, I pause to reflect on the examples set by my mentors, teachers, and colleagues. The ones that I respect most are those that prioritize the patient's well-being, possess a broad knowledge base, and display mastery of a wide range of procedures that are readily available to expertly diagnose and treat the next patient—and teach the next student. I would not mention their names, because if you are reading this, you already know them. They are the ones who spark your curiosity, inspire your journey, and show you what true caring and compassion is all about. We have met the same souls—yours just have different names.

Primary care providers are faced with a broad spectrum of medical conditions and patient presentations, with musculoskeletal disorders comprising a substantial portion of their clinical workload. This has been quantified at a prevalence of 33% by St. Sauver et al at the Mayo Clinic in 2013[1] and 21% by Keavy in 2025.[2] Proficiency in procedural care achieved during residency is a major driver of family physician scope of practice. In a 2024 survey of family medicine residency faculty published in the STFM journal, Family Medicine, Newman et al showed that 83% of respondents endorsed performing and teaching joint injections.[3] Although the report did not reveal the scope of these aspiration and injection procedures, the result suggests that this skill is being taught to most incoming family physicians. Recently, Ferderber and colleagues detailed how a successful musculoskeletal (MSK) ultrasound training workshop might be designed in a family medicine clerkship.[4] Encouragingly, family medicine residents have been shown to require relatively few clinical procedures to demonstrate competence and gain confidence in performing these.[5] Evidence now supports the benefit of primary care physicians performing musculoskeletal procedures, demonstrating advantages in cost-effectiveness, accessibility, and patient satisfaction—without compromising clinical outcomes, safety, or complication rates.[6]

Despite release of this text's fourth edition, a significant educational and practice gap persists in the areas of MSK conditions, MSK ultrasound, the use of orthobiologic applications, and other advanced and adjunctive injection techniques. For this reason, this text builds on the work of other, more competent physicians. It is my privilege to know COL (ret) Francis G. O'Connor, MD, MPH. Trained as a family physician, he is widely recognized as a leader in sports medicine, education, and research. Dr. O'Connor is professor and past chair of military and emergency medicine at the Uniformed Services University of the Health Sciences in Bethesda, Maryland. We have worked together for many years though our mutual faculty appointments with the American Academy of Family Physicians and the National Procedures Institute. Dr. O'Connor brings unique knowledge, a set of procedural skills, and teaching mastery regarding these issues. It was only natural that we combine resources, and I am very proud to continue to have him as co-author of this updated and greatly expanded text. I was fortunate that Dr. O'Connor introduced me to COL Chad Hulsopple, DO. He is the Director of the NCC Sports Medicine Fellowship and Associate Professor, Department of Family Medicine at the Uniformed Services University of the Health Sciences. Also trained as a family physician, he is a leader in sports medicine education and regarded as a leading expert in MSK ultrasound.

While teaching musculoskeletal and dermatology procedure courses, all three of us have found that primary care providers' learning needs include procedures that extend beyond traditional musculoskeletal injections. For this reason, we continue to take this project in a different direction from other injection textbooks with the inclusion of dermal anesthesia, nerve blocks, dermatology applications, and advanced techniques. The result of this collaboration represents the spectrum of useful, straightforward, effective, injection and aspiration procedures that can be performed with simple, inexpensive equipment in a full spectrum of medical settings. Although written from the perspective of practicing primary care providers in busy offices, these procedures cross specialty lines into emergency medicine, orthopedics, dermatology, anesthesia, radiology, pediatrics, and geriatrics. They may be employed in settings as diverse as outpatient offices, urgent care centers, nursing homes, emergency rooms, and inpatient facilities. This text is also commonly used for teaching purposes in medical schools, residency, and fellowship training programs.

The challenge of writing this new 5th edition lies in building on the success of previous texts by expanding content and stimulating thought, while keeping the work truly relevant and accessible to practicing clinicians. We have continued the text's focus on practically every needle-based procedure that can be performed in the primary care setting, except for spinal injections and cosmetic procedures. This entire edition has been updated and rewritten to add even more value. A major upgrade is the clinical application of MSK ultrasound. Dr. Hulsopple has made this contribution even better by developing "live" videos of ultrasound-guided needle injections for almost all MSK conditions. The inclusion of high-definition videos of landmark-guided injections and the addition of MSK ultrasound with associated videos truly sets this project apart from others. These videos are all case-based films that were recorded in real-time on actual patients, not models. Each gave their permission to use the images to advance medical education. A unique feature is that all videos were taken from the operator's viewpoint. The videos solidify learning after the user reviews the background information, local anatomy, landmarks, and techniques for each procedure. We remain grateful to Wolters Kluwer Health for their continued commitment to improving the quality of this work including the beautiful anatomic drawings in all chapters. This text is meant to serve as an extensively researched, current evidence-based, yet practical point of care resource for those clinicians who wish to learn and apply the techniques and finer details of these useful procedures.

I would like to acknowledge the following people and organizations who taught, encouraged, and helped me write this text. This project is a culmination of my 40 years of private family medicine practice and teaching. First, I must again thank my wife, Liz, for her support during my medical education, training, years of practice, teaching, and finally during the research and writing of this and previous texts. Without you, we could never have done this. The leadership and faculty of family medicine residency training programs at the University of Wyoming–Casper, Scottsdale HealthCare in Arizona and Cabarrus Family Medicine in North Carolina were instrumental in allowing me to expand my knowledge base, develop sports medicine and procedural curricula, and build expertise in evidence-based medicine. My office staff at Full Circle Family Medicine of Piedmont HealthCare in Mooresville, North Carolina, have been great—putting up with my demands and politely getting out of my way when I rush down the hall with "another great idea" or carrying video camera equipment. Without the confidence of my patients, I would never have been able to achieve mastery of these techniques—for that I am privileged to have served as your family physician. I am indeed blessed and truly continue to regard myself as a simple country doctor. I must acknowledge the opportunity to teach the Joint Injections workshops for the American Academy of Family Physicians, numerous state academies, and the Dermatologic Procedures workshops for National Procedures Institute over the years. Many thanks are directed to workshop and lecture participants for their involvement and honest feedback. Deserved recognition is extended to teaching faculty and colleagues who have provided encouragement, support, and stimulated my thinking. These physicians include Drs. Jack Pfenninger, Grant Fowler, Roy "Chip" Watkins, Kevin Burroughs, Chad Hulsopple, and of course, Francis O'Connor. Finally, a big thank you to those at Wolters Kluwer Health. In particular, Cindy Yoo—Development Editor, Anthony Gonzalez—Editorial Coordinator, and Joe Cho—Senior Acquisitions Editor. They have treated us with the utmost professionalism, support, and patience during the extremely long process of writing this fifth edition. To all involved, and so many more unintentionally left unnamed—Thank you and be healthy!

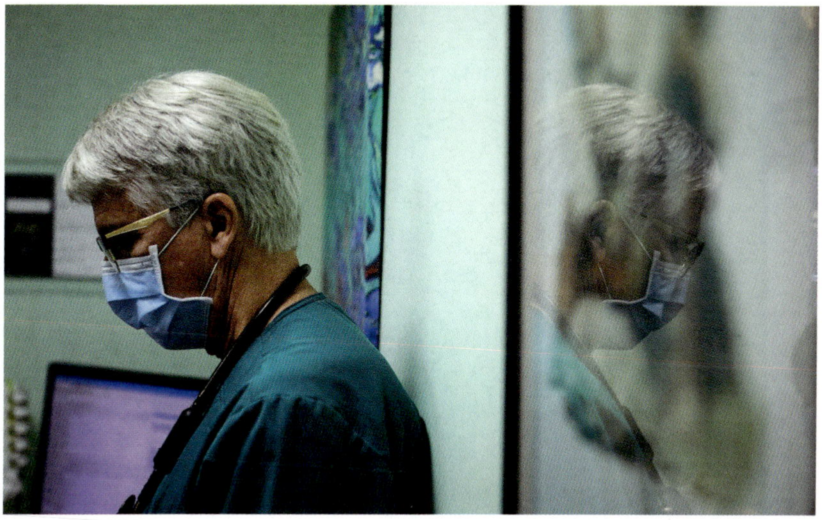

From Rowland C. Diagnosis for small family doctors: Less money, greater hardship, and patients on video. The Washington Post, 8 September, 2020. https://www.washingtonpost.com/business/2020/09/08/family-doctors-financial-crisis-coronavirus/. Used with permission.

James W. McNabb, MD

REFERENCES

1. St. Sauver JL, Warner DO, Yawn BP, et al. Why patients visit their doctors: assessing the most prevalent conditions in a defined American population. *Mayo Clin Proc.* 2013;88(1):56-67.
2. Keavy R, Horton R, Al-Dadah O. The prevalence of musculoskeletal presentations in general practice: an epidemiological study. *Fam Pract.* 2023;40(1):68-74.
3. Newman AR, Heidelbaugh JJ, Klemenhagen K, Michelfelder AJ, Power DV, Hougas JE III. Current procedural practices of family medicine teaching physicians. *Fam Med.* 2024;56(3):156-162.
4. Ferderber ML, Vann K, Tzaras A, Hadadi N, Gilbird RM. Evaluation of a musculoskeletal ultrasound workshop in the family medicine clerkship. *Fam Med.* 2022;54(1):54-57.
5. Sy J, Bloom J, Mizdrak N, Moaveni A, Toubassi D. Procedural skills training during residency: Introduction of a procedure clinic to improve technical competencies. *Can Fam Physician.* 2023;69(4):292-294.
6. Mohanty S, Mohanty A, Fainstad B, Parks ET, Irene WY. Joint efforts: a review of large joint and bursa steroid injections and aspirations by primary care physicians. *J Gen Intern Med.* 2025;40(13):3194-3206.

Contents

Videos

Videos of the following landmark-based and ultrasound-guided procedures (where available) can be found in the companion eBook edition.

ADVANCED AND ADJUNCTIVE TECHNIQUES

Auricular Battlefield Acupuncture Injection
Barbotage Injection
Tendon Brisement/High-Volume Injection
Fenestration Injection
Nerve Hydrodissection Injection
Capsular Hydrodilatation/Hydroplasty Injection
Tenotomy With Débridement Injection

SKIN ANESTHESIA

Direct Local Injection
Field Block Injection
Supraorbital and Supratrochlear Nerve Block Injection
Greater Occipital Neuralgia Injection
Headache Nerve Block Injection

SKIN AND SKIN STRUCTURES

Chalazion Injection
Keloid Scar Injection
Common Warts Injection
Granuloma Annulare and Other Thin, Benign, Inflammatory Dermatoses Injection

HEAD AND TRUNK

Temporomandibular Joint Injection
Suprascapular Neuropathy Injection
Scapulothoracic Syndrome Injection
Sacroiliac Joint Injection

UPPER EXTREMITIES

Landmark-Based Subacromial Space Injection—Posterior Approach
Ultrasound-Guided Subacromial-Subdeltoid Bursa Injection
Landmark-Based Glenohumeral Joint Injection—Posterior Approach
Ultrasound-Guided Glenohumeral Joint Injection
Landmark-Based Acromioclavicular Joint Injection
Ultrasound-Guided Acromioclavicular Joint Injection
Sternoclavicular Joint Ultrasound-Guided Injection

LOWER EXTREMITIES

Ultrasound-Guided Patellar Tendon Injection
Landmark-Based Pes Anserine Syndrome Injection
Ultrasound-Guided Pes Anserine Injection
Ultrasound-Guided Iliotibial Band Bursa Injection
Ultrasound-Guided Achilles Tendon Insertion Injection
Ultrasound-Guided Achilles Tendon Midsubstance Injection
Landmark-Based Tibialis Posterior Tendon Injection
Ultrasound-Guided Tibialis Posterior Tendon Sheath Injection
Ultrasound-Guided Tarsal Tunnel Syndrome Injection
Ankle Joint Injection—Anterolateral Approach
Landmark-Based Ankle Joint Injection—Anteromedial Approach
Ultrasound-Guided Tibiotalar Joint Injection (Ankle Joint)
Landmark-Based Fibularis Brevis Tendonitis Injection
Ultrasound-Guided Fibularis Tendon Sheath Injection
Landmark-Based Plantar Fascia Injection
Ultrasound-Guided Plantar Fascia Injection
Landmark-Based Midfoot joint Injection
Ultrasound-Guided Mid-foot Joint Injection
Landmark-Based First Metatarsophalangeal Joint Injection
Ultrasound-Guided Metatarsophalangeal Joint Injection
Morton Interdigital Neuroma Injection

1

Introduction

James W. McNabb

"Family Physicians trained to provide in-office procedures for their patients offer expertise, affordability, and convenience in a familiar, comfortable, and trusted setting."

—Dr. Thomas White, past president North Carolina Academy of Family Physicians, and rural family physician

The performance of joint and soft tissue injections and aspirations is a valuable skill that can be mastered by primary care physicians and qualified medical providers. These procedures help relieve pain and improve function for the patient, while at the same time, empowering the clinician, improving continuity of care, and decreasing health care costs. It is essential that these techniques be used thoughtfully and precisely—only after making the correct clinical diagnosis. This can be quite challenging at times but is no more difficult than diagnosing and treating any of the many other medical conditions that the primary care provider encounters on a daily basis. Learning how to accurately diagnose these conditions is beyond the scope of this text.

Our primary consideration is always the welfare of the patient. We must endeavor to provide the best medical care at the least risk of harm. This can be achieved by developing a cognitive knowledge base along with an accompanying set of complementary procedural skills. In addition, our focus must remain on providing a positive patient experience. This starts with active patient engagement and shared decision-making. It is then incumbent on us to provide a safe and supportive environment while ensuring a pain-free procedural experience. Patient satisfaction from a positive experience along with an excellent clinical outcome is our primary goal.

An important concept is that aspiration and injection therapy is not an end in itself. It is only one treatment option. The precise deposition of a therapeutic agent is a temporary measure that generally should be used as adjunctive therapy to other modalities. In many conditions, corticosteroid injection therapy used alone has been demonstrated to give only short- to intermediate-term pain/functional relief, with no difference in long-term results. In these cases, initial injection treatment in combination with other modalities and activity modification gives patients optimal long-lasting results. Additional therapeutic options may include relative rest, compression, splinting/casting, ice, heat, ultrasound, stretching, physical therapy, acupressure, administration of other medications, or even surgery. The performance of aspirations or injections alone, without correcting the underlying factors, is likely to result in recurrence if used without complementary treatments.

In this text, the following primary learning objectives are identified:

- Describe the indications and contraindications for each procedure.
- Review the current evidence-based medical literature.
- Select appropriate equipment/products for each procedure.
- Illustrate pertinent anatomic landmarks for each procedure.

- Perform injections and/or aspirations safely and effectively.
- Use ultrasound needle guidance to improve the safety, accuracy, and effectiveness of injections.
- Properly document and code the procedures.

The authors strongly recommend that all providers thoroughly read, study, and understand the information presented in the initial sections of this text BEFORE attempting to perform ANY of the procedures described in the subsequent technique chapters.

James W. McNabb, MD

2

Foundation Concepts

James W. McNabb

"It is more important to know what sort of person has a disease than to know what sort of disease a person has."

—Hippocrates

THOUGHTFUL CONSIDERATION

The evaluation and treatment of musculoskeletal conditions is a vital element of modern medical practice. With advancing insights into anatomy, biomechanics, pathophysiology, and cutting edge treatment options, primary care providers are equipped to make meaningful contributions to their patient's outcomes. The era of defaulting to nonsteroidal anti-inflammatory drugs (NSAIDs) and passive management with the hope that the condition would heal itself is behind us. Today's and tomorrow's care must be proactive, informed, and intentional.

This text serves as a guide to enhance the clinical understanding of techniques useful in treating common musculoskeletal disorders, as well as select dermatologic conditions, and anesthetic nerve blocks. As with any medical procedure, performing injections and aspirations places a great responsibility on the clinician. All invasive procedures should be done with a clear differential diagnosis and treatment plan in mind. They should never be performed indiscriminately.

Primum non nocere or "first, do no harm" is a fundamental principle of medicine. Before proceeding with any injection, the physician is obligated to consider the indications, contraindications, weight of evidence in the medical literature, expected benefits, possible side effects, anticipated outcomes, diagnostic certainty, his or her personal experience with the procedure, clinical experience, biases, the patient's response to previous interventions, and above all, the patient's values. Shared decision-making is a nuanced, individualized process requiring honest dialogue and reflective judgment with each patient. Furthermore, it is imperative that the clinician uses common sense and has self-awareness to know their limits before performing any medical procedure. In some cases, it may be preferable to use an alternative approach or request specialty consultation, rather than performing an invasive procedure. Put another way, just because one can do a procedure does not mean that one should do the procedure.

WHEN TO REFER TO A SUBSPECIALIST

While the majority of patients with musculoskeletal disorders can be competently managed by primary care providers, certain cases warrant referral to subspecialists. Standard indications include instances of diagnostic uncertainty, the provider feels uncomfortable performing a procedure, treatment has not produced the expected results, or the affected anatomical structures are difficult to access—particularly the spine, hip, or sacroiliac joints. Other referral indications include unsuccessful procedure attempts, possible septic arthritis, suspected inflammatory polyarthritis, recurrent monoarthritis unresponsive to treatment, or chronic monoarthritis of unknown origin. In such instances, appropriate referral options may include specialists in sports medicine, rheumatology, orthopedics, interventional radiology, or pain management. If an acute septic joint is suspected, the patient requires emergent inpatient hospitalization for joint drainage, débridement, irrigation, intravenous antibiotics, and possibly an infectious disease consultation in the case of an atypical infection.

STANDARD MEDICATION MANAGEMENT

Primary care providers commonly encounter musculoskeletal disorders. Traditionally, many of these have been managed using oral medications. While pharmacologic treatments play a key role, prescribers must remain vigilant regarding potential side effects and toxicities. Optimal pain management often requires a multimodal approach. In addition to drug treatment, psychosocial interventions to reduce anxiety, as well as physical interventions such as physical therapy, acupressure, and transcutaneous electrical nerve stimulation, can reduce pain, enhance pain coping skills, and restore function.

Clinical guidelines, regarding the management of acute pain from non–low back, musculoskeletal injuries in adults, were published by the American College of Physicians (ACP) and American Academy of Family Physicians (AAFP) in 2020.[1] The recommendations in the guidelines are based on a systematic review of the comparative safety and efficacy of drug and nondrug management of acute pain lasting less than 4 weeks. The review included 207 trials that enrolled 32,959 participants and evaluated 45 treatments. Their strongest recommendation with overall moderate-certainty evidence supports the first-line use of topical NSAIDs with or without menthol gel. This was the only intervention that documented positive effects in all three areas of pain relief, improvement in physical function, and patient satisfaction with treatment. A network meta-analysis incorporating randomized controlled trials and real-world data published in 2021 demonstrated that topical NSAIDs are equally effective as oral NSAIDs in managing knee osteoarthritis pain and outperform oral acetaminophen in terms of efficacy. Furthermore, topical NSAIDs were associated with reduced risks of all-cause mortality, cardiovascular diseases, and gastrointestinal (GI) bleeding compared to both oral NSAIDs and acetaminophen.[2]

Oral nonselective NSAIDs and selective cyclooxygenase-2 (COX-2) inhibitors are a very commonly employed class of medication used in the treatment of inflammatory conditions. However, many of the musculoskeletal conditions treated by primary care clinicians do not actually involve active inflammation in their pathogenesis. Nevertheless, these medications are commonly employed. The ACP/AAFP guidelines noted above give a conditional recommendation with moderate-certainty evidence to oral NSAIDs to reduce or relieve symptoms, including pain, and to improve physical function, or with oral acetaminophen to reduce pain.[1]

Unfortunately, NSAIDs and COX-2 inhibitors have significant side effects that extend beyond their well-recognized GI side effects, hepatotoxicity, nephrotoxicity, edema, increase in blood pressure, and exacerbation of congestive heart failure. A meta-analysis of 754 trials in 353,809 patients with greater than 233,798 pt years of follow-up was reported in 2013. COX-2 inhibitors and diclofenac were found to increase major vascular events by a third—primarily due to an increase in coronary events. Ibuprofen exhibited a comparable vascular risk profile, while high-dose naproxen was linked to comparatively lower risk.[3] A high-quality meta-analysis of four studies including 61,460 cases was published in 2017 in the BMJ. This showed that all NSAIDs, including naproxen, were found to be associated with an increased risk of acute myocardial infarction. Risk of myocardial infarction with celecoxib was comparable to that of traditional NSAIDs. Risk was greatest during the first month of NSAID use and with higher doses.[4] All NSAIDs double the risk of heart failure and increase the risk of upper GI complications.[3] A nationwide cohort study determined that even short-term treatment with most NSAIDs is associated with an increase in the risk of death and recurrent myocardial infarction in patients with prior myocardial infarction. Therefore, neither short- nor long-term treatment with NSAIDs is advised in this population. Any NSAID use should be limited from a cardiovascular safety point of view.[5]

Two large European population-based studies show that traditional NSAIDs and COX-2 inhibitors increase the incidence of atrial fibrillation.[6,7] A subsequent metanalysis confirmed this association.[8] The risk of atrial fibrillation seems to be particularly elevated in the initial 30 days of medication use. Since NSAIDs inhibit cyclooxygenase enzymes expressed in the kidneys, it is thought that this mechanism causes fluid retention, increases blood pressure, and leads to enlargement in both end-diastolic and end-systolic dimensions of the heart. Alternatively, the cardiac effects may stem not directly from the drugs themselves but from the inflammatory conditions and pain for which NSAIDs are commonly prescribed.

A large systematic review and meta-analysis published in 2015 showed that NSAIDs and COX-2 inhibitors also nearly double the risk of venous thromboembolism.[9] It is postulated that the inhibition of the COX-2 enzyme inhibits synthesis of prostacyclin leading to platelet activation and also stimulates the release of thromboxane causing platelet aggregation.

Although mild to moderately effective for pain relief, acetaminophen toxicity occurs on a frequent basis. In 2023, there were 78,993 acetaminophen-related exposures reported to the US National Poison Data System. Analgesics were the second most common substance category implicated in pediatric exposures and the most common in adult exposures.[10] About 2,000 cases of acute liver failure occur each year in the United States. Although not directly published in a Centers for Disease Control and Prevention-specific annual report, this figure is based on data from studies and expert consensus, including the Acute Liver Failure Study Group.[11] Unfortunately, approximately 500 people die each year in the United States from acetaminophen poisoning. A black box warning emphasizing the potential for severe liver injury and a warning highlighting the potential for allergic reactions (eg, swelling of the face, mouth, and throat, difficulty breathing, itching, or rash) are present on the label of all acetaminophen prescription drug products. Other reported side effects include anaphylaxis, acute renal tubular necrosis, anemia, thrombocytopenia, nausea, rash, and headache. A systematic literature review of eight studies by Roberts et al,[12] four showed an increase in cardiovascular adverse events (AE), one documented gastrointestinal AEs or bleeds, three showed renal AEs, and two reported increases in all-cause mortality. In 2013, the United States Food and Drug Administration published a news release informing the public of the potential of rare but severe skin reactions reported in individuals following acetaminophen ingestion. These reactions include Stevens-Johnson syndrome, toxic epidermal necrolysis, and acute generalized exanthematous pustulosis. All of these skin conditions are potentially fatal and can occur with even first exposure.[13]

Oral corticosteroid bursts are frequently prescribed. However, they may pose significant risks that are unrecognized by many practitioners. In a 2020 population-based study from Taiwan, over 15 million patients received oral steroids for a median duration of 3 days. The incidence of GI bleeding increased by a factor of 1.8, sepsis doubled, and heart failure increased by 2.4 times the controls. These AEs were noted within 5 to 30 days after steroid initiation.[14]

A Cochrane Database systematic review in 2019 downgraded the benefit of tramadol. Compared to placebo, tramadol alone or in combination with acetaminophen probably has no important benefit on pain or function in people with osteoarthritis. Moderate quality evidence shows that AEs probably cause substantially more participants to stop taking this medication.[15]

According to the 2020 ACP/AAFP guidelines,[1] opioids including tramadol should not be prescribed for managing acute pain from non–low back musculoskeletal causes, except in cases of severe injury or when first-line therapies are not effective. This class of medication is associated with little to no benefit in patients with acute non–low back pain. There are substantial harms, such as the potential for longer-term addiction and overdose. Avoiding prescribing opioids for acute musculoskeletal injuries to patients with past or current substance use disorder and restricting duration to 7 days or less and using lower doses when they are prescribed are potentially important targets to reduce rates of persistent opioid use.[16] A number of AEs, including serious events, are associated with the medium- and long-term use of opioids for chronic noncancer pain. A Cochrane review published in 2017 showed that the absolute event rate for any AE with opioids in trials using a placebo as comparison was 78%, with an absolute event rate of 7.5% for any serious AE.[17] Based on the AEs identified, clinically relevant benefit would need to be clearly demonstrated before long-term use could be considered in people with chronic noncancer pain in clinical practice.

Duloxetine, a serotonin and norepinephrine reuptake inhibitor, is often used for adjunctive treatment of chronic musculoskeletal pain. It has been shown to produce modest to moderate relief of pain, functional improvement, better mood regulation, and improvement in quality of life. This medication is usually well tolerated with mild AEs in the treatment of osteoarthritis and chronic low back pain. Side effects include nausea, fatigue, dizziness, and dry mouth. A recent review confirmed low cardiovascular risk.[18]

Glucosamine and chondroitin sulfate are over-the-counter dietary supplements that are commonly taken by patients in an effort to reduce pain from osteoarthritis. Unfortunately, despite their popularity, the data showing any benefit are weak and the data showing efficacy are conflicting. A meta-analysis of 18 articles published in 2018 by Ogata found a marginally favorable effect of glucosamine on pain and a small, nonsignificant effect on knee joint function.[19]

Given the relatively low efficacy and considerable toxicity of standard pharmacologic oral medications to control pain and progression of common musculoskeletal disorders, it is incumbent on medical practitioners to consider the use of other treatment options that may be more effective and pose less toxicity. There is often a good response to conservative measures of weight loss, relative rest, acupressure,[1] and utilization of devices such as casts, splints, orthotics, transcutaneous electrical nerve stimulation units, extracorporeal shock wave therapy, and others. Formal physical therapy is also quite helpful in those patients who are able to fully participate but is commonly underutilized.[20] Other treatment options include many of the needle-based injection and aspiration procedures in this text.

INDICATIONS FOR INJECTIONS AND ASPIRATIONS

There are numerous diagnostic and therapeutic indications for performing injection and aspiration procedures. Diagnostically, injecting local anesthetic into a joint or soft tissue structure can temporarily relieve pain, allowing for a more thorough clinical evaluation. Pain often restricts musculoskeletal assessment due to both voluntary and involuntary guarding of the affected area. Muscle spasm commonly develops in response, further limiting the range of motion of the area examined. By alleviating pain, the clinician can more effectively assess the area of interest, which is crucial for evaluating the underlying structures including muscles, tendons, ligaments, and cartilage.

Important clinical management decisions may be made based on the results of a diagnostic injection. For example, a patient may present with acute shoulder pain. Upon examination, the patient complains of moderately severe pain, holds the shoulder at her side, and is unable to demonstrate shoulder abduction. The clinical question may be whether the patient has a complete tear of the shoulder rotator cuff complex or if subacromial impingement of the rotator cuff is the culprit. The clinician may elect to perform a subacromial space injection of 1 to 2 mL of the local anesthetic, 1% mepivacaine. If after 1 minute, the patient is now able to demonstrate full range of motion including unrestricted abduction, then this "impingement test" indicates that pain was the limiting factor in her inability to abduct the shoulder. Consequently, there is not a complete tear of the rotator cuff structures. The patient may be able to continue to receive conservative care directed by the primary medical provider without a requirement for specialty referral at that particular time.

Fluid may also be obtained upon aspiration of a joint or soft tissue space. If so, then it should be grossly examined for color, clarity, and the presence of blood. Normal synovial fluid is clear and transparent. The fluid may contain blood that indicates a hemorrhagic cause—most commonly acute trauma. It may also be yellow due to xanthochromia from the breakdown of hemoglobin due to trauma or inflammation. The clarity of the fluid may be altered by the presence of white blood cells (WBCs). Crystals and cellular debris can also decrease clarity. Microscopic examination of the fluid—used to evaluate for cells, crystals, bacteria, and blood—is essential for accurate assessment and will be discussed in a subsequent section.

Therapeutically, injections and aspirations serve a wide range of clinical purposes. Simply removing excess fluid from a joint can provide substantial pain relief and restore joint range of motion. With relatively small joints such as the elbow, this can occur with the removal of as little as 3 to 5 mL of fluid. In a large knee joint, the clinician may remove as much as 100 to 150 mL of fluid in chronic conditions!

Indications for therapeutic injections include crystal arthropathies, synovitis, rheumatoid arthritis, other nonseptic inflammatory arthritides, osteoarthritis, and osteoarthrosis. Soft tissue indications include bursitis, tendonitis, tendinosis, epicondylitis, trigger points, ganglion cysts, neuromas, nerve entrapment syndromes, and fasciitis. In these cases, relief is often achieved through the precise delivery of a corticosteroid/local anesthetic mixture.

Corticosteroid injections may also be given directly into lesions in patients with skin diseases as diverse as hypertrophic scars, keloids, lichen planus, lichen simplex chronicus, psoriasis, prurigo nodularis, alopecia areata, and discoid lupus.

Injection of local anesthetics into skin structures or around nerves temporarily blocks pain. This is clinically important in order to allow the performance of otherwise painful surgical procedures.

CONTRAINDICATIONS TO INJECTIONS AND ASPIRATIONS

While understanding the indications of aspirations and injections is important, it is perhaps even more valuable to recognize the situations in which these procedures should not be performed. Absolute contraindications include performance of a procedure on an uncooperative patient, history of true allergy to the proposed injected medication, injection through infected tissues, and injection of corticosteroid into critical weight-bearing tendons. In particular, the injection of steroid into and around the Achilles, patellar, and quadriceps tendons may result in catastrophic rupture of these vital structures. Recovery from such rupture is often difficult, prolonged, and incomplete.

Many relative contraindications exist. These are variable and may apply only to certain patients or situations. Some of these include procedures near critical structures such as arteries, veins, nerves, or pleural surfaces. Also, caution must be exercised in patients with coagulation disorders, immunocompromised states, complicated diabetes, history of avascular necrosis, previous joint replacement at the injection site, allergy to the preservative in the injected solution, and excessive anxiety concerning the procedure and in patients who may not follow postprocedure instructions.

Patients receiving corticosteroids may experience activation of latent disease or an exacerbation of infections caused by amoeba, *Borrelia burgdorferi* (Lyme disease), *Candida*, *Cryptococcus*, *Mycobacterium*, *Nocardia*, *Pneumocystis*, *Strongyloides* (threadworm), *Toxoplasma*, or others.

The Society of Interventional Radiology 2020 consensus guidelines stratify musculoskeletal percutaneous procedures as having a low risk of bleeding.[21] However, there are many clinical situations where the risk of bleeding may be increased. A review of each patient's comorbidities, medications, and coagulation parameters should be considered prior to proceeding with a procedure. Coagulopathies such as hemophilia and von Willebrand disease predispose patients to bleeding complications including hemarthrosis and compartment syndrome. Certain conditions such as cirrhosis, chronic liver disease, chronic kidney disease, and vitamin K deficiency can increase the possibility of bleeding. In addition, anticoagulant, antiplatelet, acetylsalicylic acid (aspirin), and nonsteroidal anti-inflammatory medications all increase bleeding risk. The patient's coagulation profile including prothrombin time/international normalized ratio (INR), hemoglobin, and platelet count may need to be evaluated and any corrections made prior to an invasive procedure.

In patients treated with anticoagulants, the practitioner must weigh the risk of bleeding associated with a needle-based procedure against the possibility of thrombosis occurring if the anticoagulation therapy is withheld or reversed. Patients taking the oral anticoagulant medication, warfarin, do not represent an absolute contraindication to injection or aspiration. In the journal *Arthritis and Rheumatism* in 1998, Thumboo and O'Duffy reported the results of a prospective cohort study of 32 joint and soft tissue injections and aspirations involving patients attending a rheumatology clinic taking warfarin with an INR less than 4.5. Patients followed up for 4 weeks after the procedure showed no significant hemorrhages.[22] This has also been the author's experience in many more patients (unpublished). In a systematic review and meta-analysis by Tarar et al in 2023, eight studies involving 871 procedures were included. There were only five reported cases of bleeding. On meta-analysis, the estimated bleeding complication rate was 1.5% (95% CI 0.5%-4.5%). This meta-analysis supports the safety of performing joint injections and aspirations in patients receiving warfarin therapy without the need for routine preprocedural INR testing.[23] No clinical trials involving injection procedures have been reported to date on patients receiving antiplatelet drugs, thrombolytics, fibrinolytics, low molecular weight heparin, or the newer oral anticoagulant medications including direct thrombin inhibitors (dabigatran and others) and factor Xa inhibitors (apixaban, betrixaban, edoxaban, rivaroxaban, and others). Data on the safety of the performance of injection procedures in patients taking warfarin should not be extended to these anticoagulation agents.

SPECIAL MEDICAL CONDITIONS

Several medical conditions deserve special consideration. Diabetes is a very common and increasingly prevalent medical condition in the primary care patient population. Because of the frequent association with obesity, these patients often place metabolic and mechanical stress on joint and soft tissues that may be amenable to treatment using therapeutic injections. While elevated blood glucose levels are a concern, research indicates that the temporary increase following intra-articular steroid injections is typically not clinically significant. In patients with well-controlled diabetes, a single steroid injection into the knee may cause acute hyperglycemia lasting from 2 to 3 days.[24,25] Injections into the shoulder can also lead to a brief rise in postprandial glucose levels, especially with higher or repeated doses, though average glucose levels generally remain unaffected.[26] These short-term elevations in blood sugars can usually be well controlled with carbohydrate restriction, continuation of the usual diabetes treatment regimen, and close monitoring of blood sugars for a few days following injection. However, the presence of diabetes may reduce the overall effectiveness of injected corticosteroid treatment.

There is concern about the risk of bleeding when administering injections to patients taking oral anticoagulants including aspirin, NSAIDs, antiplatelet agents, warfarin, direct thrombin inhibitors (dabigatran and others), and factor Xa inhibitors (apixaban, betrixaban, edoxaban, rivaroxaban, and others). This issue was discussed above in the section on Contraindications.

Septic arthritis is a medical emergency. A joint infection is a very serious condition with dire consequences to the integrity of the joint and surrounding structures. All efforts must be made to diagnose septic arthritis as soon as possible and to provide emergent hospitalization. The patient requires treatment including surgical drainage with irrigation of the affected joint, administration of intravenous antibiotics, and pain control. This is best done in a coordinated fashion by the primary care physician with an orthopedic surgeon, and possibly an infectious disease subspecialist. Common organisms causing joint infections are *Streptococcus/Staphylococcus* species, *Neisseria gonorrhoeae*, and, increasingly, methicillin-resistant *Staphylococcus aureus.*

Rheumatoid arthritis presents unique challenges to the primary care provider. This is a destructive, rapidly progressive inflammatory arthritis. Lytic enzymes quickly degrade the joint surfaces, synovium, and supporting structures unless the process is interrupted and controlled. Joint and soft tissue injections play an important role in medical care because they can be used to deliver relatively small doses of corticosteroids locally in the affected joint(s) to augment the overall systemic management of this condition.

Management of pain involving joint replacement devices demands special consideration. Pain involving a joint replacement often occurs because the normal biomechanics are altered. Other causes of pain may include excessive postoperative scar tissue and poorly fitting or loose components of prostheses. Simple injections of corticosteroids or other substances often do not lead to meaningful improvement in the patient's pain and certainly do not correct any underlying biomechanical abnormality. There is also the possibility that an injection may be complicated by an infection of the prosthetic joint with catastrophic outcomes. In these patients, it is usually more prudent to not perform injections and to immediately refer the patients back to their orthopedic surgeon for the management of this challenging problem.

COMPLICATIONS

Complications from needle-based procedures used in injections and aspirations fall into two categories—systemic and local.[27] Systemic complications include vasovagal reactions, local anesthetic-related complications, and corticosteroid-related complications. Patients can develop allergic reactions including anaphylaxis. Other serious toxicities of local anesthetics may involve cardiac arrhythmias and seizures—but usually with inadvertent intravascular administration of doses far in excess of the amounts used with soft tissue and joint injections. Systemic complications linked to corticosteroid injections include vascular flushing, elevated blood sugar levels in patients with diabetes, impaired immune response, psychological disturbances, hypothalamic pituitary adrenal axis suppression, irregular menses, abnormal vaginal bleeding, and osteoporosis. Patients receiving corticosteroid therapy are also at an increased risk of acute infections or reactivation of an old infection due to decreased immune resistance with an inability to localize infections. This risk of infection exists with any pathogen (viral, bacterial, fungal, protozoan, or helminthic) at any location of the body. Infections may be mild or severe, and the risk of complications increases with greater doses of corticosteroid. In addition, corticosteroid therapy may mask the signs and symptoms of an active infection.

Local complications from corticosteroid injections may involve bleeding, infection, osteonecrosis of juxta-articular bone, ligament rupture, or tendon rupture. Intratendinous corticosteroid injection can lead to tendon rupture.[28-30] This is likely to occur through the inhibition of tenocyte proliferation[31] and the reduction in the strength of isolated collagen fascicles. Alternatively, the injection may attenuate pain-mediated protective mechanisms, thereby permitting excessive tensile loading of the tendon and increasing the likelihood of structural failure or rupture. Pneumothorax has been reported as a complication of trigger point injections of back muscles.[32] Injuries to the radial artery can occur with attempted aspiration of large volar wrist ganglion cysts.[33]

Localized skin complications may include depigmentation, dermal atrophy, and subcutaneous fat atrophy. These are most noticeable after injection of superficial structures but can also be seen after an intra-articular injection. This is presumably due to inadvertent superficial injection of corticosteroid or reflux of corticosteroid along the needle track back into the subcutaneous fat or dermis. It can take up to 2 months for skin effects to manifest. Skin depigmentation normalizes in most patients over a period of 1 year.[34] Although skin atrophy usually resolves, effects lasting longer than 5 years have been reported.[35] The extent and duration of such skin complications is likely related to the solubility and concentration of the corticosteroid preparation. Interestingly, normal saline infiltration has been shown to rapidly reverse local corticosteroid skin atrophy.[36]

Postinjection flare is a local phenomenon commonly believed to be due to a reaction to steroid crystals in the soft tissue and/or synovial space. The reaction occurs 6 to 24 hours following corticosteroid injection. Although the flare has been attributed in the past to crystalline corticosteroids, this is controversial and has no support in the medical literature. However, a clinically identical reaction occurs from local inflammation mediated through TRPA1 cation channels expressed in peripheral neurons. TRPA1 is sensitive to many irritants including the commonly used preservative, methylparaben.[37,38] Multidose vials of plain lidocaine, lidocaine with epinephrine, and bupivacaine all contain 1 mg of methylparaben. If a patient has a history of a "postinjection flare," "steroid flare," or "lidocaine allergy," then single use vials of 1% lidocaine that do not contain a preservative might be carefully used instead. In either case, an acute postinjection reaction can be managed using oral NSAIDs, and ice application after a repeat aspiration confirms that there is no infection.

There has been increasing concern following recent reports of toxicity of amide local anesthetics on chondrocytes. This effect has been reported with lidocaine and bupivacaine with in vitro studies[39,40] and confirmed with in vivo trials.[41-43] Of these, mepivacaine and ropivacaine may be the least toxic agents.[44] The evidence suggests that there is a greater risk for chondrolysis with longer exposure to a high concentration of local anesthetic, such as with the use of a continuous infusion of anesthetic via a pain pump following orthopedic surgery.[45] However, toxic late cellular and metabolic changes are seen even after a single injection of local anesthetic in animal models.[46] Some studies suggest that the preservatives and the pH of the local anesthetic solution may also play a role in chondrotoxicity.[47]

Intra-articular injection of local anesthetics differs from that of continuous intra-articular infusion. Chondrocyte toxicity to the anesthetic directly correlates with the length of exposure to the product. The uptake and clearance of the anesthetic in the joint or soft tissues is dependent on several factors related to the physiochemical properties of the local anesthetic and local blood flow. Uptake tends to be delayed for local anesthetics with high lipophilicity and protein binding.[48] Of the amide local anesthetics, bupivacaine has the greatest values for these properties and probably has the longest residence time in tissues.[49] In a systematic review of the effects of a single dose of local anesthetics on cartilage in 2017, Kreuz et al included 12 studies with 4 different anesthetics. They found a toxic effect on chondrocytes and cartilage that increased in a type-, dose-, and time-dependent fashion, especially on osteoarthritic cartilage. In this review, bupivacaine and lidocaine were more chondrotoxic than mepivacaine and ropivacaine.[44]

There is evidence that corticosteroids may also have deleterious effects on cartilage. In 2017, McAlindon et al[50] published the results of a randomized clinical trial in JAMA. They injected the knees of 140 patients with symptomatic knee osteoarthritis with corticosteroids every 3 months and measured the volume of knee cartilage with MRI scans. They showed that at the end of 2 years, there was a loss of 0.29 mm of cartilage thickness in patients injected with triamcinolone versus 0.13 mm in the saline group, with no significant difference on knee pain severity between treatment groups. Further, a systematic review by Wernecke et al[51] showed that corticosteroids have a time- and dose-dependent effect on articular cartilage, with beneficial effects occurring at low doses and durations and detrimental effects at high doses and durations.

SAFETY

To ensure the safety of both patient and operator, specific procedural protocols must be followed. First, the provider should clearly identify local anatomic landmarks. This step is critical to confirm that needle advancement is performed with a knowledge of the underlying structures. Next, universal precautions must be observed at all times to prevent inadvertent exposure to blood and body fluids. The use of personal protective equipment is mandatory. However, for the majority of injections and aspirations, nonsterile examination gloves are sufficient. For almost all outpatient clinical situations, the use of sterile gloves, drapes, gowns, or masks is typically unnecessary—provided that strict adherence to medical antiseptic technique is maintained throughout the procedure.

In order to decrease the chance of needle stick injury, there are a variety of safer-sharps needle systems available for use. It is the practitioner's responsibility to utilize one of these safer designs to avoid injury and maintain compliance with OSHA regulations. After use, all sharps must be placed immediately in a puncture-resistant sharps container. Filled sharps containers are then disposed in accordance with state-regulated medical waste rules.

Medical antiseptic techniques are always used when performing invasive procedures. Common antiseptic products commercially available as prep pads include 10% povidone-iodine aqueous and 2% chlorhexidine-alcohol solutions. Both are broad spectrum antiseptics with activity against gram-positive bacteria, gram-negative bacteria, fungi, and enveloped viruses. Chlorhexidine-alcohol has been shown to be significantly more effective than povidone-iodine in preventing postoperative superficial and deep surgical site infections.[52,53] In patients undergoing neuraxial blockade procedures, alcohol-based chlorhexidine-alcohol significantly lowers the incidence of insertion site colonization compared with the use of povidone-iodine.[54] These studies are consistent with others demonstrating superior clinical efficacy of chlorhexidine versus povidone-iodine in reducing the bacterial concentration in the operative field in foot and ankle surgery.[55,56] Further, chlorhexidine gluconate is not inactivated by blood or serum proteins, whereas this occurs with iodophors.[57,58] Lower postoperative infection rates with chlorhexidine-alcohol is thought to be related to chlorhexidine's more rapid action, persistent activity, and residual antimicrobial effect.[59] Antiseptics should be allowed to dry according to the manufacturer's recommendation.

Using a medical aseptic technique does not imply that the procedure must be done in a sterile operating room environment. However, it does require that the provider takes the necessary precautions to ensure a minimal chance that infectious organisms are carried into the tissues by the needle. When performing injections and aspirations, the operator must always follow the antiseptic, "no-touch" technique. This procedure does not allow for any contact of the injection site after sterile preparation of the skin. Following identification of the local landmarks, the injection site is marked with ink. Then, an impression in the skin is made at that site by applying firm pressure with the retracted tip of a ballpoint pen. Next, the injection site is cleansed with alcohol, followed by application of an antiseptic agent (10% povidone-iodine aqueous or 2% chlorhexidine-alcohol). After these steps are completed, there is no further contact or touching of the site with any nonsterile objects. The only object that comes into contact with this site is the tip of the sterile needle.

It is important to use needles and syringes for only a single, individual patient. These must never be used on other patients or reused on the same patient. If single-dose (single-use) medication vials are used, then they must only be used for only one patient. Because these vials do not contain preservative, they can never be reused, even at a later time with the same patient. The rubber stopper on a medication vial must be cleaned with alcohol prior to piercing it. Medication vials are entered with a new needle and a new syringe even when obtaining additional doses for the same patient.

Always attempt to aspirate before injecting any substance into tissues. This will confirm that the needle tip is not inside a blood vessel. Performing this simple maneuver ensures that inadvertent intravascular injection of the injection solution does not occur.

Place the injection *within* a joint or bursa and *around* a tendon. An injection into the substance of a tendon is likely to weaken that structure. Rupture may follow—especially if it is a weight-bearing tendon such as the Achilles, patellar, or quadriceps tendons. Also, avoid injecting directly into nerves. Such an injection is often evident since the patient usually reports pain, paresthesias, or numbness at the instant of needle contact with a nerve. In this case, simply withdraw the needle slightly and attempt to reposition it before proceeding with the injection.

After the injection has been completed, sterile gauze is used to wipe the site, and if necessary, apply direct pressure. Finally, a sterile adhesive dressing is applied. The needles are immediately disposed in a puncture-resistant sharps container. Following the procedure, the patient should remain in the office for a period of time in which the office staff observes the patient for any signs of systemic or local reactions.

ANATOMY

It is critical that the clinician has a complete understanding of the three-dimensional anatomy and the structure's function in each area that is selected for injection and/or aspiration. A thorough knowledge of the target area brings a deeper understanding of the pathologic process causing the patient's symptoms. This makes the physical examination maneuvers meaningful. Finally, it enables the provider to develop a list of alternative diagnostic possibilities. With this knowledge, the physician is able to take the next step. They can understand structural relationships beneath the surface of the skin. The physician is then able to think in three dimensions. While advancing the needle, it is important to "visualize" the location of the needle as it passes through the anatomic structures. Performing these thought processes enables the clinician to clinically determine the location of the needle tip in "real time." This results in improved clinical outcomes through the accurate placement of a therapeutic product or the insertion of a large-bore needle for fluid aspiration. Complications from needle trauma are also minimized by avoidance of critical structures.

LANDMARKS

For each injection or aspiration procedure, the physician must identify the pertinent local anatomic landmarks. These are areas that represent underlying bony prominences or easily identifiable soft tissues. The landmarks are specific to each injection site. After identification, the structures should be marked on overlying skin with ink by using either a ballpoint pen or a surgical marker. Next, the entry site for the needle is indicated with ink. Then an indentation in the skin is created by applying firm pressure over the ink mark using the retracted tip of a ballpoint pen. An indentation must be done since aseptic preparation of the area will remove ink marks. This process gives the clinician a visual frame of reference and standardizes the procedure from one patient to the next. No matter how much experience a physician has with a procedure, the process of identifying and marking the landmarks and entry site should not be skipped. After committing the landmarks to a surface drawing, the patient is instructed not to move that area of the body. Repositioning may change the relationships between the skin markings and the underlying anatomy.

TOPICAL ANESTHESIA

Providing the patient a pain-free experience is the responsibility of the primary care provider.[60] In select injections, such as the posterior approach to the subacromial space, techniques such as stretching/pinching the skin and other dermal stimulation may give adequate distraction to the patient so that pain from needle insertion is not experienced.

Painless local anesthesia via percutaneous needle introduction can be achieved by use of either skin cooling or application of a topical local anesthetic agent. A topical vapocoolant spray can be used to give rapid onset of brief, but effective, skin numbness. These skin refrigerants cause a brief period of noncytotoxic cooling of the epidermis. This provides up to 30 seconds of local anesthetic effect, which blocks the pain associated with needle injections. The mechanism of action for anesthesia is to decrease nerve conduction velocity of the A-delta fibers and C fibers of the peripheral nervous system, thus interrupting nociceptive input to the spinal cord. A meta-analysis by Zhu et al[61] in 2018 documented that a vapocoolant spray significantly decreases pain during intravenous cannulation when compared with placebo spray or no treatment in both adults and children.

The classic vapocoolant agent, Gebauer's Ethyl Chloride, is available in glass bottle and metal can containers. Both vessels are held at 3 to 9 in away from the treatment area in a well-ventilated space. The bottle is held upside down, while the Accu-Stream 360 canister may be held in any position. The stream of Ethyl Chloride is sprayed continuously to the site for 3 to 7 seconds from the bottle and for 4 to 10 seconds from the can, or until the skin just turns white—whichever occurs first. The needle is then immediately inserted into the skin. Extra caution must be exercised when using Ethyl Chloride as this product is flammable. It should never be used in the setting of open flames or sparks—including cautery units, hyfrecators, electrosurgical machines, radiofrequency devices, intense pulsed light generators, or lasers.

Alternatively, Gebauer's Pain Ease (a proprietary mixture of 1,1,1,3,3-pentafluoropropane and 1,1,1,2-tetrafluoroethane) is available both as a medium stream spray and as an aerosolized mist spray. These products are distributed in pressurized metal cans and are nonflammable products. Both Pain Ease products are administered at a distance of 3 to 7 in from the target site by holding the can in an upright position. They are sprayed for 4 to 10 seconds until the skin begins to frost. Do not spray for longer than 10 seconds. The medium stream produces a pinpoint stream in a smaller target site. The fine droplets of mist are dispersed in a 3-cm diameter circular pattern. Adequate local anesthesia for needle injection or minor surgical procedures lasts up to 30 seconds. Pain Ease is not carcinogenic or teratogenic and, thus, may be used safely in pregnancy when used as directed. Furthermore, this product offers advantages over Ethyl Chloride, including a larger field of anesthesia and lack of "running" of liquid down the skin (with use of the mist spray) and no fire hazard. In contrast to Ethyl Chloride which is only approved for use on intact skin, Pain Ease may also be used on minor skin wounds and intact mucous membranes. With prolonged contact, both Ethyl Chloride and Pain Ease may damage polyvinylchloride coverings used to upholster examination tables. Barrier pads used during injections effectively keep the vapocoolant fluid from contact with the upholstery.

Ethyl Chloride and Pain Ease do not claim to be sterile, but the products have passed the Microbial Limit Test in accordance with the United States Pharmacopeia. These tests are designed to demonstrate that a substance is free from *S aureus*, *Escherichia coli*, *Pseudomonas aeruginosa*, and *Salmonella* species. Those tests also measure total bacteria, mold, and yeast growth.[62] A 2012 study showed that Ethyl Chloride may be an effective disinfectant alone and may improve skin disinfection when used with povidone-iodine compared to povidone-iodine alone.[63] Thus, there does not appear to be a need to wipe the field with an antiseptic agent again following the application of a topical vapocoolant spray. In addition, ethyl chloride bottles used in the clinical settings show no bacterial or fungal contamination through their shelf life and routine use.[64]

EQUIPMENT

It is strongly recommended that medical providers prepare and organize all equipment and supplies required for injections and aspirations in advance. Proper organization ensures that materials are readily accessible, streamlining the procedure and minimizing the time spent gathering items. This proactive approach also helps reduce the risk of unintended medical errors. All necessary tools should be arranged well before the procedure begins to support efficiency and patient safety.

Based on provider or organization preference, four options can be utilized.

1. A dedicated cabinet
2. An injection tray
3. An injection cart
4. Injection packs

A cabinet works well in a setting where the provider consistently works out of the same room. It keeps the supplies centralized and visible but requires collection of the various components at the time a procedure is performed. A large plastic tray or an injection cart provides a portable option for organizing materials. These may work well in a large clinic or teaching setting. Another option is to create "injection packs" that include all of the supplies used universally in these procedures.

After many years of performing these procedures, the author's preferred option in his private medical office is to store materials in a central location. Then, individual injection packs are organized by medical office assistants prior to patient visits. These are placed with associated medications and various syringe and needle options inside a secure cabinet in each examination room. When a patient presents with a condition that requires an injection or aspiration, a pack is simply retrieved from the cabinet and placed on the counter in the examination room. The author uses those materials but is also free to select other syringe sizes and/or needle lengths from the cabinet. At the time of the injection, the author or his staff fills the injection syringe with the appropriate medication(s) and secures the correct needle. This preprocedure organization enhances office efficiency and reduces the possibility of a medical mistake.

Items that should be collected and organized (Fig. 2.1):

- Gloves—nonsterile exam gloves
- Barrier "chucks" pads—nonsterile

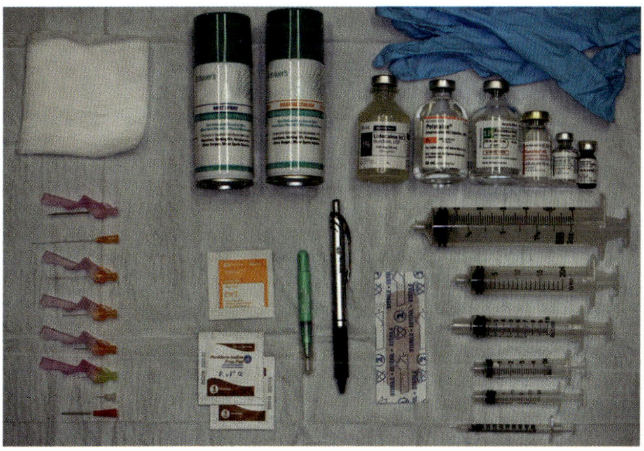

FIGURE 2.1 • Equipment for injections and aspirations.

- Alcohol pads
- 10% povidone-iodine pads or 2% chlorhexidine-70% alcohol pads
- Gauze pads—nonsterile
- Adhesive bandages
- Hemostat surgical clamp (optional)
- Syringes
  - 3 mL
  - 5 mL
  - 10 mL
  - 20 mL
  - 60 mL
- Needles
  - 18 to 20 gauge—1-in blunt tip fill needle—for drawing medications
  - 20 gauge—1 in—for aspiration of small joints
  - 18 gauge—1½ in—for aspiration of large joints and bursa
  - 25 gauge—5/8, 1, 1½, and 2 in—for injections
  - 20 gauge—3½ in spinal needles—for deep injections/aspirations
- Pain Ease mist or medium stream vapocoolant spray
- Lidocaine: 1% plain
- Mepivacaine: 1% plain
- Steroid of choice (usually triamcinolone 40 mg/mL)
- Viscosupplementation agent of choice (ordered as needed)

LANDMARK-GUIDED INJECTION TECHNIQUE

When performing injections and/or aspirations, it is important that the medical provider follows a standardized routine. This helps organize the clinician, prepares the patient, and reduces the possibility of procedural omissions. The following steps should be done in the order presented:

1. Determine the medical diagnosis and consider relevant differential diagnoses.
2. Consider all contraindications to the procedure.
3. Discuss the proposed procedure and alternatives with the patient and/or responsible party.
4. Obtain written informed consent from the patient and/or responsible party. (See Appendix 1.)
5. Collect and prepare the required materials.
6. Correctly position the patient for the procedure.
7. Identify and mark the anatomic landmarks and injection site with ink. (Do not allow the patient to move the affected area from the time that the marks are placed until after the procedure is completed.)
8. Press firmly on the skin with the retracted tip of a ballpoint pen to further identify the injection site.
9. Put on clean examination gloves.
10. Prepare clean skin with an alcohol pad followed by either a 10% povidone-iodine prep pad or a 2% chlorhexidine-70% alcohol prep pad. Then allow this to dry according to the manufacturer's recommendations.
11. Provide local anesthesia as indicated through the use of tactile distraction, vapocoolant spray (Pain Ease), and/or injected local anesthesia.
12. Using the no-touch technique, introduce the needle at the insertion site and advance it precisely into the treatment area.

13. If using ultrasound guidance, follow the instructions in each individual chapter (optional).
14. Aspirate synovial or bursa fluid (optional) and send it for laboratory examination if indicated. If injecting corticosteroid solution or viscosupplement immediately following aspiration, do not remove the needle from the joint or bursa. In this case, grasp the needle hub firmly (with a hemostat clamp if necessary), twist off the original syringe, and then immediately attach the second syringe that contains the corticosteroid.
15. Inject the proper corticosteroid solution or viscosupplement into the target site. Always aspirate before injecting to avoid intravascular administration. Do not inject the medication against resistance.
16. Withdraw the needle.
17. Apply direct pressure over the injection site with a sterile gauze pad.
18. Apply a sterile adhesive bandage.
19. Provide the patient with specific postinjection aftercare instructions. (See Appendix 2.)
20. Document the procedure. (See Appendix 3.)

ULTRASOUND-GUIDED INJECTION TECHNIQUE

When performing ultrasound-guided injections and/or aspirations, the preparation and performance of the procedure largely follows the landmark-guided format. Again, it is important that the medical provider follows a standardized routine. This helps organize the clinician, prepares the patient, and reduces the possibility of procedural omissions. The following steps should be done in the order presented:

1. Determine the medical diagnosis and consider relevant differential diagnoses.
2. Consider all contraindications to the procedure.
3. Discuss the proposed procedure and alternatives with the patient and/or responsible party.
4. Obtain written informed consent from the patient and/or responsible party. (See Appendix 1.)
5. Collect and prepare the required materials.
6. Correctly position the patient and the ultrasound machine for the procedure.
7. Perform a preliminary ultrasound scan.
8. Identify and mark the anatomic landmarks and injection site with ink. (Do not allow the patient to move the affected area from the time that the marks are placed until after the procedure is completed.)
9. Press firmly on the skin with the retracted tip of a ballpoint pen to further identify the injection site.
10. Put on clean (or sterile) examination gloves.
11. Prepare clean skin with an alcohol pad followed by 2% chlorhexidine-70% alcohol prep pad. Then allow this to dry according to the manufacturer's recommendations.
12. Prepare the ultrasound probe.
13. Attach syringe to needle.
14. Provide local anesthesia as indicated through use of tactile distraction, vapocoolant spray (Pain Ease), and/or injected local anesthesia.
15. Using the no-touch technique, introduce the needle at the insertion site and advance it precisely into the treatment area.

16. Place needle under the ultrasound probe and advance it to the desired target.
17. Follow the ultrasound instructions in each individual chapter.
18. Aspirate synovial or bursa fluid (optional) and send it for laboratory examination if indicated. If injecting corticosteroid solution or viscosupplement immediately following aspiration, do not remove the needle from the joint or bursa. In this case, grasp the needle hub firmly (with a hemostat clamp if necessary), twist off the original syringe, and then immediately attach the second syringe that contains the corticosteroid.
19. Inject the proper corticosteroid solution or viscosupplement into the target site. Always aspirate before injecting to avoid intravascular administration. Do not inject the medication against resistance.
20. Withdraw the needle.
21. Apply direct pressure over the injection site with a sterile gauze pad.
22. Apply a sterile adhesive bandage.
23. Provide the patient with specific postinjection aftercare instructions. (See Appendix 2.)
24. Document the procedure. (See Appendix 3.)

SYNOVIAL FLUID ANALYSIS

The acquisition of a sample of synovial fluid for microscopic analysis is a primary objective of arthrocentesis. Examination of the fluid can provide information critical to the diagnosis of the condition that has caused the joint effusion.[65,66] This is especially important in the case of acute monoarthritis in which either septic or crystal arthritis may be present. After arthrocentesis has been successfully performed, the appearance of the fluid is observed. The gross appearance of the fluid should be noted. Normal synovial fluid is clear and transparent. This provides a quick clinical estimation of the amount of inflammation present in the joint. Totally transparent fluid originates in normal joints and is observed with noninflammatory conditions such as osteoarthritis. The degree of turbidity generally parallels the amount of inflammation. Most turbid to purulent synovial fluid usually occurs in septic joints, but exceptions are not uncommon. Next, the fluid is either immediately examined under a microscope or transferred as quickly as possible to a laboratory capable of providing diagnostic testing. When the specimen is sent for synovial fluid analysis, it is placed in a glass tube anticoagulated with liquid ethylenediaminetetraacetate. Do not use tubes that contain heparin, oxalate, or lithium since these anticoagulants confound crystal analysis. However, for best practices, contact the local laboratory to determine the preferred method for transportation of the fluid. Fluid submitted for culture is transferred from the syringe to appropriate culture media. A general bacterial culture medium is appropriate for most cases of septic arthritis. However, if gonorrhea is suspected in a patient with acute monoarthritis, then transport the sample in Thayer-Martin medium under carbon dioxide. If a fungal infection is considered, plate the specimen for growth in Sabouraud dextrose agar.

In the past, a number of tests for glucose, pH, and lactic acid were routinely performed, but evidence-based investigations have disproved their value. Traditionally, joint effusions have been classified as normal, noninflammatory, inflammatory, septic, and hemorrhagic. The absolute cell count is the major discriminating factor between inflammatory and noninflammatory fluid. Fluids with cell counts less than 2,000 cells/mm^3 are likely to be noninflammatory, and inflammatory fluids generally have more than 2,000 cells/mm^3. The differential leukocyte count may add further information. Noninflammatory fluid generally contains less than 50% polymorphonuclear cells, and an inflammatory fluid has considerably more. The only clinically useful synovial tests in the setting of septic arthritis are the WBC count, percentage of polymorphonuclear cells, Gram stain, and culture.

Crystal analysis can be performed in any office equipped with a microscope. A single drop of fluid is placed on a clean slide and examined under a cover slip. Crystals can be observed with plain microscopy and preliminary identification made for crystals, WBCs, and bacteria. A polarizing light microscope provides the gold standard for crystal identification.[67] This examination is usually only available in a referral laboratory. Monosodium urate crystals found in gout appear needle shaped and are strongly negatively birefringent when examined under polarization. Calcium pyrophosphate dihydrate crystals are found in pseudogout. These are strongly refractile, short, rhomboid-shaped, and weakly positively birefringent. The presence of intracellular crystals is an even more specific predictor for gout or pseudogout (Table 2.1).

AFTERCARE

Immediately following the aspiration and/or injection procedure, apply firm pressure to the sterile bandage, covering the site. Once the provider is assured that the patient is stable and is not at risk of falling, assist them in safely getting down from the examination/procedure table. Gentle massage and slow, controlled range of motion are encouraged to help distribute the corticosteroid throughout the joint space or soft tissues. After discharge from the office, patients should be advised to look for and immediately report any adverse reactions. Early detection of an infection is critical. Therefore, any swelling, redness, increased warmth, proximal red streaking, or fever greater than 100 °F should be reported immediately.

Patients often experience immediate and complete resolution of pain following an injection that includes a local anesthetic. However, this temporary relief can mask

TABLE 2.1

Synovial Fluid Properties

	Appearance	Viscosity	Cells/mm^3	% PMNs	Crystals
Normal	Transparent	High	<180	<10%	None
Osteoarthritis	Transparent	High	200-2,000	<10%	None
Rheumatoid arthritis	Translucent	Low	2,000-50,000	Variable	None
Psoriatic arthritis	Translucent	Low	2,000-50,000	Variable	None
Reactive arthritis	Translucent	Low	2,000-50,000	Variable	None
Gout	Translucent to cloudy	Low	2,000-50,000	>90%	Needle-like + birefringence
Pseudogout	Translucent to cloudy	Low	2,000-50,000	>90%	Rhomboid-like – birefringence
Septic arthritis	Cloudy	Variable	2,000-50,000+	>90%	None
Hemarthrosis	Red	Low	2,000-50,000	<10%	None

PMN, polymorphonuclear cell.

symptoms and eliminate the body's natural protective feedback, increasing the risk of further injury to the treated area. They should be informed that the initial pain relief is provided by the injected local anesthetic and that its effect will only be temporary. For example, plain 1% lidocaine typically provides relief for approximately 1 hour. The anti-inflammatory effect of the injected corticosteroid usually has a 24- to 48-hour onset of action. Thus, patients should be informed that the pain is expected to return in about an hour and decrease again within 1 to 2 days as the corticosteroid takes effect.

Additional instructions may be given following aspiration and/or injection. The patient might be directed to apply ice to the affected area, although current evidence does not support its effectiveness. NSAIDs may be prescribed depending on the clinical situation—but with full knowledge and considerations of the side effects and potential toxicities discussed earlier in this chapter. Research indicates that immobilization of the affected area is not necessary.[68,69] However, temporary reduction in use and modification of activity can be beneficial. While some patients may prefer a compressive elastic wrap or splint for comfort, routine splinting of injected areas is not supported by medical literature. Providing patients with an aftercare education handout that outlines specific instructions and the most common possible adverse reactions is highly recommended (see Appendix 3).

DOCUMENTATION OF THE PROCEDURE

A very important step in the provision of medical services is the full and accurate description of the events that occurred before, during, and after the procedure. This serves not only as the official medical record but also as a billing record and a legal document. The note should affirm that discussion of the proposed procedure and the alternative treatments occurred, possible complications were discussed, and all questions were answered. The note must include the fact that written informed consent was obtained (Appendix 1). Then, it should document patient position, anesthesia, supplies used, and the physical steps involved in performing the procedure. The record should also include any pertinent findings, any complications encountered, and the patient's postprocedure condition. Finally, a list of patient instructions, treatment plan, and follow-up care should be documented and signed by the medical provider and any supervisors if necessary.

See the example of documentation for a knee joint aspiration and injection in Appendix 2. This may be modified as needed to meet the needs of the specific aspiration/injection procedure, patient, provider, and medical organization. A review of this document by legal counsel prior to implementation is recommended.

BILLING AND CODING

In order to receive appropriate payment for services provided, it is essential that the clinician assigns the proper code(s) for the procedure(s) performed. This ensures fair payment for the work done at the visit and reimbursement for any eligible supplies. A complete description of the procedure(s) performed during the patient encounter must be documented in the medical record in order to support the level of coding. Specific Current Procedural Terminology (CPT) codes are employed to bill for skin, perineural, and musculoskeletal injections and aspirations. The practitioner should consult an up-to-date CPT manual for a list of the applicable procedural codes.

The current CPT manual defines small joints as those in the fingers and toes. Temporomandibular, acromioclavicular, sternoclavicular, wrist, elbow, ankle, and olecranon bursae are defined as intermediate joints or bursa. Large structures are the glenohumeral joint, sacroiliac joint, hip joint, knee joint, and the subacromial bursa.

According to their definitions, the CPT codes are used once for each tendon, joint, or bursa injected. If more than one tendon, joint, or bursa is injected at a visit, then the codes are listed multiple times for each separate structure that is injected. In addition, the modifiers –51 or –59 should be used to indicate when multiple procedures are performed. Usually –59 is used to code for multiple injections at different sites, but the specific modifier used is determined by the preference of each insurance carrier. Note that trigger point injection CPT codes are used only once each session regardless of the number of injections performed. The CPT manual gives specific instructions when reporting multiple ganglion cyst aspirations/injections.

Be aware that Medicare and most commercial insurance companies apply the multiple surgery rule when paying for multiple injections. They generally pay 100% of the allowable fee for the first procedure, 50% for the second, and 25% for the third and subsequent procedures.

Diagnostic codes must also be submitted in order for an insurance company to justify payment for the injection/aspiration procedure. These codes follow the standard International Classification of Diseases (ICD) system.

J codes are used to charge for the injected medication/device used during the procedure. Therapeutic injectable products, such as corticosteroids and viscosupplementation agents, are billed in addition to the injection administration CPT codes. The J codes are not used for local anesthetics since their use is considered a necessary part of the procedure—much like the needle and syringe. The charge is reflected as the number of units used during the procedure. For instance, the J code for Kenalog is expressed in 10 mg units. If 40 mg of Kenalog was injected, then the patient is charged 4 units.

An evaluation and management (E&M) code can be billed only if the documentation of the visit supports the necessity and completeness of the evaluation. In the setting of performing a procedure, this requires the –25 modifier and may be used only if there is a "significant, separately identifiable evaluation and management service by the same physician or other qualified health care professional on the same day of the procedure or other service."[70] Otherwise, only the CPT code and associated J code can be used if the evaluation is not performed or does not meet those conditions.

INFORMED CONSENT

As with any invasive procedure, informed consent must be obtained from the patient. For the purpose of documentation, this should be done in a written format. The patient must also have an adequate opportunity to ask questions, including a discussion of alternative methods of diagnosis and treatment. An example of an informed consent form is included in Appendix 1.

EVIDENCE-BASED MEDICINE

Intra-articular and soft tissue corticosteroid injections are common procedures performed by primary care physicians. They are accepted interventions and are frequently used to treat various musculoskeletal conditions. Although significant therapeutic efficacy is claimed from over 50 years of published research, a closer examination of the literature yields less convincing evidence of significant long-term improvement of specific, measured outcomes. The available data support short- to medium-term benefit from most corticosteroid injections. There is currently insufficient high-quality data to provide a definitive answer on the efficacy of corticosteroid injections. However, lack of discrete medical evidence does not necessarily mean that these procedures are ineffective. Even gold standard, evidence-based, medical resources such as Cochrane Database of Systematic Reviews suffer from performing meta-analysis on studies with data that are themselves flawed. New investigations that are methodologically sound are needed to measure outcomes of corticosteroid injections given for the treatment of specific conditions.

REFERENCES

1. Qaseem A, McLean RM, O'Gurek D, et al. Nonpharmacologic and pharmacologic management of acute pain from non-low back, musculoskeletal injuries in adults: a clinical guideline from the American College of Physicians and American Academy of Family Physicians. *Ann Intern Med.* 2020;173(9):739-748.
2. Zeng C, Doherty M, Persson MSM, et al. Comparative efficacy and safety of acetaminophen, topical and oral non-steroidal anti-inflammatory drugs for knee osteoarthritis: evidence from a network meta-analysis of randomized controlled trials and real-world data. *Osteoarthritis Cartilage.* 2021;29(9):1242-1251.
3. Bhala N, Emberson J, Merhi A, et al. Vascular and upper gastrointestinal effects of non-steroidal anti-inflammatory drugs: meta-analyses of individual participant data from randomised trials. *Lancet.* 2013;382(9894):769-779.
4. Bally M, Dendukuri N, Rich B, et al. Risk of acute myocardial infarction with NSAIDs in real world use: bayesian meta-analysis of individual patient data. *BMJ.* 2017;357:j1909.
5. Olsen AS, Fosbøl EL, Lindhardsen J, et al. Duration of treatment with nonsteroidal anti-inflammatory drugs and impact on risk of death and recurrent myocardial infarction in patients with prior myocardial infarction. A nationwide cohort study. *Circulation.* 2011;123:2226-2235.
6. Schmidt M, Christiansen CF, Mehnert F, Rothman KJ, Sørensen HT. Non-steroidal anti-inflammatory drug use and risk of atrial fibrillation or flutter: population based case-control study. *BMJ.* 2011;343:d3450.
7. Krijthe BP, Heeringa J, Hofman A, Franco OH, Stricker BH. Non-steroidal anti-inflammatory drugs and the risk of atrial fibrillation: a population-based follow-up study. *BMJ Open.* 2014;4(4):e004059.
8. Chokesuwattanaskul R, Chiengthong K, Thongprayoon C, et al. Nonsteroidal anti-inflammatory drugs and incidence of atrial fibrillation: a meta-analysis. *QJM.* 2020;113(2):79-85.
9. Ungprasert P, Srivali N, Wijarnpreecha K, Charoenpong P, Knight EL. Non-steroidal anti-inflammatory drugs and risk of venous thromboembolism: a systematic review and meta-analysis. *Rheumatology.* 2015; 54(4):736-742.
10. Poisoning Statistics. *National Data.* 2023. Accessed August 8, 2025. https://www.poison.org/poison-statistics-national
11. MacDonald AJ, Speiser JL, Ganger DR, et al; US Acute Liver Failure Study Group. Clinical and neurologic outcomes in acetaminophen-induced acute liver failure: a 21-year multicenter cohort study. *Clin Gastroenterol Hepatol.* 2021;19(12):2615-2625.e3.
12. Roberts E, Delgado Nunes V, Buckner S, et al. Paracetamol: not as safe as we thought? A systematic literature review of observational studies. *Ann Rheum Dis.* 2016;75(3):552-559.
13. FDA Drug Safety Communication. *FDA Warns of Rare but Serious Skin Reactions With the Pain Reliever/Fever Reducer Acetaminophen.* Accessed December 29, 2013. http://www.fda.gov/Drugs/DrugSafety/ucm363041.htm
14. Yao TC, Huang YW, Chang SM, Tsai S-Y, Wu AC, Tsai H-J. Association between oral corticosteroid bursts and severe adverse events: a nationwide population-based cohort study. *Ann Intern Med.* 2020;173(5):325-330.
15. Toupin April K, Bisaillon J, Welch V, et al. Tramadol for osteoarthritis. *Cochrane Database Syst Rev.* 2019;(5):CD005522. doi:10.1002/14651858.CD005522.pub3
16. Riva JJ, Noor ST, Wang L, et al. Predictors of prolonged opioid use after initial prescription for acute musculoskeletal injuries in adults: a systematic review and meta-analysis of observational studies. *Ann Intern Med.* 2020;173(9):721-729.
17. Els C, Jackson TD, Kunyk D, et al. Adverse events associated with medium- and long-term use of opioids for chronic non-cancer pain: an overview of Cochrane Reviews. *Cochrane Database Syst Rev.* 2017;10(10):CD012509.
18. Park K, Kim S, Ko YJ, Park BJ. Duloxetine and cardiovascular adverse events: a systematic review and meta-analysis. *J Psychiatr Res.* 2020;124:109-114.
19. Ogata T, Ideno Y, Akai M, et al. Effects of glucosamine in patients with osteoarthritis of the knee: a systematic review and meta-analysis. *Clin Rheumatol.* 2018;37(9):2479-2487.

20. Allen KD, Choong PF, Davis AM, et al. Osteoarthritis: models for appropriate care across the disease continuum. *Best Pract Res Clin Rheumatol.* 2016;30(3):503-535.
21. Patel IJ, Rahim S, Davidson JC, et al. Society of Interventional Radiology Consensus Guidelines for the periprocedural management of thrombotic and bleeding risk in patients undergoing percutaneous image-guided interventions—Part II: recommendations: endorsed by the Canadian Association for Interventional Radiology and the Cardiovascular and Interventional Radiological Society of Europe. *J Vasc Interv Radiol.* 2019;30(8):1168-1184.e1.
22. Thumboo J, O'Duffy JD. A prospective study of the safety of joint and soft tissue aspiration and injections in patients taking warfarin sodium. *Arthritis Rheum.* 1998;4:736-739.
23. Tarar MY, Malik RA, Charalambous CP. Bleeding complications in patients on warfarin undergoing joint injection/aspiration: systematic review and meta-analysis. *Rheumatol Int.* 2023;43(2):245-251.
24. Habib GS, Bashir M, Jabbour A. Increased blood glucose levels following intra-articular injection of methylprednisolone acetate in patients with controlled diabetes and symptomatic osteoarthritis of the knee. *Ann Rheum Dis.* 2008;67:1790-1791.
25. Habib G, Safia A. The effect of intra-articular injection of betamethasone acetate/betamethasone sodium phosphate on blood glucose levels in controlled diabetic patients with symptomatic osteoarthritis of the knee. *Clin Rheumatol.* 2009;28:85-87.
26. Habib GS, Abu-Ahmad R. Lack of effect of corticosteroid injection at the shoulder joint on blood glucose levels in diabetic patients. *Clin Rheumatol.* 2007;26:566-568.
27. Kamel SI, Rosas HG, Gorbachova T. Local and systemic side effects of corticosteroid injections for musculoskeletal indications. *AJR Am J Roentgenol.* 2024;222(3):e2330458.
28. Clark SC, Jones MW, Choudhury RR, Smith E. Bilateral patellar tendon rupture secondary to repeated local steroid injections. *J Accid Emerg Med.* 1995;12:300-301.
29. Ford LT, DeBender J. Tendon rupture after local steroid injection. *South Med J.* 1979;72:827-830.
30. Chen SK, Lu C-C, Chou P-H, Guo L-Y, Wu W-L. Patellar tendon ruptures in weight lifters after local steroid injections. *Arch Orthop Trauma Surg.* 2009;129:369-372.
31. Scutt N, Rolf CG, Scutt A. Glucocorticoids inhibit tenocyte proliferation and tendon progenitor cell recruitment. *J Orthop Res.* 2006;24:173-182.
32. Paik NC, Seo JW. CT-guided needle aspiration of pneumothorax from a trigger point injection. *Pain Med.* 2011;12(5):837-841.
33. Jalul M, Humphrey AR. Radial artery injury caused by a sclerosant injected into a palmar wrist ganglion. *J Hand Surg Eur.* 2009;34(5):698-699.
34. Rogojan C, Hetland ML. Depigmentation: a rare side effect to intra-articular glucocorticoid treatment. *Clin Rheumatol.* 2004;23:373-375.
35. Lund IM, Donde R, Knudsen EA. Persistent local cutaneous atrophy following corticosteroid injection for tendinitis. *Rheumatol Rehabil.* 1979;18:91-93.
36. Shumaker PR, Rao J, Goldman MP. Treatment of local, persistent cutaneous atrophy following corticosteroid injection with normal saline infiltration. *Dermatol Surg.* 2005;31:1340-1343.
37. Fujita F, Moriyama T, Higashi T, et al. Methyl p-hydroxybenzoate causes pain sensation through activation of TRPA1 channels. *Br J Pharmacol.* 2007;151(1):153-160.
38. Mager ML, Ciotu CI, Gold-Binder M, Heber S, Fischer MJM. TRPA1-dependent and -independent activation by commonly used preservatives. *Front Pharmacol.* 2023;14:1248558.
39. Dragoo JL, Braun HJ, Kim HJ, Phan HD, Golish SR. The in vitro chondrotoxicity of single-dose local anesthetics. *Am J Sports Med.* 2012;40(4):794-799.
40. Jacobs TF, Vansintjan PS, Roels N, et al. The effect of lidocaine on the viability of cultivated mature human cartilage cells: an in vitro study. *Knee Surg Sports Traumatol Arthrosc.* 2011;19(7):1206-1213.
41. Wiater BP, Neradilek MB, Polissar NL, Matsen FA III. Risk factors for chondrolysis of the glenohumeral joint: a study of three hundred and seventy-five shoulder arthroscopic procedures in the practice of an individual community surgeon. *J Bone Joint Surg Am.* 2011;93(7):615-625.
42. Scheffel PT, Clinton J, Lynch JR, Warme WJ, Bertelsen AL, Matsen FA III. Glenohumeral chondrolysis: a systematic review of 100 cases from the English language literature. *J Shoulder Elbow Surg.* 2010;19(6):944-949.
43. Jayaram P, Kennedy DJ, Yeh P, Dragoo J. Chondrotoxic effects of local anesthetics on human knee articular cartilage: a systematic review. *PM R.* 2019;11(4):379-400.
44. Kreuz PC, Steinwachs M, Angele P. Single-dose local anesthetics exhibit a type-, dose-, and time-dependent chondrotoxic effect on chondrocytes and cartilage: a systematic review of the current literature. *Knee Surg Sports Traumatol Arthrosc.* 2018;26(3):819-830.
45. Grishko V, Xu M, Wilson G, Pearsall AW IV. Apoptosis and mitochondrial dysfunction in human chondrocytes following exposure to lidocaine, bupivacaine, and ropivacaine. *J Bone Joint Surg Am.* 2010;92(3):609-618.
46. Piper SL, Kramer JD, Kim HT, Feeley BT. Effects of local anesthetics on articular cartilage. *Am J Sports Med.* 2011;39(10):2245-2253.
47. Dragoo JL, Korotkova T, Kim HJ, Jagadish A. Chondrotoxicity of low pH, epinephrine, and preservatives found in local anesthetics containing epinephrine. *Am J Sports Med.* 2010;38(6):1154-1159.
48. Pardo MC Jr. *Miller's Basics of Anesthesia.* 8th ed. American Dental Society of Anesthesiology; c2022:146.
49. Becker DE, Reed KL. Local anesthetics: review of pharmacological considerations. *Anesth Prog.* 2012;59(2):90-101.
50. McAlindon TE, LaValley MP, Harvey WF, et al. Effect of intra-articular triamcinolone vs saline on knee cartilage volume and pain in patients with knee osteoarthritis: a randomized clinical trial. *JAMA.* 2017;317(19):1967-1975.

51. Wernecke C, Braun HJ, Dragoo JL. The effect of intra-articular corticosteroids on articular cartilage: a systematic review. *Orthop J Sports Med.* 2015;3(5).
52. Darouiche RO, Wall MJ Jr, Itani KMF, et al. Chlorhexidine-alcohol versus povidone-iodine for surgical-site antisepsis. *N Engl J Med.* 2010;362:18-26.
53. Wade RG, Burr NE, McCauley G, Bourke G, Efthimiou O. The comparative efficacy of chlorhexidine gluconate and povidone-iodine antiseptics for the prevention of infection in clean surgery: a systematic review and network meta-analysis. *Ann Surg.* 2021;274(6):e481-e488.
54. Krobbuaban B, Diregpoke S, Prasan S, Thanomsat M, Kumkeaw S. Alcohol-based chlorhexidine vs. povidone iodine in reducing skin colonization prior to regional anesthesia procedures. *J Med Assoc Thai.* 2011;94(7):807-812.
55. Ostrander RV, Botte MJ, Brage ME. Efficacy of surgical preparation solutions in foot and ankle surgery. *J Bone Joint Surg Am.* 2005;87:980-985.
56. Bibbo C, Patel DV, Gehrmann RM, Lin SS. Chlorhexidine provides superior skin decontamination in foot and ankle surgery: a prospective randomized study. *Clin Orthop Relat Res.* 2005;438:204-208.
57. Mangram AJ, Horan TC, Pearson ML, Silver LC, Jarvis WR. CDC: guideline for prevention of surgical site infection, 1999. *Infect Control Hosp Epidemiol.* 1999;20(4):250-266. http://www.cdc.gov/hicpac/pdf/guidelines/SSI_1999.pdf
58. Brown TR, Ehrlich CE, Stehman FB, Golichowski AM, Madura JA, Eitzen HE. A clinical evaluation of chlorhexidine gluconate spray as compared with iodophor scrub for preoperative skin preparation. *Surg Gynecol Obstet.* 1984;158:363-366.
59. Denton GW. Chlorhexidine. In: Block SS, ed. *Disinfection, Sterilization, and Preservation.* 5th ed. Lippincott Williams & Wilkins; 2001:321-336.
60. Berry PH, Dahl JD. The new JCAHO pain standards: implications for pain management nurses. *Pain Manag Nurs.* 2000;1(1):3-12.
61. Zhu Y, Peng X, Wang S, et al. Vapocoolant spray versus placebo spray/no treatment for reducing pain from intravenous cannulation: a meta-analysis of randomized controlled trials. *Am J Emerg Med.* 2018;36(11):2085-2092.
62. Gebauer's Pain Ease® Topical Anesthetic Skin Refrigerant Technical Data Document. Accessed August 2, 2025. https://www.gebauer.com/hs-fs/hub/150313/file-68341047-pdf/docs/pe_medical_device_statement.pdf
63. Azar FM, Lake JE, Grace SP, Perkinson B. Ethyl chloride improves antiseptic effect of betadine skin preparation for office procedures. *J Surg Orthop Adv.* 2012;21(2):84-87.
64. Sandrowski K, Graham J, Knott S, et al. Sterility of ethyl chloride spray after use in the clinic. *Hand (N Y).* 2021;16(2):210-212.
65. Courtney P, Doherty M. Joint aspiration and injection and synovial fluid analysis. *Best Pract Res Clin Rheumatol.* 2013;27(2):137-169.
66. Oliviero F, Mandell BF. Synovial fluid analysis: relevance for daily clinical practice. *Best Pract Res Clin Rheumatol.* 2023;37(1):101848.
67. Pascual E, Sivera F, Andrés M. Synovial fluid analysis for crystals. *Curr Opin Rheumatol.* 2011;23(2):161-169.
68. Charalambous C, Paschalides C, Sadiq S, Tryfonides M, Hirst P, Paul AS. Weight bearing following intra-articular steroid injection of the knee: survey of current practice and review of the available evidence. *Rheumatol Int.* 2002;22(5):185-187.
69. Chatham W, Williams G, Moreland L, et al. Intraarticular corticosteroid injections: should we rest the joints? *Arthritis Care Res.* 1989;2(2):70-74.
70. American Medical Association. *CPT® 2025 Professional Edition.* October 2024. 1344 p. ISBN-13#: 978-1640163041.

3

Injectable Agents

James W. McNabb

LOCAL ANESTHETICS

Local anesthetics are membrane stabilizing drugs. They act by inhibiting sodium influx through sodium-specific ion channels in the neuronal cell membrane. They reversibly decrease the rate of depolarization and repolarization of excitable membranes in nociceptors—thus interrupting pain impulses.

Local anesthetics are commonly injected either alone or with another compound, such as a corticosteroid, when treating painful conditions. The injection of local anesthetic into joints or soft tissues serves several purposes. Administration of the local anesthetic provides short-term pain relief. This allows for patient feedback. It may provide a more comprehensive examination of the affected area without the limitation of pain. Although mixing steroids with local anesthetics is not recommended by the manufacturers of injectable corticosteroids, it is common clinical practice to mix a local anesthetic in the same syringe as the corticosteroid solution prior to injection. By convention, the clear liquid (local anesthetic) is drawn up in the syringe first, followed by the cloudy fluid (steroid). The added volume of the local anesthetic helps dilute the corticosteroid. This enables dispersion of steroid in a large joint space, bursa, tendon sheath, or soft tissue plane. Pain relief following injection confirms proper placement of corticosteroid both to the clinician and to the patient. Although pain often returns after the effect of the anesthetic agent wears off, the patient can be assured that the injected corticosteroid is properly placed and should begin to exert its clinical effect within 24 to 48 hours.

There are several commercially available choices of local anesthetics. Most commonly, the amide class of local anesthetics is used. The clinically significant characteristics of the amides are summarized in Table 3.1. Lidocaine (lignocaine, Xylocaine) for local anesthetic injection is commercially available as 0.5%, 1%, and 2% concentrations with or without epinephrine. The duration of action for infiltration anesthesia without epinephrine is 30 to 120 minutes. For soft tissue injections, the author exclusively uses 1% lidocaine without epinephrine. This is commonly available in multiuse bottles containing the preservative, methylparaben. Lidocaine is also available in 2-mL single-use preservative-free vials. The 2% solution of lidocaine confers no clinically important advantages and increases the risk of toxicity following administration of large amounts of greater than 4.5 mg/kg. The inclusion of epinephrine likewise offers no clinical advantages with musculoskeletal injections/aspirations and is not used in these procedures to dilute the corticosteroid. Importantly, lidocaine with epinephrine is acidic (pH = 4.5) and causes significant transient local burning pain upon injection.

Bupivacaine (Marcaine, Sensorcaine, and others) is another commonly used local anesthetic. It has a longer onset of action but offers extended anesthetic effect. Duration of action for infiltration anesthesia without epinephrine is 120 to 240 minutes. Multidose

TABLE 3.1

Characteristics of Common Local Anesthetics

Anesthetic	Onset of Action (min)	Duration Without Epinephrine (min)	Max. Dosage w/o Epinephrine (mg/kg)
Lidocaine	<1	30-120	4.5
Mepivacaine	3-20	30-120	6.0
Bupivacaine	2-10	120-240	2.5
Ropivacaine	3-15	120-240	2.5

Data from Kouba DJ, LoPiccolo MC, Alam M, et al. Guidelines for the use of local anesthesia in office-based dermatologic surgery. *J Am Acad Dermatol.* 2016;74(6):1201-1219; Park KK, Sharon VR. A review of local anesthetics: minimizing risk and side effects in cutaneous surgery. *Dermatol Surg.* 2017;43(2):173-187.

vials also contain 1 mg of methylparaben as a preservative. Many clinicians prefer to mix 1% lidocaine with 0.25% bupivacaine in order to give the patient rapid onset of local anesthesia with an extended duration. However, there is no proven clinical benefit using this approach. Because of the additional steps required to draw up the separate anesthetics, preparation of this combination may increase the chance of contamination and needle stick injury. It may also give the patient a false sense of security since there is prolonged initial pain relief before the tissues have healed. Since the negative feedback from pain is absent for an extended period of time, the patient might suffer further injury such as tendon rupture through inadvertent use of the affected body area.

Mepivacaine (Carbocaine, Polocaine) is a newer agent that is a shorter-acting homolog of bupivacaine. It is available as 1%, 1.5%, and 2% solutions for injection. It has a shorter onset of action and anesthetic effect. Duration of action for infiltration anesthesia without epinephrine is 30 to 120 minutes. This is available in multiuse bottles containing the preservative, methylparaben, and also as single-use preservative-free vials.

Ropivacaine (Naropin) is a newer agent that is also a long-acting homolog of bupivacaine. It is available as a 0.5% and 0.75% solutions for injection. It also has a longer onset of action and offers extended anesthetic effect. Duration of action for infiltration anesthesia without epinephrine is extended at 120 to 240 minutes for the 0.5% solution. Ropivacaine is available in multiuse bottles containing the preservative, methylparaben, and also as single-use preservative-free vials.

Levobupivacaine (Chirocaine) is the levo-enantiomer of bupivacaine. It is also a recently developed option for local anesthesia. Levobupivacaine is commercially available as 2.5, 5.0, and 7.5 mg/mL solutions. Both of these stereoisomers display less cardiovascular and central nervous system toxicity than racemic bupivacaine.[1]

The pH of local anesthetics can be buffered to decrease local pain. The pH of 1% lidocaine without epinephrine is 6.5, while the pH of 1% lidocaine with epinephrine is 4.5. Bupivacaine is isotonic. Adding sterile 8.4% sodium bicarbonate to lidocaine with epinephrine at a ratio of 1:10 neutralizes the mixture and has been shown to provide significant pain relief. However, this is not a clinically important issue with joint injections because plain lidocaine is used and not lidocaine with epinephrine.

In general, the amount of local anesthetic injected is dependent on the injection site and disease process. The smallest volume of the lowest concentration of the anesthetic with the least side effect profile should be used. For instance, large volumes (5-10 mL) of lidocaine were commonly used in the past for the treatment of large joints such as shoulders, sacroiliac joints, hips, and knees. More recently, the author has found equivalent anesthetic effect with much small volumes (0.5-1 mL) of mepivacaine or other anesthetics. This recommendation to limit anesthetic administration is made to decrease the possibility of local and systemic toxicity.

A discussion of chondrocyte toxicity of the amide class of local anesthetics is included in the Complications section of Chapter 2.

CORTICOSTEROIDS

Corticosteroids used for injection purposes are synthetic derivatives of hydrocortisone. The exact mechanism of action of corticosteroids is complex with various sites of action. They bind to glucocorticoid receptors regulating gene transcription. By altering the production of protein annexin-1, corticosteroids reduce cytokines and other inflammatory mediators.[2-4] They lead to downregulation of immune function,[5] inhibition of cell-mediated immunity, and reduction in the number of macrophages and polymorphonuclear cells accumulating at inflammatory sites. There is also a vascular stabilizing effect by the inhibition of endothelial expression of adhesion molecules for neutrophils. Capillary dilation and vascular permeability are therefore reduced.[2,3] The end effect is to reduce the amount of inflammation, thereby reducing swelling and pain.

Several corticosteroids are commercially available for joint and soft tissue injections (Table 3.2). These include triamcinolone acetonide (Kenalog), triamcinolone diacetate (Aristocort), triamcinolone hexacetonide (Aristospan), methylprednisolone acetate (Depo-Medrol), betamethasone acetate and sodium phosphate (Celestone Soluspan), and dexamethasone acetate (Decadron-LA). The agents differ with regard to their solubility, biological half-life, and potency as compared to hydrocortisone (Table 3.2). Different products have varying effects and solubility in the tissues. The solubility is inversely proportional to the biologic duration of effect of the agent. Hydrocortisone is

TABLE 3.2

Properties of Injectable Corticosteroids

Corticosteroid	Relative Anti-inflammatory Potency	Solubility (%Wt/Vol)	Biologic Half-life (h)
Hydrocortisone acetate (Hydrocortone)	1	High 0.002	8-12
Triamcinolone acetonide (Kenalog)	5	Intermediate 0.004	12-36
Triamcinolone hexacetonide (Aristospan)	5	Intermediate 0.0002	12-36
Methylprednisolone acetate (Depo-Medrol)	5	Intermediate 0.0014	12-36
Betamethasone acetate and sodium phosphate (Celestone Soluspan)	25	Low/high	26-54
Dexamethasone acetate (Decadron-LA)	25	Low	26-54

almost never used because of its high solubility and very short duration of action. It also has significant mineralocorticoid activity that is not shared by the other agents.

The common synthetic corticosteroids used in musculoskeletal procedures are derivatives of prednisolone. Corticosteroid preparations are either soluble or insoluble. Most corticosteroid preparations contain corticosteroid esters, which are highly insoluble in water and thus form microcrystalline suspensions.[6] The more insoluble, esterified corticosteroids remain at the injection sites far longer than the soluble forms.

Dexamethasone preparations, however, are not esters and are freely soluble in water; hence, the preparation is clear (ie, nonparticulate). The potential advantage of corticosteroid ester preparations is that they require hydrolysis by cellular esterases to release the active moiety and consequently should last longer in the joint than do nonester preparations.[7] On the other hand, freely water-soluble preparations, such as dexamethasone sodium phosphate and betamethasone sodium phosphate, are taken up rapidly by cells and thus have a quicker onset of effect but with a concomitant reduced duration of action.[4]

Notably, the betamethasone formulation, Celestone Soluspan, contains a combination of betamethasone salt and betamethasone ester and, therefore, may provide a dual action of quick onset and long duration of therapy. However, most studies have not shown a clinically significant difference between this product and other corticosteroid ester preparations in terms of onset or duration.[8,9]

Few studies have been conducted that directly compare the various agents in terms of their efficacy. A comparison of intra-articular administration of triamcinolone acetonide, triamcinolone hexacetonide, and a combination of betamethasone phosphate and acetate was conducted by Derendorf et al. They demonstrated complete absorption of all corticosteroids from the site of injection over a period of 2 to 3 weeks. Because of its lower solubility, triamcinolone hexacetonide was absorbed more slowly than triamcinolone acetonide, thus maintaining synovial levels for a longer time and creating lower systemic corticoid levels. Endogenous hydrocortisone suppression correlated with exogenous steroid levels.[10] A systematic review of the relative efficacy of various corticosteroids was published by Garg et al in 2014. This included seven good quality trials that overall showed no difference in long-term efficacy between the medications that included triamcinolone acetate, triamcinolone hexacetonide, methylprednisolone, and betamethasone.[11] Similar results were reported by Cushman et al in 2018.[12] In a double-blind study utilizing corticosteroid injections of knee joints in patients with rheumatoid arthritis, Hajialilo et al[13] found no difference in pain outcomes comparing triamcinolone hexacetonide and dexamethasone. Another recent double-blind, randomized controlled trial including patients with rheumatoid arthritis or spondyloarthritis with an acutely swollen knee joint found no difference in pain at 24 weeks when injected with either triamcinolone acetonide or methylprednisolone acetate.[14]

No studies have been done that conclusively determine which corticosteroid is preferred for injection of joints versus soft tissues. Without good data, the selection of the particular corticosteroid agent is left to the preference of the individual clinician. Despite lack of literature support, some clinicians prefer to choose a relatively insoluble preparation for intra-articular use and a more soluble form for use in soft tissues and peritendinous injections.

The dose of corticosteroid to be used generally depends on the injection site, disease process, and degree of inflammation. Unfortunately, there is no high-quality published medical literature to help in the determination of dosing. In general, the lowest possible dose should be used, at least with the initial injection of a structure. This recommendation

TABLE 3.3

Equivalent Dosages of Injectable Corticosteroids

Corticosteroid Preparation	Trade Name	Equivalent Dose/Volume (mg/mL)
Triamcinolone acetonide	Kenalog	40
Triamcinolone hexacetonide	Aristospan	40
Methylprednisolone acetate	Depo-Medrol	40
Dexamethasone acetate	Decadron-LA	8
Betamethasone acetate and sodium phosphate	Celestone Soluspan	6

is made to balance the effectiveness of an injection with the desire to minimize the possibility of local and systemic toxicity. Suggested doses of corticosteroids are listed in each individual injection chapter. Table 3.3 presents equivalent dosages of corticosteroids used for injection. For the purposes of this book, all doses are expressed in milligrams of triamcinolone acetonide suspension (Kenalog). If the practitioner chooses to use another steroid, then the comparative dosage can be simply calculated from the table. For instance, if the chapter in this text indicates that 20 mg of triamcinolone is to be used for injection into the wrist joint, then one could use 20 mg of Kenalog, 20 mg of Aristospan, 20 mg of Depo-Medrol, 4 mg of Decadron-LA, or 3 mg of Celestone Soluspan.

Information concerning the frequency of intra-articular corticosteroid injection appears to be primarily based upon professional opinion. An article published in 2015 reviewed this issue.[15] Hypothalamic-pituitary-adrenal axis (HPAA) suppression is the most common and dangerous, although often unrecognized and untreated, side effect of glucocorticoid administration. The risk and duration depend both on patient and treatment characteristics. A review by Whelan et al[16] found that appendicular skeleton corticosteroid injections are less likely to cause adrenal insufficiency than spinal injections. However, Guaraldi et al[17] determined that a single 40-mg intrabursal injection of methylprednisolone acetate or triamcinolone acetate is sufficient to suppresses the HPAA up to 45 days. Although typically asymptomatic, patients should be instructed to recognize and report symptoms suggestive for hypocortisolism, to provide prompt diagnosis, and eventually, treatment, thus avoiding severe complications. The exact effect of repeated dosing and higher dosing is unknown. In general, most experts advocate that corticosteroid injections should be performed no more often than every 3 months. This non–evidence-based guide is an attempt to prevent potential steroid-related complications, including HPAA suppression, osteoporosis, and local articular degradation.

The author typically uses only a small syringe when injecting solutions of anesthetic/corticosteroid. A 3-mL syringe is used in almost all joint and soft tissue injection sites. This accommodates up to 1 mL of local anesthetic (lidocaine or mepivacaine without epinephrine) and up to 1 mL of corticosteroid. Each syringe is prepared at the time of the procedure by drawing up the volume of local anesthetic first followed by corticosteroid. Prior to injecting a patient with the mixture, a common observation is that the insoluble corticosteroid often precipitates along the dependent aspect of the syringe. Immediately before the injection, 1 mL of air is aspirated into the syringe creating a "mixing bubble" (Fig. 3.1). The syringe is then rapidly rotated in order to disperse the corticosteroid evenly within the volume of local anesthetic. The needle of the syringe is

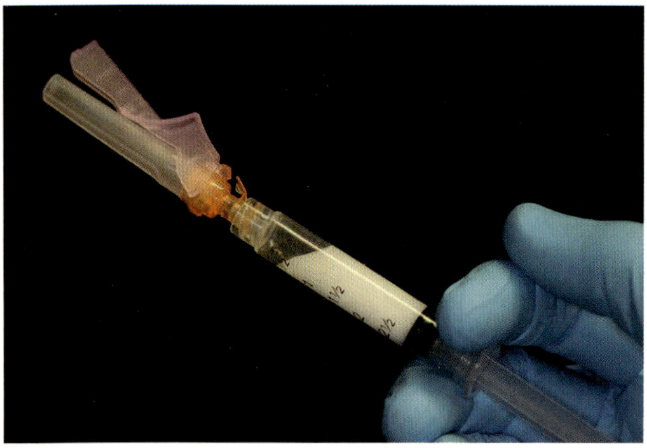

FIGURE 3.1 ● Mixing bubble.

then pointed upward and the small volume of air expelled before the needle is inserted into the skin at the target site.

There is a common misconception that distributing the corticosteroid over a wide area enhances the effect from soft tissue injections. Practitioners frequently use a "fanning" or "peppering" technique to distribute the solution across the area of concern. However, this practice is almost always unnecessary. The volume of anesthetic/corticosteroid solution injected as a bolus will passively move along tendon sheaths and local fascia planes. However, consideration might be given to "fanning" the injection when treating trochanteric pain syndrome because the involved area is frequently quite large.

VISCOSUPPLEMENTS

Hyaluronan (sodium hyaluronate) is a natural complex sugar of the glycosaminoglycan family. The concentration and size of endogenous hyaluronan are reduced in the joint fluid of patients with osteoarthritis. There are many commercially available products for injection that can be used to supplement this substance in joint fluid. These agents are high molecular weight derivatives of hyaluronan, which are synthetically derived from rooster combs or produced by bacterial fermentation and extraction. Injection of exogenous, high molecular weight hyaluronic acid into a joint can interrupt the osteoarthritis cascade by downregulating the production of the inflammatory cytokines and enzymes, restoring production of native hyaluronic acid, and slowing the progression of osteoarthritis. The exact mechanism of action of viscosupplements is unknown but results in improved physical cushioning of the joint, restoration of favorable viscosity, stimulation of production of endogenous hyaluronan by synoviocytes, decreased inflammation, less pain, and improved joint function. Furthermore, a recent study demonstrated a marked decrease in intra-articular friction in diseased joints treated with hyaluronic acid.[18]

In the United States, the Food and Drug Administration (FDA) has approved the clinical use of viscosupplements only for the treatment of knee osteoarthritis. Knee osteoarthritis is a chronic disease state that has a number of therapeutic options. Of these, viscosupplements serve an important, but often underutilized, role. Body weight reduction and physical therapy are the most effective measures. However, when pain persists, pharmacologic options may be utilized. Unfortunately, oral nonsteroidal anti-inflammatory drugs and acetaminophen are only modestly effective and possess significant toxicity. Opioids should not be used on a chronic basis in this condition. Corticosteroid injections are effective for short- to medium-term use, especially in patients experiencing an acute flare in pain and swelling. In the author's opinion, viscosupplements are unfortunately not commonly utilized until very late in the disease process.

Viscosupplements occupy an important position in the mid-term (3 months) to long-term (6 months) treatment of knee osteoarthritis. Their use may allow appropriate postponement of knee replacement surgery. They have a documented record of effectiveness and long-term safety. In addition, there may be specific advantages of viscosupplements in the treatment of patients who have brittle diabetes mellitus, those who have failed corticosteroid injections, patients who have received frequent corticosteroids and are in danger of the significant side effects from repeated administration, or those who have a rare allergy to corticosteroids.

Injectable hyaluronan is commercially available in the United States as several products as listed in Table 3.4. They are classified by the FDA not as medications, but

TABLE 3.4

FDA-Approved Viscosupplementation Products

Viscosupplementation products—synthetically derived from rooster combs
Gel-One (Zimmer) http://gelone.zimmerbiomet.com/
30 mg/mL—3-mL syringe given as a single injection
Synvisc (Sanofi-Aventus) www.synvisc.com
8 mg/mL—2-mL syringe given as 3 weekly injections
Synvisc-One (Sanofi-Aventus) www.synviscone.com
8 mg/mL—6-mL syringe given as a single injection
Hyalgan (Fidia Pharma) www.hyalgan.com
10 mg/mL—2-mL syringe given as three to 5 weekly injections
Supartz (Seikagaku/Bioventus) www.supartz.com
10 mg/mL—2.5-mL syringe given as 5 weekly injections
Viscosupplementation products—produced by bacterial fermentation and extraction
Euflexxa (Ferring) www.euflexxa.com
10 mg/mL—2-mL syringe given as 3 weekly injections
Durolane (Bioventus) www.durolane.com
20 mg/mL—3-mL syringe given as a single injection
Gelsyn-3 (Bioventus) https://www.oakneepainrelief.com/gelsyn_3/
16.8 mg/mL—2-mL syringe given as 3 weekly injections
Orthovisc (Anika) https://anika.com/medical/products/orthovisc/
15 mg/mL—2-mL syringe given as three to 4 weekly injections
Monovisc (Anika) https://anika.com/medical/products/monovisc/
22 mg/mL—4-mL syringe given as a single injection
GenVisc-850 (OrthogenRx) https://genvisc850.com/
10 mg/mL—2.5-mL syringe given as 5 weekly injections
Hymovis (Fidia Pharma) https://hymovis.com/
8 mg/mL—3-mL syringe given as 2 weekly injections
Triluron (OrthogenRx) https://triluron.com/
10 mg/mL—2-mL syringe given as 3 weekly injections
TriVisc (OrthogenRx) https://orthogenrx.com/products/oa-knee-pain/
4 mg/mL—2.5-mL syringe given as 3 weekly injections
Visco-3 (Zimmer Biomet) https://www.zimmerbiomet.com/en/products-and-solutions/products/restorative-therapies/visco-3.html
10 mg/mL—2.5-mL syringe given as 3 weekly injections

FDA, United States the Food and Drug Administration.

rather as medical devices. These agents are approved only for the treatment of pain in osteoarthritis of the knee joint in patients who have failed to respond adequately to conservative nonpharmacologic therapy and simple analgesics, such as acetaminophen. Despite an increasing body of literature, the use of these viscosupplements in other joints besides the knee has not been approved to date by the FDA.

In a 2013 guideline based on consensus, the American Academy of Orthopaedic Surgeons deemed the use of intra-articular injections of hyaluronic acid as not an appropriate treatment modality.[19] On the other hand, the European-based, Osteoarthritis Research Society International consensus guidelines, published in 2019, place hyaluronic acid injections as a Level 1B recommendation.[20] Evidence-based support in the medical literature for the use of hyaluronan derivatives is inconsistent, although there is an increasing body of literature documenting positive outcomes. The primary reason for the professional disagreement is due to differences in the studied hyaluronic acid products and especially the significant variations in the quality of trial designs and conduct. In an effort to address this, Xing et al[21] performed a PRISMA-compliant systematic review of overlapping meta-analyses that demonstrated hyaluronic acid injections are an effective intervention in treating knee osteoarthritis without increased risk of adverse events. Furthermore, Altman et al[22] showed that repeated courses of intra-articular injections of hyaluronic acid are an effective and safe treatment for knee osteoarthritis. There may be value in injecting viscosupplements in combination with other agents—especially platelet-rich plasma.[23] Finally, injected viscosupplements have been shown to be a cost-effective intervention for the treatment of knee osteoarthritis. In 2024, Ranawat et al[24] showed a favorable cost profile, decreased opioid and corticosteroid use as rescue medication, and a delay to the need for total knee replacement surgery.

Although the viscosupplements are similar in many respects, there are significant differences in the physical properties of each one (Table 3.5). Some hyaluronate products are derived from processing of rooster combs. Others are extracted from bacteria that have been genetically engineered to produce exact copies of human hyaluronic acid. More important from a clinical standpoint is the molecular weight of the agent and cross-linking of the molecules. A higher molecular weight and the presence of cross-linking increase the residence time in the joint and generally predict a longer-term response to treatment. Research suggests that there is an optimal molecular weight range that maximizes the ability of how hyaluronic acid interacts with cell surface receptors on synoviocytes, thereby maximizing the synthesis of native hyaluronic acid.[25] Optimal molecular weight molecules (between 500,000 and 4 million Daltons) bind strongly to cell surface receptors, maximizing the stimulation of native hyaluronic acid biosynthesis. In addition, the commercially available products also differ in their duration of effect (13-26 weeks) and in the number of injections needed for a treatment course (single injection vs 3-5 weekly procedures). Single-injection hyaluronic acid therapies for the treatment of knee pain due to osteoarthritis offer similar efficacy to multi-injection regimens, reduce the exposure of patients to invasive procedures, decrease potential side effects, maximize the probability of treatment completion/compliance, decrease costs, and increase convenience for patients.[26] All of these preparations are prepackaged in sterile syringes. However, these products are expensive, and provider knowledge of the preauthorization and reimbursement process is essential.

Administration of intra-articular viscosupplements is contraindicated in patients with known hypersensitivity to hyaluronan products or patients with current infections in or around the target knee. It is of paramount importance to ensure that the viscosupplement product is accurately injected entirely within the knee joint. Thus, when

TABLE 3.5

FDA-Approved Viscosupplements: Physical Properties

Product	Mol. Wt. (MDa)	Elasticity (Pa s)	Viscosity (Pa)	Cross-linked	Injections	Duration
Healthy young synovial fluid	6	117	45	No	N/A	
Osteoarthritic synovial fluid	1.1-1.9	1.9	1.4	No	N/A	
Durolane	10-15	~100-300	~200-300	Yes—100%	1	26 wk
Euflexxa	2.4-3.6	~1.0-2.0	~40-50	No	3	26 wk
Gel-One	N/A	Unknown	Unknown	Yes—100%	1	26 wk
Gelsyn-3	1.1	~1.0-2.0	~40-60	No	3	26 wk
GenVisc-850	0.62-1.2	~1.0-1.5	~30-40	No	5	30 wk
Hyalgan	0.5-0.7	~0.5-1.0	~20-30	No	5	26 wk
Hymovis	2.5	~80-120	~150-200	No	2	26 wk
Monovisc	1.0-2.9	~45-60	~100-150	Yes—partial	1	26 wk
Orthovisc	1.0-3.6	~2.5-3.0	~50-60	No	3-4	22 wk
Supartz	0.6-1.2	~1.0-1.5	~30-40	No	5	26 wk
Synvisc	~6	~100-200	25	Yes—partial	3	26 wk
Synvisc-One	~6	~100-200	25	Yes—partial	1	26 wk
Triluron	0.5-0.7	~1.5-2.0	~40-50	No	1	26 wk
TriVisc	0.85	~1.5-2.0	~40-50	No	1	26 wk
Visco-3	0.6-1.2	~1.5-2.0	~40-50	No	1	26 wk

FDA, United States the Food and Drug Administration.

TABLE 3.6

Botulinum Neurotoxin

Botulinum neurotoxin type A products
Botox (Allergan) https://www.botox.com/main
100 units/vial
Dysport (Ipsen) https://dysport.com
500 units/vial
Xeomin (Merz) https://xeomin.com
50, 100, and 200 units/vial
Botulinum neurotoxin type B product
MyoBloc (Solstice Neurosciences) http://www.myobloc.com
5,000 units/mL

performing an intra-articular knee injection of any viscosupplement, the operator must aspirate synovial fluid in order to document successful entry through the knee joint capsule. Ultrasound guidance of the aspiration and injection procedure is strongly recommended to ensure a successful procedure. Inadvertent injection extra-articularly into the perisynovial tissues, into the fat pad, or intravascularly greatly increases the risk of adverse reactions. The most commonly reported adverse effects of the viscosupplements' injections are transient local pain, arthralgia, joint stiffness, joint swelling, joint warmth, and gait disturbance. Use caution when injecting the rooster comb–derived products in patients allergic to avian proteins, feathers, or egg products.

BOTULINUM TOXIN

Botulinum neurotoxin is a group of seven related proteins produced by *Clostridium botulinum.* Of these, only type A and type B neurotoxins are approved for use in the United States. Botulinum toxin irreversibly binds to the presynaptic nerve membrane and blocks formation and transmission of acetylcholine at the neuromuscular junction. Botulinum toxin causes flaccid paralysis of the injected muscles. It effectively creates "medical splinting" of the target musculotendinous unit that prevents activation of the muscle. This functional forced rest of the target area for approximately 3 months allows the pathologic tissue an opportunity to heal.

Injections are performed using anatomic landmarks, ultrasound, or with electromyographic guidance. Those affected muscles with highest clinical and EMG activity are injected. Therapeutic effect from the injection usually occurs in the first 7 days, and the response lasts for an average of 12 weeks. Injections may be repeated every 3 to 4 months. Recovery occurs through proximal axonal sprouting and muscle reinnervation by formation of new neuromuscular junctions.

Effective treatment using botulinum toxin has been demonstrated in clinical studies to be effective in the treatment of various musculoskeletal disorders, including cervical dystonia, cervicogenic headache, migraine headache, temporomandibular joint disorders associated with increased muscle activity, myofascial pain disorder, piriformis syndrome, limb dystonia (writer's cramp), lateral epicondylitis, and plantar fasciitis. A list of the botulinum toxin products currently approved for use in the United States is displayed in Table 3.6. At this time of publication, the use of botulinum neurotoxin for the treatment of musculoskeletal pain is approved by the U.S. FDA only for cervical dystonia in adult patients, muscle stiffness in those with spasticity, and for prophylaxis of headaches in adult patients with chronic migraine (≥15 days per month with headache lasting 4 hours a day or longer).[27] Use of botulinum toxin for other painful conditions is considered off-label use. An individual practitioner, however, may consider it appropriate for use in patients with a condition that does not respond to, or is judged inappropriate for, other treatment options.

OTHER

Other investigational agents may earn a future role in the practice of medicine and be delivered via intra-articular injections. These include nonsteroidal anti-inflammatory drug injections including ketorolac (Toradol)[28-30] and biologic agents such as Sprifermin (recombinant human fibroblast growth factor 18). This intra-articularly injected disease-modifying osteoarthritis drug has shown promising results with increasing knee joint cartilage thickness.[31,32] A very exciting developing treatment involves gene transfer by delivering appropriate viral vectors to synoviocytes in joints for the treatment of rheumatoid arthritis, psoriatic arthritis, other inflammatory arthritis, and osteoarthritis.[33]

REFERENCES

1. Miller RD, Pardo MC Jr. *Basics of Anesthesia*. 6th ed. Elsevier; c2011:140-141.
2. Schramm R, Thorlacius H. Neutrophil recruitment in mast cell-dependent inflammation: inhibitory mechanisms of glucocorticoids. *Inflamm Res*. 2004;53:644-652.
3. Malemud CJ. Cytokines as therapeutic targets for osteoarthritis. *BioDrugs*. 2004;18:23-35.
4. Barnes PJ. Anti-inflammatory actions of glucocorticoids: molecular mechanisms. *Clin Sci (Lond)*. 1998;94:557-572.
5. Eymontt MJ, Gordon GV, Schumacher HR, Hansell JR. The effects on synovial permeability and synovial fluid leukocyte counts in symptomatic osteoarthritis after intraarticular corticosteroid administration. *J Rheumatol*. 1982;9:198-203.
6. MacMahon PJ, Eustace SJ, Kavanagh EC. Injectable corticosteroid and local anesthetic preparations: a review for radiologists. *Radiology*. 2009;252(3):647-661.
7. Wright JM, Cowper JJ, Page Thomas DP, Knight CG. The hydrolysis of cortisol 21-esters by a homogenate of inflamed rabbit synovium and by rheumatoid synovial fluid. *Clin Exp Rheumatol*. 1983;1:137-141.
8. Blankenbaker DG, De Smet AA, Stanczak JD, Fine JP. Lumbar radiculopathy: treatment with selective lumbar nerve blocks—comparison of effectiveness of triamcinolone and betamethasone injectable suspensions. *Radiology*. 2005;237:738-741.
9. Stanczak J, Blankenbaker DG, De Smet AA, Fine J. Efficacy of epidural injections of Kenalog and Celestone in the treatment of lower back pain. *AJR Am J Roentgenol*. 2003;181:1255-1258.
10. Derendorf H, Möllmann H, Grüner A, Haack D, Gyselby G. Pharmacokinetics and pharmacodynamics of glucocorticoid suspensions after intra-articular administration. *Clin Pharmacol Ther*. 1986;39(3):313-317.
11. Garg N, Perry L, Deodhar A. Intra-articular and soft tissue injections, a systematic review of relative efficacy of various corticosteroids. *Clin Rheumatol*. 2014;33(12):1695-1706.
12. Cushman DM, Bruno B, Christiansen J, Schultz A, McCormick ZL. Efficacy of injected corticosteroid type, dose, and volume for pain in large joints: a narrative review. *PM R*. 2018;10(7):748-757.
13. Hajialilo M, Ghorbanihaghjo A, Valaee L, et al. A double-blind randomized comparative study of triamcinolone hexacetonide and dexamethasone intra-articular injection for the treatment of knee joint arthritis in rheumatoid arthritis. *Clin Rheumatol*. 2016;35(12):2887-2891.
14. Kumar A, Dhir V, Sharma S, Sharma A, Singh S. Efficacy of methylprednisolone acetate versus triamcinolone acetonide intra-articular knee injection in patients with chronic inflammatory arthritis: a 24-week randomized controlled trial. *Clin Ther*. 2017;39(1):150-158.
15. Johnston PC, Lansang MC, Chatterjee S, Kennedy L. Intra-articular glucocorticoid injections and their effect on hypothalamic-pituitary-adrenal (HPA)-axis function. *Endocrine*. 2015;48(2):410-416.
16. Whelan G, Sim J, Smith B, Moffatt M, Littlewood C. Are corticosteroid injections associated with secondary adrenal insufficiency in adults with musculoskeletal pain? A systematic review and meta-analysis of prospective studies. *Clin Orthop Relat Res*. 2022;480(6):1061-1074.
17. Guaraldi F, Gori D, Calderoni P, et al. Comparative assessment of hypothalamic-pituitary-adrenal axis suppression secondary to intrabursal injection of different glucocorticoids: a pilot study. *J Endocrinol Invest*. 2019;42(9):1117-1124.
18. Mederake M, Trappe D, Jacob C, et al. Influence of hyaluronic acid on intra-articular friction—a biomechanical study in whole animal joints. *BMC Musculoskelet Disord*. 2022;23(1):927.

19. Sanders JO, Murray J, Gross L. Non-arthroplasty treatment of osteoarthritis of the knee. *J Am Acad Orthop Surg.* 2014;22(4):256-260.
20. Bannuru RR, Osani MC, Vaysbrot EE, et al. OARSI guidelines for the non-surgical management of knee, hip, and polyarticular osteoarthritis. *Osteoarthritis Cartilage.* 2019;27(11):1578-1589.
21. Xing D, Wang B, Liu Q, et al. Intra-articular hyaluronic acid in treating knee osteoarthritis: a PRISMA-compliant systematic review of overlapping meta-analysis. *Sci Rep.* 2016;6:32790.
22. Altman R, Hackel J, Niazi F, Shaw P, Nicholls M. Efficacy and safety of repeated courses of hyaluronic acid injections for knee osteoarthritis: a systematic review. *Semin Arthritis Rheum.* 2018;48(2):168-175.
23. Palco M, Fenga D, Basile GC, et al. Platelet-rich plasma combined with hyaluronic acid versus leucocyte and platelet-rich plasma in the conservative treatment of knee osteoarthritis. A retrospective study. *Medicina (Kaunas).* 2021;57(3):232.
24. Ranawat A, Guo K, Phillips M, et al. Health economic assessments of hyaluronic acid treatments for knee osteoarthritis: a systematic review. *Adv Ther.* 2024;41(1):65-81.
25. Smith MM, Ghosh P. The synthesis of hyaluronic acid by human synovial fibroblasts is influenced by the nature of the hyaluronate in the extracellular environment. *Rheumatol Int.* 1987;7(3):113-122.
26. McElheny K, Toresdahl B, Ling D, Mages K, Asif I. Comparative effectiveness of alternative dosing regimens of hyaluronic acid injections for knee osteoarthritis: a systematic review. *Sports Health.* 2019;11(5):461-466.
27. Botox prescribing information. Accessed August 1, 2025. https://www.rxabbvie.com/pdf/botox_medguide.pdf
28. Min KS, St Pierre P, Ryan PM, Marchant BG, Wilson CJ, Arrington ED. A double-blind randomized controlled trial comparing the effects of subacromial injection with corticosteroid versus NSAID in patients with shoulder impingement syndrome. *J Shoulder Elbow Surg.* 2013;22(5):595-601.
29. Lee SC, Rha DW, Chang WH. Rapid analgesic onset of intra-articular hyaluronic acid with ketorolac in osteoarthritis of the knee. *J Back Musculoskelet Rehabil.* 2011;24(1):31-38.
30. Rhim HC, Ruiz J, Taseh A, et al. Nonsteroidal anti-inflammatory drug injections versus steroid injections in the management of upper and lower extremity orthopedic conditions: a systematic review with meta-analysis. *J Clin Med.* 2024;13(4):1132.
31. Hochberg MC, Guermazi A, Guehring H, et al. Effect of intra-articular sprifermin vs placebo on femorotibial joint cartilage thickness in patients with osteoarthritis: the FORWARD randomized clinical trial. *JAMA.* 2019;322(14):1360-1370.
32. Eckstein F, Hochberg MC, Guehring H, et al. Long-term structural and symptomatic effects of intra-articular sprifermin in patients with knee osteoarthritis: 5-year results from the FORWARD study. *Ann Rheum Dis.* 2021;80(8):1062-1069.
33. Evans CH, Ghivizzani SC, Robbins PD. The 2024 OREF clinical research award: progress toward a gene therapy for arthritis. *J Am Acad Orthop Surg.* 2024;32(23):1052-1060.

4

Orthobiologics

Francis G. O'Connor

Orthobiologics are biologically derived substances that are utilized to enhance or accelerate the body's natural healing process of musculoskeletal injuries. Biotherapeutic agents employed in the realm of orthobiologics, not uncommonly referred to and identified as regenerative medicine, include prolotherapy, autologous blood, platelet-rich plasma (PRP), stem cells, and others. "Regenerative medicine" describes an emerging field of musculoskeletal medicine that employs the precise application of autologous, allogeneic, or proliferative injectable agents that focus on augmenting the body's endogenous repair capabilities at the specific injury site.[1]

The growth of regenerative medicine has emerged from increasing evidence that has challenged the efficacy of conventional treatment options for the care of common musculoskeletal ailments. In 1999, Kraushaar and Nirschl, using electron microscopy of surgical sections from tennis elbow procedures, demonstrated the absence of inflammatory cells, questioning the role of inflammation, and paving the way for the identification of a degenerative pathway for overuse injuries by coining the term "angiofibroblastic tendinosis."[2] This identification of a degenerative process raised concern over the role of anti-inflammatory medication.[2] Traditionally, nonsteroidal anti-inflammatory medications have been prescribed by medical providers for the management of these disorders, but with the increasing recognition of degenerative tendinopathy, their role has been called to question.[3] Corticosteroid injections, in particular, have been the subject of several systematic reviews that have identified that while in musculoskeletal soft tissue injuries they may provide short-term relief, there are concerns that these effects may in the long term be no better than placebo and, in some cases, harmful.[4] In the case of spine injections, including epidural steroid injections in the setting of subacute and chronic lumbar pain, an updated Cochrane review concluded that "there is currently insufficient evidence to support the use of [corticosteroid] injection therapy in subacute and chronic low-back pain."[5]

In addition to injectable agents for many joint and soft tissue disorders, conventional surgical procedures have also been challenged for their efficacy. Arthroscopic surgery for the repair of knee meniscal tears in patients over the age of 40 has been shown in a recent meta-analysis to be no better than sham surgery or conservative treatment,[6,7] while surgery for rotator cuff impingement has been challenged for failing to provide improved patient outcomes.[8] In the management of arthritis, joint replacement surgery has resulted in profound improvement in the quality of life for many patients, but these procedures are management techniques and not without their own complications and risks.[9] These publications in the peer-reviewed medical literature have raised not only provider, but also patient, concern in the current approach to treating common musculoskeletal disorders, and focused consideration on other potential alternative treatments that are minimally invasive, to include the regenerative medicine model.[10]

Mulvaney et al[1] have described the regenerative medicine treatment model as a paradigm shift from catabolism and tissue degeneration to anabolism and tissue repair.

In the setting of chronic injury, there are several postulated mechanisms for failed self-tissue repair, as described by Mulvaney et al:

1. "The body fails to recognize an injury and mounts an ineffective healing response.
2. The repair mechanism is overwhelmed by ongoing tissue insults such as chronic repetitive movements without adequate recovery, ligamentous laxity resulting in pathologic joint movement, and functional movement disorders resulting in pathologic movement.
3. The repair mechanisms are inhibited by a suboptimal healing milieu. Factors contributing to a catabolic, suboptimal healing milieu include, but are not limited to, exposure to toxins (including many pharmaceuticals), poor diet, obesity, lack of regular exercise, chronic systemic inflammation, chronic infection, poor sleep, hormonal deficiencies, and chronic stress."[11,12]

The aforementioned etiologies for a failure of self-repair are potential targets and opportunities for regenerative medicine and counseling. The objective of regenerative medicine treatment is to promote and augment native and natural processes.[1] While there is an abundance of regenerative therapies currently available to providers, this review focuses on some of the more common therapies with the most robust evidence-based literature: prolotherapy, autologous blood, PRP therapy, and autologous stem cells. Importantly, while the field of orthobiologics holds exciting promise, recent expert consensus leaders have identified considerable challenges, including cost and ethical considerations, the need for standardized communication, improved regulatory frameworks, and enhanced safety measures.[13]

PROLOTHERAPY

Prolotherapy, initially described by Hackett,[14] has been used as a treatment modality since the 1950s. The theory supporting prolotherapy as an intervention is that accumulated ligamentous laxity (through acute trauma or chronic microtrauma) allows the joints to move beyond their intended physiologic parameters. This disproportionate motion can then lead to pathologic responses, including annular ligament tears resulting in vertebral disc bulges, or cartilage degradation resulting in osteoarthritis (OA). Prolotherapy has generally been used as a regional modality, insofar as many ligaments work in concert to prevent abnormal joint motion. Prolotherapy is also used in the management of degenerative tendinopathies.[15]

The most studied "proliferant" solution is 15% dextrose, although other agents have been used (eg, sodium morrhuate). When injected in or very proximal to a ligament or tendon, the hypertonic dextrose is thought to induce a mild cellular injury via a rapid osmotic shift of fluid, which in turn initiates an inflammatory response.[16] This focused initiation of the healing cascade is postulated to heal the previously unrecognized ligamentous injury and restore the damaged ligament to its ideal length and structure. By healing all or most of the major ligaments in a painful joint or section of spine, normal motion parameters will be restored, allowing the area to heal over time. Because the healing cascade is initiated by induction of inflammation, patients need to refrain from using anti-inflammatory medications for 7 days prior to treatment and in the posttreatment recovery period.

For years, the scientific evidence supporting the use of prolotherapy lagged behind its use in clinical practice. In the last decade, however, this lack of medical evidence has been effectively addressed by dedicated researchers. High-quality studies currently support the use of prolotherapy in many chronic injuries. One of the most significant of these studies was a multicenter randomized clinical trial (RCT) by Rabago et al, in which the investigators followed 90 patients for 1 year and concluded that prolotherapy resulted in clinically meaningful improvement of pain, function, and stiffness scores for knee OA when compared to saline injections or at-home exercise programs. The protocol used in the study targeted both intra-articular and ligament structures around the knee.[17] Hauser et al published a systematic review of dextrose prolotherapy for chronic musculoskeletal pain. Their paper reviewed 14 RCTs and concluded that the "use of dextrose prolotherapy is supported for treatment of tendinopathies, knee and finger joint OA, and spinal/pelvic pain due to ligament dysfunction."[18] Dumais et al[19] conducted a randomized crossover study for the treatment of knee OA and concluded that "the use of prolotherapy is associated with a marked reduction in symptoms, which was sustained for over 24 weeks." There are now many high-quality statistically significant studies supporting the use of prolotherapy in joint OA, tendinopathies, and chronic spine pain.[15,20-24] Finally, a recently performed systematic review evaluating prolotherapy in sports medicine, that included over 20 articles and 1,136 patient encounters, found that prolotherapy was not only safe but also appears to be a promising alternative treatment for common tendinopathies.[25]

AUTOLOGOUS BLOOD

Autologous blood injections (ABI) contain platelets with growth factors that may help in the healing process of chronic injuries. Specifically identified in platelets are transforming growth factor-β, platelet-derived growth factor, insulinlike growth factor, vascular endothelial growth factor, and epidermal growth factor. These platelet growth factors stimulate the healing process and are thought to lead to repair of the damaged tissue. The hypothesis is that these growth factors stimulate angiogenesis and cell proliferation and increase tensile strength and the recruitment of repair cells.

The ABI procedure is easily performed in the clinical setting. A variable amount of blood is withdrawn from the patient by standard venipuncture; usually about 2 to 3 mL into a syringe with a variable amount of anesthetic. The combination of the blood and anesthetic is injected into and around the damaged tendon, usually with ultrasound guidance. A "peppering" technique is sometimes used to inject the autologous blood; this involves inserting the needle into the tendon, injecting some of the blood, withdrawing without emerging from the skin, slightly redirecting, and reinserting (see Chapter 6 on Advanced and Adjunctive Techniques that addresses fenestration). After the procedure, patients are usually advised to avoid strenuous or excessive use of the tendon for a few weeks, after which physical therapy is initiated. Although the procedure is minimally invasive, there are still potential side effects. These include a small risk of the area becoming infected and temporary pain at the injection site. ABI are advantageous over other procedures that involve the use of blood products; however, as due to the patient's own blood being injected, there is no risk of transfusion-transmitted infection or reactions.

The evidence is limited on the efficacy of ABI as a regenerative therapy. While ABI is utilized for a wide variety of tendinopathies, one of the common uses is for recalcitrant tennis elbow. In one study, 28 patients with lateral epicondylitis were injected with 2 mL of autologous blood under the extensor carpi radialis brevis. All patients had failed previous nonsurgical treatments, including all or combinations of physical therapy, splinting, nonsteroidal anti-inflammatory medication, and prior steroid injections. After ABI therapy, 22 patients (79%) in whom nonsurgical modalities had failed were relieved completely of pain even during strenuous activity.[26] A subsequent meta-analysis by Chou et al[27] concluded that ABI is more effective than corticosteroid injection but not more effective than PRP injection in treating lateral epicondylitis. Finally, while ABI is promising, a systematic review by de Vos et al commented that there are currently limited high-quality clinical studies. Future clinical studies should use a proper control group, randomization, blinding, or validated disease-specific outcome measures to assess for pain and function. In addition, the authors note that a good experimental model for studying tendinopathy would be helpful for basic research.[28]

PLATELET-RICH PLASMA

PRP, defined as a concentration of platelets above baseline, has been in clinical use since the 1990s.[29] PRP is prepared from autologous blood by using centrifuge density separation with removal of the red blood cells and then further concentrating the platelet-rich fraction of the remaining plasma. Platelets activate (degranulate) when they contact air, broken fragments of collagen (such as at the site of damaged tissue), or sense another platelet in proximity undergoing degranulation. When platelets degranulate, they release alpha granules that contain the aforementioned growth factors that signal for inflammation and stimulate the body's endogenous repair mechanisms.

PRP has been shown to be an effective treatment modality in many well-done RCTs,[30-35] although some of the evidence had shown mixed results.[36] Laver et al published a systematic review of the literature looking at 29 studies (11 RCTs) comparing PRP against hyaluronic acid for both knee and hip OA. They concluded that current clinical evidence supports the benefit of PRP treatment for knee and hip OA compared to several alternative treatments.[37] One issue that continues to confound the results of many RCTs comparing the tested substance to a saline-injected control is that there is reasonable evidence indicating that a saline injection is not a control but a treatment.[38] Another confounding issue in PRP research may be attributed to the fact that it is difficult to statistically account for, and to appropriately power studies for, variations in even similar types of injuries, posttreatment recovery regimes, method of injection, skill of the clinician, and concomitant pharmaceutical use (and many other factors). Also, there is not one homologous preparation of PRP that is being compared in the literature.[39] There are many commercially available systems and lab-based preparation protocols for the preparation of PRP. Furthermore, optimal platelet concentrations have not been established for musculoskeletal repair. The qualitative differences in PRP also is a confounding variable in research. The presence and concentrations of the various blood components—red blood cells, white blood cells, and platelets—all have been proposed to have either beneficial or deleterious effects. For example, there are some data to support that leukocyte-poor PRP is more beneficial than leukocyte-rich PRP for intra-articular applications, while leukocyte-rich PRP may be superior for intratendon applications.[40,41] Nonetheless, the clinical superiority of any one preparation has not been the subject of ongoing research.[42] Mautner et al[39] have described a comprehensive PRP nomenclature paper designed to define PRP based on the variable components to accurately and quickly describe the type of PRP being used in the prospective study.

STEM CELLS

Autologous mesenchymal stems cells (MSCs) appear to facilitate musculoskeletal repair not so much by differentiating into the required target tissue but by binding to the injury site and acting in a paracrine fashion to facilitate tissue repair.[43] Autologous stem cell preparations can be created from adipose-derived MSCs and from bone marrow–derived MSCs. Currently, there is ongoing debate regarding which source is more optimal for musculoskeletal applications. Marrow-derived stem cells have been shown to have a higher osteogenic and chondrogenic potential with in vitro studies. But human studies investigating the use of adipose-derived stem cells for the treatment of OA have shown comparable results to those for marrow-derived treatments. Furthermore, adipose has a significantly greater number of stem cells than bone marrow per equivalent unit of measurement. However, it remains to be seen whether any of these differences result in clinically meaningful differences in improved outcomes in human studies. All that being stated, the number of stem cells derived from both bone marrow and fat is exceedingly small; estimated at approximately 1 in 10,000. In addition, the number of viable cells that are actually delivered and survive with an injection is currently unknown.

Mulvaney et al[1] performed a review of the medical literature and found six RCTs using bone marrow–derived and adipose-derived stem cells to treat knee arthritis, which concluded the following: there were no serious adverse events and there were superior radiological outcomes favoring stem cell injections. Two trials reported improved histological outcomes, improved arthroscopically scored healing rates, and superior patient-reported outcomes. However, the level of evidence in some of the studies was reduced to level 3 due to perceived risk of bias.[44] Emadedin et al[45] published a randomized, triple-blind, placebo-controlled trial using bone marrow aspirate concentrate for knee OA of 43 patients and concluded that bone marrow aspirate concentrate was safe and provided clinically significant relief of pain for over 6 months versus placebo. Centeno et al[46] published a study of 840 OA knees with long-term follow-up treated with bone marrow–derived stem cells and found this application to be both safe and efficacious. Centeno et al[47] also published a prospective multisite study of 115 shoulder OA and rotator cuff tears treated with bone marrow–derived stem cells, which showed statistically significant improvement in Disabilities of the Arm, Shoulder and Hand scores. Hernigou et al recently published their landmark RCT comparing total knee arthroplasty with subchondral bone marrow injections for severe knee OA, with a 12-year follow-up. Both groups had similar favorable improvement. The cell therapy group showed improvement in both cartilage and bone marrow lesions. There were significantly greater medical and surgical complications following total knee arthroplasty compared to the cell injection group.[48] Although there is ongoing debate about which source of MSCs is superior for orthopedic regenerative applications, both need further high-quality RCT level evidence to support their clinical efficacy.

The Australasian College of Sports Physicians published a position statement in 2016 stating that autologous MSC stem cell therapy should have the same four-phase trial safety testing as a new drug before being considered safe; their position statement was also covering the potential use of culture-expanded MSCs.[49] Regarding the safety of non–culture-expanded MSCs from either bone marrow or adipose tissue, current medical literature supports that both sources appear to be safe and reasonably efficacious for the treatment of knee and hip OA and some tendinopathies and tendon tears; however, more high-quality research is needed.

SUMMARY

Regenerative medicine offers promising new approaches to musculoskeletal injuries. These therapies have been shown to be largely safe; however, there are limited evidence-based data to guide their utilization at this time. Importantly, a critical observation is that there is currently no evidence that current orthobiologic therapies available in the United States can lead to any tissue regeneration. It is critical that providers are honest with the data when discussing these approaches with patients and proceed with caution; more evidence and guidance will develop with time. The National Football League recently published guidance with key summary points that best addresses where we are currently with the routine utilization of orthobiologic therapies[50]:

- "Orthobiologic treatments, such as PRP and 'stem cells,' offer promise for pain relief and potentially improved healing of certain conditions affecting tendons, ligaments, and joints.
- The indications for use and the claims reporting tissue regeneration after PRP or stem cell therapy are not supported by the available evidence at this time.
- Indiscriminate use of orthobiologic treatments and/or lack of rigorous protocols for tissue processing and delivery can paradoxically put athlete health and safety at risk.
- Active research studies by scientists will help define the best indications and applications for biologic therapies that maximize both the benefit and safety for the athletes."

All that being stated, it is important to maintain perspective on the limited supporting medical evidence for many currently accepted treatments and surgeries. Regenerative options may be a safer and more physiologic treatment choice for many injuries and long-term patient health. Clinicians need to carefully and continuously assess the literature and do what they think is the best for their patient.

REFERENCES

1. Mulvaney SW, Tortland P, Shiple B, Curtis K. Regenerative medicine options for chronic musculoskeletal conditions: a review of the literature. *Endurance Sports Med.* 2018;(Fall/Winter):6-15.
2. Kraushaar BS, Nirschl RP. Tendinosis of the elbow (tennis elbow). Clinical features and findings of histological, immunohistochemical, and electron microscopy studies. *J Bone Joint Surg Am.* 1999;81(2):259-278.
3. Kane SF, Olewinski LH, Tamminga KS. Management of chronic tendon injuries. *Am Fam Physician.* 2019;100(3):147-157.
4. Coombes BK, Bisset L, Vicenzino B. Efficacy and safety of corticosteroid injections and other injections for management of tendinopathy: a systematic review of randomised controlled trials. *Lancet.* 2010;376(9754):1751-1767.
5. Staal JB, de Bie RA, de Vet HC, Hildebrandt J, Nelemans P. Injection therapy for subacute and chronic low back pain: an updated Cochrane review. *Spine (Phila Pa 1976).* 2009;34(1):49-59.
6. Lee DY, Park YJ, Kim HJ, et al. Arthroscopic meniscal surgery versus conservative management in patients aged 40 years and older: a meta-analysis. *Arch Orthop Trauma Surg.* 2018;138(12):1731-1739.
7. Siemieniuk RAC, Harris IA, Agoritsas T, et al. Arthroscopic surgery for degenerative knee arthritis and meniscal tears: a clinical practice guideline. *BMJ.* 2017;357:j1982.
8. Khan M, Alolabi B, Horner N, Bedi A, Ayeni OR, Bhandari M. Surgery for shoulder impingement: a systematic review and meta-analysis of controlled clinical trials. *CMAJ Open.* 2019;7(1):E149-E158.
9. Skou ST, Roos EM, Laursen MB, et al. A randomized, controlled trial of total knee replacement. *N Engl J Med.* 2015;373(17):1597-1606.
10. Jeyaraman M, Jeyaraman N, Ramasubramanian S, Balaji S, Muthu S. Evidence-based orthobiologic practice: current evidence review and future directions. *World J Orthop.* 2024;15(10):908-917.
11. Anderson K, Hamm RL. Factors that impair wound healing. *J Am Coll Clin Wound Spec.* 2012;4(4):84-91.
12. Gosling CM, Forbes AB, Gabbe BJ. Health professionals' perceptions of musculoskeletal injury and injury risk factors in Australian triathletes: a factor analysis. *Phys Ther Sport.* 2013;14(4):207-212.
13. Gilat R, Muth SA, Hurley ET, et al; Biologic Association Member Organization Representatives. Experts achieve consensus on a majority of statements regarding ethics, transparency, regulation and best practices for the use of orthobiologics. *Arthroscopy.* 2025;41(9):3611-3621.
14. Hackett GS. Joint stabilization through induced ligament sclerosis. *Ohio State Med J.* 1953;49(10):877-884.
15. Yelland MJ, Sweeting KR, Lyftogt JA, Ng SK, Scuffham PA, Evans KA. Prolotherapy injections and eccentric loading exercises for painful Achilles tendinosis: a randomised trial. *Br J Sports Med.* 2011;45(5):421-428.
16. Jensen KT, Rabago DP, Best TM, Patterson JJ, Vanderby R Jr. Early inflammatory response of knee ligaments to prolotherapy in a rat model. *J Orthop Res.* 2008;26(6):816-823.

17. Rabago D, Patterson JJ, Mundt M, et al. Dextrose prolotherapy for knee osteoarthritis: a randomized controlled trial. *Ann Fam Med.* 2013;11(3):229-237.
18. Hauser RA, Lackner JB, Steilen-Matias D, Harris DK. A systematic review of dextrose prolotherapy for chronic musculoskeletal pain. *Clin Med Insights Arthritis Musculoskelet Disord.* 2016;9:139-159.
19. Dumais R, Benoit C, Dumais A, et al. Effect of regenerative injection therapy on function and pain in patients with knee osteoarthritis: a randomized crossover study. *Pain Med.* 2012;13(8):990-999.
20. Smigel LR, Reeves KD, Lyftogt J, Rabago DP. Poster 385 caudal epidural dextrose injections (D5W) for chronic back pain with accompanying buttock or leg pain: a consecutive patient study with long-term follow-up. *PM R.* 2016;8(9S):S286-S287.
21. Dwivedi S, Sobel AD, DaSilva MF, Akelman E. Utility of prolotherapy for upper extremity pathology. *J Hand Surg Am.* 2019;44(3):236-239.
22. Watson JD, Shay BL. Treatment of chronic low-back pain: a 1-year or greater follow-up. *J Altern Complement Med.* 2010;16(9):951-958.
23. Kim WM, Lee HG, Jeong CW, Kim CM, Yoon MH. A randomized controlled trial of intra-articular prolotherapy versus steroid injection for sacroiliac joint pain. *J Altern Complement Med.* 2010;16(12):1285-1290.
24. Ryan M, Wong A, Taunton J. Favorable outcomes after sonographically guided intratendinous injection of hyperosmolar dextrose for chronic insertional and midportion Achilles tendinosis. *AJR Am J Roentgenol.* 2010;194(4):1047-1053.
25. Capotosto S, Nazemi AK, Komatsu DE, Penna J. Prolotherapy in the treatment of sports-related tendinopathies: a systematic review of randomized controlled trials. *Orthop J Sports Med.* 2024;12(11):23259671241275087.
26. Calandruccio JH, Steiner MM. Autologous blood and platelet-rich plasma injections for treatment of lateral epicondylitis. *Orthop Clin North Am.* 2017;48(3):351-357.
27. Chou LC, Liou TH, Kuan YC, Huang YH, Chen HC. Autologous blood injection for treatment of lateral epicondylosis: a meta-analysis of randomized controlled trials. *Phys Ther Sport.* 2016;18:68-73.
28. de Vos RJ, van Veldhoven PL, Moen MH, Weir A, Tol JL, Maffulli N. Autologous growth factor injections in chronic tendinopathy: a systematic review. *Br Med Bull.* 2010;95:63-77.
29. Marx RE, Carlson ER, Eichstaedt RM, Schimmele SR, Strauss JE, Georgeff KR. Platelet-rich plasma: growth factor enhancement for bone grafts. *Oral Surg Oral Med Oral Pathol Oral Radiol Endod.* 1998;85(6):638-646.
30. Smith PA. Intra-articular autologous conditioned plasma injections provide safe and efficacious treatment for knee osteoarthritis: an FDA-sanctioned, randomized, double-blind, placebo-controlled clinical trial. *Am J Sports Med.* 2016;44(4):884-891.
31. Dai WL, Zhou AG, Zhang H, Zhang J. Efficacy of platelet-rich plasma in the treatment of knee osteoarthritis: a meta-analysis of randomized controlled trials. *Arthroscopy.* 2017;33(3):659-670.e1.
32. Peerbooms JC, Lodder P, den Oudsten BL, Doorgeest K, Schuller HM, Gosens T. Positive effect of platelet-rich plasma on pain in plantar fasciitis: a double-blind multicenter randomized controlled trial. *Am J Sports Med.* 2019;47(13):3238-3246.
33. Gosens T, Peerbooms JC, van Laar W, den Oudsten BL. Ongoing positive effect of platelet-rich plasma versus corticosteroid injection in lateral epicondylitis: a double-blind randomized controlled trial with 2-year follow-up. *Am J Sports Med.* 2011;39(6):1200-1208.
34. Mishra AK, Skrepnik NV, Edwards SG, et al. Efficacy of platelet-rich plasma for chronic tennis elbow: a double-blind, prospective, multicenter, randomized controlled trial of 230 patients. *Am J Sports Med.* 2014;42(2):463-471.
35. Laudy AB, Bakker EW, Rekers M, Moen MH. Efficacy of platelet-rich plasma injections in osteoarthritis of the knee: a systematic review and meta-analysis. *Br J Sports Med.* 2015;49(10):657-672.
36. Yerlikaya M, Talay Çaliş H, Tomruk Sütbeyaz S, et al. Comparison of effects of leukocyte-rich and leukocyte-poor platelet-rich plasma on pain and functionality in patients with lateral epicondylitis. *Arch Rheumatol.* 2018;33(1):73-79.
37. Laver L, Marom N, Dnyanesh L, Mei-Dan O, Espregueira-Mendes J, Gobbi A. PRP for degenerative cartilage disease: a systematic review of clinical studies. *Cartilage.* 2017;8(4):341-364.
38. Bar-Or D, Rael LT, Brody EN. Use of saline as a placebo in intra-articular injections in osteoarthritis: potential contributions to nociceptive pain relief. *Open Rheumatol J.* 2017;11:16-22.
39. Mautner K, Malanga GA, Smith J, et al. A call for a standard classification system for future biologic research: the rationale for new PRP nomenclature. *PM R.* 2015;7(4 Suppl):S53-S59.
40. Xu Z, Yin W, Zhang Y, et al. Comparative evaluation of leukocyte- and platelet-rich plasma and pure platelet-rich plasma for cartilage regeneration. *Sci Rep.* 2017;7:43301.
41. Zhou Y, Zhang J, Wu H, Hogan MV, Wang JH. The differential effects of leukocyte-containing and pure platelet-rich plasma (PRP) on tendon stem/progenitor cells—implications of PRP application for the clinical treatment of tendon injuries. *Stem Cell Res Ther.* 2015;6(1):173.
42. Andia I, Martin JI, Maffulli N. Advances with platelet rich plasma therapies for tendon regeneration. *Expert Opin Biol Ther.* 2018;18(4):389-398.
43. Caplan AI. Why are MSCs therapeutic? New data: new insight. *J Pathol.* 2009;217(2):318-324.
44. Pas HI, Winters M, Haisma HJ, Koenis MJ, Tol JL, Moen MH. Stem cell injections in knee osteoarthritis: a systematic review of the literature. *Br J Sports Med.* 2017;51(15):1125-1133.
45. Emadedin M, Labibzadeh N, Liastani MG, et al. Intra-articular implantation of autologous bone marrow-derived mesenchymal stromal cells to treat knee osteoarthritis: a randomized, triple-blind, placebo-controlled phase 1/2 clinical trial. *Cytotherapy.* 2018;20(10):1238-1246.

46. Centeno C, Pitts J, Al-Sayegh H, Freeman M. Efficacy of autologous bone marrow concentrate for knee osteoarthritis with and without adipose graft. *Biomed Res Int.* 2014;2014:370621.
47. Centeno CJ, Al-Sayegh H, Bashir J, Goodyear S, Freeman MD. A prospective multi-site registry study of a specific protocol of autologous bone marrow concentrate for the treatment of shoulder rotator cuff tears and osteoarthritis. *J Pain Res.* 2015;8:269-276.
48. Hernigou P, Auregan JC, Dubory A, Flouzat-Lachaniette CH, Chevallier N, Rouard H. Subchondral stem cell therapy versus contralateral total knee arthroplasty for osteoarthritis following secondary osteonecrosis of the knee. *Int Orthop.* 2018;42(11):2563-2571.
49. Osborne H, Anderson L, Burt P, Young M, Gerrard D. Australasian College of Sports Physicians-position statement: the place of mesenchymal stem/stromal cell therapies in sport and exercise medicine. *Br J Sports Med.* 2016;50(20):1237-1244.
50. Rodeo S, Bedi A. 2019-2020 NFL and NFL physician society orthobiologics consensus statement. *Sports Health.* 2020;12(1):58-60.

5

Musculoskeletal Ultrasound

Francis G. O'Connor

INTRODUCTION

The utilization of ultrasound (US) in musculoskeletal medicine has been transformative in the last decade; procedures previously exclusively done by interventional radiologists are now readily performed in the hands of the primary care provider at the point-of-care (see Fig. 5.1).[1,2] Interventional US is routinely taught in residency and fellowship education, and US is increasingly being integrated into anatomy instruction as a part of undergraduate medical education.[3] The American Medical Society for Sports Medicine (AMSSM) has recently published curricular guidelines for musculoskeletal US education.[4] Importantly, the Association for Medical Ultrasound (American Institute of Ultrasound in Medicine [AIUM]), a multidisciplinary association and leader dedicated to advancing the safe and effective use of US in medicine through research and professional and public education, has developed clinical practice guidelines and practice parameters that guide the performance of musculoskeletal US examinations.[5-8]

Evidence to support the "value added" of US guidance continues to accumulate.[1,2,9,10] Multiple publications have documented concerning variability in the accuracy of palpation-guided injections.[11,12] Eustace reported that only 29% of subacromial injections reached the intended target, while Bum Park et al found that in a study of patients with knee osteoarthritis, 83% of palpation-guided injections were successful in finding the intra-articular space compared to 96% of ultrasound-guided injections (USGIs). US needle guidance clearly has an advantage over palpation-guided injections in its real-time capability, and the ability to visualize soft targets helps the clinician avoid surrounding neurovascular structures. Publications continue to emerge supporting the observation that USGIs are more accurate, more efficacious, and potentially more cost-effective. In 2015, the AMSSM published a consensus position stand on interventional musculoskeletal US. The document concluded: there is **strong** evidence that USGIs are more accurate; **moderate** evidence that USGIs are more efficacious; and finally, **preliminary** evidence that USGIs are more cost-effective.[9]

INDICATIONS

USGIs follow comparable guidance already discussed for palpation-guided injections; however, there are several other indications that favor the utilization of US (see Table 5.1). There are several technically challenging injections described in this fifth edition that warrant consideration for improved accuracy to facilitate either a more precise diagnosis or administer a medication in a specific location. An example of such an injection would be to the piriformis muscle, where a palpation-guided injection may be unable to delineate the location among multiple muscle groups in the deep posterior hip.

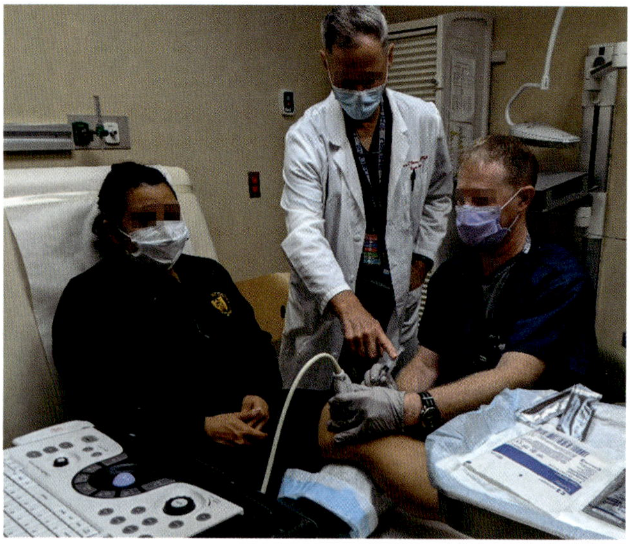

FIGURE 5.1 ● Primary care provider performing office-based ultrasound-guided suprapatellar knee injection.

A second clear indication is where local standard of care recommends that an injection be performed under fluoroscopic or US guidance, for matters of either safety or accuracy. Examples where guidance may be required include intra-articular hip, sacroiliac, or facet joint injections (see Fig. 5.2).

Another common scenario for transitioning from a palpation-guided injection to an USGI is failure of the former injection to provide clinical improvement. An injection failure is not uncommonly associated in a patient with comorbid obesity. US guidance may also be warranted for injection targets in close proximity to vulnerable neurovascular structures (eg, femoral artery while performing an iliopsoas injection) or where a high-risk procedure in close proximity to a structure where needle puncture may be potentially harmful (eg, sternoclavicular joint with proximity to the lung with the potential complication of a pneumothorax).

CONTRAINDICATIONS

Contraindications for USGIs follow the identical precautions previously identified for palpation-guided injections. Importantly, however, it should be noted that using an US requires a three-dimensional recognition of anatomical relationships and reasonable hand-eye coordination in order to successfully employ real-time needle guidance. It is

TABLE 5.1

Ultrasound-Guided Injection Indications

Ultrasound Guidance Indication	Example
Accuracy	Piriformis
Recommended guidance	Intra-articular hip
Palpation-guided failure	Subacromial impingement (obesity)
Assess anatomy	Iliopsoas bursa—femoral artery
High-risk procedure	Proximity to the lung

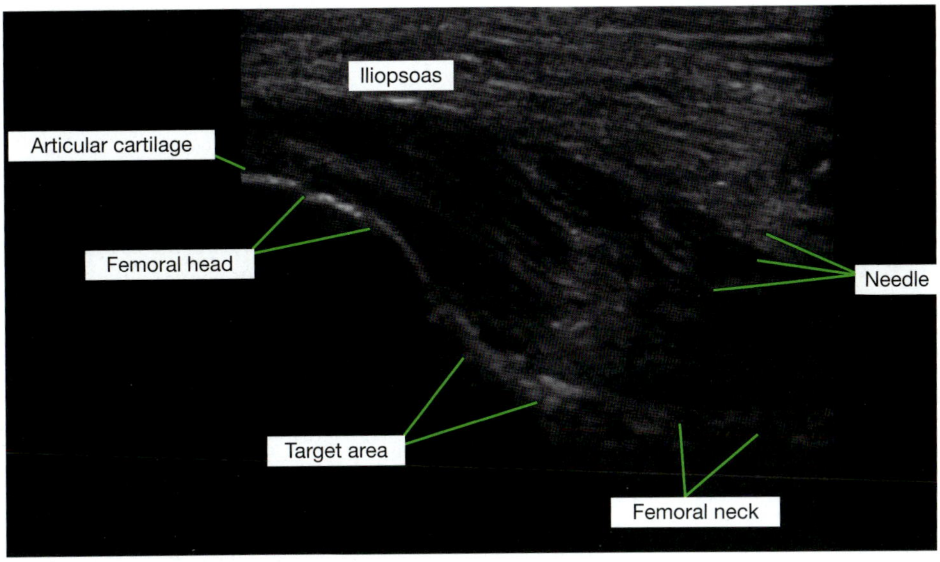

FIGURE 5.2 ● Needle approaching anterior hip capsule during intra-articular hip joint injection.

critically important that the provider recognize their limitations, as the skillful use of US guidance requires considerable investment in training and practice.

NORMAL ULTRASOUND ANATOMY SIGNALS

Musculoskeletal US is a remarkable tool that represents a dramatic innovation in the diagnosis and management of musculoskeletal disorders. This technology, however, is associated with a "significant" learning curve with new patterns to recognize and requires integrating knowledge of three-dimensional and cross-sectional anatomy with known palpation-evident superficial anatomical structures. A complete review of US anatomical signals is beyond the scope of this introduction, and the interested reader is referred to several excellent texts.[13,14] Basic anatomical structures, however, are introduced as well as the artifactual concepts of anisotropy and acoustic shadowing.

US imaging produces four characteristic signals: hyperechoic, hypoechoic, isoechoic, and anechoic. "Hyperechoic" represents a strong reflection, with a bright echo signal on B-mode (Brightness-mode) imaging. "Hypoechoic" is interpreted as a weak or lower-intensity (less bright) echo signal, while "isoechoic" is the term used when an US finding indicates a structure has the same echogenicity, or brightness, as the surrounding tissue. Finally, "anechoic" represents a dark area, absent of echo signal. These terms are used to describe patterns characteristic of commonly encountered musculoskeletal structures (see Table 5.2), muscle (see Fig. 5.3), tendon (see Fig. 5.4), ligament (see Fig. 5.5), nerve (see Fig. 5.6), and bone (see Fig. 5.7).

In addition to understanding normal US signaling, it is critical to understand sonographic artifacts in order to properly interpret an image. While there are many artifacts that affect musculoskeletal US imaging and needle guidance,[13,14] two warrant specific attention here: anisotropy and acoustic shadowing.

Anisotropy, a term commonly used in musculoskeletal US, is used to describe the artifact produced in certain tissues with tilting of the probe and resultant changes in observed echogenicity. Certain musculoskeletal structures, for example, tendons, as a result of angular dependence, will demonstrate changes in echogenicity (hyperechoic

TABLE 5.2

Ultrasound Signals for Common Anatomic Structures

Anatomical Structure	Ultrasound Signal
Muscle	• Hypoechoic with multiple hyperechoic lines, which represent fibro adipose septa or perimysium • Transverse—loosely arranged hyperechoic foci, resulting in a "starry night" appearance • Longitudinal—obliquely fascicular, "multipennate" appearance
Tendon	• Hyperechoic with anisotropy • Tightly arranged, bright lines longitudinally or bright dots transversely at right angles—compact fibrillary pattern
Nerve	• Linearly fascicular pattern with hypoechoic fascicles and hyperechoic connective tissue longitudinally • Transversely, clustered fascicles—"honeycomb," "cluster-of-grapes," or "speckled" appearance
Ligament	• Hyperechoic striated appearance that are more compact than tendons • Trilaminar appearance—central hypoechoic layer • Connect two osseous structures
Bone	• Intense hyperechoic appearance of cortical bone • Hyaline cartilage is hypoechoic or anechoic

to hypoechoic) with a change in the angle of the incident US beam (see Fig. 5.8). Recognition of this US artifact is critical as to not misinterpret this phenomenon as demonstrating pathology. Tendons are susceptible to anisotropy to a greater degree than nerves.

Acoustic shadowing is another commonly seen artifact key to understand for the provider utilizing musculoskeletal US. The US image relies on beam reflection for the production of an US image; when the beam encounters a highly reflective interface, for example, bone or calcifications, there is no beam to further penetrate with resultant shadowing (see Fig. 5.9). This artifact may also occur when air or gas is in a tissue.

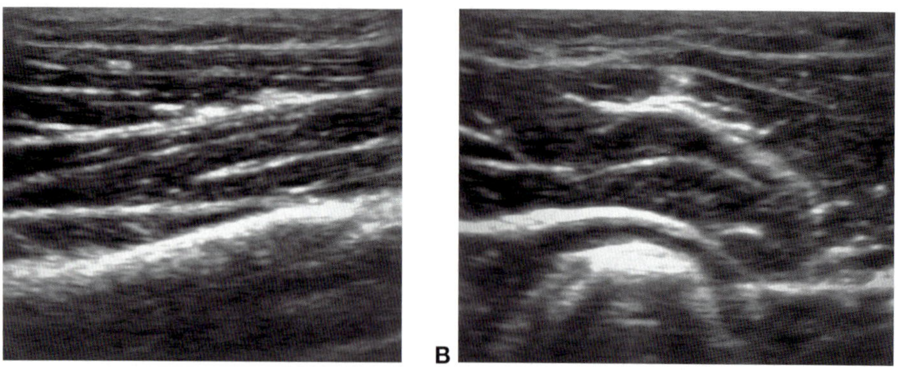

A B

FIGURE 5.3 ● **A.** Muscle, long axis (multipennate). **B.** Muscle, short axis (starry night).

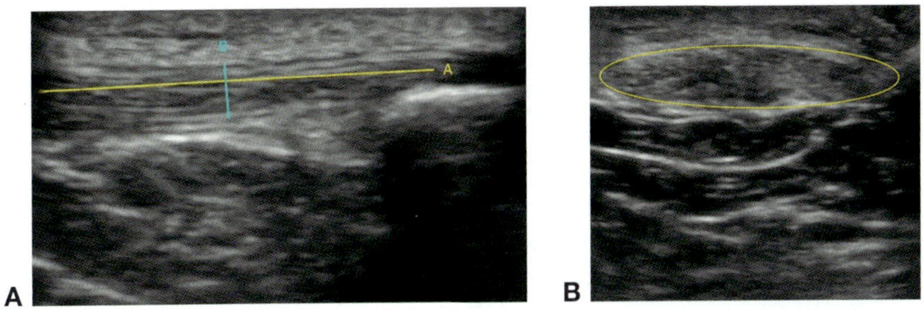

FIGURE 5.4 ● **A.** Tendon, long axis (patellar tendon). *Lines* indicated by *A* and *B* illustrate borders of the patellar tendon. **B.** Tendon, short axis (patellar tendon) (*yellow circle*).

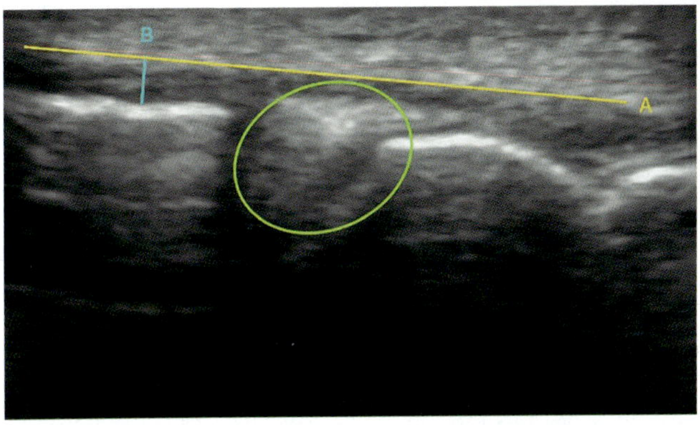

FIGURE 5.5 ● Ligament, long axis (medial collateral ligament). *Lines A* and *B* outline the width and length borders of the medial collateral ligament; the *circle* identifies the medial meniscus.

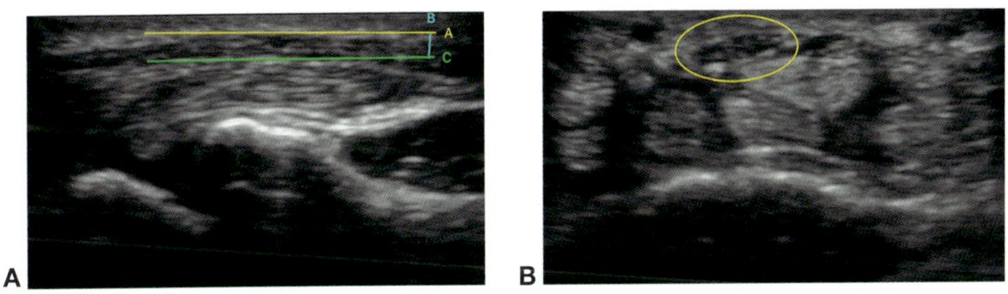

FIGURE 5.6 ● **A.** Nerve, long axis (median nerve). *Lines A, B,* and *C* outline the width and long-axis borders of the median nerve. **B.** Nerve, short axis (median nerve), and tendons, short axis. The *yellow circle* outlines the median nerve in short axis.

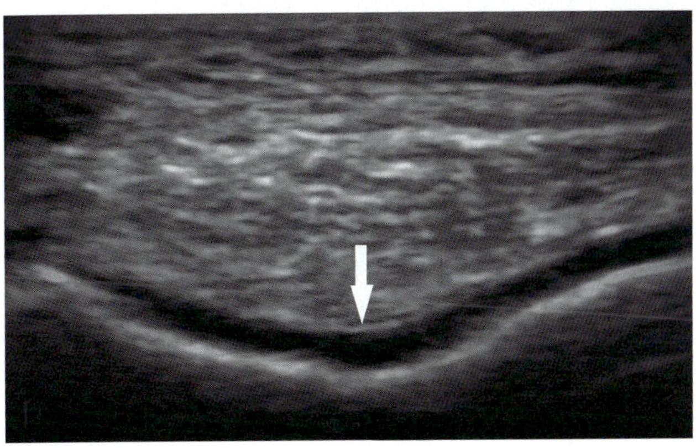

FIGURE 5.7 ● Bone and overlying articular cartilage (femoral sulcus). The *arrow* points directly to the femoral cartilage.

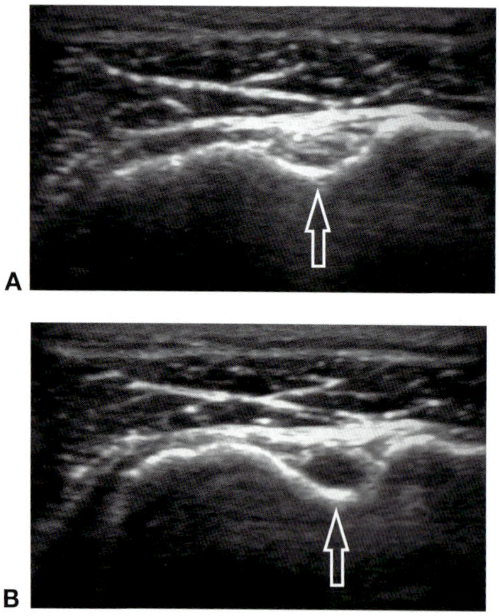

FIGURE 5.8 Short-axis view of biceps tendon demonstrating anisotropy. The *arrow* in **(A)** and **(B)** points directly to the biceps tendon in short axis. **A** illustrates hyperechoic signal with the probe perpendicular to the tendon. **B** illustrates anechoic signal when the probe is not directly perpendicular to the tendon.

Importantly, musculoskeletal US imaging is noted for the utilization of mnemonics and metaphors to describe common normal patterns as well as sonopathologies. As an example, the appearance of a normal supraspinatus as it inserts into the greater tuberosity is identified as the characteristic "bird's beak" appearance with the convexity of the bursal surface noting a normal tendon. This contrasts with the "crocodile mouth" appearance of a torn supraspinatus identifying a concavity of the bursal surface and loss of tissue integrity (see Fig. 5.10). The interested reader is referred to references that identify commonly utilized terminologies and demonstrative videos.[15,16]

ULTRASOUND TRANSDUCER MANIPULATION TERMINOLOGY

The US probe can be manipulated in multiple directions to enhance both target and needle image acquisition. A useful pneumonic that identifies the various aspects of probe manipulation is "P.A.R.T.": pressure, alignment, rotation, and tilt (see Fig. 5.11).[17]

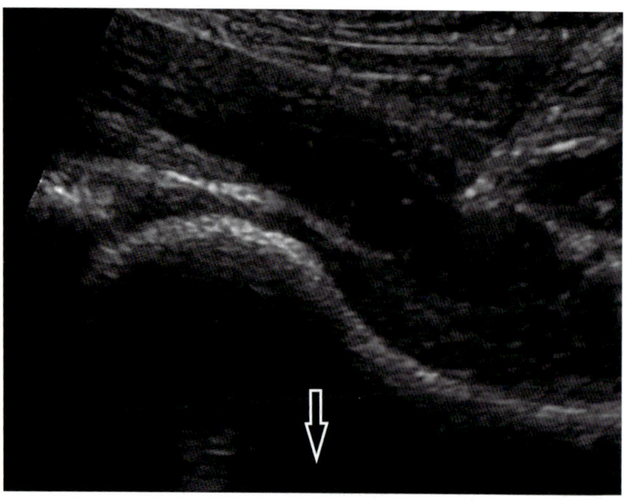

FIGURE 5.9 Long-axis view of an intra-articular hip injection. *Arrow* illustrates the acoustic shadowing deep to the cortex of the femoral neck.

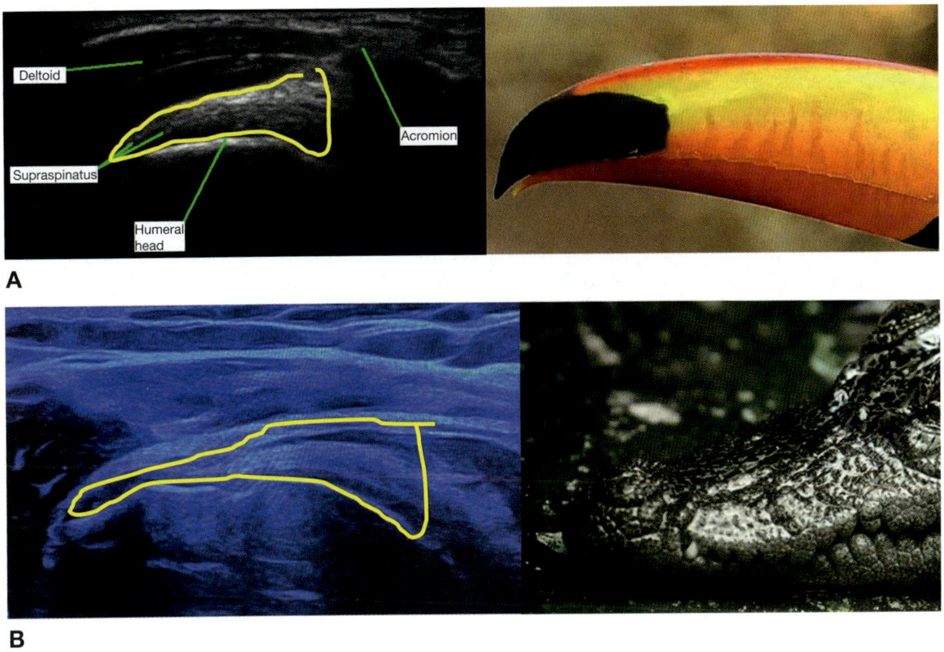

FIGURE 5.10 ● Normal supraspinatus "bird's beak" **(A)** in contrast with abnormal "crocodile mouth" appearance suggesting a rotator cuff tear **(B)**.

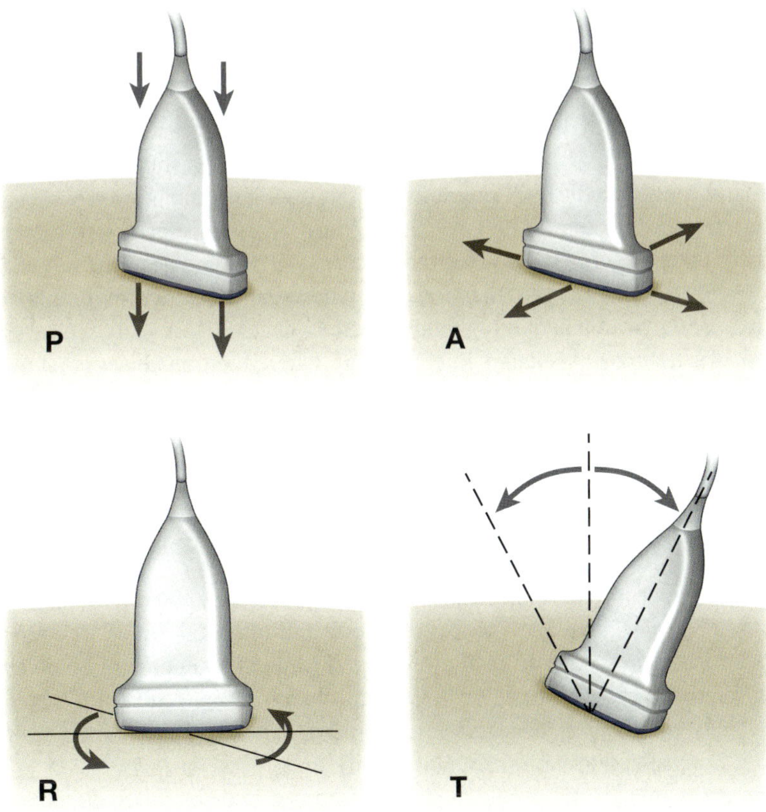

FIGURE 5.11 ● The PART pneumonic for probe motion: pressure, axial slide, rotation, and tilt.

The pressure applied with the probe by the provider can considerably impact image quality, the echogenicity of the tissue, and can shorten the distance to the structure of interest. Pressure is generally applied evenly across the probe, but the provider may apply asymmetric pressure on one side in order to direct the US beam in the desired direction to facilitate a target or create more room for needle entrance. Axial relocation, or "translation," can be either in a long-axis or short-axis direction in relation to the transducer probe footprint. This axial motion has the principal goal of finding the structure of interest and positioning it optimally on the screen for needle advancement. Axial translation is also referred to as a "slide" in either the long or short axis. "Rotation" is where the transducer is spun around the center axis of the probe; this facilitates an axial view of the target with its long axis parallel to the surface but not perpendicular to the current US plane. By continuous rotation of the probe to 90° of the initial probe position, one can change the image of a structure from its short-axis to its long-axis view. Finally, "tilt" is where the transducer is angled in the plane of its short axis; this is also described as "sweeping," "toggling," or "fanning" the probe. Tilting of the probe can facilitate a preview before the probe is engaged in a short-axis slide.

Recently a Delphi-based consensus statement, led by AIUM and AMSSM, was published to standardize terminology in musculoskeletal US. The document defined musculoskeletal US as the use of US to diagnose and/or guide treatment of conditions involving bones, joints, tendons, muscles, bursae, ligaments, cartilage, nerves, fascia, and related soft tissue structures, while sports US is used to diagnose and/or guide treatment for injuries and medical conditions associated with sport and exercise. Table 5.3 provides the consensus terminology for probe manipulation.[18]

ULTRASOUND NEEDLE GUIDANCE TERMINOLOGY

The performance of USGIs introduces specific terminology and definitions. Core to these definitions are understanding and describing the relationship of the transducer to the target and to the needle.[11] "Long-axis" ("longitudinal") images are where the long axis of the transducer is parallel to the anatomic target (see Fig. 5.12), while "short-axis" ("transverse") alignment is where the transducer is perpendicular to the target structure (see Fig. 5.13). "Out-of-plane" injections are where the transducer is perpendicular to the long axis of the needle and only the hyperechoic needle tip or shaft can be visualized (see Fig. 5.14), whereas "in-plane" injections are where the transducer is parallel to the needle, and the entire segment of the needle shaft and tip are seen approaching the target (see Fig. 5.15). In-plane injections are preferred in clinical practice.

ULTRASOUND AND NEEDLE GUIDANCE

Performing an USGI successfully requires the integration of three factors: patient selection with appropriate indications, knowledge of US anatomy (sonoanatomy), and the ability to visualize and drive a needle to the intended target. The first two of these factors are addressed with the cultivation of clinical acumen and knowledge. The third task requires practice aimed at both visuospatial and psychomotor development. Simultaneously controlling, visualizing, and guiding a needle is a complex task, requiring hand-eye coordination with manual dexterity.

Learning to image the needle while performing real-time US guidance can be challenging and requires practiced hand-eye coordination with both the needle and probe hands simultaneously. One group of educators developed the "**S.T.A.R.** technique"

TABLE 5.3

Transducer Manipulation Terminology

Slide	Motion of the transducer across the body surface in any direction
Heel-toe	Motion in the long axis of the transducer along a fixed point changing the angle of insonation away from 90° to the skin surface while maintaining contact with the skin surface, often used to achieve an angle of insonation at 90° to the target structure to optimize visualization and eliminate anisotropy
Tilt	Motion in the short axis of the transducer along a fixed point changing the angle of insonation away from 90° to the skin surface while maintaining contact with the skin surface, often used to achieve an angle of insonation at 90° to the target structure to optimize visualization and eliminate anisotropy
Compression	Force is applied by the sonographer or sonologist on the transducer toward the patient's body
Rotation	Motion along a fixed center axis point of the transducer in the clockwise or counterclockwise direction
Pivot	Motion along a fixed axis point at the end of the transducer in the clockwise or counterclockwise direction
Stand off	The transducer does not touch the skin surface but rests on a layer of acoustic coupling gel or other acoustic medium with angle of insonation at 90° to the skin surface
Oblique stand off	The transducer does not touch the skin surface but rests on a layer of acoustic coupling gel or other acoustic medium with angle of insonation away from 90° to the skin surface
Sonopalpation	Force is applied on the transducer toward the patient's body to elicit symptom provocation (eg, pain)

Adapted from Hall MM, Allen GM, Allison S, et al. Recommended musculoskeletal and sports ultrasound terminology: a Delphi-based consensus statement. *J Ultrasound Med.* 2022;41(10):2395-2412.

(See, Tilt, Align, Rotate) to assist novice users in acquiring the necessary skills to perform USGIs (see Table 5.4 and Fig. 5.16).[19]

In addition to utilizing the STAR technique, a short-axis injection poses unique challenges, compared to a long-axis injection, as the needle is not seen the entire path during its approach to the intended target. When using an out-of-plane technique, the hyperechoic needle tip or shaft is only identified once it begins to cross the plane of the US beam. Accordingly, as the needle is advanced, the provider will be unable to image the needle tip until it has passed by this transducer plane. The technique required to see the needle tip during the entire injection is termed the "walk down" technique. This technique involves a series of transverse probe linear slides as the needle tip is progressively introduced, and followed by US imaging, more deeply into the soft tissue in the direction of the target. This out-of-plane technique can additionally be used to direct a needle deeper without moving the probe. The needle is introduced out-of-plane under

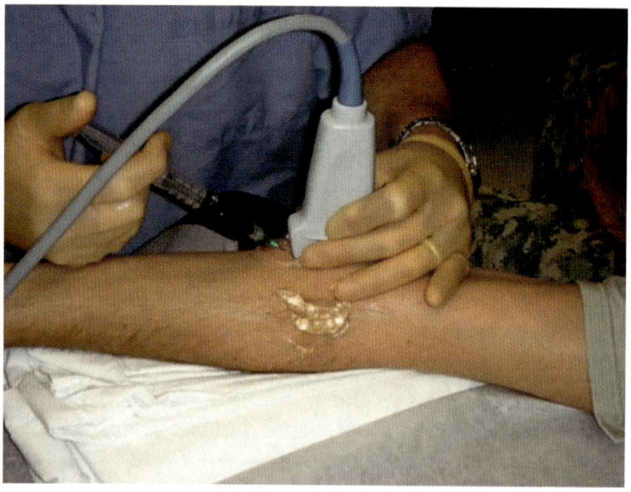

FIGURE 5.12 ● Long-axis orientation, in-plane injection (cubital tunnel).

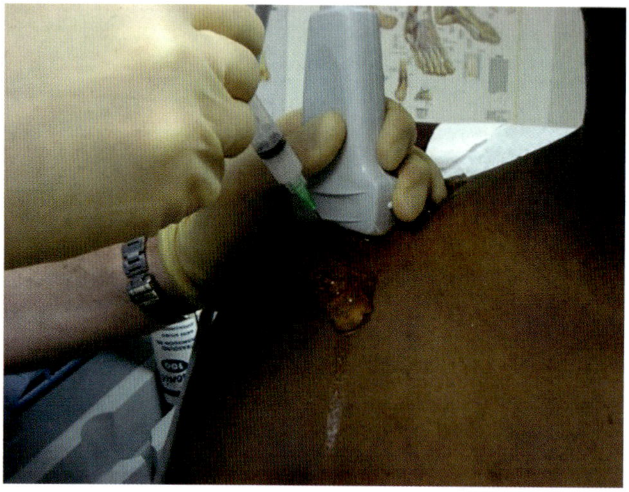

FIGURE 5.13 ● Short-axis orientation, out-of-plane injection (acromioclavicular joint).

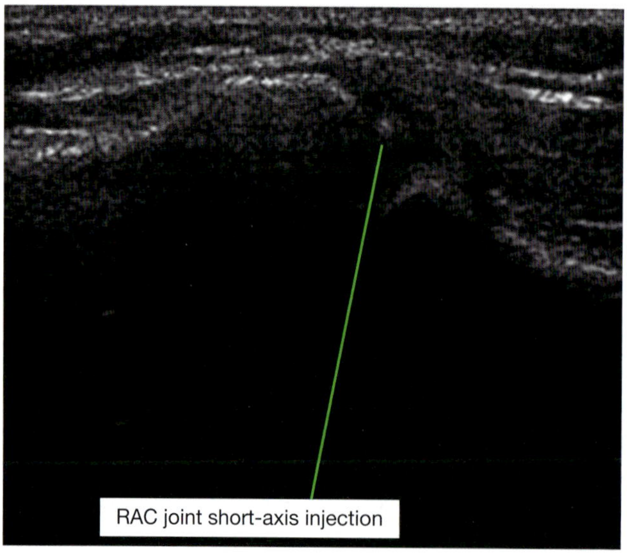

FIGURE 5.14 ● Out-of-plane injection (acromioclavicular joint). RAC, right acromioclavicular.

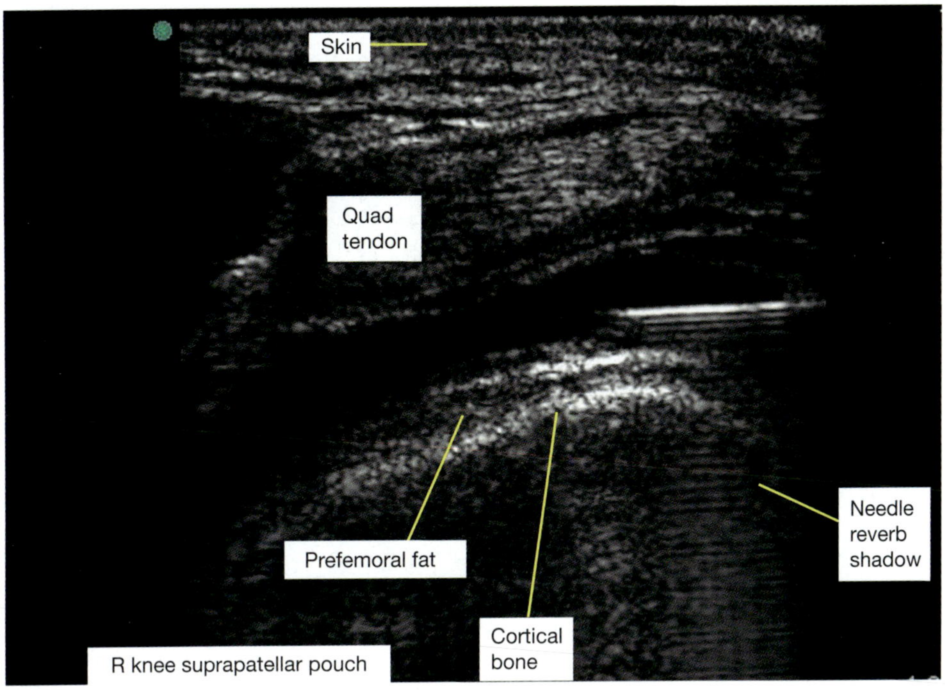

FIGURE 5.15 ● In-plane injection, short-axis (transverse) target image (suprapatellar recess).

the center of the probe in order to see the tip over the intended target, and then partially withdrawn to redirect deeper, and advanced again until the needle tip, deeper than before, is closer to the target. This is repeated until the needle tip arrives at the target. The repeated redirects are like taking steps as you walk the needle to the target. The critical observation is that once the needle tip comes in to view, it should not be advanced, as there is no reference as to where the needle tip is in the soft tissues.

ULTRASOUND GUIDANCE OF PROCEDURES

USGIs proceed in a comparable fashion to palpation-guided procedures with several distinct steps; these steps as originally described by Lento, with addition of adding documentation and several modifications.[20,21]

TABLE 5.4

The STAR Technique for Needle Ultrasound Acquisition and Guidance

See	S	The participant is taught to look directly at the transducer and needle instead of the ultrasound screen, without moving the probe or needle.
Tilt	T	The participant tilts the transducer back and forth on a horizontal axis to achieve maximal brightness of the needle.
Align	A	The participant kept the same tilt and slide the transducer toward the needle (in the direction identified during "see") until the needle came into view.
Rotate	R	The participant turned the transducer on its long axis until full needle visualization was achieved.

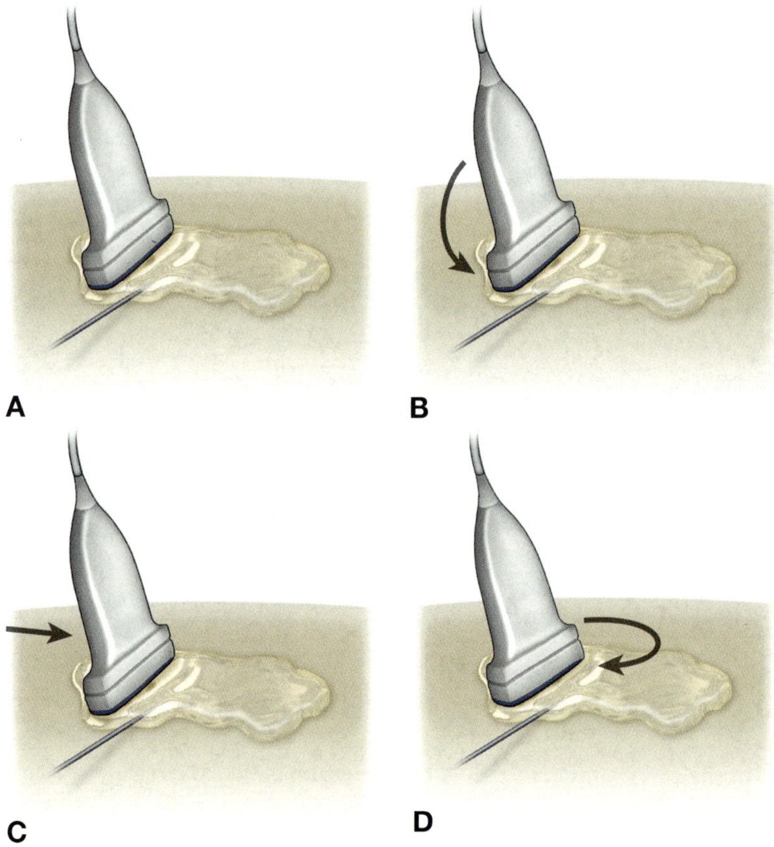

FIGURE 5.16 ● The STAR technique for needle ultrasound acquisition and guidance. **A.** See. **B.** Tilt. **C.** Align. **D.** Rotate.

Step 1: History and Physical

An USGI's success depends upon a proper diagnosis; the history and physical examination, to include a review of diagnostic imaging tests, should be completed prior to commencing with an injection.

Step 2: Obtain Consent

As previously described, consent for all injections should be witnessed and documented in the medical record. Unique to an USGI, there should be a careful discussion of the role of the US as compared to a standard palpation-guided injection. Patients should additionally be asked if they would like to visualize the injection during the procedure. While the technology is of interest to most patients, some patients may become anxious and potentially vagal when witnessing a needle in their own body.

Step 3: Assemble Equipment

A sterile field should be considered to hold supplies for the injection. This step in the procedure is comparable to that discussed for palpation-guided injections.

Step 4: Position Patient and Machine

The US machine should be placed in-line, at eye level, and in most cases directly across from the injector, on the other side of the patient; this limits head motion and facilitates greater accuracy in needle placement and direction. The patient should be comfortable and relaxed, and if at all possible, in a supine position to limit the possibility of a vasovagal reaction. When holding the probe, the provider should learn to scan with the nondominant hand, as the dominant hand should be used to direct the needle. In addition, when holding the probe, the provider's fourth and fifth fingers should maintain skin contact to limit unintended motion and anchor the probe on the patient.

Step 5: Preliminary Scan

This preliminary scan confirms the diagnosis, identifies the target, and assists the provider in best determining whether an in-plane versus out-of-plane needle approach is optimal. The preliminary scan also assists the provider in determining the appropriate needle length as well as planning for modifications to the planned procedure (eg, aspiration of a joint effusion prior to injection).

Step 6: Demarcate Skin

Marking the skin during the preliminary scan will assist in identifying the appropriate target and in allowing facilitation of demarcating the location of the probe after the sterile preparation of the skin. The skin can be marked with an appropriate skin-marking pen on either end of the probe so that correct replacement can occur.

Step 7: Don Sterile Gloves

The appropriate gloves should be selected prior to performing the injection. Sterile gloves are only required if the provider intends to touch the location of the intended needle injection, which in this text a "no-touch" technique is preferred for both landmark and US-guided procedures. The issue of sterile versus nonsterile gloves has previously been discussed in detail.

Step 8: Clean Skin

An appropriate skin cleaning agent (eg, chlorhexidine gluconate) should be selected prior to performing the injection. Agents have been previously discussed, however, with US, a key variable will be ensuring compliance with the probe manufacturer's recommendations to avoid damage to the probe head.

Step 9: Draw Up Medications; Local Anesthesia as Needed

The procedure of drawing up medications and preparing the skin with local anesthesia prior to the injection are comparable to those utilized for palpation-guided injections.

Step 10: Prepare Probe

Preparation of the probe prior to performing an USGI is an area of active controversy and has been addressed by the AIUM Practice Parameter.[8] Most importantly, US-guided procedures should be performed in accordance with the provider's facility infection control guidelines. The patient's skin should appropriately be cleansed with an antiseptic cleanser. The US transducer also represents a potential source of contamination; accordingly, probes should be disinfected between each procedure according to manufacturer's recommendations and facility-specific infection control guidelines.[8]

The use of sterile US gel, drapes, and probe covers/condoms may provide the best method to reduce the risk of contamination and infection. Alternatives include the use of a sterile glove covering the transducer combined with sterile gel, the use of a sterile condom covering the transducer combined with sterile gel, or the use of a sterile occlusive dressing, for example Tegaderm, directly applied to the transducer face combined with sterile gel. Providers who use the "no-touch" technique, as previously described, place the transducer over the target region but away from the prepared skin entry site. The needle is passed through the prepared skin region, and it passes under the transducer within the body. This technique should only be used by experienced clinicians due to the risk of cross-contamination secondary to inadvertent transducer or needle movement.[8]

Step 11: Attach Syringe to Needle

Alternatively, the needle can be attached directly to the extension tubing which is then attached to the syringe. This technique can be useful because the provider can focus on stabilizing the needle tip during the injection, while the medical assistant depresses the plunger.

Step 12: Place Needle Under Probe

Using the STAR technique, the actual needle (as opposed to the needle on the image screen) should be observed being introduced into the tissue deep to the probe. Once the actual needle is visualized as under the probe, the provider can then look to the screen and identify the needle on the US image. Short-axis slides in an orthogonal plane are then utilized to maintain normal recognized anatomic relationships during the injection.

Step 13: Documentation

The AIUM Practice Parameter specifies clear guidance for proper procedure documentation.[7] "Adequate documentation is essential and should be permanently documented in the patient's medical record. Retention of the ultrasound examination should be consistent both with clinical needs and with relevant legal and local health care facility requirements. The procedure documentation should include the following: (a) Patient identification, (b) Facility identification, (c) Procedure date, (d) Requested procedure, including side of body, (e) Indication for the procedure, (f) Justification for ultrasound guidance, (g) Description of the target and relevant associated structures, both normal and abnormal, (h) Description of the use of ultrasound to localize the target and the essential elements of the procedure, including transducer position, approach to the target, and method of needle tracking (in plane or out of plane). Deviations from standard techniques are described and justified, (i) The type and amount of medication, if used, (j) Needle/device type and gauge, and (k) Specimens removed, if any, as well as their disposition."[7] The choice of aseptic technique used during the US-guided procedure should be documented in the report.

The AIUM Practice Parameter also provides guidance for proper image utilization and documentation.[7] "Preprocedural, intraprocedural, and post procedure still image(s) or videos: (a) Images should be labeled with the patient identification, facility identification, procedure date, and side (right or left) of the procedure site. (b) Inclusion of at least one image demonstrating the needle or device placed into the target region is required unless the indirect technique is used. (c) All images should be permanently archived and easily retrievable. (d) Variations from normal size or morphology should be recorded and accompanied by measurements."[7]

NEW ULTRASOUND TECHNOLOGY

US technology continues to improve, with advancements in quality imaging in tools that have smaller interfaces and are more mobile in a variety of care settings. Integrated functions additionally make it easier for the user to produce high-caliber and clinically useful imaging. With continued improvements in high-resolution imaging, procedural interventions in and around finer structures (eg, nerves), previously challenging in the best of hands, are becoming more common place. Finally, newer technologic advancements are moving US from station-based machines to handheld portable devices. Handheld US systems can attach to a smart phone, provide excellent resolution and penetration, and conveniently drop into the end-user's lab coat. Accompanied by decreasing costs over time, these devices will provide primary care providers with wide accessibility to use musculoskeletal US and other point-of-care office and hospital applications.

REFERENCES

1. Sorensen B, Hunskaar S. Point-of-care ultrasound in primary care: a systematic review of generalist performed point-of-care ultrasound in unselected populations. *Ultrasound J.* 2019;11(1):31.
2. Sconfienza LM, Albano D, Allen G, et al. Clinical indications for musculoskeletal ultrasound updated in 2017 by European Society of Musculoskeletal Radiology (ESSR) consensus. *Eur Radiol.* 2018; 28:5338-5351.
3. Berko NS, Goldberg-Stein S, Thornhill BA, Koenigsberg M. Survey of current trends in postgraduate musculoskeletal ultrasound education in the United States. *Skeletal Radiol.* 2016;45:475-482.
4. Finnoff JT, Berkoff DJ, Brennan F, et al. American Medical Society for Sports Medicine (AMSSM) recommended sports ultrasound curriculum for sports medicine fellowships. *Br J Sports Med.* 2015;49:145-150.
5. The Association for Medical Ultrasound. American Institute of Ultrasound Medicine. Accessed February 12, 2025. https://www.aium.org/
6. The AIUM practice parameter for the performance of the musculoskeletal ultrasound examination. *J Ultrasound Med.* 2023;42(9):E23-E35.
7. AIUM practice parameter for documentation of an ultrasound examination. *J Ultrasound Med.* 2020; 39(1):E1-E4.
8. AIUM practice parameter for the performance of selected ultrasound-guided procedures. *J Ultrasound Med.* 2016;35(9):1-40.
9. Finoff J, Hall MM, Adams E; American Medical Society for Sports Medicine. American Medical Society for sports medicine position statement: interventional musculoskeletal ultrasound in sports medicine. *Clin J Sports Med.* 2015;25:6-22.
10. Daniels EW, Cole D, Jacobs B, Phillips SF. Existing evidence on ultrasound-guided injections in sports medicine. *Orthop J Sports Med.* 2018;6(2):2325967118756576.
11. Bum Park Y, Ah Choi W, Kim YK, Chul Lee S, Hae Lee J. Accuracy of blind versus ultrasound guided suprapatellar bursal injection. *J Clin Ultrasound.* 2012;40(1):20-25.
12. Eustace JA, Brophy DP, Gibney RP, Bresnihan B, FitzGerald O. Comparison of accuracy of steroid placement with clinical outcomes in patients with shoulder symptoms. *Ann Rheum Dis.* 1995;38:59-63.
13. Jacobsen JA. *Fundamentals of Musculoskeletal Ultrasound.* 3rd ed. Elsevier; 2018.
14. Bianchi S, Martinoli C, Abdelwahad IF, et al. *Ultrasound of the Musculoskeletal System.* Springer-Verlag Berlin Heidelberg; 2008.
15. Jačisko J, Ricci V, Mezian K, et al. Mnemonics and metaphorical videos for detecting/diagnosing musculoskeletal sonopathologies. *Am J Phys Med Rehabil.* 2023;102(2):184-190.

16. Kim SY, Cheon JH, Seo WJ, Yang GY, Choi YM, Kim KH. A pictorial review of signature patterns living in musculoskeletal ultrasonography. *Korean J Pain.* 2016;29(4):217-228.
17. Ihnatsenka B, Boezaart AP. Ultrasound: basic understanding and learning the language. *Int J Shoulder Surg.* 2010;4(3):55-62.
18. Hall MM, Allen GM, Allison S, et al. Recommended musculoskeletal and sports ultrasound terminology: a Delphi-based consensus statement. *Br J Sports Med.* 2022;56:310-319. doi:10.1136/bjsports-2021-105114
19. Lam NC, Fishburn SJ, Hammer AR, Petersen TR, Gerstein NS, Mariano ER. A randomized controlled trial evaluating the See, Tilt, Align, and Rotate (STAR) maneuver on skill acquisition for simulated ultrasound-guided interventional procedures. *J Ultrasound Med.* 2015;34(6):1019-1026.
20. Lento PH. Preparation and setup for musculoskeletal ultrasound-guided procedures. In: Malanga G, Mautner K, eds. *Atlas of Ultrasound-Guided Musculoskeletal Injections.* McGraw Hill; 2014.
21. Visco CJ. Introduction to interventional ultrasound. In: Malanga G, Mautner K, eds. *Atlas of Ultrasound-Guided Musculoskeletal Injections.* McGraw Hill; 2014.

Advanced and Adjunctive Techniques

6

Francis G. O'Connor

Injections have empowered primary care providers to deliver a number of evidence-based therapies to directly treat soft tissue and articular disorders in musculoskeletal medicine.[1] The ability to precisely target injuries to not only maximize potential benefit but also limit adverse systemic side effects, has been of great benefit to the delivery of patient-centered care. With the increased level of comfort and utilization of injections, importantly with the addition of ultrasound (US) guidance, there has been a propagation of additional unique techniques and tools that can be utilized in musculoskeletal medicine.[2] The last decade has furthermore added considerable evidence-based literature to support the "value added" of these interventions in improving cost-effective clinical outcomes when in the hands of point-of-care providers.[3] These advanced techniques can assist in achieving pain relief, affect mechanical change in soft tissue structures, and ultimately provide improved clinical care. The techniques discussed in this chapter include battlefield auricular acupuncture (pain management); barbotage (calcific tendinopathy); high-volume injection (HVI) tendon brisement (tendinopathy/tenosynovitis); needle fenestration (tendinopathy); hydrodissection (nerve entrapment); hydrodilatation/hydroplasty (adhesive capsulitis); trigger point dry needling (myofascial pain); and percutaneous tenotomy with débridement (tendinopathy). While these techniques are reviewed and evidence is introduced to support their incorporation in clinical practice, it should be emphasized that these are considered advanced skills that require additional training and practice to employ skillfully.

Auricular Battlefield Acupuncture

Battlefield acupuncture (BFA) was developed by US Air Force physician Dr. Richard Niemtzow in 2001.[4] The technique was specifically developed to provide pain relief during a period when an opiate analgesic may not be typically utilized or appropriate, secondary to systemic effects that may interfere with mission completion. BFA is an extension of the longstanding technique of auriculotherapy and designed for the rapid relief of pain.[5] Utilizing specific acupoints on the outer ear that are thought to interact with central nervous system pain processing, auricular BFA can provide a quick and convenient method to provide pain relief (see Fig. 6.1). The technique employs ASP (Aiguille Semi-Permanente) needles, which are semipermanent, and have the characteristics of remaining in the ear acupoints for up to 3 to 4 days before being pushed out toward the surface by the previous flattened epidermis. This pain relief has a variable duration from minutes to days, depending upon the individual and the pathology being addressed. While the technique was originally developed to assist in the management of wounded warfighters on the battlefield, BFA has widely grown in popularity and offers an alternative or adjunct to systemic analgesics.

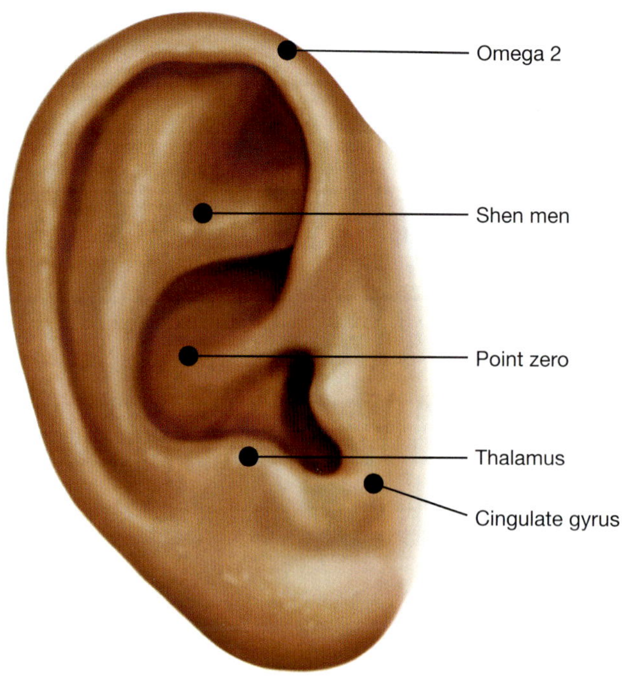

FIGURE 6.1 ● Auricular acupoints.

EVIDENCE

BFA has been utilized on the battlefield by medical acupuncturists and nonacupuncturists alike. While BFA has been increasingly employed, research has been limited in the field of auriculotherapy. A small randomized controlled trial ($n = 94$) of female patients with acute migraines demonstrated that auriculotherapy provided short-term pain relief when specific auricular acupoints were utilized.[6] A more recent systematic review conducted on 43 articles evaluating BFA for migraine therapy demonstrated a role for both abortive and prophylactic treatment.[7] A pilot study of emergency room (ER) patients ($n = 87$) with a wide variety of pain complaints demonstrated a 23% reduction in pain for those receiving auriculotherapy before leaving the ER as compared to standard care, while both groups had the same level of pain reduction at 24 hours after the ER visit.[8] BFA has additionally demonstrated efficacy in the management of perioperative pain.[9] Finally, a recent meta-analysis was performed to assess the efficacy of auriculotherapy for pain relief in an emergency setting. The meta-analysis used data from several randomized studies and included 286 patients. There were no observed significant adverse effects, and patient satisfaction was significantly improved. Results regarding if acupuncture reduced pain medication use, however, were equivocal. While study numbers were limited, ear acupuncture, either as a stand-alone or as an adjunctive technique, significantly reduced pain scores.[10] While current evidence is limited, BFA is becoming widely employed in the military and emergency medicine communities and is proving to be a useful adjunct in managing acute pain.

CONTRAINDICATIONS

Active skin infection, needle phobia, and pregnancy are considered to be the only contraindications.

EQUIPMENT

- ASP or acupuncture needles (see Fig. 6.2)
- Alcohol pads

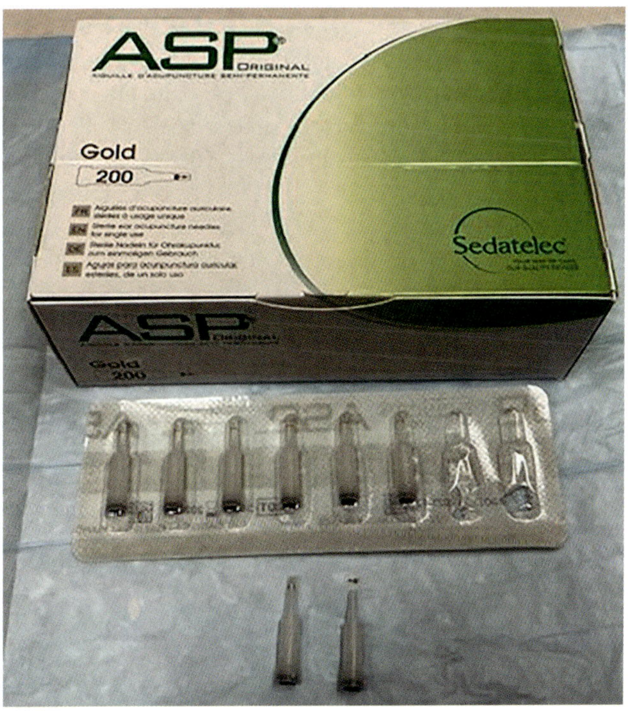

FIGURE 6.2 • ASP (Aiguille Semi-Permanente) needle. (ASP from Sedatelec.)

PREPROCEDURAL INSTRUCTIONS

The patient should be informed that the indwelling needles or pins may be mildly uncomfortable but are generally well tolerated. The needles can be self-removed at any time; however, they will typically fall out in 2 to 10 days in most patients. Patients are additionally informed that pain relief may not be immediate and may take several days to achieve. Patients are instructed after initial placements that they should not engage in vigorous activity until they know the response they will get from the ASP needles.

ANESTHESIA

Typically, no local anesthesia is required for BFA administration.

TECHNIQUE

The technique of BFA has been developed and described by Niemtzow.[4] The clinician performing the BFA "technique" first conducts an appropriate history and physical examination. The five acupoints are sequentially identified, and needles are subsequently administrated as indicated: cingulate gyrus, thalamic nuclei (anterior), omega 2, point zero, and shen men. This order of needle administration is commonly taught with acronym "CTOPS" or "CCTTOOPPSS" indicating the process of alternating between the ears.

1. Either the left or right ear is chosen for the placement of the needles; if the pain is not clearly lateralized, use the ear on the nondominant hand.
2. An ASP needle is first inserted into the cingulated gyrus.
3. The patient is allowed to ambulate for about 2 minutes to determine whether pain attenuation has occurred. If no pain attenuation has occurred, an ASP needle is inserted into the cingulate gyrus of the opposite ear and the patient ambulates to determine the new pain level.
4. If pain attenuation is less than 20% via the cingulated gyrus, another ASP needle is placed in the anterior thalamic in the ear that has produced the most pain attenuation. The patient ambulates and the new pain level is determined.
5. Whichever ear insertion produces pain attenuation, ASP needles are placed in a similar sequential manner into omega 2, shen men, and point zero (Fig. 6.3). Indications to stop advancing to other sites include complete pain relief, or the patients desire to stop.
6. After the dominant ear has received ASP needles in all the "battlefield acupuncture" points, the pain level is evaluated. If the pain level is 0-1/10, the therapeutic goal is achieved. In the case where the pain level is above 1/10, the contralateral ear is needled in a similar manner.

AFTERCARE

The clinician should observe for ear irritation or infection; mild erythema after the procedure is to be expected. Typical postprocedure instructions include the following advice to patients:

- Do not be surprised if the pain increases over the first few days; this can be a normal reaction and should not be considered a failed treatment.

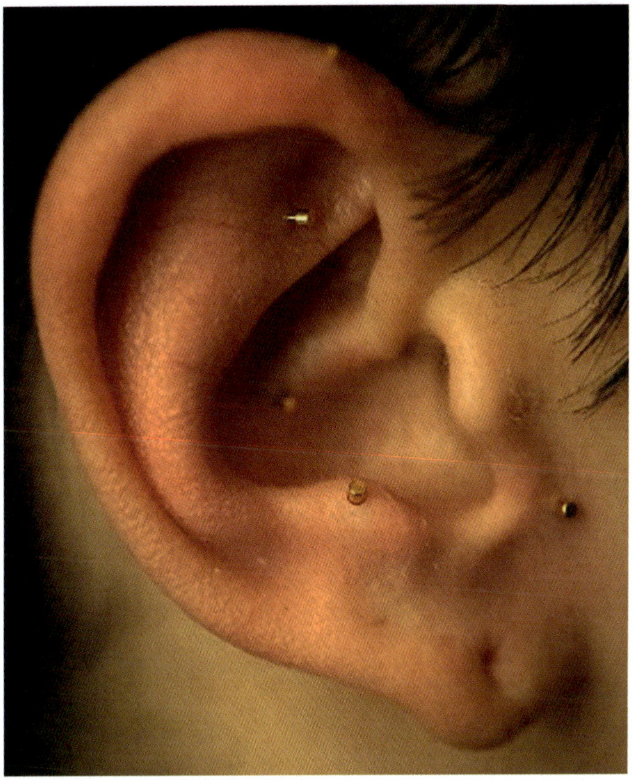

FIGURE 6.3 ● Auricular acupoints with ASP (Aiguille Semi-Permanente) needles inserted.

- The needles may be uncomfortable during sleep or when brushing against another object. If they are uncomfortable, they may be removed before failing out on their own, or one may use the Band-Aid that is provided in the BFA kit.
- Watch for signs of infection, to include redness, discharge, or marked pain.
- Avoid excessive activity after the initial procedure and thereafter tailor activity based upon the initial response.
- Plan your activities to include some rest after the procedure; do not plan for a peak performance immediately after the procedure.
- Continue to take prescription medications as prescribed by one's regular physician.
- Keep written notes on the response to the procedure to be shared with the treating provider at follow-up visits.

PEARLS

- BFA is a great adjunct to other treatments and also can be a guide to see if the patient will respond to more advanced acupuncture.
- BFA can be repeated at any interval, but the usual protocol for an acute pain is as follows: initial, repeat in 3 to 6 days as efficacy wanes and then spread out time from there.
- For chronic pain, there will be a finite response, that is, every 1 to 2 weeks.
- If the pain is not clearly lateralized, use the ear on the nondominant hand; normal phone use may irritate ASP needles.
- If the pain has been significantly reduced, consider treating only one ear. This may facilitate the patient being able to achieve a comfortable sleeping position.

A video showing auricular battlefield acupuncture with insertion of ASP needles can be found in the companion eBook.

REFERENCES

1. Stephens MB, Beutler AI, O'Connor FG. Musculoskeletal injections: a review of the evidence. *Am Fam Physician.* 2008;78(8):971-976.
2. Finnoff JT, Hall MM, Adams E, et al. American Medical Society for Sports Medicine (AMSSM) position statement: interventional musculoskeletal ultrasound in sports medicine. *PM R.* 2015;7(2):151-168.e12.
3. Daniels EW, Cole D, Jacobs B, Phillips SF. Existing evidence on ultrasound-guided injections in sports medicine. *Orthop J Sports Med.* 2018;6(2):2325967118756576.
4. Niemtzow RC. Battlefield acupuncture: my story. *Med Acupunct.* 2018;30(2):57-58.
5. Nogier R. History of auriculotherapy: additional information and new developments. *Med Acupunct.* 2021;33(6):410-419.
6. Allais G, Romoli M, Rolando S, et al. Ear acupuncture in the treatment of migraine attacks: a randomized trial on the efficacy of appropriate versus inappropriate acupoints. *Neurol Sci.* 2011;32(Suppl 1):S173-S175.
7. Williams KA. Auricular therapy for migraine. *Curr Pain Headache Rep.* 2024;28(8):835-841.
8. Goertz CMH, Niemtzow R, Burns SM, Fritts MJ, Crawford CC, Jonas WB. Auricular acupuncture in the treatment of acute pain syndromes: a pilot study. *Mil Med.* 2006;171(10):1010-1014.
9. Zhang G, Xu G, Tang Y, et al. The analgesic effectiveness of auriculotherapy for acute postoperative pain: a systematic review and meta-analysis. *Complement Ther Med.* 2025;88:103112.
10. Jan AL, Aldridge ES, Rogers IR, Visser EJ, Bulsara MK, Niemtzow RC. Does ear acupuncture have a role for pain relief in the emergency setting? A systematic review and meta-analysis. *Med Acupunct.* 2017;29(5):276-289.

Barbotage

US-guided barbotage, a procedure of repeated injection and aspiration, is commonly used in the management of soft tissue calcific deposits.[1] Calcific tendinopathy has been identified and treated in a number of locations including the patellar and gluteal tendons but is most commonly identified in the tendons of rotator cuff about the shoulder. Rotator cuff calcific tendinopathy (RCCT), a common disease that occurs in up to 7.5% of asymptomatic adults and up to 20% of painful shoulders, is frequently diagnosed in women in their 40s and 50s. RCCT, which is not uncommonly disabling, can be treated conservatively with excellent results.[2]

The exact etiology of calcific tendinopathy is currently not understood but postulated to be the result of a local tissue degenerative cascade. The calcification process is specifically thought to be related to a cell-mediated disease in which metaplastic transformation of tenocytes into chondrocytes induces calcification inside the tendon.[3] Uhthoff and Sarkar[4] describe the pathogenesis in three stages: (1) precalcific stage with fibrocartilaginous transformation within the tendon; (2) calcific stage with calcium deposition; and finally, the (3) postcalcific phase, in which self-healing and repair of the affected tendon occurs which can last several months. In the calcific stage, a resorptive phase occurs, which is characterized by vascular invasion, edema, and increased intratendinous pressure with possible extravasation of calcium crystals in the subacromial bursa. This phase is usually associated with the development of acute pain that can be highly disabling and unresponsive to common analgesics.[2] The acute phase is generally associated with "softer" deposits with poorly defined borders, while the more chronic "harder" lesions tend to appear more granular with sharply defined borders.

EVIDENCE

US-guided barbotage is a safe technique, with a high success rate and low complication rate.[5] There is currently limited evidence assessing its effectiveness compared with other major treatment modalities including extracorporeal shock wave (ESWT) therapy, subacromial corticosteroid injections, dry needling, and arthroscopic calcific deposit excision. A recently performed systematic review of 908 patients, however, recommended US-guided barbotage.[6] Interestingly, de Witte et al have two publications looking at 1-year and 5-year follow-up results of US-guided barbotage with a subacromial corticosteroid injection versus US-guided subacromial corticosteroid injection alone. While the results demonstrated a clear benefit at 1 year, there were no significant clinical or radiologic differences at the 5-year mark.[7,8] In a second systematic review, US-guided barbotage was directly compared with ESWT; after 12 months of follow-up, the US group demonstrated improved pain relief when compared with those treated with

ESWT.[9] Minimally invasive US-guided barbotage for the treatment of RCCT is a well-established treatment option.[10]

As will be described, barbotage can be performed with both one- and two-needle techniques. There is one published study evaluating the efficacy of the one-needle technique versus the two-needle technique and found no significant difference in clinical outcomes at 1-year follow-up. However, the data suggested that a double-needle approach might be more appropriate to treat harder deposits, while one needle may be more useful in treating fluid, or softer calcifications.[11] In addition, recent evidence suggests that the utilization of warm saline has been shown both to reduce procedure duration and improve calcium deposit dissolution, particularly in cases of hard calcifications.[12] Finally, if US-guided barbotage is utilized, the evidence suggests that the procedure is optimally followed by a subacromial corticosteroid injection.[13]

CONTRAINDICATIONS

The barbotage procedure has comparable contraindications that apply to all bursal injections as previously described. In addition, US-guided barbotage is not indicated when patients are asymptomatic, the calcification is very small (≤5 mm), or the calcifications have migrated into the bursal space. There is additional evidence that patients with intraosseous migration of calcification experience worse results.[14]

EQUIPMENT

- One or two 18-guage needles (depending on the technique chosen: single or double needle)
- Two 25-guage needles for subacromial injections prior to and after the barbotage procedure
- Two syringes (20 and 3 mL)
- One 10-cm 18- or 20-guage spinal needle (optional)
- Bowl (to collect the washing fluid)
- Sterile saline solution (100-200 mL, warmed to 38-40 °C)
- Lidocaine 1% or mepivacaine (10 mL)
- Steroid (1 mL, 40 mg/mL)
- US machine with high-frequency linear array transducer

PREPROCEDURAL INSTRUCTIONS

The patient should be placed in a supine position, to prevent patient movement during the procedure. The arm of the affected shoulder should lie completely extended along the body with a slight internal or external rotation, according to calcification location. The procedural guidance for utilization of US guidance, to include sterile technique, is detailed in the previous chapter of **Introduction to Ultrasound**.

ANESTHESIA

Using US guidance with an in-plane approach, inject up to 10-mL lidocaine or mepivacaine along the path of the needles into the subacromial bursa and around the calcification.

TECHNIQUE

US-guided barbotage is performed with patients in the supine position on a table; the two-needle and one-needle techniques are described by Messina et al.[14]

1. After sterile preparation of the skin and US probe as previously described, the target calcification is visualized with a high-frequency linear array transducer.
2. Using a 25-guage needle, local anesthesia (up to 10 mL of lidocaine or mepivacaine) is injected in the subacromial bursa and around the calcification with an in-plane approach.
3. When using the two-needle technique, the first needle is inserted into the lowest portion of the calcification with needle bevel open toward the probe.
4. The second needle is then inserted into the calcification parallel and superficial to the first needle, with its bevel opposite to the first needle, 25° to 30° of angulation, in order to create a correct washing circuit.
5. The calcification is then filled with saline solution, applying a gentle intermittent pressure in order to dissolve its core and allowing the calcific fluid to exit through the second needle, until a complete internal emptying is visualized.
6. As calcium fills the syringe, exchange is made with new syringes until no further calcium is expelled.
7. Remaining observed calcification can be fenestrated with the needle.
8. The procedure is then concluded with a subacromial steroid injection.

The single-needle technique is comparable to the two-needle technique, with the caveat being that the calcification is punctured with one needle only. Washing is performed by pushing the syringe plunger to hydrate the deposit. Calcium then refluxes back together with the saline solution within the same syringe as the plunger is released.

The single-needle technique has been thought to have a lower risk of infection and bleeding. On the other hand, the use of two needles ensures an in–out flow of the saline solution outside the calcification, reducing the risk of calcification disruption and subsequent postprocedural bursitis.

AFTERCARE

- There are currently no evidence-based guidelines for postprocedural care, however, Messina et al[11,14] have published their protocol.
- They have suggested a short course of nonsteroidal anti-inflammatory drugs and relative rest (ie, no elevation of the arm over the shoulder) for up to 2 weeks.
- This is followed by a short treatment of physical therapy.
- Imaging is not routinely used during follow-up.
- Patients are instructed to call if pain persists for more than a few days after treatment or in case of fever, or in case of pain recurrence after 2 months posttreatment.

PEARLS

- The initial subacromial injection should involve 5 to 10 mL of lidocaine to facilitate comfort for the patient during the procedure; corticosteroid into the subacromial space following the procedure decreases postprocedure pain.
- Warm saline to facilitate the barbotage has been demonstrated to reduce procedure duration and improve calcium deposit dissolution.

- Data suggest that that a double-needle approach might be more appropriate to treat harder deposits, while a one-needle approach may be more useful in treating fluid.
- Air infiltration into the soft tissues should be avoided as this may obscure visualization of the calcific deposit and surrounding sonoanatomy.
- Additional tips and tricks have been published and are available for the interested reader.[11]

A video showing barbotage can be found in the companion eBook.

REFERENCES

1. Davidson J, Jayaraman S. Guided interventions in musculoskeletal ultrasound: what's the evidence? *Clin Radiol.* 2011;66(2):140-152.
2. Speed CA, Hazleman BL. Calcific tendinitis of the shoulder. *N Engl J Med.* 1999;340(20):1582-1584.
3. De Carli A, Pulcinelli F, Rose GD, Pitino D, Ferretti A. Calcific tendinitis of the shoulder. *Joints.* 2014;2(3):130-136.
4. Uhthoff HK, Sarkar K. Calcifying tendinitis. *Baillieres Clin Rheumatol.* 1989;3(3):567-581.
5. Lanza E, Banfi G, Serafini G, et al. Ultrasound-guided percutaneous irrigation in rotator cuff calcific tendinopathy: what is the evidence? A systematic review with proposals for future reporting. *Eur Radiol.* 2015;25(7):2176-2183.
6. Gatt DL, Charalambous CP. Ultrasound-guided barbotage for calcific tendonitis of the shoulder: a systematic review including 908 patients. *Arthroscopy.* 2014;30(9):1166-1172.
7. de Witte PB, Selten JW, Navas A, et al. Calcific tendinitis of the rotator cuff: a randomized controlled trial of ultrasound-guided needling and lavage versus subacromial corticosteroids. *Am J Sports Med.* 2013;41(7):1665-1673.
8. de Witte PB, Kolk A, Overes F, Nelissen RGHH, Reijnierse M. Rotator cuff calcific tendinitis: ultrasound-guided needling and lavage versus subacromial corticosteroids: five-year outcomes of a randomized controlled trial. *Am J Sports Med.* 2017;45(14):3305-3314.
9. Zhang T, Duan Y, Chen J, Chen X. Efficacy of ultrasound-guided percutaneous lavage for rotator cuff calcific tendinopathy: a systematic review and meta-analysis. *Medicine (Baltimore).* 2019;98(21):e15552.
10. Moya D, Rashid M, Rowinski S, et al. Therapeutic options in rotator cuff calcific tendinopathy. *SICOT J.* 2025;11:9.
11. Sconfienza LM, Viganò S, Martini C, et al. Double-needle ultrasound-guided percutaneous treatment of rotator cuff calcific tendinitis: tips & tricks. *Skeletal Radiol.* 2013;42(1):19-24.
12. Sconfienza LM, Bandirali M, Serafini G, et al. Rotator cuff calcific tendinitis: does warm saline solution improve the short-term outcome of double-needle US-guided treatment? *Radiology.* 2012;262(2):560-566.
13. Arirachakaran A, Boonard M, Yamaphai S, Prommahachai A, Kesprayura S, Kongtharvonskul J. Extracorporeal shock wave therapy, ultrasound-guided percutaneous lavage, corticosteroid injection and combined treatment for the treatment of rotator cuff calcific tendinopathy: a network meta-analysis of RCTs. *Eur J Orthop Surg Traumatol.* 2017;27(3):381-390.
14. Messina C, Banfi G, Orlandi D, et al. Ultrasound-guided interventional procedures around the shoulder. *Br J Radiol.* 2016;89(1057):20150372.

Tendon Brisement High-Volume Injection

Tendon brisement—as opposed to fenestration and tenotomy, which directly approaches degenerative tendinopathy with intratendinous needling and débridement of abnormal angiofibroblastic tissue—focuses on disrupting adherent peritendinous neovessels and neonerves. Brisement was first described in 1997 and was initially meant to interrupt the degenerative cycle of the tendon proper by initiating a healing cascade, but in essence seems equivalent to currently described high volume injections (HVIs).[1] Brisement specifically is the injection of fluid into the space between a tendon and its lining, peritenon, or peritendinous fat pad. While the exact mechanism of efficacy is unknown, this procedure is thought to potentially break up scar tissue, disrupt associated neovessels and neonerves, and ultimately stimulate the healing of the tendon. Tendon brisement and HVI procedures essentially perform a hydrostatic decompression of soft tissues. Brisement procedures, or HVIs, are most commonly described with the Achilles tendon and patellar tendon but have also been described in other tendons with associated synovial sheaths, for example, the peroneal tendons.

EVIDENCE

There have been several manuscripts that have addressed HVI therapy. US-guided HVI therapy for patellar tendinopathy was first described by Crisp et al in 2008.[2] Nine patients with recalcitrant patellar tendinopathy, with associated neovascularity demonstrated by US, were treated with HVI between the patellar tendon and Hoffa's fat pad. The injection consisted of 10 mL of 0.5% bupivacaine, 25 mg of cortisone, and between 20 and 40 mL of normal saline, based upon the resistance encountered by the treating provider. Subjects reported significant improvement 2 weeks following the procedure.

A study by Chan et al[3] included 30 patients with refractory Achilles tendinopathy. All patients underwent an HVI injection that included 10-mL 0.5% bupivacaine, 25-mg hydrocortisone, and 4 to 10 mL of normal saline that was administered between the anterior aspect of the Achilles tendon and Kager's fat pad. Vascularity was assessed with power Doppler, and eccentric loading was subsequently prescribed. The results from visual pain scores showed a significant improvement in the short term (2 weeks), with a mean change of 50 mm, from a mean of 76 mm to a mean of 25 mm. There was also a statistically significant improvement in function with a mean gain of 50 mm, as well as a significant reduction demonstrated at a 30-week follow-up assessment.

In addition to the aforementioned studies, where HVI incorporated the utilization of a corticosteroid, there are a limited number of studies that employed fluid volume alone, generally a combination of lidocaine and normal saline.[4,5] While these studies demonstrated positive results, they involved limited numbers and lacked a control group for comparison. In a review of available literature, Davidson et al[6] classified the level of evidence as a 2 (including prospective comparative studies), but opined that further work was required. The HVI technique, while promising, and a potentially useful procedure in those who have otherwise failed conservative rehabilitative therapy, is limited by a lack of strong evidence at this time.

CONTRAINDICATIONS

The brisement/HVI procedure has comparable contraindications that apply to all bursal and peritendinous injections as previously described. The provider in particular should be cautious in an area where either a partial- or full-thickness tear in a tendon is evident, as either pain relief or an inappropriate intratendinous corticosteroid injection may propagate the tear.

EQUIPMENT

- One 21- to 22-guage needle
- Sterile saline solution (20-100)
- Lidocaine 1% (10 mL)
- Steroid (1 mL, 40 mg/mL) (optional)
- US machine with high-frequency linear array transducer

PREPROCEDURAL INSTRUCTIONS

The patient should be placed in a supine position to prevent patient movement during the procedure. The limb of the affected extremity should lie completely extended along the body to facilitate optimal visualization. The procedural guidance for utilization of US guidance, to include sterile technique, is detailed in the previous chapter of **Introduction to Ultrasound**.

ANESTHESIA

Using US guidance with an in-plane approach, inject up to 10-mL lidocaine along the path of the needle's track through the skin and soft tissue proximal to the intended area of the brisement procedure.

TECHNIQUE

1. After the patient is placed in the appropriate position (eg, prone for Achilles tendinopathy) and appropriately prepped and draped, the involved tendon is examined by US to identify the area of tendinopathy.
2. The skin and subcutaneous tissue is anesthetized utilizing a 25-gauge needle.
3. A brisement or HVI can be performed, utilizing a 21- or 22-guage needle.
4. The tendon is identified, or the tendon fat pad interface, using the linear probe being held perpendicular to the effected region.
5. The needle then enters the area of interest, and a combination of lidocaine and normal saline is injected to tolerance and/or resistance. The amount injected is variable, with the literature describing 5 to 100 mL. Some authors argue that exceedingly large volumes may risk tendon rupture and/or compartment syndrome.

AFTERCARE

- After tendon brisement or HVI, in particular for the Achilles or patellar tendon, the patient is asked to avoid excessive activity for several days.
- For the Achilles tendon, a walking boot is often used and, for the patellar tendon, a knee brace may be used.
- Such mechanical braces are not typically used for the upper extremity or greater trochanteric regions.
- The timing of stretching and physical therapy after tendon brisement is also variable in the literature.

PEARLS

- Patients should be supine for the procedure to carefully observe for vasovagal syncope.
- Patients who have brisement or HVI near a weight-bearing tendon should have the limb protected for at least 48 to 72 hours.
- Physical therapy should commence after the procedure to facilitate optimal healing.

A video showing tendon brisement can be found in the companion eBook.

REFERENCES

1. Johnston E, Scranton P Jr, Pfeffer GB. Chronic disorders of the Achilles tendon: results of conservative and surgical treatments. *Foot Ankle Int.* 1997;18(9):570-574.
2. Crisp T, Khan F, Padhiar N, et al. High volume ultrasound guided injections at the interface between the patellar tendon and Hoffa's body are effective in chronic patellar tendinopathy: a pilot study. *Disabil Rehabil.* 2008;30(20-22):1625-1634.
3. Chan O, O'Dowd D, Padhiar N, et al. High volume image guided injections in chronic Achilles tendinopathy. *Disabil Rehabil.* 2008;30(20-22):1697-1708.
4. Wheeler PC, Tattersall C. Novel interventions for recalcitrant Achilles tendinopathy: benefits seen following high-volume image-guided injection or extracorporeal shockwave therapy—a prospective cohort study. *Clin J Sport Med.* 2020;30(1):14-19.
5. Maffulli N, Del Buono A, Oliva F, Testa V, Capasso G, Maffulli G. High-volume image-guided injection for recalcitrant patellar tendinopathy in athletes. *Clin J Sport Med.* 2016;26(1):12-16.
6. Davidson J, Jayaraman S. Guided interventions in musculoskeletal ultrasound: what's the evidence? *Clin Radiol.* 2011;66(2):140-152.

Fenestration (Percutaneous Tenotomy)

The use of a needle to produce multiple punctate incisions or openings in a tendon for tendinopathy is termed tendon fenestration; the procedure is importantly distinguished by the absence of the use of an injectable agent.[1] Tenotomy, or percutaneous needle tenotomy, has also been used as a synonymous term in the literature and is often applied where the intervention results in tendon lengthening, release, or débridement. The theory behind this procedure is that repetitively passing the needle though the area of tendinosis disrupts the chronic degenerative process, causes bleeding and inflammation, and locally increases growth factors and other substances that promote healing. The primary goal of tendon fenestration is to convert a chronic tendon abnormality into an acute condition to facilitate improved healing. Needle fenestration is commonly utilized for tendinopathy in multiple structures including the patellar, elbow, gluteus medius, and Achilles tendons.

EVIDENCE

There have been multiple publications in the peer-reviewed literature to support the role of fenestration in treating common tendinopathies.[1-3] One of the first to report on the benefit of needle fenestration was McShane et al.[4] In a study involving 52 patients, and a 22-month follow-up, they reported that 92% of subjects reporting good to excellent results. Krey et al[2] performed a recent systematic review of the literature on needle fenestration, finding only four manuscripts that met their inclusion criteria. However, they did conclude that the current evidence suggests that tendon needling improves patient-reported outcome measures in patients with tendinopathy. They also concluded that there is a trend that shows that the addition of autologous blood products may further improve these outcomes. A recently performed systematic review by Maag et al included a total of 10 studies, representing 11 tendon sites. The authors concluded that US-guided needle fenestration was both efficacious and safe, in particular for lateral elbow tendinopathy, medial elbow tendinopathy, and gluteal tendinopathy. The authors noted, however, that higher quality studies were needed to assess the effectiveness of these interventions for different types of tendinopathy.[5]

CONTRAINDICATIONS

There are several contraindications to consider when performing any US-guided percutaneous procedure. These include (1) patients with a bleeding disorder; (2) patients who are anticoagulated; and (3) the presence of local infection. The presence of an underlying tendon tear deserves discussion because the risk of tendon rupture as a complication of the procedure increases with the degree of a preexisting tendon tear. While there are no evidence-based guidelines, most authorities advocate fenestration with tendinosis, interstitial tearing, or partial-thickness tearing up to 50% of the tendon thickness, while avoiding fenestration if a tear is greater than 50% of the tendon thickness.[1,2]

EQUIPMENT

- 27-guage needle
- 22-guage needle
- 5- to 10-mL lidocaine 1%
- US machine with high-frequency linear array transducer

PREPROCEDURAL INSTRUCTIONS

Prior to the fenestration procedure, the patient is instructed to avoid nonsteroidal anti-inflammatory medication for 2 weeks before and after the procedure. Avoidance of such medications theoretically may increase the chance of healing in that inflammation, growth factors, and the healing cascade will not be altered.

ANESTHESIA

Using US guidance with an in-plane approach, inject up to 10-mL lidocaine along the path of the needles into the peritendinous tissue of the intended needle fenestration procedure. Some patients have significant pain when the needle is at the surface of the tendon. Injection of an anesthetic agent at the tendon surface is often effective in significantly reducing symptoms. The amount of anesthetic agent should be minimized because it may potentially interfere with the healing process after fenestration.

TECHNIQUE

1. US imaging is first performed to confirm the presence of tendinosis and to plan the optimal approach to needle guidance. The area of tendinosis is targeted, which is usually near its enthesis or attachment to bone.
2. The skin is then marked to indicate the proposed needle puncture site as well as the position of the transducer. This indicates the area that needs to be cleansed prior to the procedure, and additionally, it allows the transducer to be returned to the exact imaging plane.
3. First, the skin is scrubbed with an appropriate cleansing agent, and sterile drapes are placed around the puncture site.
4. The US probe is then inserted into a sterile probe cover with gel, and sterile gel is used on the skin surface.
5. Using a 27-gauge needle, the subcutaneous tissues are infiltrated with local anesthetic (Fig. 6.4).
6. Regarding the size of the needle used for fenestration, the authors use a 20-gauge needle for the shoulder, hip, and knee, and a 22-gauge needle for tendons about smaller joints. The length of the needle may be either 1.5 or 3 cm. The needle typically is inserted along the long-axis of the tendon, parallel to the transducer. Passing the needle in-plane, or parallel to the long-axis of the transducer, is often preferred for US guidance because the needle is visualized in its entirety. The needle can then be angle corrected during the procedure to provide real-time visualization of the fenestration.

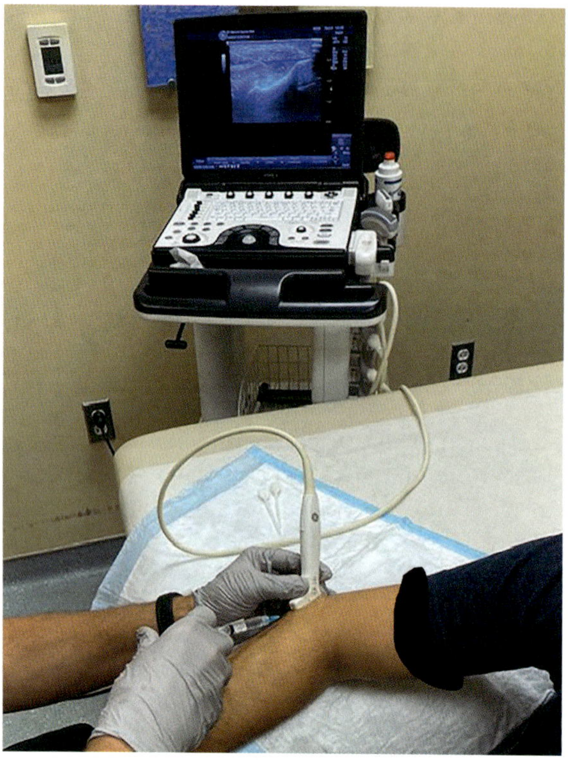

FIGURE 6.4 ● Needle fenestration of the tendon of the extensor carpi radialis brevis.

7. A few technical aspects should be considered prior to entering the tendon to minimize any patient discomfort. First, the needle should be positioned in-plane, along the long axis of the transducer and tendon. Second, the needle should be placed at the proper angle while the needle is still at a very superficial level within the subcutaneous tissues. It is much easier to make changes in the needle trajectory while the needle is superficial. After entering deeper structures, such as muscle or tendon, the needle becomes more difficult to redirect.
8. Once the needle is identified in-plane and the target visualized, the needle is advanced to the tendon abnormality.
9. If the needle has a stylet, it should be removed prior to fenestration. The needle is then passed into the tendon, within the area of tendinosis, subsequently partially withdrawn and redirected, sequentially redirecting shallower or deeper to cover the area of tendinosis within the plane of the transducer. If the tendon abnormality is adjacent to bone, the needle is advanced to make contact with the bone. The transducer is turned 90° to determine if the needle needs to be positioned or redirected medially or laterally relative to the short axis of the tendon. The needle is again partially retracted and then redirected and advanced medially or laterally, sequentially redirecting to cover the short-axis area of tendinosis. The transducer is then turned 90° again, in-plane with the needle, and the fenestration continues in a similar manner, repeating until the target area has been satisfactorily fenestrated. If the patient is having symptoms, additional anesthetic agent may be injected into the tendon, although this should be minimized. The number of times the needle passes through the tendon varies but often ranges from 15 to 50 passes, depending on the size of the tendon abnormality. As the needle passes through the abnormal tendon, the tendon tends to soften.

10. The procedure is terminated when the entire area of tendinosis is treated and feels soft during needle advancement.

AFTERCARE

- After the tendon fenestration, the patient is asked to avoid nonsteroidal anti-inflammatory drugs for 2 weeks so as not to interfere with the healing process. For similar reasons, ice is avoided so as to not inhibit the induced inflammation, which is a precursor for tendon healing.
- For weight-bearing tendons, precautions should be considered to enhance healing and avoid the complication of tendon tear. For the Achilles tendon, a walking boot is often used and, for the patellar tendon, a knee brace is used. Such mechanical braces are not typically used for the upper extremity or greater trochanteric regions.
- The timing of stretching and physical therapy after tendon fenestration is also variable in the literature, although many authors advocate waiting 2 weeks after fenestration.

PEARLS

- In addition to needle fenestration, it may be useful to consider the addition of either a prolotherapy injectant, autologous blood, or another regenerative agent.
- Advise the patient that it may take up to 6 weeks postprocedure to see clinical benefits.
- Nonsteroidal anti-inflammatory drugs should be avoided postprocedure as this negates the intent of inducing an inflammatory response.

A video showing fenestration (percutaneous tenotomy) can be found in the companion eBook.

REFERENCES

1. Chiavaras MM, Jacobson JA. Ultrasound-guided tendon fenestration. *Semin Musculoskelet Radiol.* 2013;17(1):85-90.
2. Krey D, Borchers J, McCamey K. Tendon needling for treatment of tendinopathy: a systematic review. *Phys Sportsmed.* 2015;43(1):80-86.
3. Mattie R, Wong J, McCormick Z, Yu S, Saltychev M, Laimi K. Percutaneous needle tenotomy for the treatment of lateral epicondylitis: a systematic review of the literature. *PM R.* 2017;9(6):603-611.
4. McShane JM, Shah VN, Nazarian LN. Sonographically guided percutaneous needle tenotomy for treatment of common extensor tendinosis in the elbow: is a corticosteroid necessary? *J Ultrasound Med.* 2008;27(8):1137-1144.
5. Maag L, Linder S, Hackett L, et al. Effectiveness of percutaneous needle tenotomy for tendinopathies: a systematic review. *Sports Health.* 2025;17(4):834-842.

Nerve Hydrodissection

Nerve hydrodissection, also identified as adhesiolysis neuroplasty, procedures have emerged in musculoskeletal medicine with the increasing utilization of US.[1,2] Nerve hydrodissection can be defined as the introduction of a solution under pressure between tissue planes to create separation and detach adhesions with the goal of releasing a potential soft tissue tethers or obstruction from an entrapped peripheral nerve.[1,3] Hydrodissection has been suggested as a safe and proven procedure for the blunt dissection of tissue planes. That being stated, guiding a needle along a small to medium size nerve in two axial planes is a high-skill level procedure.

While the use of hydrodissection in the treatment of peripheral nerve entrapment syndromes is a relatively new and emerging concept, the concept itself has been used for many years in a variety of settings. Hydrodissection has been used in urologic oncology to preserve the neurovascular bundle during radical prostatectomy and to prevent nerve damage during radiofrequency ablation of kidney tumors.[4,5] It has been used to preserve perforating arteries during breast reconstruction, as well as to define surgical planes during ophthalmologic procedures.[6,7] The most oft-cited risk associated with peripheral nerve hydrodissection has been that of intraneural injection and resultant nerve damage. However, a study of 257 patients receiving peripheral nerve blocks before shoulder arthroscopy reported a 17% incidence of intraneural injection with zero patients experiencing postoperative neurologic complications.[8] A second study evaluated 72 cases of apparent intraneural injection, none of which resulted in any permanent nerve injury.[9] These findings suggest that while unintentional intraneural injections should be avoided, the complication of intraneural injection does not pose as ominous a risk as once thought.

EVIDENCE

Case reports have been published reporting successful treatment of peripheral neuropathies using hydrodissection techniques, such as a case of meralgia paresthetica as described by Mulvaney in 2011,[10] and a case of foot drop as described by Tabor et al in 2017.[11] However, these cases used local anesthetic or corticosteroid as part of the injectate solution. Improvement in radial nerve palsy signs and symptoms after US-guided perineural injection of D5W was noted in a single case report.[12] One recent study compared the use of corticosteroid injection versus D5W perineural injections of the median nerve in carpal tunnel syndrome patients. This study showed increased benefit in the D5W group compared with the corticosteroid group at 4 to 6 months of follow-up.[13] While US-guided nerve hydrodissection is a promising minimally invasive intervention, a recent retrospective review of 204 cases demonstrated that although nearly 50% of interventions resulted in moderate to significant improvement at 6 months, the remaining half of patients had minimal improvement. The authors identified the need for further research in this potentially exciting intervention for nerve entrapments.[14]

CONTRAINDICATIONS

There are several contraindications to consider when performing any US-guided percutaneous procedure. These include (1) patients with a bleeding disorder; (2) patients who are anticoagulated; and (3) the presence of local infection. When approaching a nerve hydrodissection procedure, the provider should insure an accurate diagnosis of an entrapment neuropathy. In addition, patients with demonstrated distal evidence of atrophy or progressive weakness should be considered for surgical evaluation and consultation.

EQUIPMENT

- One 21- to 22-guage needle
- D5W solution (20-100 mL)
- Lidocaine 1% (10 mL)
- Steroid (1 mL, 40 mg/mL) (optional)
- US machine with high-frequency linear array transducer

PREPROCEDURAL INSTRUCTIONS

The patient should be placed in a supine position, to prevent patient movement during the procedure. The patient should be instructed to report any numbness or tingling during the procedure as this would warrant retraction and redirection of the needle. The procedural guidance for utilization of US guidance, to include sterile technique, is detailed in the previous chapter of **Introduction to Ultrasound**.

ANESTHESIA

The overlying skin is anesthetized using lidocaine 1% with epinephrine.

TECHNIQUE

Plan the procedure to hydrodissect the nerve in the direction of distal to proximal.

1. The procedural area just proximal and distal to the site of entrapment is appropriately prepped by cleaning the skin overlying the path of the nerve with a single-use chlorhexidine sponge followed by application of sterile US gel. The transducer is cleansed with appropriate bactericidal wipes.
2. The affected nerve is then visualized in the short axis where the nerve is most superficial and easy to visualize.
3. Using a two-provider technique, the first provider uses US guidance to advance a 21- to 25-gauge US needle to a point just superficial and medial or lateral to the nerve in the surrounding connective tissue, dependent upon the related vascular anatomy.
4. Advance the needle initially in short axis (out-of-plane) to ensure you are over the correct nerve, then switch to long axis (in-plane) for precise depth control when approaching the nerve.
5. The needle is attached to connector tubing, which is attached to a 10- to 20-mL syringe held by the second provider. The syringe is filled with 5% dextrose in water (D5W) solution as the sole injectate for this procedure.

6. As the needle is approximated to the perineural connective tissue, the D5W is slowly injected to bluntly dissect the surrounding connective tissue from the nerve.
7. Using fluid to maintain distance between the needle and the nerve, the needle is maneuvered superficially, deep, and circumferentially while injecting aliquots of fluid around the nerve until a complete hypoechoic ring (aka: halo) of fluid is visualized in both the short and long axes (Fig. 6.5).
8. At this point, the nerve is visualized in long axis and further injectate is pushed through the syringe along the superficial aspect of the nerve, traveling along the length of the nerve segment and extending the area of hydrodissection through the site of entrapment.
9. If at any time during the procedure the nerve appears to be getting larger: STOP, as you are injecting intraneurally and high volumes may damage the nerve. If at any time during the procedure you see concentric rings of tissue expanding away from the nerve: STOP, you are injecting into the perineurium, and high volumes may compress and damage the nerve.

AFTERCARE

- Following the procedure, pressure should be applied as well as a surface bandage.
- A pressure dressing should be avoided as it may increase friction and accentuate the tissues that caused the entrapment.
- Immediate physical therapy is recommended to reinforce physiologic nerve gliding.

PEARLS

- Consider the utilization of buffered lidocaine; additionally, consider the use of 2% lidocaine if the patient is a known "slow metabolizer" of local anesthetics by history.
- Before starting the hydrodissection procedure, measure and document the nerve cross-sectional area and record comments on the appearance of the nerve (eg, the nerve was 14 mm^2, and anechoic with the loss of the normal "bundle of grapes" appearance in cross section).
- A one-provider approach (hand on syringe approach) has the advantage of maintaining the sense of "injection pressure" during injection but requires greater skill, while the two-provider approach (hand on needle approach) affords greater precision in needle handling at the cost feeling injection pressure.

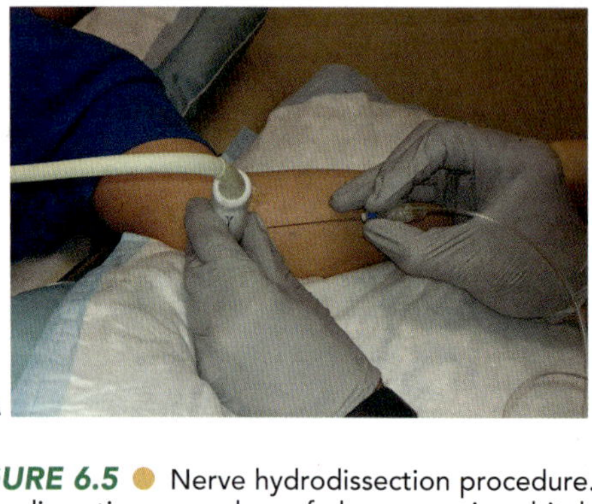

A

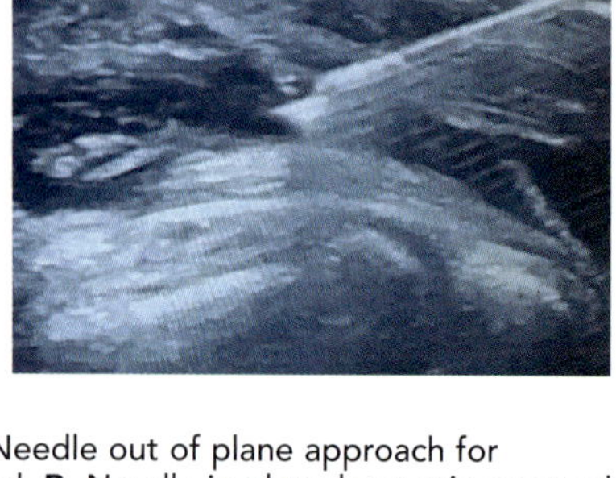

B

FIGURE 6.5 ● Nerve hydrodissection procedure. **A.** Needle out of plane approach for hydrodissection procedure of ulnar nerve in cubital tunnel. **B.** Needle in-plane long-axis approach for hydrodissection procedure of ulnar nerve in cubital tunnel.

- 10- or 20-mL syringes are recommended for hydrodissection procedures. A larger syringe (eg, 60 mL) is too large to have any sense of injection pressure with two providers and is too cumbersome to handle for one provider. Instead, have multiple full syringes available to support the planned procedure.
- Physical therapy and home exercise should emphasize nerve glide exercises.

A video showing a nerve hydrodissection procedure can be found in the companion eBook.

REFERENCES

1. Cass SP. Ultrasound-guided nerve hydrodissection: what is it? A review of the literature. *Curr Sports Med Rep.* 2016;15(1):20-22.
2. Norbury JW, Nazarian LN. Ultrasound-guided treatment of peripheral entrapment mononeuropathies. *Muscle Nerve.* 2019;60(3):222-231.
3. Bokey EL, Keating JP, Zelas P. Hydrodissection: an easy way to dissect anatomical planes and complex adhesions. *Aust N Z J Surg.* 1997;67(9):643-644.
4. Guru KA, Perlmutter AE, Butt ZM, Peabody JO. Hydrodissection for preservation of neurovascular bundle during robot-assisted radical prostatectomy. *Can J Urol.* 2008;15(2):4000-4003.
5. Lee SJ, Choyke LT, Locklin JK, Wood BJ. Use of hydrodissection to prevent nerve and muscular damage during radiofrequency ablation of kidney tumors. *J Vasc Interv Radiol.* 2006;17(12):1967-1969.
6. Ting J, Rozen WM, Morsi A. Improving the subfascial dissection of perforators during deep inferior epigastric artery perforator flap harvest: the hydrodissection technique. *Plast Reconstr Surg.* 2010;126(2):87e-89e.
7. Malavazzi GR, Nery RG. Visco-fracture technique for soft lens cataract removal. *J Cataract Refract Surg.* 2011;37(1):11-12.
8. Liu SS, YaDeau JT, Shaw PM, Wilfred S, Shetty T, Gordon M. Incidence of unintentional intraneural injection and postoperative neurological complications with ultrasound-guided interscalene and supraclavicular nerve blocks. *Anaesthesia.* 2011;66(3):168-174.
9. Bigeleisen PE. Nerve puncture and apparent intraneural injection during ultrasound-guided axillary block does not invariably result in neurologic injury. *Anesthesiology.* 2006;105(4):779-783.
10. Mulvaney SW. Ultrasound-guided percutaneous neuroplasty of the lateral femoral cutaneous nerve for the treatment of meralgia paresthetica: a case report and description of a new ultrasound-guided technique. *Curr Sports Med Rep.* 2011;10(2):99-104.
11. Tabor M, Emerson B, Drucker R, Brunk E. High-stepping cross-country athlete: a unique case of foot drop and a novel treatment approach. *Curr Sports Med Rep.* 2017;16(5):314-316.
12. Chen S-R, Shen Y-P, Ho T-Y, Chen L-C, Wu Y-T. Ultrasound-guided perineural injection with dextrose for treatment of radial nerve palsy: a case report. *Medicine (Baltimore).* 2018;97(23):e10978.
13. Wu Y-T, Ke M-J, Ho T-Y, Li T-Y, Shen Y-P, Chen L-C. Randomized double-blinded clinical trial of 5% dextrose versus triamcinolone injection for carpal tunnel syndrome patients. *Ann Neurol.* 2018;84(4):601-610.
14. Sabbineni M, Ajmera P, Wang B, Varma V, Mbuagbaw L, Choudur HN. Exploring the therapeutic potential of ultrasound-guided nerve hydrodissection: a comprehensive retrospective analysis. *Clin Radiol.* 2025;85:106863.

Capsular Hydrodilatation/Hydroplasty

Capsular hydrodilatation, also known as hydroplasty, is a nonsurgical intervention used in the management of adhesive capsulitis, also known as frozen shoulder.[1] Adhesive capsulitis is a common disorder encountered by primary care providers with an estimated prevalence of 2% to 5% of the general population. Most patients diagnosed with adhesive capsulitis are women between 40 and 60 years of age, with the disorder commonly associated with both diabetes mellitus and hypothyroidism. Adhesive capsulitis is defined as a pathologic process in which contracture of the glenohumeral capsule is a hallmark, where there is restriction of both active and passive range of motion. Clinically, it presents as pain, stiffness, and dysfunction of the affected shoulder; the natural history of frozen shoulder has been described as a progression through three phases: painful, stiffness, and recovery, also known as freezing, frozen, and thawing. Adhesive capsulitis is generally considered self-limited; however, it can persist for years with some patients never regaining full function of their shoulder.[2]

EVIDENCE

Hydrodilatation (capsular distension) is a nonoperative treatment that involves an injection of local anesthetic into the shoulder capsule at high pressure to distend, stretch, or rupture the joint capsule. Although therapeutic regimens will differ between units, common to most is the instillation of a large volume of saline containing steroid, local anesthetic, and contrast material into the glenohumeral joint under imaging guidance, typically around 30 mL. A randomized controlled study of 46 patients compared hydrodilatation with placebo and demonstrated statistically and clinically significant improvement in functional outcome scores at 6 weeks following intervention.[3] One study comparing hydrodilatation, to glenohumeral and subacromial injections, found that while there was no significant difference at 6 months, that hydrodilatation provided faster relief.[4] A Cochrane review found that there is "silver" level evidence that capsular distension with saline and steroid provides short-term benefits in pain, range of movement, and function in adhesive capsulitis; however, it is uncertain whether this is better than alternative interventions.[5] Ramirez[2] in their recent review in *American Family Physician* assigned B level evidence (inconsistent or limited-quality patient-oriented evidence) to the procedure, concluding that the combination of hydrodilatation and corticosteroid injection may expedite recovery of pain free range of motion compared with corticosteroid injection alone. In addition to utility for shoulder adhesive capsulitis, a recent case report demonstrated efficacy of capsular distention for the management of a postoperative capsulitis after an arthroscopic hip labral repair.[6]

CONTRAINDICATIONS

- Anticoagulation/coagulopathy
- Systemic sepsis
- Allergies to contrast, steroid, or local anaesthetic
- Acute trauma

EQUIPMENT

- One 22-guage needle for the hydrodilatation procedure
- One 25-guage needle for soft tissue injection prior to the hydrodilatation procedure
- Four syringes ([2] 20 mL and [2] 3 mL)
- Surgical tubing and three way stop cock (optional)
- Bowl (to collect the washing fluid)
- Sterile saline solution (100-200 mL)
- Lidocaine 1% or mepivacaine (10 mL)
- Steroid (1 mL, 40 mg/mL)
- High-frequency linear array transducer

PREPROCEDURAL INSTRUCTIONS

For the preferred, posterior approach (see below), the patient should be placed in a lateral decubitus position, with the target shoulder up and non–weight bearing. The arm of the affected shoulder should lie in a neutral-adducted position. The procedural guidance for utilization of US guidance, to include sterile technique, is detailed in the previous chapter of **Introduction to Ultrasound**.

ANESTHESIA

Using US guidance with an in-plane approach, inject up to 10-mL lidocaine along the path of the needles into the glenohumeral joint.

TECHNIQUE

Hydrodilatation, also known as hydroplasty, can be performed from an anterior or a posterior approach. The posterior approach is the preferred approach and is accomplished with the following steps:

1. The patient is positioned in a side lying position with the affected shoulder up. The forearm should be internally rotated to facilitate opening the posterior glenohumeral joint.
2. A high-frequency linear or curvilinear probe can then be used to identify the infraspinatus and posterior glenohumeral joint.
3. After a sterile site preparation, an in-plane injection proceeds with the 25-guage needle, providing track local anesthesia.
4. The injection then proceeds with a 22-guage spinal needle along the previous identified track, until the joint capsule is penetrated (Fig. 6.6).
5. At this point, local anesthetic and corticosteroid is injected into the joint (eg, 1 mL Kenalog 40 mg in combination with 4 mL 1% lidocaine).
6. The syringe is then changed to a 20-mL syringe of normal saline; optionally, an extension tubing with a three way stop cock can be attached.

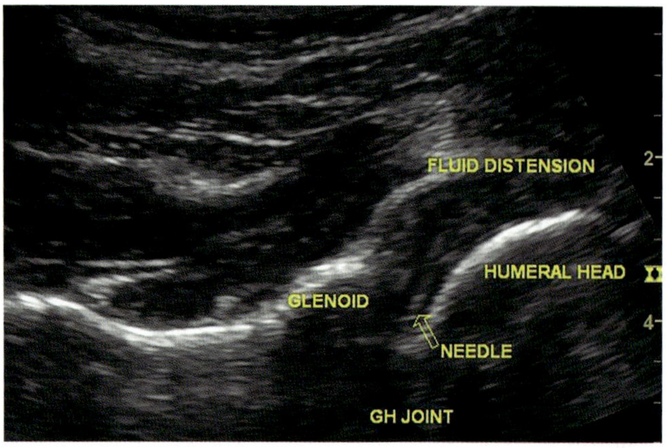

FIGURE 6.6 Hydrodilatation procedure of the posterior glenohumeral (GH) joint.

7. Normal saline 0.9% is then introduced into the joint (10-40 mL) to produce a hydraulic distention of the joint.

AFTERCARE

- Following the procedure, pressure should be applied as well as a bandage.
- Immediate physical therapy is recommended to reinforce capsular range of motion.

PEARLS

- Patients should be supine following the procedure to carefully observe for vasovagal syncope.
- A suprascapular nerve block can be considered prior to the procedure to facilitate patient comfort.
- Physical therapy immediately after the procedure is highly recommended to optimally leverage the hydrodilatation procedure.

A video showing capsular hydrodilatation/hydroplasty can be found in the companion eBook.

REFERENCES

1. Halverson L, Maas R. Shoulder joint capsule distension (hydroplasty): a case series of patients with "frozen shoulders" treated in a primary care office. *J Fam Pract.* 2002;51(1):61-63.
2. Ramirez J. Adhesive capsulitis: diagnosis and management. *Am Fam Physician.* 2019;99(5):297-300.
3. Buchbinder RGS, Green S, Forbes A, Hall S, Lawler G. Arthrographic joint distension with saline and steroid improves function and reduces pain in patients with painful stiff shoulder: results of a randomized, double blind, placebo-controlled trial. *Ann Rheum Dis.* 2004;63(3):302-309.
4. Yoon JP, Chung SW, Kim J-E, et al. Intra-articular injection, subacromial injection, and hydrodilatation for primary frozen shoulder: a randomized clinical trial. *J Shoulder Elbow Surg.* 2016;25(3):376-383.
5. Buchbinder R, Green S, Youd JM, Johnston RV, Cumpston M. Arthrographic distension for adhesive capsulitis (frozen shoulder). *Cochrane Database Syst Rev.* 2008;(1):CD007005.
6. Cox R, Bowers RL, Wright S, et al. Ultrasound-guided high-volume pressure hydrodilatation for postoperative adhesive capsulitis of the hip: case report and literature review. *Clin J Sport Med.* 2025;36(2):211-214.

Myofascial Trigger Point Dry Needling

Myofascial pain syndrome is a common condition that arises from muscles or related fascia and is associated with painful myofascial trigger points (MTrPs). Each trigger point is a highly localized, hyperirritable focal area in a palpable, taut band of skeletal muscle fibers. Patients present frequently to primary care physicians with this condition. Although the trigger points may be injected with corticosteroids or local anesthetics, the nodules are also commonly treated with multiple needle piercings without the introduction of an injectant. This practice of "dry needling" is attributed to Simons et al[1] who empirically developed techniques involving the passage of needles into isolated trigger points for the treatment of myofascial pain syndrome. This therapeutic modality, also known as intramuscular stimulation, is based on theories similar, but not exclusive, to traditional acupuncture. However, dry needling targets discrete trigger points, which are the direct and palpable source of pain, rather than traditional meridians.

Dry needling is an invasive procedure in which a standard hollow hypodermic needle or a solid core acupuncture needle is inserted through the skin and directly into an MTrP (Fig. 6.7). Proper dry needling of an MTrP will elicit both referred pain and a "local twitch response." This is an involuntary spinal cord reflex in which the muscle fibers in the taut band quickly contract. The local twitch response indicates the proper placement of the needle in a trigger point. At the site of an active trigger point, there are elevated levels of inflammatory mediators, known to be associated with persistent pain states and myofascial tenderness. This local milieu positively changes with the occurrence of a local twitch response.[2] Lewit[3] demonstrated that the therapeutic effect from passage of a needle is distinct from that of the injected substance.

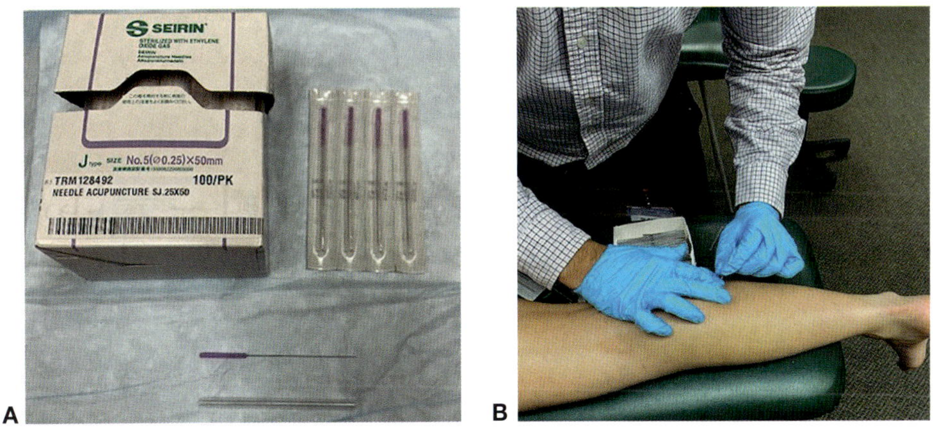

FIGURE 6.7 ● Myofascial trigger point dry needling procedure. **A.** Dry needles. (Lhasa OMS.) **B.** Dry needling technique to lateral gastrocnemius.

EVIDENCE

An examination of the peer-reviewed literature regarding the benefit of dry needling is inconclusive. There are randomized clinical trials indicating both positive effects and no difference.[4-7] The use of US may improve the accuracy, clinical response, and safety of the procedure.[8] A recent systematic review, however, indicated no difference in outcomes in patients treated with dry needling when compared with placebo for the treatment of myofascial pain syndrome.[9] Another comprehensive review yielded insufficient evidence to make any recommendations about acupuncture or dry needling for acute low back pain.[10] For chronic low back pain, however, results show that acupuncture is more effective for pain relief and improving function than no treatment or sham treatment in the short term. The technique has a small incremental effect when added to other conventional therapies but is not more effective than are other conventional and "alternative" treatments.

Most reported studies suffer from significant methodologic limitations and may not be generalizable.[10,11] Furthermore, rigorous evidence regarding the potential physiologic mechanisms of actions and effects of this modality is sparse and incomplete. Studies performed in an acupuncture setting do not necessarily apply to dry needling.[12] Since it appears that significant symptomatic improvement occurs in some patients who are treated with injection of MTrPs, further high-quality research is required to determine the proper place of this intervention in the treatment of myofascial pain syndrome. Areas that need to be addressed include proper study design that include blinding, randomization, use of controls, and sufficient numbers of patients. A recently published systematic review including 24 studies and over 500 athletes, identified that while promising, significant gaps remain in the treatment of elite, world-class, and Paralympic athletes, as well as understanding long-term effects.[13]

Several adverse effects associated specifically with dry needling have been reported. These include pain, hematoma, syncopal episodes, and pneumothorax.[14] Overall, the rate of complications is low, and dry needling/acupuncture provided by experienced physicians is considered a safe treatment.[15]

CONTRAINDICATIONS

There are few contraindications to dry needling; however, there are some concerns that would preclude dry needling. Patients with either a needle phobia, a belief the technique will not help, or an unwillingness to participate in the procedure, or consent, present clear contraindications. Dry needling should not be performed over an area with either evidence of cellulitis or lymphedema as both may potentially worsen with needle intervention. Relative contraindications include, but are not limited to, abnormal bleeding tendencies, a severely compromised immune system (eg, cancer, HIV, hepatitis, etc.), vascular disease, diabetes mellitus, pregnancy, frail patients, epilepsy, allergy to metals or latex, children, and individuals taking certain prescriptive medications (eg, significant mood-altering medication, blood thinning agents, etc.). Additional relative contraindications include an altered psychological status, anatomic considerations (extreme caution must be taken over the pleura and lungs, blood vessels, nerves, organs, joints, prosthetic implants, implantable electrical devices, etc.), needling near a surgical site within 4 months of the surgical procedure, and a decreased ability to tolerate the procedure.

EQUIPMENT

- 3-mL syringe
- Needle choices:
  - 25-gauge, 1- to 2-in needle (standard hollow hypodermic needle)
  - A 0.30 × 50-mm solid core acupuncture needle. The 0.30 corresponds to the gauge, or diameter, of the needle, and the 50 corresponds to length
- (Optional) 0.5 to 1 mL of 1% lidocaine without epinephrine per trigger point
- One alcohol prep pad
- Two povidone-iodine or chlorhexidine prep pads
- Sterile gauze pads
- Sterile adhesive bandage

PREPROCEDURAL INSTRUCTIONS

The patient should be placed in a comfortable position, to prevent patient movement during the procedure. The patient should be instructed to report any numbness or tingling during the procedure as this would warrant retraction and redirection of the needle. The procedural guidance for percutaneous injections, to include sterile technique, is detailed in the previous chapter of **Introduction to Ultrasound**.

ANESTHESIA

Skin distraction or local anesthesia of the skin using topical vapocoolant spray.

TECHNIQUE

Standard Hollow Hypodermic Needle

1. The needle entry point is located directly over the MTrP nodule(s). At that site, press firmly on the skin with the retracted tip of a ballpoint pen. This indention represents the entry point for the needle.
2. After the landmarks are identified, the patient should not move.
3. Prep the insertion site with alcohol. Current standards of care in the United States recommend preparing the skin with 70% isopropyl alcohol prior to needling, as well the practitioner utilizing gloves during the intervention.[16]
4. Achieve good local anesthesia by using topical vapocoolant spray.
5. With the nondominant hand, firmly press on either side of the nodule with the index and long fingers in order to "fix" the position of the muscular nodule.
6. Position the needle and syringe at a 30° to 45° angle to the skin with the tip of the needle directed toward the trigger point.
7. Using the no-touch technique, quickly introduce the needle at the insertion site.
8. Advance the needle carefully into the nodule until the needle tip is located in the center of the trigger point. Successful entry into the nodule will be accompanied by a quick muscle contraction known as the local twitch response. There may also be increased pain at the site of the trigger point or referred pain. Leave the needle in place until the muscle twitch (spasm) relaxes.
9. If performing dry needling, partially withdraw the needle from the nodule and back to the subcutaneous fat before advancing again into the trigger point. Repeat the process 5 to 10 times or until the twitch response is extinguished.

10. If desired, 0.5 to 1 mL of 1% lidocaine without epinephrine may be injected slowly into the nodule during the final entry of the needle—though it should be noted that this would constitute a trigger point injection, rather than dry needling alone.
11. Finally, withdraw the needle through the skin.
12. Apply a sterile adhesive bandage.
13. Massage and stretch each of the injection sites.
14. Reexamine the area of involvement in 5 minutes to confirm pain relief and observe for any complications.

Solid Core Acupuncture Needle

In addition to the hollow needle technique, solid core acupuncture needles can be utilized, with some modifications to the aforementioned technique.

1. The trigger point is identified using palpation methods previously described.
2. A pincer grip technique is employed to gently lift the skin. Additionally, flat palpation can be utilized to take up the slack of the skin.
3. A high-quality, sterile, disposable, solid filament needle is then inserted directly through the skin or using a guide tube that is then removed.[17] The depth of needle penetration must be sufficient to engage the MTrP.
4. Once the needle has penetrated the skin and is inserted into the muscle, techniques vary: the practitioner may utilize a slow, steady, lancing, or pistoning motion in and out of the muscle (termed, "dynamic needling"); he or she may leave the needle in situ (termed, "static needling"); or the needle may be rotated several revolutions in order to draw the fascia or soft tissues.[17] Baldry[18] recommends leaving the needle in situ for 30 to 60 seconds for "average responders," or up to 2 to 3 minutes in "weak responders." While there is no consensus as to which technique is ideal using a solid core needle, it is the opinion of the author that dynamic needle is superior to static needling (without intramuscular electrical stimulation) in most cases.

AFTERCARE

- Ice, heat, stretching, and/or physical therapy as indicated.
- Treatment of the underlying condition.
- Consider follow-up examination in 2 weeks.

PEARLS

- The key objective with this procedure is to elicit the local twitch response when directing a needle into an MTrP.
- Avoid advancing the needle so deeply as to risk complications including pneumothorax.

REFERENCES

1. Simons DG, Travell JG, Simons LS. *Travell and Simons' Myofascial Pain and Dysfunction: The Trigger Point Manual.* 2nd ed. Lippincott Williams & Wilkins; 1999.
2. Vulfsons S, Ratmansky M, Kalichman L. Trigger point needling: techniques and outcome. *Curr Pain Headache Rep.* 2012;16(5):407-412.

3. Lewit K. The needle effect in the relief of myofascial pain. *Pain.* 1979;6(1):83-90.
4. Tekin L, Akarsu S, Durmuş O, Cakar E, Dinçer U, Kıralp MZ. The effect of dry needling in the treatment of myofascial pain syndrome: a randomized double-blinded placebo-controlled trial. *Clin Rheumatol.* 2013;32(3):309-315.
5. Ga H, Choi J-H, Park C-H, Yoon H-J. Acupuncture needling versus lidocaine injection of trigger points in myofascial pain syndrome in elderly patients—a randomised trial. *Acupunct Med.* 2007;25(4):130-136.
6. Barbagli P, Bollettin R, Ceccherelli F. Acupuncture (dry needle) versus neural therapy (local anesthesia) in the treatment of benign back pain. Immediate and long-term results. *Minerva Med.* 2003;94(4 Suppl 1): 17-25.
7. Hong CZ. Lidocaine injection versus dry needling to myofascial trigger point. The importance of the local twitch response. *Am J Phys Med Rehabil.* 1994;73(4):256-263.
8. Chiavaras MM, Jacobson JA. Ultrasound-guided tendon fenestration. *Semin Musculoskelet Radiol.* 2013;17(1):85-90.
9. Cummings TM, White AR. Needling therapies in the management of myofascial trigger point pain: a systematic review. *Arch Phys Med Rehabil.* 2001;82(7):986-992.
10. Furlan AD, van Tulder MW, Cherkin DC, et al. Acupuncture and dry-needling for low back pain. *Cochrane Database Syst Rev.* 2005;(1):CD001351.
11. Tough EA, White AR, Cummings TM, Richards SH, Campbell JL. Acupuncture and dry needling in the management of myofascial trigger point pain: a systematic review and meta-analysis of randomised controlled trials. *Eur J Pain.* 2009;13(1):3-10.
12. Cagnie B, Dewitte V, Barbe T, Timmermans F, Delrue N, Meeus M. Physiologic effects of dry needling. *Curr Pain Headache Rep.* 2013;17(8):348.
13. Kużdżał A, Trybulski R, Muracki J, Klich S, Clemente FM, Kawczyński A. Dry needling in sports and sport recovery: a systematic review with an evidence gap map. *Sports Med.* 2025;55(4):811-844.
14. Witt CM, Pach D, Brinkhaus B, et al. Safety of acupuncture: results of a prospective observational study with 229,230 patients and introduction of a medical information and consent form. *Forsch Komplementmed.* 2009;16(2):91-97.
15. White A, Hayhoe S, Hart A, Ernst E. Adverse events following acupuncture: prospective survey of 32,000 consultations with doctors and physiotherapists. *BMJ.* 2001;323(7311):485-486.
16. Stephens MB, Beutler AI, O'Connor FG. Musculoskeletal injections: a review of the evidence. *Am Fam Physician.* 2008;78(8):971-976.
17. Finnoff JT, Hall MM, Adams E, et al. American Medical Society for Sports Medicine (AMSSM) position statement: interventional musculoskeletal ultrasound in sports medicine. *PM R.* 2015;7(2):151-168.e12.
18. Baldry P. Superficial versus deep dry needling. *Acupunct Med.* 2002;20(2-3):78-81.

Tenotomy With Débridement

US-guided percutaneous tenotomy with débridement is a recently FDA-approved procedure that is indicated for recalcitrant tendinopathy. Current specific indications include extensor and flexor tendinopathy at the elbow; patellar and Achilles tendinopathy; and plantar fasciopathy. One technique (Tenex) relies on the concept of "phacoemulsification," which is a technique utilized during cataract surgery. In this technique, an ultrasonic vibrating needle tip emulsifies the area of tendinopathy, while a second lumen in the needle system suctions the débrided tissue. The system requires real-time US guidance and a handheld instrument that utilizes an 18-gauge double-lumen needle.[1] A second technique (TenJet) involves a pressurized, high-velocity stream of saline and suction, which offers an alternative to ultrasonic débridement.[2] Yet another device (Ocelot Nano) functions by rapidly oscillating a stainless-steel needle to mechanically debride and fragment a targeted area of diseased tendon.

EVIDENCE

There are several published studies that have looked at the role and efficacy of percutaneous ultrasonic tenotomy (PUT) with débridement.[3,4] Barnes et al[3] prospectively studied 19 patients, aged 38 to 67 years, in whom greater than 6 months of conservative management for medial (7) or lateral (12) elbow tendinopathy had failed. They demonstrated that PUT appeared to be a safe and effective treatment option for chronic, refractory lateral, or medial elbow tendinopathy up to 1 year after the procedure. In a second study evaluating the efficacy of TenJet, authors included 100 patients with tennis elbow.[4] Patients were evaluated with the Oxford Elbow Score prior to the procedure and at 1-year follow-up and demonstrated a statistically significant difference in baseline to 1 year ($P < .001$). No complications were reported and zero patients went on to require open surgical intervention. These studies, however, like other published studies to date, are limited to case series; accordingly, the efficacy of PUT compared to other treatment options is limited at this time.

Maag et al[5] recently published a systematic review evaluating percutaneous needle tenotomy, and both Tenex and TenJet efficacy; a total of 10 studies, representing 11 tendon sites, were included (of note, no studies involving TenJet met criteria for inclusion). The authors concluded that these minimally invasive modalities were both efficacious and safe. However, the authors noted that both patients and practitioners would benefit from higher quality studies in a greater number of body regions to assess the effectiveness of these interventions for different types of tendinopathy. While this is a promising new technology, that offers yet another alternative to surgical intervention, further study is warranted to assess the role of this intervention.

CONTRAINDICATIONS

There are several contraindications to consider when performing any US-guided percutaneous procedure. These include (1) patients with a bleeding disorder; (2) patients who are anticoagulated; and (3) the presence of local infection. The presence of underlying tendon tear deserves discussion because the risk of tendon rupture as a complication of the procedure increases with the degree of a preexisting tendon tear.

EQUIPMENT

- 27-guage needle
- 22-guage needle
- 5- to 10-mL lidocaine 1% or mepivacaine
- Handheld device with equipment kit (depends on system used)
- High-frequency linear array transducer

PREPROCEDURAL INSTRUCTIONS

The patient should be placed in a supine position, to prevent patient movement during the procedure. The limb of the affected extremity should lie completely extended along the body to facilitate optimal visualization. The procedural guidance for utilization of US guidance, to include sterile technique, is detailed in the previous chapter of **Introduction to Ultrasound**.

ANESTHESIA

Using US guidance with an in-plane approach, inject up to 10-mL lidocaine along the path of the needle's track through the skin and soft tissue proximal to the intended area of the brisement procedure.

TECHNIQUE

1. US is first performed to confirm the presence of tendinosis and to plan the optimal approach to needle guidance. The area of tendinosis is targeted, which is usually near its enthesis or attachment to bone.
2. The needle typically is inserted along the long axis of the tendon, parallel to the transducer. Passing the needle in-plane, or long axis to the transducer, is the preferred method for US guidance because the needle is visualized in its entirety. The needle can then be angled corrected during the procedure to provide real-time visualization of the débridement.
3. The skin is then marked to indicate the proposed needle puncture site as well as the position of the transducer. This indicates the area that needs to be cleansed prior to the procedure, and additionally, it allows the transducer to be returned to the exact imaging plane.
4. The skin is scrubbed with an appropriate cleansing agent, and sterile drapes are placed around the puncture site. The US probe is then inserted into a sterile probe cover with gel, and sterile gel is used on the skin surface.
5. Using a 27-gauge needle, the subcutaneous tissues are infiltrated local anesthetic.

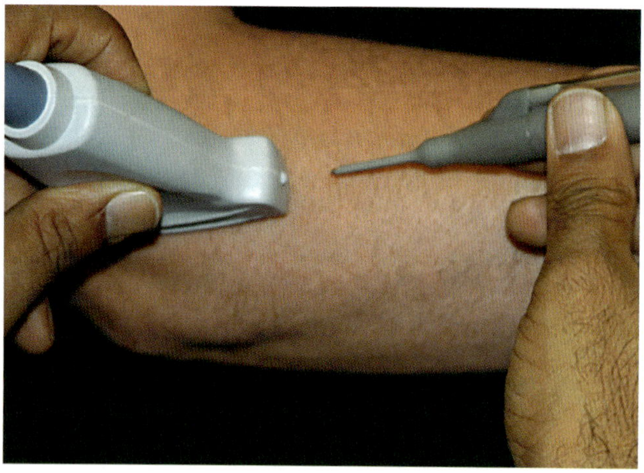

FIGURE 6.8 ● Equipment and location for ultrasound-guided elbow percutaneous tenotomy with ultrasonic débridement procedure.

6. A no. 11-blade scalpel is then utilized to make a stab incision to permit entry of the PUT device.
7. The PUT device is then introduced to the area of tendinopathy, where it can be activated with the use of a foot pedal (Fig. 6.8).
8. The PUT device is redirected over the area of tendinopathic tissue comparable to a needle fenestration procedure (see above). The procedure is considered complete when the identified damaged tissue has been broken down or removed.
9. When the procedure is concluded, wound closure is accomplished with a sterile adhesive dressing.

AFTERCARE

- Postprocedure care and rehabilitation is highly variable dependent upon the area and degree of clinical débridement.
- Comparable to the fenestration procedure, the patient is asked to avoid nonsteroidal anti-inflammatory drugs for 2 weeks so as not to interfere with the healing process. For similar reasons, ice is avoided so as to not inhibit the induced inflammation, which is a precursor for tendon healing.
- For weight-bearing tendons, precautions should be considered to enhance healing and avoid the complication of tendon tear. For the Achilles tendon, a walking boot is often used and, for the patellar tendon, a knee brace is used. Such mechanical braces are not typically used for the upper extremity or greater trochanteric regions.
- The timing of stretching and physical therapy after tendon débridement is also variable in the literature, although many authors advocate waiting 2 weeks after débridement.

PEARLS

- Advise the patient it may take up to 6 weeks postprocedure to see clinical benefits.
- Nonsteroidal anti-inflammatory drugs should be avoided postprocedure as this negates the intent of inducing an inflammatory response.

A video showing tenotomy with débridement can be found in the companion eBook.

REFERENCES

1. Peck E, Jelsing E, Onishi K. Advanced ultrasound-guided interventions for tendinopathy. *Phys Med Rehabil Clin N Am.* 2016;27(3):733-748.
2. Wong AK, Swami PN, Reed TF, Bitterman A, Grande DA. Efficacy and safety of a percutaneous tenotomy system for debridement of tendinopathic tissues. *J Long Term Eff Med Implants.* 2018;28(3):199-203.
3. Barnes DE, Beckley JM, Smith J. Percutaneous ultrasonic tenotomy for chronic elbow tendinosis: a prospective study. *J Shoulder Elbow Surg.* 2015;24(1):67-73.
4. Dakkak M, Patel V, King D, Genin J. Ultrasound-guided tenotomy for lateral epicondylitis with TenJet improves physical functional and decreased pain outcomes at 1 year: a case series review. *JSES Int.* 2023;7(5):872-876.
5. Maag L, Linder S, Hackett L, et al. Effectiveness of percutaneous needle tenotomy for tendinopathies: a systematic review. *Sports Health.* 2025;17(4):834-842.

7 Direct Local Injection

James W. McNabb

Direct injection by infiltration of an anesthetic into the skin is a valuable method to provide precise local anesthesia. This injection is done in a discrete area so that a minor skin procedure may be performed painlessly. Generally, 1% lidocaine *with epinephrine* at a concentration of 1:100,000 (5 mg/mL) is the anesthetic choice for most skin procedures—whereas 1% lidocaine without epinephrine or 1% mepivacaine without epinephrine is used for musculoskeletal injections. If anesthesia is required for more than 60 minutes, bupivacaine 0.25% with or without epinephrine used alone or mixed with lidocaine may be considered. The addition of epinephrine to the local anesthetic provides certain advantages, including prolongation of anesthetic duration of action and vasoconstriction to provide some hemostasis. Due to dermal vasoconstriction, blanching of the skin will occur in the affected area. This affords the advantage of allowing visual estimation of the area of anesthesia—thus decreasing the possibility of operating on skin that is not anesthetized. The epinephrine-induced vasoconstriction also delays absorption of lidocaine. The prolongation in the rate of absorption decreases the risk of toxicity and increases the maximum recommended dose of lidocaine from 4 to 7 mg/kg.[1] The addition of epinephrine also permits the use of larger volumes of the local anesthetic, if needed.

Several techniques may be employed to reduce the pain of injection caused by insertion of the needle and infiltration of the anesthetic into the skin. Ideally, the smallest needle, usually 30 gauge, should be used. Adjunctive techniques include the use of topical vapocoolant spray or creating a skin distraction by lightly scratching or inducing vibrations in the skin around the injection site. Both of these techniques equally decrease the pain associated with needle insertion.[2] Quick insertion of the needle into the skin, warming the injection fluid,[3] and injecting the anesthetic solution slowly[4] all decrease pain. If clinically indicated, injecting into the subcutaneous tissue is less painful than infiltrating directly into the dermis. However, placement subcutaneously without concomitant intradermal injection increases the time to full-skin anesthesia to approximately 5 minutes.

The pH of lidocaine with epinephrine is 4.5. Thus, it is acidic and causes intense burning pain upon injection. As an option, lidocaine/epinephrine buffered with sodium bicarbonate to achieve a neutral pH above 6.8[5] significantly decreases the injection pain.[6,7] Buffering of the solution is particularly useful in circumstances where the pain of local anesthetic injection is poorly tolerated, such as in large areas of infiltration, in sensitive areas such as the face or genitalia, and in children.[8] To buffer the anesthetic, mix one part of 8.4% sodium bicarbonate to nine parts of 1% lidocaine with epinephrine immediately prior to the procedure. Mixing of the solutions may be done within the syringe that is to be used for the injection. Simply, draw up both solutions, add 0.5 mL of air, and rotate the syringe to mix. Then, invert the syringe and expel the air bubble before proceeding. Raising the pH reduces the pain of injection without affecting the onset or efficacy of local anesthesia.

PATIENT POSITION

- Any, but generally recumbent on the examination/procedure table with the area of concern presented to the clinician.

ANESTHESIA

- Use topical vapocoolant spray to decrease the pain associated with injection. Use topical vapocoolant spray or create manual skin distraction (see below).

EQUIPMENT

- Topical vapocoolant spray
- 3-mL syringe
- 30-gauge ½-in needle
- 1% lidocaine with epinephrine
- 8.4% sodium bicarbonate (optional)
- One alcohol prep pad
- Sterile gauze pads

TECHNIQUE

1. Draw up 2 to 3 mL of 1% lidocaine/epinephrine in a 3-mL syringe.
2. If desired, mix a nine part volume of 1% lidocaine/epinephrine with one part volume of 8.4% sodium bicarbonate within the syringe.
3. Prep the insertion site with the alcohol pad.
4. Use topical vapocoolant spray or create manual skin distraction by lightly scratching or inducing vibrations in the skin around the injection site to achieve transient local anesthesia.
5. Using the no-touch technique, quickly insert the needle through the skin at the injection site (Fig. 7.1).

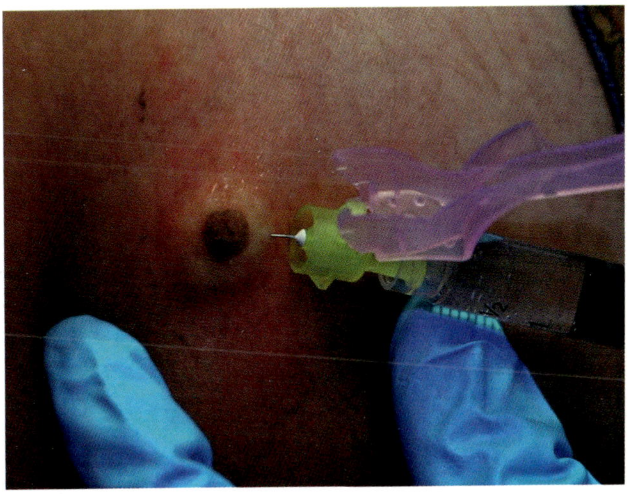

FIGURE 7.1 • Direct local injection.

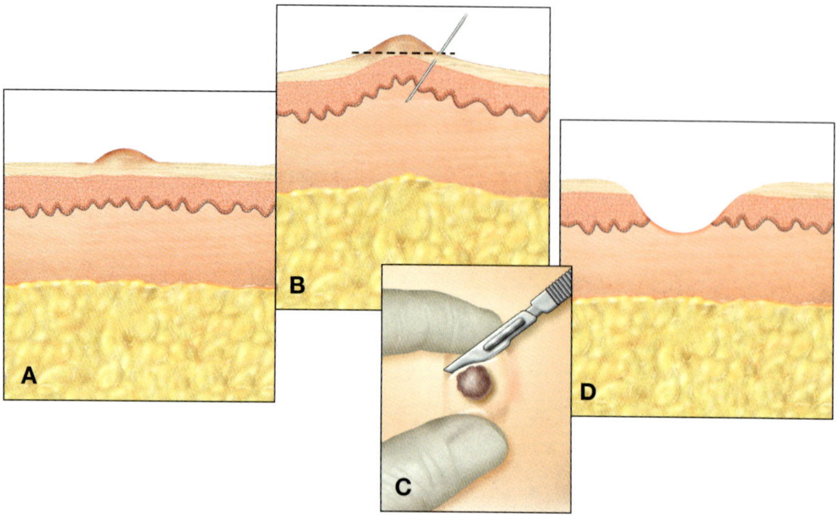

FIGURE 7.2 ● Steps in direct local injection.

6. Advance the needle at an angle below the center of the lesion in the subdermal tissue. Withdraw the syringe plunger to ensure that there is no blood return in the syringe to suggest intravascular needle placement. Inject approximately 1 mL of the anesthetic solution.
7. Then, withdraw the needle slightly while keeping it in the skin and then readvance the needle to a point in the deep dermis that is directly under the center of the skin lesion. Inject approximately 1 mL of the anesthetic solution. This intradermal injection produces a wheal directly underneath the lesion.
8. The lesion is thus "floated" upward. This adds to procedure safety by increasing tissue depth and separating subcutaneous structures (vessels, nerves, tendons) from the surgical instrument (Fig. 7.2).
9. Remove the needle and apply direct pressure with the gauze pad.
10. Proceed with the skin procedure only after complete anesthesia is ensured in the target area.

AFTERCARE

- None needed.

A video showing a direct local anesthetic injection can be found in the companion eBook.

REFERENCES

1. Tetzlaff JE. The pharmacology of local anesthetics. *Anesthesiol Clin North Am.* 2000;18:217-233.
2. Charalambides M, Yannoulias B, Gnanappiragasam D, Veitch D, Wernham A. Local anaesthetics in dermatological surgery: a review of adjuncts and pain reduction techniques. *Clin Exp Dermatol.* 2022;47(10):1781-1793.
3. Hogan ME, vanderVaart S, Perampaladas K, Machado M, Einarson TR, Taddio A. Systematic review and meta-analysis of the effect of warming local anesthetics on injection pain. *Emerg Med.* 2011;58(1):86-98.
4. Hamelin ND, St-Amand H, Lalonde DH, Harris PG, Brutus JP. Decreasing the pain of finger block injection: level II evidence. *Hand (N Y).* 2013;8:67-70.

5. Bancroft JW, Benenati JF, Becker GJ, Katzen BT, Zemel G. Neutralized lidocaine: use in pain reduction in local anesthesia. *J Vasc Interv Radiol.* 1992;3(1):107-109.
6. Masters JE. Randomised control trial of pH buffered lignocaine with adrenaline in outpatient operations. *Br J Plast Surg.* 1998;51(5):385-387.
7. Hanna MN, Elhassan A, Veloso PM, et al. Efficacy of bicarbonate in decreasing pain on intradermal injection of local anesthetics: a meta-analysis. *Reg Anesth Pain Med.* 2009;34(2):122-125.
8. Davies RJ. Buffering the pain of local anaesthetics: a systematic review. *Emerg Med (Fremantle).* 2003;15(1):81-88.

Field Block Injection

The injection of local anesthetic into skin around an area of a planned surgical procedure is termed a field block. This procedure is a useful method to provide anesthesia to a larger area than that achieved with a direct local injection. It is commonly used to provide anesthesia immediately prior to surgical excision of a skin lesion. It is also used when direct injection into or distortion of the surgical site is not desired. Use of a field block allows the use of a smaller volume of anesthetic to affect a larger area. In this procedure, the local anesthetic is injected into the dermis circumferentially around the surgical site using only two points of needle entry. Infiltration of the anesthetic creates a diamond-shaped "virtual fence" that prevents the nerve impulses from leaving the targeted field of skin. For the reasons noted in "Direct Local Injection," 1% lidocaine with epinephrine (optionally buffered with sodium bicarbonate) is the anesthetic choice for this skin procedure. If anesthesia is required for more than 60 minutes, bupivacaine 0.25% with or without epinephrine used alone or mixed with lidocaine may be considered.

Instead of inserting the needle oriented perpendicularly to the skin, this procedure is performed in a horizontal plane to the skin surface. The operator identifies the area of excision that requires anesthesia, which includes the lesion and surrounding surgical margins. Excisions are usually performed using a fusiform shape. The insertion sites of the needle are located just beyond the corners of the fusiform outline. A longer needle (usually a 1-in 30-gauge needle for use on the face or a 2-in 25-gauge needle for other areas) is inserted into the skin and advanced within the dermis (without injection) to a point that is outside of the margin of the excision and just past the midpoint of the lesion. The local anesthetic solution is then injected into the dermis as the needle is slowly withdrawn. Before the needle is removed from the skin, the tip is redirected and advanced to the opposite side of the planned excision. After the local anesthetic is injected, the needle is withdrawn and the process repeated on the other side of the lesion.

PATIENT POSITION

- Any, but generally recumbent on the examination/procedure table with the area of concern presented to the clinician.

ANESTHESIA

- Use topical vapocoolant spray or create manual skin distraction (see below).

EQUIPMENT

- Topical vapocoolant spray
- 5-mL or 10-mL syringe
- 1-in 30-gauge needle for face or a 2-in 25-gauge needle for other areas

- 1% lidocaine with epinephrine
- 8.4% sodium bicarbonate (optional, but recommended)
- Alcohol prep pad(s)
- Sterile gauze pads

TECHNIQUE

1. Draw up 5 to 10 mL of 1% lidocaine/epinephrine in a 5-mL or 10-mL syringe.
2. If desired, mix a nine part volume of 1% lidocaine/epinephrine with one part volume of 8.4% sodium bicarbonate within the syringe.
3. Identify the needle insertion sites located just beyond the points of the fusiform outline (Fig. 7.3).
4. Prep the insertion sites with the alcohol pad(s).
5. Use topical vapocoolant spray or create manual skin distraction by lightly scratching or inducing vibrations in the skin around the injection site to achieve transient local anesthesia.
6. Using the no-touch technique, quickly insert a long needle (usually a 1-in 30-gauge needle for use on the face or a 2-in 25-gauge needle for other areas), oriented in a horizontal plane, through the skin using a single, rapid needle stick.
7. Advance the long needle within the dermis (without injection) to a point that is outside of the margin of the excision and just past the midpoint of the lesion. The location of the needle tip can usually be observed as it is advanced.
8. The local anesthetic is injected and infused into the dermis as the needle is slowly withdrawn. The intradermal injection produces a linear wheal along the needle tract (Fig. 7.4).
9. Before the needle is removed from the skin, the tip is redirected and advanced to the opposite side of the width of the excision.
10. After the local anesthetic is injected, the needle is withdrawn completely and the process repeated on the other side of the lesion.
11. After the intradermal anesthetic infusion has been completed, remove the needle and apply direct pressure with the gauze pad.
12. Proceed with the skin procedure only after complete anesthesia is ensured in the target area.

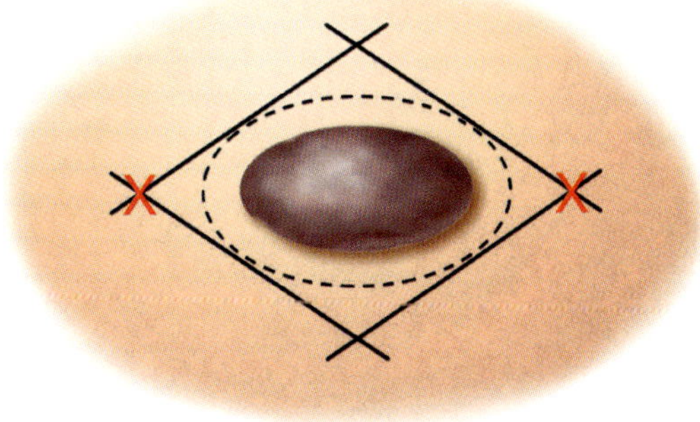

FIGURE 7.3 • Location for field-block local anesthesia injection.

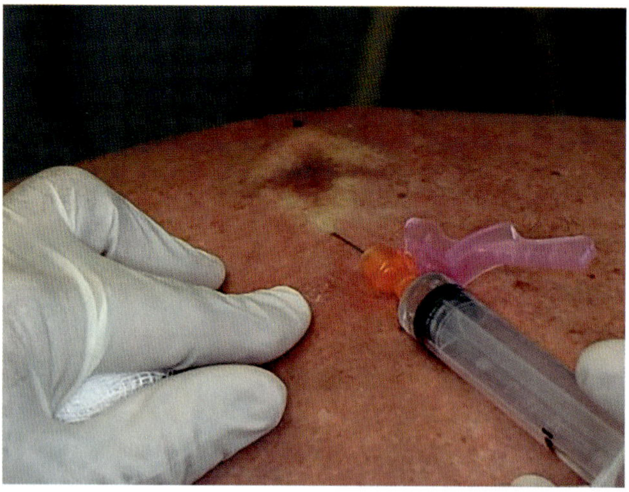

FIGURE 7.4 ● Field block.

AFTERCARE

- None needed.

A video showing a field-block injection can be found in the companion eBook.

Digital Nerve Block

Injection of local anesthetic around the digital nerves is a useful procedure to provide anesthesia of the thumbs, fingers, and toes so that surgical procedures may be conducted on those digits. The addition of epinephrine in the local anesthetic is desirable to extend the time of action of the anesthetic and to decrease bleeding in the operative field. For many years, conventional teaching was that epinephrine should be avoided in acral areas that contain end arterioles, such as fingers, toes, penis, tip of nose, and earlobes, or skin flaps with marginal viability. However, there is now a large body of evidence that withholding epinephrine in patients with normal vascular flow is not necessary and is in fact a "medical myth."

The idea that epinephrine should never be injected into fingers originated between 1920 and 1940, when procaine was used with and without epinephrine, with resulting reports of finger necrosis. Nearly all of the 48 reported cases of finger necrosis attributable to procaine local anesthesia occurred before 1950, with most implicating procaine injected without epinephrine.[1] Procaine is very acidic, with a pH of 3.6, and it further acidifies to a pH as low as 1 with prolonged storage. This acidity, not the addition of epinephrine, is likely responsible for the historical reports of finger necrosis.[2]

An extensive review of the literature from 1880 to 2000, a prospective series in 3,110 patients[3] retrospective reviews of 1,111 cases[4] and 1,334 cases,[5] as well as another review of 4,953 cases involving surgery of the nose, ears, extensive flaps, and skin grafts,[6] have definitively documented that it is safe to use lidocaine with epinephrine in acral areas and digits. Remarkably, there were no instances of vascular complications associated with the use of epinephrine reported in any of these published articles. Ultimately, the decision whether or not to use lidocaine with epinephrine rests with the medical provider. This may be particularly important in patients with medical conditions that may lead to vascular compromise, including Raynaud phenomenon, connective tissue disease, advanced diabetes, peripheral vascular disease, and Buerger disease (thromboangiitis obliterans).

The thumbs, fingers, and toes are innervated by two sets of nerves that course through the medial and lateral aspect of each digit. There are pairs of dorsal and palmar/plantar nerves. Each nerve is associated with a corresponding artery. The objective of a digital nerve block is to bathe each of the four nerves in local anesthetic with epinephrine to achieve operative anesthesia while avoiding injury to the vascular structures and digit. Traditionally this procedure has been performed utilizing a two-injection dorsal technique and more recently a web space two-injection technique. However, there is a growing body of evidence that demonstrates preference, and at least equivalent efficacy, for a single-injection technique into the volar subcutaneous tissues at the proximal digit.[7-11]

Lidocaine (1%) with epinephrine has a similar onset of action but is significantly less painful and has a shorter duration of action than bupivacaine (0.5%).[12-14] Therefore, the current preferred method to perform a digital nerve block is a single injection of

2 mL of 1% lidocaine with epinephrine (1:100,000) into the volar subcutaneous tissue at the proximal digit to create a firm, turgid feel to the tissue. This technique is referred to as the SIMPLE block (Single, subcutaneous, Injection, at the Middle, of the Proximal phalanx, using Lidocaine, with Epinephrine).[8]

Relevant Anatomy: (Fig. 7.5)

PATIENT POSITION

- Recumbent on the examination/procedure table with the hand or foot extended to the clinician.

ANESTHESIA

- Use topical vapocoolant spray or create manual skin distraction (see below).

EQUIPMENT

- Topical vapocoolant spray
- 3-mL syringe
- 30-gauge ½-in needle
- 2 mL of 1% lidocaine with epinephrine
- One alcohol prep pad
- Sterile gauze pads

TECHNIQUE

1. Locate the needle insertion site over the palmar/plantar crease at the junction of the digit and the palm or sole of the foot.[4]
2. Prep the insertion site with the alcohol pad.

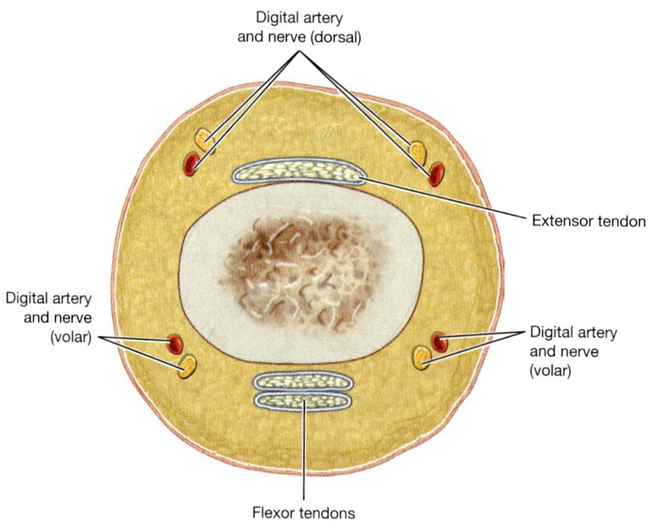

FIGURE 7.5 ● Digital anatomy.

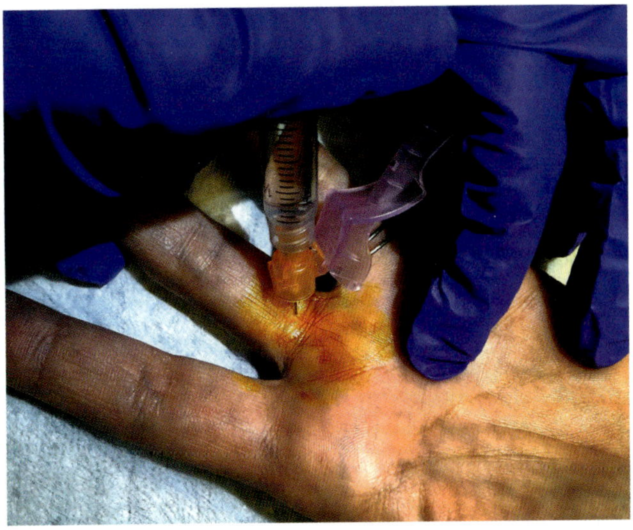

FIGURE 7.6 • Digital nerve block.

3. Use topical vapocoolant spray or create manual skin distraction by lightly scratching or inducing vibrations in the skin around the injection site to achieve transient local anesthesia.[11]
4. Using the no-touch technique, insert the 30-gauge ½-in needle perpendicularly through the skin using a single, quick needle stick. Advance the needle in a few millimeters through the skin into the subcutaneous tissue (Fig. 7.6).
5. Withdraw the plunger of the syringe to ensure that there is no blood return.
6. Inject 2 mL of lidocaine with epinephrine as a bolus in the subcutaneous tissue.
7. Remove the needle and apply direct pressure with a gauze pad—spreading the local anesthetic up to the digital nerves.
8. Allow at least 5 to 10 minutes for the anesthesia to take effect.
9. Repeat the procedure if necessary.
10. Proceed with the procedure only after complete anesthesia is ensured in the digit.

AFTERCARE

- None needed.

REFERENCES

1. Denkler K. A comprehensive review of epinephrine in the finger: to do or not to do. *Plast Reconstr Surg.* 2001;108(1):114-124.
2. Thomson CJ, Lalonde DH, Denkler KA, Feicht AJ. A critical look at the evidence for and against elective epinephrine use in the finger. *Plast Reconstr Surg*. 2007;119(1):260-266.
3. Lalonde D, Bell M, Benoit P, Sparkes G, Denkler K, Chang P. A multicenter prospective study of 3,110 consecutive cases of elective epinephrine use in the fingers and hand: the Dalhousie Project clinical phase. *J Hand Surg Am.* 2005;30(5):1061-1067.
4. Chowdhry S, Seidenstricker L, Cooney DS, Hazani R, Wilhelmi BJ. Do not use epinephrine in digital blocks: myth or truth? Part II. A retrospective review of 1111 cases. *Plast Reconstr Surg.* 2010;126(6):2031-2034.
5. Chapeskie H, Juliao A, Payne S, Koichopolos J. Evaluation of the safety of epinephrine in digital nerve blockade: retrospective case series analysis of 1334 toe surgeries. *Can Fam Physician.* 2016;62(6):e334-e339.
6. Häfner HM, Röcken M, Breuninger H. Epinephrine-supplemented local anesthetics for ear and nose surgery: clinical use without complications in more than 10,000 surgical procedures. *J Dtsch Dermatol Ges.* 2005;3(3):195-199.

7. Hung VS, Bodavula VK, Dubin NH. Digital anaesthesia: comparison of the efficacy and pain associated with three digital nerve block techniques. *J Hand Surg Br.* 2005;30(6):581-584.
8. Williams JG, Lalonde DH. Randomized comparison of the single-injection volar subcutaneous block and the two-injection dorsal block for digital anesthesia. *Plast Reconstr Surg.* 2006;118(5):1195-1200.
9. Bashir MM, Khan FA, Afzal S, Khan BA. Comparison of traditional two injections dorsal digital block with volar block. *J Coll Physicians Surg Pak.* 2008;18(12):768-770.
10. Tzeng YS, Chen SG. Tumescent technique in digits: a subcutaneous single-injection digital block. *Am J Emerg Med.* 2012;30(4):592-596.
11. Martin SP, Chu KH, Mahmoud I, Greenslade JH, Brown AF. Double-dorsal versus single-volar digital subcutaneous anaesthetic injection for finger injuries in the emergency department: a randomised controlled trial. *Emerg Med Australas.* 2016;28(2):193-198.
12. Schnabl SM, Unglaub F, Leitz Z, Breuninger H, Häfner HM. Skin perfusion and pain evaluation with different local anaesthetics in a double blind randomized study following digital nerve block anaesthesia. *Clin Hemorheol Microcirc.* 2013;55(2):241-253.
13. Alhelail M, Al-Salamah M, Al-Mulhim M, Al-Hamid S. Comparison of bupivacaine and lidocaine with epinephrine for digital nerve blocks. *Emerg Med J.* 2009;26(5):347-350.
14. Thomson CJ, Lalonde DH. Randomized double-blind comparison of duration of anesthesia among three commonly used agents in digital nerve block. *Plast Reconstr Surg.* 2006;118(2):429-432.

Facial Nerve Blocks

Facial nerve blocks are utilized to achieve anesthesia of various regions of the face. The technique is used when direct injection into the surgical field or distortion of the surgical site is not desired. In this case, a small volume of the local anesthetic is injected around the specific nerve that innervates a defined area of skin. Therefore, a small volume affects a much larger area than would otherwise be possible using local injections. This decreases excessive pain and bruising associated with multiple injections. It also reduces the total amount of local anesthetic required, thus minimizing the potential for medication toxicity. There are three classic nerve blocks that are commonly performed to provide anesthesia to most of the face. These are the supraorbital/supratrochlear, infraorbital, and mental nerve blocks. Each of these nerves is a terminal sensory branch of the fifth cranial nerve, and each has its own discrete foramen to exit the bony structures. Once the foramen is located, a small amount of anesthetic (0.5-1 mL) can be injected at that site to provide the desired effect. As shown in Figure 7.7, all of the three facial foramina are located along a line drawn in a vertical (sagittal) orientation from the center of the patient's pupil.

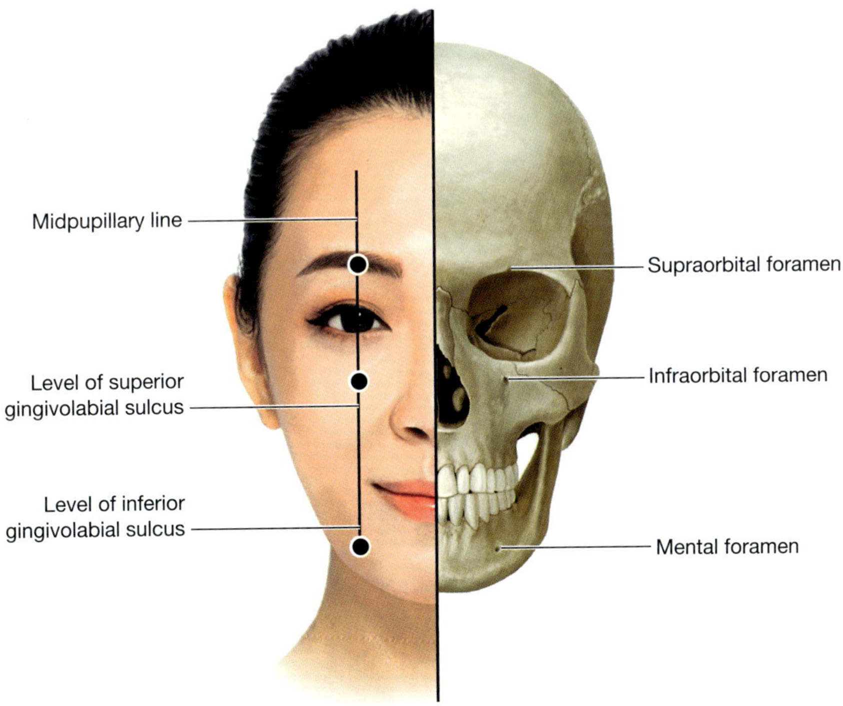

FIGURE 7.7 ● Foramina for nerve blocks.

The supraorbital foramen is the easiest to identify. It is located superior to the center of the pupil and palpated as a subtle depression in the supraorbital ridge underneath the eyebrow. The supratrochlear nerve is commonly injected along with the supraorbital nerve to extend the anesthetic effect to the midline of the forehead. This nerve is located at the supraorbital ridge immediately superior to the inner canthus of the eye. In most people, this is located at the medial aspect of the eyebrow.

The infraorbital foramen may be found in the maxilla about 1.5 cm inferior to the infraorbital rim—and in line with the pupil. A depression in the maxilla cannot be palpated.

Finally, the mental nerve is located along the same line drawn in a vertical (sagittal) orientation from the center of the patient's pupil. It is positioned at the midpoint of the height of the mandible. A discrete depression is also not palpable.

To confirm the correct location, firm palpation directly over each of the foramen elicits a sensation of intense, dull pain, not found in adjacent areas. From a coding standpoint, all injections to establish local anesthesia for a surgical procedure are considered part of that procedure. As such, they are included in the Current Procedural Terminology procedural code and not billed separately.

Supraorbital and Supratrochlear Nerve Blocks

The supraorbital and supratrochlear nerves are perhaps the easiest of the facial nerve blocks to perform. These nerves are terminal sensory branches of the ophthalmic trunk of the fifth cranial nerve. The blocks are used to administer reversible local anesthesia to the forehead and anterior scalp. Various procedures including laceration repair, skin lesion removal, photodynamic therapy, or laser facial skin resurfacing of the forehead may be performed utilizing these blocks. Headache disorders including cluster, tension, and migraine headaches may also be treated in part by performing these blocks.[1-3]

Relevant Anatomy: (Fig. 7.8)

PATIENT POSITION

- With the patient supine on the examination table and the patient's head rotated toward the clinician, the clinician stands lateral to the side of the face that is being injected.

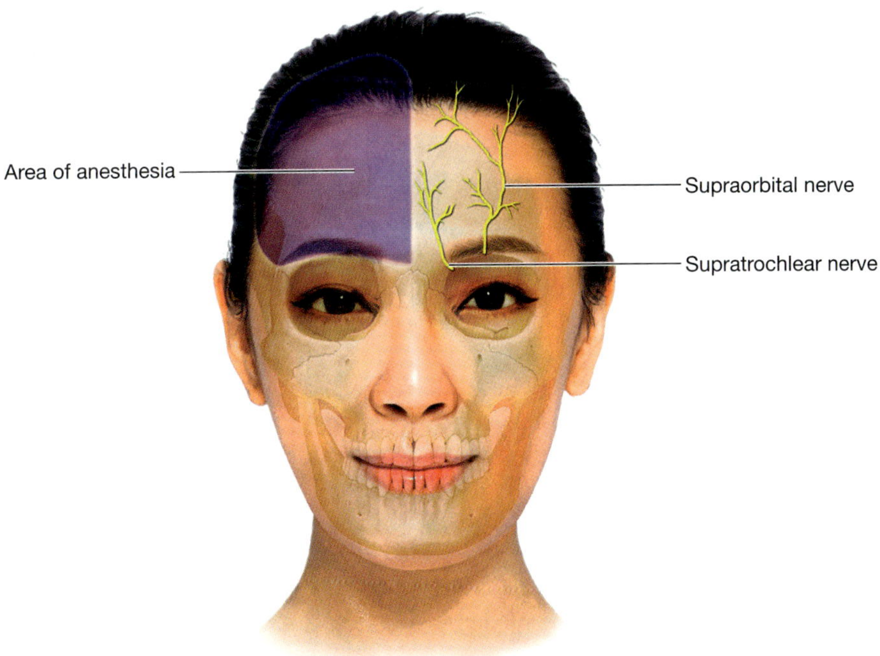

FIGURE 7.8 ● Supraorbital and supratrochlear nerves and innervated areas.

LANDMARKS

1. The supraorbital foramen is located superior (sagittal) to the center of the pupil and is palpated as a subtle depression in the supraorbital ridge underneath the eyebrow.
2. In an anatomic study of skulls, supraorbital foramina were found to be approximately 25 mm lateral to the midline, 30 mm medial to the temporal crest of the frontal bone, and 2 to 3 mm superior to the supraorbital rim. Additional exits for branches of the supraorbital nerve were present in 14% of skulls.[4]
3. The supratrochlear nerve is located at the supraorbital ridge superior (sagittal) to the inner canthus of the eye. In most people, this is located at the medial aspect of the eyebrow.
4. At sites located immediately superior to the eyebrow over each nerve location, press firmly on the skin with the retracted tip of a ballpoint pen. This indention represents the entry point(s) for the needle.

ANESTHESIA

- Preinjection use of topical vapocoolant sprayed directly over the injection site is contraindicated due to the close proximity to the eyes. However, PainEase mist may be applied indirectly over the point of injection (see below).
- Alternatively, skin distraction techniques may be employed by lightly scratching or inducing vibrations in the skin around the injection site.

EQUIPMENT

- Topical vapocoolant spray
- 3-mL syringe
- 30-gauge ½-in needle
- 1 mL of 1% lidocaine with or without epinephrine
- One alcohol prep pad
- Sterile gauze pad

TECHNIQUE

1. Prep the insertion site with the alcohol pad.
2. Firmly place the tip of the nondominant hand index finger over the edge of the orbital rim just below the location of the supraorbital foramen. This helps to prevent accidental passage of the needle below the rim and keeps the anesthetic up in proper position around the nerve.
3. Position the needle at a 90° angle to the skin just above the eyebrow with the tip of the needle directed toward the supraorbital foramen.
4. Consider preinjection skin anesthesia by spraying PainEase mist onto a sterile cotton swab until saturated. Then, apply the swab over the point of injection. Alternatively, skin distraction techniques may be employed by lightly scratching or inducing vibrations in the skin around the injection site.
5. Using the no-touch technique, quickly introduce the needle at the insertion site.
6. Advance the needle directly over the supraorbital foramen, touch the bone, and withdraw about 1 mm.
7. Withdraw the plunger of the syringe to ensure that there is no blood return.

8. Inject 1/2 to 1 mL of 1% lidocaine with or without epinephrine directly over the supraorbital foramen (depending on anticipated procedure time).
9. Following injection, withdraw the needle.
10. Repeat the process for the supratrochlear nerve with the needle positioned over the supraorbital ridge immediately superior to the inner canthus of the eye.
11. Proceed with the skin procedure only after complete anesthesia is ensured in the target area.

AFTERCARE

- None needed.

A video showing supraorbital/supratrochlear nerve block injections can be found in the companion eBook.

REFERENCES

1. Blumenfeld A, Ashkenazi A, Napchan U, et al. Expert consensus recommendations for the performance of peripheral nerve blocks for headaches—a narrative review. *Headache.* 2013;53(3):437-446.
2. Ilhan Alp S, Alp R. Supraorbital and infraorbital nerve blockade in migraine patients: results of 6-month clinical follow-up. *Eur Rev Med Pharmacol Sci.* 2013;17(13):1778-1781.
3. Wahab S, Kataria S, Woolley P, et al. Literature review: pericranial nerve blocks for chronic migraines. *Health Psychol Res.* 2023;11:74259.
4. Gupta T. Localization of important facial foramina encountered in maxillo-facial surgery. *Clin Anat.* 2008;21(7):633-640.

Infraorbital Nerve Block

The infraorbital nerve is a terminal sensory branch of the maxillary trunk of the fifth cranial nerve. This block is used to administer reversible local anesthesia to the medial midface excluding the central nose. Various procedures including skin and upper lip laceration repair, photodynamic therapy, laser facial skin resurfacing of the midface/upper lip, skin and upper lip filler placement, or skin lesion removal may be performed following this block.

Relevant Anatomy: (Fig. 7.9)

PATIENT POSITION

- With the patient supine on the examination table and the patient's head rotated toward the clinician, the clinician stands lateral to the side of the face that is being injected.

LANDMARKS

1. In an anatomic study of skulls, infraorbital foramina were found to be 28.5 mm lateral to the midline and approximately 7 mm inferior to the inferior orbital rim and along

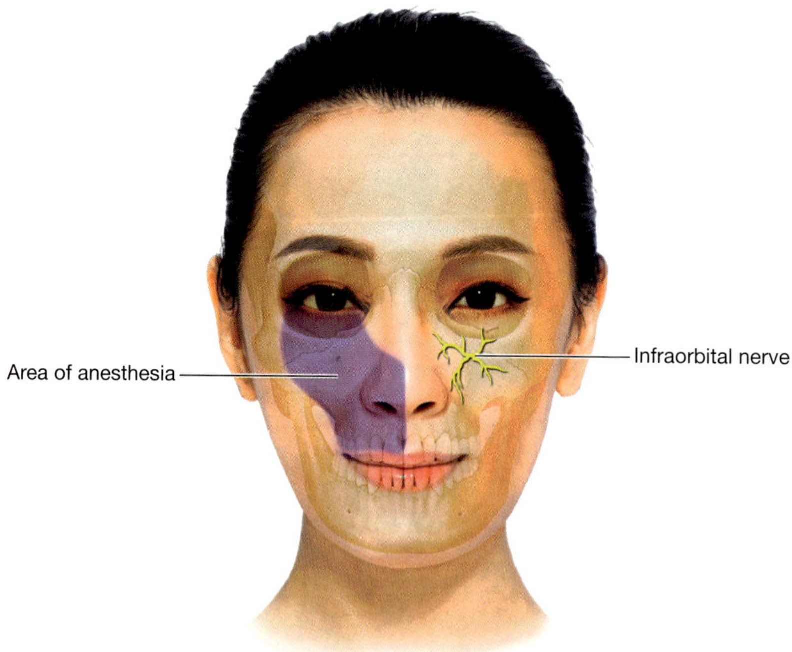

FIGURE 7.9 ● Infraorbital nerve and innervated area.

a line drawn in a vertical (sagittal) orientation from the center of the patient's pupil.[1] A depression in the maxilla at the site of the foramen is not palpable. To confirm the location, firm pressure directly over the foramen elicits the sensation of intense, dull pain, not found in adjacent areas.
2. At that site, press firmly on the skin with the retracted tip of a ballpoint pen. This indentation represents the entry point for the needle when using the transdermal approach.

ANESTHESIA

- Preinjection use of topical vapocoolant sprayed directly over the injection site is contraindicated due to the close proximity to the eyes. However, PainEase mist may be applied indirectly over the point of injection (see below).
- Alternatively, skin distraction techniques may be employed by lightly scratching or inducing vibrations in the skin around the injection site.

EQUIPMENT

- Headlamp or other light source (for intraoral approach)
- Topical vapocoolant spray (optional)
- 3-mL syringe
- 30-gauge ½-in needle for transdermal approach or a 25-gauge 1½-in needle for intraoral approach
- 1 mL of 1% lidocaine with or without epinephrine (depending on anticipated procedure time)
- One alcohol prep pad (for transdermal approach)
- Sterile gauze pad

TECHNIQUE (TRANSDERMAL)

1. Prep the insertion site with the alcohol pad.
2. Position the needle perpendicularly to the skin at the location over the maxilla identified above. The tip of the needle is directed toward the infraorbital foramen.
3. Consider preinjection skin anesthesia by spraying PainEase mist onto a sterile cotton swab until saturated. Then, apply the swab over the point of injection. Alternatively, skin distraction techniques may be employed by lightly scratching or inducing vibrations in the skin around the injection site.
4. Using the no-touch technique, quickly introduce the needle at the insertion site.
5. Advance the needle over the infraorbital foramen, touch the bone, and withdraw about 1 mm.
6. Withdraw the plunger of the syringe to ensure that there is no blood return.
7. Inject 1/2 to 1 mL of 1% lidocaine with or without epinephrine directly over the infraorbital foramen.
8. Following injection, withdraw the needle.
9. Proceed with the skin procedure only after complete anesthesia is ensured in the target area.

TECHNIQUE (INTRAORAL)

1. Patient position is the same as described above, but with the patient's neck extended in order to tilt the head back.
2. Use a headlamp or other light source to provide good illumination for the procedure.
3. Grasp the upper lip with gauze and elevate it superiorly.
4. Identify the maxillary third to fourth tooth from midline (canine/first premolar). The infraorbital foramen is located just superior to the apex of the gingivolabial mucosal reflection between these teeth.
5. A 1½-in 25-gauge needle is positioned in the sagittal plane, directed toward the ipsilateral pupil.
6. The needle is quickly inserted at this point and advanced approximately 1 cm to a position over the infraorbital foramen.
7. Withdraw the plunger of the syringe to ensure that there is no blood return.
8. Inject 1/2 to 1 mL of 1% lidocaine with or without epinephrine directly over the infraorbital foramen.
9. Following injection, withdraw the needle.
10. Proceed with the skin procedure only after complete anesthesia is ensured in the target area.

AFTERCARE

- None needed.

REFERENCE

1. Gupta T. Localization of important facial foramina encountered in maxillo-facial surgery. *Clin Anat.* 2008;21(7):633-640.

External Nasal Nerve Block

Infraorbital nerve blocks provide reversible anesthesia to the lateral nasal skin but not to the central portion of the nose. Blocks of the external nasal nerves supplement nasal anesthesia by providing anesthesia of the skin over the cartilaginous nasal dorsum and the tip of the nose.

The external nasal nerve is a terminal sensory branch of the anterior ethmoidal nerve from the trunk of the fifth cranial nerve. It emerges 5 to 10 mm lateral to the nasal midline at the osseous junction of the distal edge of the nasal bones.

Various procedures including skin laceration repair, photodynamic therapy, laser facial skin resurfacing of the nose, or skin lesion removal may be performed following this block.

Relevant Anatomy: (Fig. 7.10)

PATIENT POSITION

- With the patient supine on the examination table and the patient's head rotated toward the clinician, the clinician stands lateral to the side of the face that is being injected.

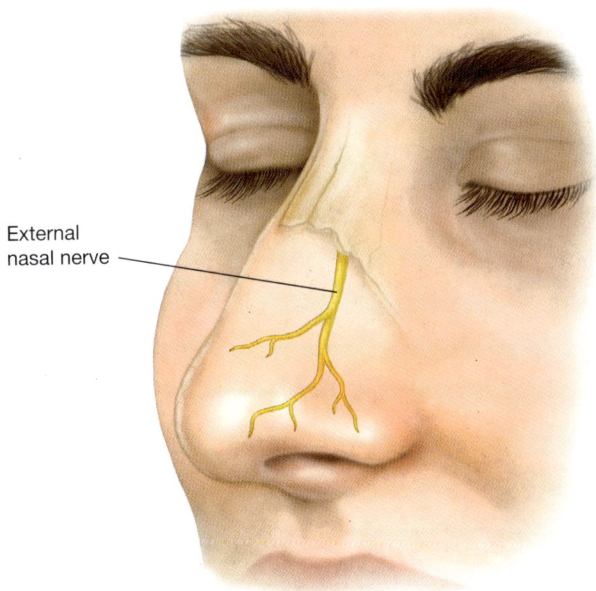

FIGURE 7.10 ● External nasal nerve and innervated area.

LANDMARKS

1. Palpate the distal rim of the nasal bone at the osseous cartilaginous junction. Select and mark an injection site 7.5 mm lateral to the midline.[1]
2. At that site, press firmly on the skin with the retracted tip of a ballpoint pen. This indentation represents the entry point for the needle.

ANESTHESIA

- Preinjection use of topical vapocoolant sprayed directly over the injection site is contraindicated due to the close proximity to the eyes. However, PainEase mist may be applied indirectly over the point of injection (see below).
- Alternatively, skin distraction techniques may be employed by lightly scratching or inducing vibrations in the skin around the injection site.

EQUIPMENT

- Topical vapocoolant spray
- 3-mL syringe
- 30-gauge ½-in needle
- 1 mL of 1% lidocaine with or without epinephrine (depending on anticipated procedure time)
- One alcohol prep pad
- Sterile gauze pad

TECHNIQUE

1. Prep the insertion site with the alcohol pad.
2. Position the needle perpendicularly to the skin over the lateral nose at the osseous cartilaginous junction as identified above.
3. Consider preinjection skin anesthesia by spraying PainEase mist onto a sterile cotton swab until saturated. Then, apply the swab over the point of injection. Alternatively, skin distraction techniques may be employed by lightly scratching or inducing vibrations in the skin around the injection site.
4. Using the no-touch technique, quickly introduce the needle at the insertion site.
5. Advance the needle only into the deep dermis. (When attempting to advance the needle into the subcutaneous tissue, it is very easy to advance the needle too far and enter the nasal cavity.)
6. Withdraw the plunger of the syringe to ensure that there is no blood return.
7. Slowly inject 1/2 to 1 mL of 1% lidocaine with or without epinephrine into the tissue.
8. Following injection, withdraw the needle.
9. Proceed with the skin procedure only after complete anesthesia is ensured in the target area.

AFTERCARE

- None needed.

REFERENCE

1. Moskovitz JB, Sabatino F. Regional nerve blocks of the face. *Emerg Med Clin North Am.* 2013;31(2):517-527.

Mental Nerve Block

The mental nerve is a terminal sensory branch of the mandibular trunk of the fifth cranial nerve. This block is used to administer reversible local anesthesia to the lower mid-face. Various procedures including skin and lower lip laceration repair, photodynamic therapy, laser facial skin resurfacing of the midface/lower lip, skin and lower lip filler placement, or skin lesion removal may be performed following this block.

Relevant Anatomy: (Fig. 7.11)

PATIENT POSITION

- With the patient supine on the examination table and the patient's head rotated toward the clinician, the clinician stands lateral to the side of the face that is being injected.

LANDMARKS

1. In an anatomic study of skulls, mental foramina were on average, 25.8 mm lateral to the midline and about 13 mm superior to the inferior mandibular margin and along a

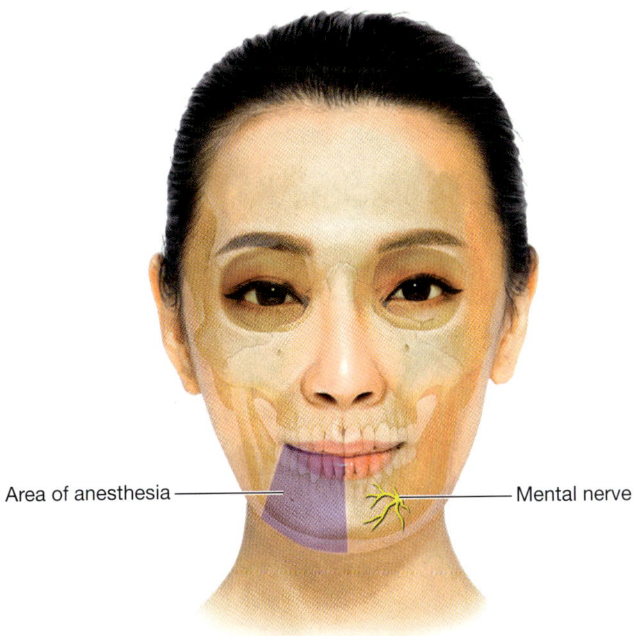

FIGURE 7.11 ● Mental nerve and innervated area.

line drawn in a vertical (sagittal) orientation from the center of the patient's pupil.[1] A depression in the mandible at the site of the foramen is difficult to palpate. To confirm the location, firm pressure directly over the foramen elicits the sensation of intense, dull pain, not found in adjacent areas.
2. At that site, press firmly on the skin with the retracted tip of a ballpoint pen. This indentation represents the entry point for the needle when using the transdermal approach.

ANESTHESIA

- Use topical vapocoolant spray or create manual skin distraction (see below).

EQUIPMENT

- Headlamp or other light source (for intraoral approach)
- 3-mL syringe
- 30-gauge ½-in needle for transdermal approach or a 25-gauge 1½-in needle for intraoral approach
- 1 mL of 1% lidocaine with or without epinephrine (depending on anticipated procedure time)
- One alcohol prep pad (for transdermal approach)
- Sterile gauze pad

TECHNIQUE (TRANSDERMAL)

1. Prep the insertion site with the alcohol pad.
2. Position the needle perpendicularly to the skin at the location over the mandible identified above. The tip of the needle is directed toward the mental foramen.
3. Use topical vapocoolant spray or create manual skin distraction by lightly scratching or inducing vibrations in the skin around the injection site to achieve transient local anesthesia.
4. Using the no-touch technique, quickly introduce the needle at the insertion site.
5. Advance the needle over the mental foramen, touch the bone, and withdraw about 1 mm.
6. Withdraw the plunger of the syringe to ensure that there is no blood return.
7. Inject 1/2 to 1 mL of 1% lidocaine with or without epinephrine directly over the mental foramen.
8. Following injection, withdraw the needle.
9. Proceed with the skin procedure only after complete anesthesia is ensured in the target area.

TECHNIQUE (INTRAORAL)

1. Use a headlamp or other light source to provide good illumination for the procedure.
2. Grasp the lower lip with gauze and retract it inferiorly.
3. Identify the mandibular third to fourth tooth from midline (canine/first premolar). The infraorbital foramen is located just inferior to the apex of the gingivolabial mucosal reflection between these teeth.

4. A 1½-in 25-gauge needle is positioned in the sagittal plane, directed inferiorly toward the mental foramen.
5. The needle is quickly inserted at this point and advanced approximately 0.5 cm to a position over the mental foramen.
6. Withdraw the plunger of the syringe to ensure that there is no blood return.
7. Inject 1/2 to 1 mL of 1% lidocaine with or without epinephrine directly over the mental foramen.
8. Following injection, withdraw the needle.
9. Proceed with the skin procedure only after complete anesthesia is ensured in the target area.

AFTERCARE

- None needed.

REFERENCE

1. Gupta T. Localization of important facial foramina encountered in maxillo-facial surgery. *Clin Anat.* 2008;21(7):633-640.

External Ear Nerve Block

The external ear has complex innervation with four nerves contributing to sensory input. As illustrated in Figure 7.12A, the auriculotemporal nerve innervates the superior aspect of the external ear, the lesser occipital nerve is responsible for the mid-posterior external ear, and the great auricular nerve innervates the inferior aspect of the ear. Importantly, the auricular branch of the vagus nerve provides sensory input for the external ear canal and the cavum concha of the external ear.

The injection of local anesthetic into skin around the external ear is traditionally termed a ring nerve block—illustrated in Figure 7.12B. This technique allows a small volume of anesthetic to affect a larger area. In this case, the points of needle entry are located immediately superior and inferior to the ear. Intradermal infiltration of the anesthetic creates a diamond-shaped "virtual fence" of anesthesia circumferentially around the ear. The local anesthetic of choice for this procedure is 1% lidocaine with epinephrine (optionally buffered with sodium bicarbonate).

If the external ear canal or the cavum concha of the external ear will be involved in the surgical procedure, then direct local injection into the affected area will be required to provide supplementary anesthesia to the skin innervated by the auricular branch of the vagus nerve.

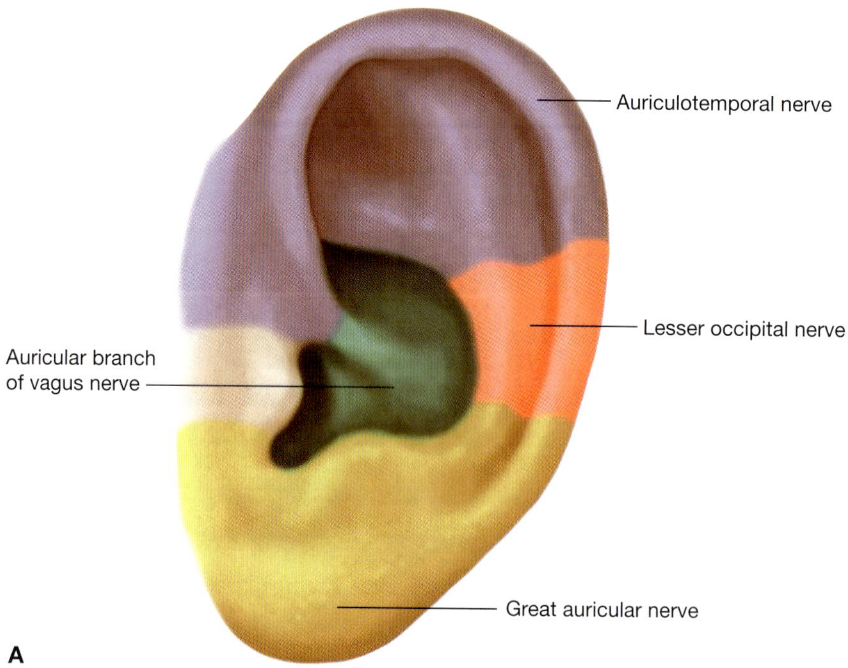

FIGURE 7.12 **A.** The auriculotemporal nerve innervates the superior aspect of the external ear, the lesser occipital nerve is responsible for the mid-posterior external ear, the great auricular nerve innervates the inferior aspect of the ear, and the auricular branch of the vagus nerve innervates the cavum concha.

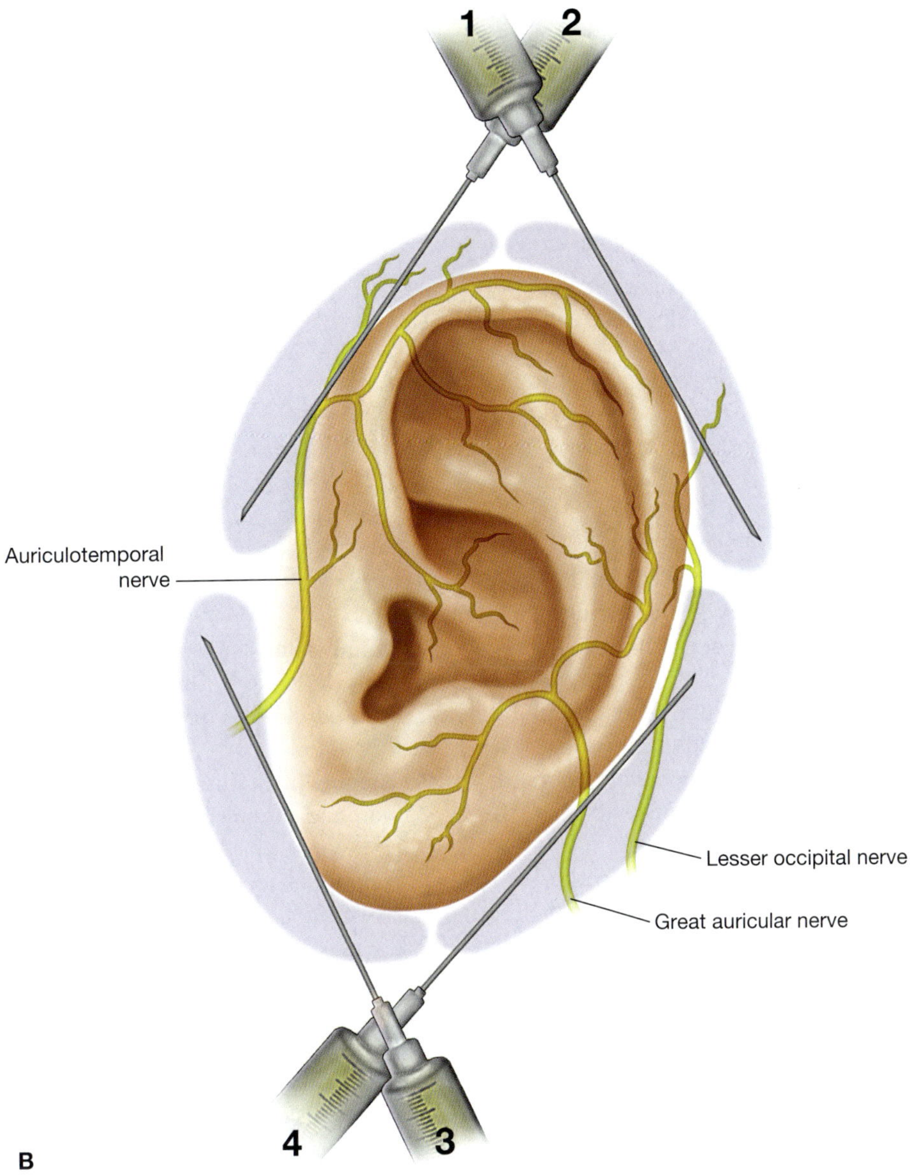

FIGURE 7.12 • (*Continued*) **B.** Identify the needle insertion sites located immediately superior and also just inferior to the external ear.

The literature demonstrates that ultrasound can help localize the great auricular nerve and the lesser occipital nerve for anesthetic blockade.[1]

The most common procedures for this type of anesthetic block involve ear laceration repair, hematoma evacuation, foreign body removal, and ear skin lesion excision/removal.

Relevant Anatomy: (Fig. 7.12A and B)

PATIENT POSITION

- Supine on the examination table with the head of the bed slightly elevated.

ANESTHESIA

- Use topical vapocoolant spray or create manual skin distraction (see below) to decrease the pain associated with injection.

EQUIPMENT

- Topical vapocoolant spray
- 10-mL syringe
- 1½-in or a 2-in 25-gauge needle
- 5 to 10 mL of 1% lidocaine with epinephrine
- 8.4% sodium bicarbonate
- Alcohol prep pad(s)
- Two povidone-iodine or chlorhexidine prep pads
- Sterile gauze pads

TECHNIQUE

1. Draw up and mix 9 mL of 1% lidocaine/epinephrine with 1 mL of 8.4% sodium bicarbonate (if desired) within the syringe.
2. Identify the needle insertion sites located immediately superior and also just inferior to the external ear (Fig. 7.12B).
3. Prep the insertion site(s) with alcohol followed by the povidone-iodine or chlorhexidine pads.
4. Use topical vapocoolant spray or create manual skin distraction by lightly scratching or inducing vibrations in the skin around the injection site to achieve transient local anesthesia.
5. Start with the superior injection site. Using the no-touch technique, quickly insert a 1½-in or a 2-in 25-gauge needle through the skin with a single, quick needle stick.
6. Advance the long needle in a horizontal plane within the dermis anterior to the ear. The location of the needle tip can be observed as it is advanced.
7. Withdraw the plunger of the syringe to ensure that there is no blood return.
8. The local anesthetic is injected and infused into the dermis as the needle is slowly withdrawn. The intradermal injection produces a wheal along the needle tract.
9. Before the needle is removed from the skin, the tip is redirected and advanced in a horizontal plane within the dermis posterior to the ear.
10. Again, withdraw the plunger of the syringe to ensure that there is no blood return.
11. After the local anesthetic is injected, the needle is withdrawn and the above process repeated at the inferior aspect of the ear.
12. After the intradermal anesthetic infusion has been completed, remove the needle and apply direct pressure to the injection sites with the gauze pad.
13. Proceed with the skin procedure only after complete anesthesia of the ear is ensured in the target area.

AFTERCARE

- None needed.

REFERENCE

1. Kravchik L, Ng M, Hsu NM, VanHoy TB. Peripheral nerve block of the external ear. 2024 Feb 26. *StatPearls [Internet]*. StatPearls Publishing; 2025 Jan-.

Greater Occipital Nerve Block

Patients occasionally present to the primary care office for the treatment of headaches caused by greater occipital neuralgia. The greater occipital nerve, which is composed of C2 sensory fibers, can become entrapped as it passes through the aponeurotic attachments of the trapezius and semispinalis capitis muscles to the occipital bone. Typically, the pain of occipital neuralgia begins in the neck and then spreads to the vertex, ear, frontal area, and even the eyes. The International Classification of Headache Disorders, 3rd edition (https://ichd-3.org/), describes occipital neuralgia as unilateral or bilateral paroxysmal, shooting or stabbing pain in the posterior part of the scalp, in the distribution(s) of the greater, lesser and/or third occipital nerves, sometimes accompanied by diminished sensation or dysesthesia in the affected area and commonly associated with tenderness over the involved nerve(s), and pain is eased temporarily by local anesthetic block of the nerve.[1] The pain of occipital neuralgia may reach the fronto-orbital area through trigeminocervical interneuronal connections in the trigeminal spinal nuclei.

There is an increasing body of evidence that greater occipital nerve block injections are a safe and effective technique to treat headache pain. They have been shown to be an efficacious treatment for migraines, trigeminal neuralgia, hemicrania continua, postlumbar puncture, postconcussive, cluster, and cervicogenic headaches but not medication overuse and chronic tension-type headaches.[2] Suboccipital steroid injections of the greater occipital nerve for the treatment of cluster headaches received a Level A recommendation in the 2016 American Headache Society Evidence-Based Guidelines.[3] In a population of 159 childhood and adolescent patients with disabling headaches of various diagnoses, unilateral injections of the greater occipital nerve were shown to be an effective treatment with rapid onset and with minimal side effects.[4] In a 5-year retrospective study of 562 patients, greater occipital nerve blocks effectively reduced pain in the acute treatment of patients with migraine headaches.[5] Also, in a single-center retrospective study of 190 adult patients with migraine headaches, occipital nerve blocks used as adjunctive therapy showed safety and efficacy measured by the reduction in pain.[6] Furthermore, ultrasound guidance has been demonstrated to increase the effectiveness of the greater occipital nerve injection procedure.[7,8]

Relevant Anatomy: (Fig. 7.13)

PATIENT POSITION

- The patient sitting on an examination stool with neck flexed and leaning forward with the forehead resting on the patient's crossed arms, which are resting on the pull-out foot tray of the examination table. The clinician stands behind the patient and slightly lateral on the side of treatment.

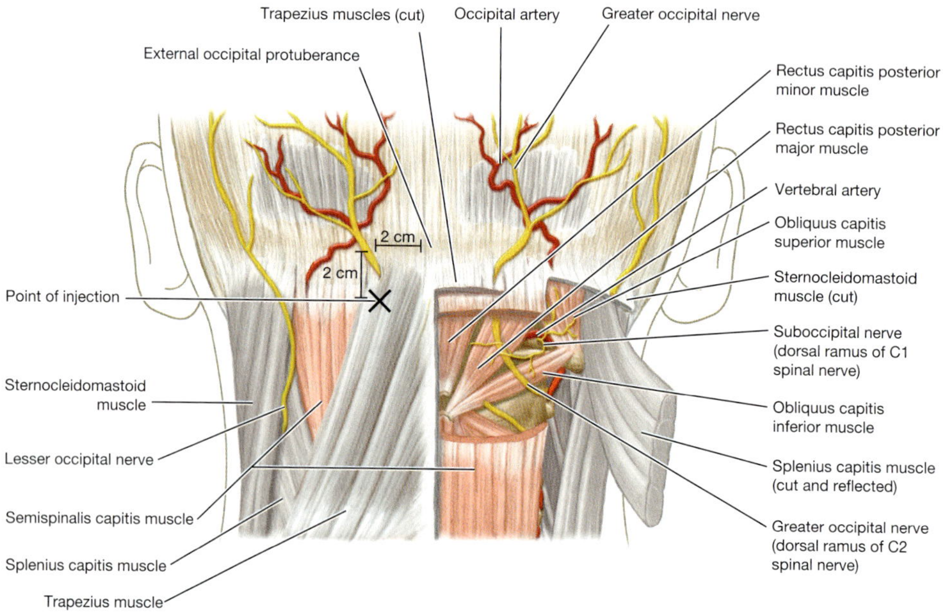

FIGURE 7.13 Suboccipital region. (Modified with permission from Gest TR. *Lippincott® Atlas of Anatomy*. 2nd ed. Wolters Kluwer; 2020.)

LANDMARKS

1. Find the inion (the most prominent projection) of the external occipital protuberance at the midline of the occipital bone.
2. The point of injection of the greater occipital nerve is 2 cm lateral to the external occipital protuberance along the superior nuchal line and then 2 cm inferior (caudal).[9]
3. At the point where the greater occipital nerve courses over the occipital bone, pressure over the nerve will elicit pain. Mark that spot with an ink pen.
4. At that site, press firmly on the skin with the retracted tip of a ballpoint pen. This indentation represents the entry point for the needle.
5. After the landmarks are identified, the patient should not move the neck.

ANESTHESIA

- Transient topical anesthesia using vapocoolant spray is difficult over the posterior occiput especially in patients who have thick hair. Consider manual skin distraction by lightly scratching or inducing vibrations in the skin around the injection site to achieve transient local anesthesia.

EQUIPMENT (FOR A SINGLE UNILATERAL INJECTION)

- 3-mL syringe
- 25-gauge 1-in needle
- 1 mL of 1% lidocaine without epinephrine
- 1 mL of 0.5% bupivacaine without epinephrine
- 1 mL of the steroid solution (40 mg of triamcinolone acetonide)
- One alcohol prep pad

- Two povidone-iodine or chlorhexidine prep pads
- Sterile gauze pads

TECHNIQUE

1. Part the hair and prep the insertion site with alcohol followed by the povidone-iodine or chlorhexidine pads.
2. Position the needle and syringe perpendicular to the skin with the tip of the needle directed anteriorly toward the inferior nuchal line of the occiput.
3. Create manual skin distraction by lightly scratching or inducing vibrations in the skin around the injection site to achieve transient local anesthesia at the same time that the needle is being inserted into the skin.
4. Using the no-touch technique, quickly introduce the needle at the insertion site (Fig. 7.14).
5. Advance the needle toward the location of the greater occipital nerve until the needle tip contacts the occiput at the inferior nuchal line. Back up the needle 1 to 2 mm.
6. Withdraw the plunger of the syringe to ensure that there is no blood return.
7. Inject the anesthetic/steroid solution as a bolus around the greater occipital nerve. The injected solution should flow smoothly into the tissues. If increased resistance is encountered, advance or withdraw the needle slightly before attempting further injection.
8. Following injection, withdraw the needle and apply direct pressure with a gauze pad until all bleeding has stopped.
9. Reexamine the greater occipital nerve in 1 to 5 minutes to assess pain relief.

AFTERCARE

- Analgesics, muscle relaxants, ice, physical therapy, musculoskeletal manipulation, and/or other modalities as indicated.
- Consider follow-up examination in 2 weeks.

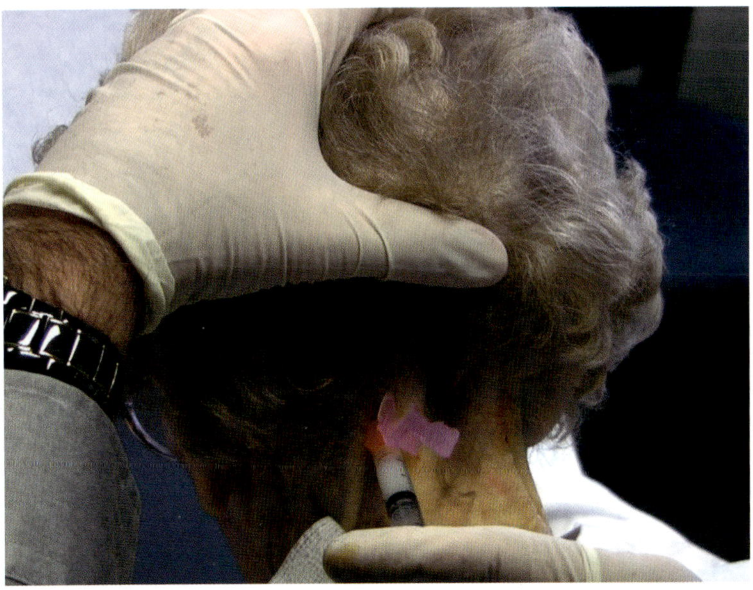

FIGURE 7.14 • Greater occipital neuralgia injection.

PEARLS

- Occipital neuralgia must be distinguished from occipital referral of pain from the atlantoaxial or upper zygapophyseal joints or from tender trigger points in neck muscles or their insertions.[1]

A video showing a landmark-guided greater occipital nerve block injection can be found in the companion eBook.

REFERENCES

1. Accessed July 2, 2025. https://ichd-3.org/13-painful-cranial-neuropathies-and-other-facial-pains/13-4-occipital-neuralgia/
2. Wahab S, Kataria S, Woolley P, et al. Literature review: pericranial nerve blocks for chronic migraines. *Health Psychol Res.* 2023;11:74259.
3. Robbins MS, Starling AJ, Pringsheim TM, Becker WJ, Schwedt TJ. Treatment of cluster headache: the American Headache Society Evidence-Based Guidelines. *Headache*. 2016;56(7):1093-1106.
4. Puledda F, Goadsby PJ, Prabhakar P. Treatment of disabling headache with greater occipital nerve injections in a large population of childhood and adolescent patients: a service evaluation. *J Headache Pain.* 2018;19(1):5.
5. Allen SM, Mookadam F, Cha SS, Freeman JA, Starling AJ, Mookadam M. Greater occipital nerve block for acute treatment of migraine headache. *J Am Board Fam Med.* 2018;31(2):211-218.
6. Ebied AM, Nguyen DT, Dang T. Evaluation of occipital nerve blocks for acute pain relief of migraines. *J Clin Pharmacol.* 2019;60:378-383.
7. Palamar D, Uluduz D, Saip S, Erden G, Unalan H, Akarirmak U. Ultrasound-guided greater occipital nerve block: an efficient technique in chronic refractory migraine without aura? *Pain Physician.* 2015;18(2):153-162.
8. Pingree MJ, Sole JS, O'Brien TG, Eldrige JS, Moeschler SM. Clinical efficacy of an ultrasound-guided greater occipital nerve block at the level of C2. *Reg Anesth Pain Med.* 2017;42(1):99-104.
9. Loukas M, El-Sedfy A, Tubbs RS, et al. Identification of greater occipital nerve landmarks for the treatment of occipital neuralgia. *Folia Morphol (Warsz).* 2006;65(4):337-342.

Headache Nerve Blocks

Headache peripheral nerve blocks are useful procedures that may be done to relieve the pain of various headaches,[1] including muscular tension, cervicogenic,[2] migraine,[3-5] cluster,[6-8] chronic daily headache, paroxysmal hemicrania, and hemicrania continua.[9,10] They may be used in patients who have failed home medications and may help patients with medication overuse headaches to wean off of acute therapy.[11] Nerve blocks also may be appropriate for children[12,13] and pregnant patients.[14]

These injection techniques are used to provide reversible local anesthesia in order to achieve effective blockade of any or all of the bilateral greater occipital, lesser occipital, auriculotemporal, zygomaticotemporal, supraorbital, and supratrochlear nerves. Selection of the single nerve or multiple nerves to be injected is clinically determined on the basis of local pain or pain radiation when the nerve of interest is compressed. Multiple cranial nerve blocks may provide an efficacious, well-tolerated, and reproducible transitional treatment for chronic headache disorders when greater occipital nerve blocks have been unsuccessful.[15] Corticosteroids may be added to the greater occipital nerve injections to provide longer-term symptomatic relief. Suboccipital steroid injections of the greater occipital nerve for the treatment of cluster headaches received a Level A recommendation in the 2016 American Headache Society Evidence-Based Guidelines.[7] On the other hand, several small studies are inconclusive regarding the efficacy of adding steroids to local anesthetics for the treatment of migraine headache.[4]

Pain relief from the headache nerve block injections commonly lasts longer than the usual expected anesthetic effect of the lidocaine and bupivacaine. Almost all patients experience pain relief after receiving anesthetic nerve blocks, but there is no way to predict which patient will experience long-term pain relief.

Contraindications to peripheral nerve blocks include a known allergy to a local anesthetic, open skull defect, and an overlying skin infection. Pregnancy is a relative contraindication.

Relevant Anatomy: (Fig. 7.15)

PATIENT POSITION

- For the greater occipital and lesser occipital nerve injections, the patient is positioned sitting on an examination stool with neck flexed and leaning forward with the forehead resting on the patient's crossed arms, which are placed on the pull-out foot tray of the examination table. The clinician stands behind the patient and slightly lateral on the side of treatment.
- For the auriculotemporal and zygomaticotemporal nerve injections, the patient is positioned lying supine on the examination table with the head of the bed slightly elevated. The clinician stands lateral to the side of the face that is being injected.

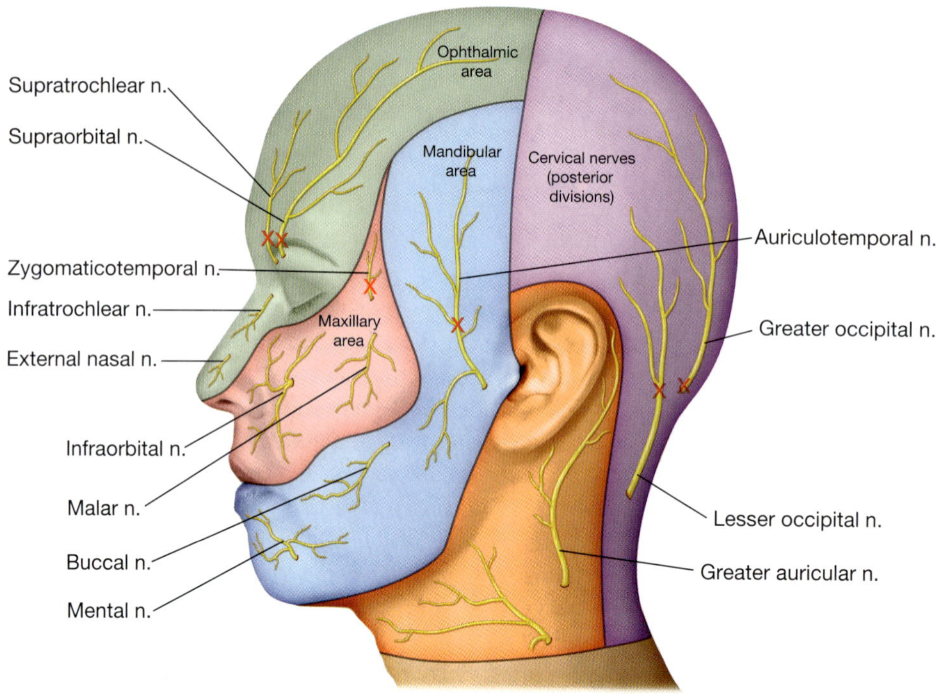

FIGURE 7.15 ● Scalp nerves and their innervated areas. The *red X* indicates the injection sites for each nerve.

- For the supraorbital and supratrochlear nerve injections, the patient is positioned lying supine on the examination table with the patient's head rotated toward the clinician. The clinician stands lateral to the side of the face that is being injected.

LANDMARKS

1. Refer to the Greater Occipital Nerve Block Chapter for the location of this nerve.
2. The point of injection of the lesser occipital nerve is over the medial border of the sternocleidomastoid muscle. The position of the injection is 1 cm inferior and over the lateral third of a line between the external occipital protuberance and the mastoid process. Pressure over the nerve will often elicit pain.
3. The point of injection of the auriculotemporal nerve is 1.5 cm anterior to the ear at the level of the tragus.
4. The point of injection of the zygomaticotemporal nerve is 1.5 cm posterior to the lateral orbital rim above the zygomatic arch.
5. Refer to the Supraorbital and Supratrochlear Nerve Blocks Chapter for location of these nerves.

ANESTHESIA

- Transient topical anesthesia of the skin using a direct spray of a vapocoolant spray is not advised for use with the supratrochlear, supraorbital, and zygomaticotemporal nerves due to the close proximity of the injection sites to the eyes. However, consider preinjection skin anesthesia by spraying PainEase mist onto a sterile cotton swab until saturated. Then, apply the swab over the point of injection. Alternatively, skin distraction techniques may be employed by lightly scratching or inducing vibrations in the skin around the injection site.

- Transient topical anesthesia using vapocoolant spray is difficult over the posterior occiput especially in patients who have thick hair. Skin distraction techniques may be employed.

EQUIPMENT (IF ALL SITES WILL BE INJECTED)

- One 5-mL syringe
- Two 10-mL syringes
- Two 30-gauge ½-in needles and one 25-gauge 1-in needle
- 10 mL of 1% lidocaine without epinephrine
- 10 mL of 0.5% bupivacaine without epinephrine
- 2 mL of the steroid solution (40 mg/mL of triamcinolone acetonide)
- Alcohol prep pads
- Sterile gauze pads

TECHNIQUE

1. Over each of the nerve block injection sites, press firmly on the skin with the retracted tip of a ballpoint pen. These indentations represent the entry points for the needles.
2. Prep each of the insertion sites with alcohol pads.
3.
    - One 10-mL syringe is used for the bilateral greater occipital and lesser occipital nerve injections. Fill the 10-mL syringe with 4 mL of 1% lidocaine without epinephrine, 4 mL of 0.5% bupivacaine without epinephrine, and 2 mL of the steroid solution (triamcinolone acetonide 40 mg/mL). Mix the contents of each syringe. Attach a 25-gauge 1-in needle.
    - One 10-mL syringe is used for bilateral auriculotemporal and zygomaticotemporal nerve injections. Fill the 10-mL syringe with 4 mL of 1% lidocaine without epinephrine and 4 mL of 0.5% bupivacaine without epinephrine. Mix the two anesthetics in each syringe. Attach a 30-gauge ½-in needle.
    - One 5-mL syringe is used for the bilateral supraorbital and supratrochlear nerve injections. Fill the 5-mL syringe with 2 mL of 1% lidocaine without epinephrine and 2 mL of 0.5% bupivacaine without epinephrine. Mix the two anesthetics in each syringe. Attach a 30-gauge ½-in needle.
4. Provide skin distraction by pinching, stretching, and/or rubbing adjacent skin at the same time that the needle is being inserted into the skin.
5. Using the no-touch technique, quickly introduce the needles at each insertion site.
6.
    - For the greater occipital nerve headache injections, follow the technique described in the dedicated chapter and infuse 2.5 mL of the lidocaine/steroid mixture at the site of each greater occipital nerve.
    - For the lesser occipital nerve headache injections, position the 25-gauge 1-in needle perpendicular to the skin at the identified point of entry. Advance the needle toward the location of that nerve until the needle tip contacts the occiput at the superior nuchal line. Back up the needle 1 to 2 mm. Withdraw the plunger of the syringe to ensure that there is no blood return. Inject 2.5 mL of the anesthetic/steroid mixture over each lesser occipital nerve site.

- For the auriculotemporal and zygomaticotemporal nerve headache injections, position the 30-gauge ½-in needle perpendicular to the skin at each of the injection sites described above. Advance it into the subcutaneous tissue under the injection site. Withdraw the plunger to ensure that there is not intravascular placement. Inject 2 mL of the anesthetic mixture at the site of each nerve.
- For the supraorbital and supratrochlear nerve headache injections, follow the technique described in the dedicated chapter and infuse 1 mL of the anesthetic mixture around each supraorbital and supratrochlear nerve.

7. Following the injections, withdraw the needles and apply direct pressure. For supraorbital and supratrochlear injections, press and push the anesthetic up the forehead and away from the eyes.
8. Reexamine the patient in 1 to 5 minutes to assess pain relief.

AFTERCARE

- None needed.

Videos showing landmark-guided headache nerve block injections can be found in the companion eBook.

REFERENCES

1. Blumenfeld A, Ashkenazi A, Napchan U, et al. Expert consensus recommendations for the performance of peripheral nerve blocks for headaches—a narrative review. *Headache.* 2013;53(3):437-446.
2. Lauretti GR, Correa SW, Mattos AL. Efficacy of the greater occipital nerve block for cervicogenic headache: comparing classical and subcompartmental techniques. *Pain Pract.* 2015;15(7):654-661.
3. Ruiz Pinero M, Mulero Carrillo P, Pedraza Hueso MI, de la Cruz Rodríguez C, López Mesonero L, Guerrero Peral AL. Pericranial nerve blockade as a preventive treatment for migraine: experience in 60 patients. *Neurologia.* 2016;31(7):445-451.
4. Allen SM, Mookadam F, Cha SS, Freeman JA, Starling AJ, Mookadam M. Greater occipital nerve block for acute treatment of migraine headache. *J Am Board Fam Med.* 2018;31(2):211-218.
5. Li W, Tang L. Influence of greater occipital nerve block on the relief of acute migraine: a meta-analysis. *Medicine (Baltimore).* 2024;103(42):e39955.
6. Gonen M, Balgetir F, Aytac E, Taşcı İ, Demir CF, Müngen B. Suboccipital steroid injection alone as a preventive treatment for cluster headache. *J Clin Neurosci.* 2019;68:140-145.
7. Robbins MS, Starling AJ, Pringsheim TM, Becker WJ, Schwedt TJ. Treatment of cluster headache: the American Headache Society Evidence-Based Guidelines. *Headache.* 2016;56(7):1093-1106.
8. Lambru G, Abu Bakar N, Stahlhut L, et al. Greater occipital nerve blocks in chronic cluster headache: a prospective open-label study. *Eur J Neurol.* 2014;21(2):338-343.
9. Cortijo E, Guerrero-Peral AL, Herrero-Velazquez S, et al. Hemicrania continua: characteristics and therapeutic experience in a series of 36 patients. *Rev Neurol.* 2012;55(5):270-278.
10. Wahab S, Kataria S, Woolley P, et al. Literature review: pericranial nerve blocks for chronic migraines. *Health Psychol Res.* 2023;11:74259.
11. Tobin J, Flitman S. Occipital nerve blocks: when and what to inject? *Headache.* 2009;49(10):1521-1533.
12. Szperka CL, Gelfand AA, Hershey AD. Patterns of use of peripheral nerve blocks and trigger point injections for pediatric headache: results of a survey of the American Headache Society Pediatric and Adolescent Section. *Headache.* 2016;56(10):1597-1607.
13. Puledda F, Goadsby PJ, Prabhakar P. Treatment of disabling headache with greater occipital nerve injections in a large population of childhood and adolescent patients: a service evaluation. *J Headache Pain.* 2018;19(1):5.
14. Govindappagari S, Grossman TB, Dayal AK, Grosberg BM, Vollbracht S, Robbins MS. Peripheral nerve blocks in the treatment of migraine in pregnancy. *Obstet Gynecol.* 2014;124(6):1169-1174.
15. Miller S, Lagrata S, Matharu M. Multiple cranial nerve blocks for the transitional treatment of chronic headaches. *Cephalalgia.* 2019;39(12):1488-1499.

8

Chalazion

James W. McNabb

A chalazion is an acute or chronic granuloma that forms due to inflammation and obstruction in the meibomian glands (tarsal glands) on the conjunctival surface of either the upper or the lower eyelids. The obstruction in these small sebaceous glands may occur due to allergy, acne in adolescence, or rosacea. A chalazion contains many steroid-responsive immune cells including macrophages, plasma cells, polymorphonuclear cells, and eosinophils. Patients with this condition occasionally present to the primary care office, and although considered self-limited, a chalazion may last for weeks to months before spontaneously resolving. Traditional conservative treatment includes the application of local heat, lubricant eye drops, and careful cleansing of the affected eyelid. Although frequently prescribed, an antibiotic is unlikely to improve the resolution of a chalazion or even a hordeolum.[1]

An often overlooked procedure is the simple injection of a small amount of corticosteroid (4 mg of triamcinolone) into or around the chalazion lesion.[2] Studies show that the procedure is quick, well tolerated, and safe. It results in greater than 80% resolution of the chalazion lesion within days of administration.[3-6] Response rates mirror that of surgical treatment with incision and curettage.[7] Additional advantages of this technique over traditional incision and curettage include its simplicity, less pain, considerably decreased cost, no requirement of special instruments, no need for postoperative eye patching, and convenience for both the provider and the patient. Lesions that persist after more than 2 months of conservative therapy should be treated with surgery or a corticosteroid injection.

Relevant Anatomy: (Fig. 8.1)

PATIENT POSITION

- Supine on the examination table with the head of the bed elevated 30°.
- The patient's hands are folded in their lap.
- The clinician stands lateral to the patient, on the same side as the chalazion.

ANESTHESIA

- Injection of local anesthetic into the skin of the eyelid prior to injection of the corticosteroid is not used because it causes local swelling that may obliterate the location of the chalazion.

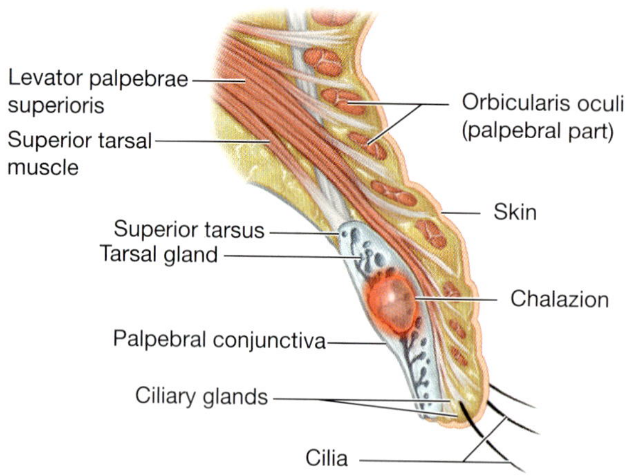

FIGURE 8.1 Superior eyelid. The tarsus forms the skeleton of the eyelid and contains the tarsal glands.

- Topical corneal anesthesia is never provided so that inadvertent introduction of the needle through the eyelid, the conjunctiva, and into the globe would be recognized by the patient experiencing significant pain.
- Topical vapocoolant spray cannot be sprayed around the eyes.
- Topical vapocoolant spray can be sprayed onto a cotton swab to saturate it. Then the swab may be applied directly to the injection site over the eyelid skin.
- Alternatively, nerve blocks can be used to provide adequate skin anesthesia of the eyelids. A supraorbital nerve block should block pain from the upper eyelid, and an infraorbital block should anesthetize the lower eyelid.

EQUIPMENT

- (Optional) Sterile corneal eye shields (Kolberg Optical Supplies, Inc. http://www.corneaprotectors.com/)
- (Optional) Chalazion clamp
- Topical vapocoolant spray and cotton swab
- 3-mL syringe
- 30-gauge ½-in needle
- 0.1 mL of the 40 mg/mL steroid solution (4 mg of triamcinolone acetonide)
- One alcohol prep pad
- Two povidone-iodine or chlorhexidine prep pads
- Sterile gauze pads

TECHNIQUE

1. (Optional) Provide adequate anesthesia to the upper eyelid by performing supraorbital and supratrochlear nerve blocks or the lower eyelid by performing an infraorbital nerve block. See Chapter 7.
2. (Optional) Corneal eye shield protectors may be used to protect the cornea and globe.
3. Identify the injection site a few millimeters lateral to the chalazion. Prep the insertion site with alcohol followed by the povidone-iodine or chlorhexidine pads.
4. (Optional) A chalazion clamp may also be used, if desired, to stabilize the lesion. However, use of this instrument requires both nerve block(s) and topical corneal anesthesia.

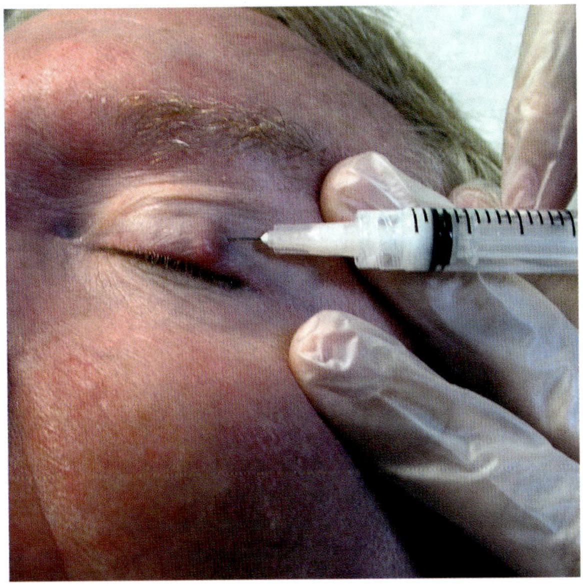

FIGURE 8.2 • Chalazion injection.

5. With your fingertips, apply lateral traction to the eyelid to stretch and fix the skin.
6. Approach the eyelid from a lateral to a medial direction.
7. To ensure safety, make sure that the needle is oriented parallel to the surface of the globe of the eye. The operator should also rest their injection hand on the patient's face to stabilize the needle.
8. In order to provide topical anesthesia, spray Pain Ease Mist onto a sterile cotton swab until saturated. Then, apply the swab just lateral to the chalazion.
9. Using the no-touch technique, carefully, quickly insert the needle through the skin external to the eyelid about 2 to 3 mm lateral to the chalazion (Fig. 8.2).
10. Advance the needle slowly and carefully into the center of the chalazion.
11. After needle insertion into the chalazion, confirm accurate placement by moving the needle slightly from side to side to ensure that the lesion moves with the needle.
12. Inject 0.1 mL (4 mg) of the steroid solution (40 mg/mL of triamcinolone acetonide) into the chalazion. Swelling of the chalazion will occur.
13. Remove the needle and apply direct pressure with the gauze pad.

AFTERCARE

- None needed.
- Consider follow-up examination in 1 week.

PEARLS

- After the needle has been inserted into the chalazion, confirm accurate placement by moving the needle slightly from side to side to ensure that the nodule moves with the needle.
- Response to the chalazion steroid injection is usually seen within days of the procedure.
- One-third of the cases may require a second injection.

- If the chalazion continues to recur after two injections, it should be evaluated for malignancy. In this case, referral to a subspecialist colleague is recommended for more aggressive measures such as primary excision or curettage through a cruciform incision.
- Potential complications may include inadvertent corneal injury, penetration of the globe, cataract from administration of steroid in the globe, persistent triamcinolone deposits,[8] and skin depigmentation.

A video showing a chalazion injection can be found in the companion eBook.

REFERENCES

1. Alsoudi AF, Ton L, Ashraf DC, et al. Efficacy of care and antibiotic use for chalazia and hordeola. *Eye Contact Lens.* 2022;48(4):162-168.
2. Wu AY, Gervasio KA, Gergoudis KN, Wei C, Oestreicher JH, Harvey JT. Conservative therapy for chalazia: is it really effective? *Acta Ophthalmol.* 2018;96(4):e503-e509.
3. Wong MY, Yau GS, Lee JW, Yuen CY. Intralesional triamcinolone acetonide injection for the treatment of primary chalazions. *Int Ophthalmol.* 2014;34(5):1049-1053.
4. Ben Simon GJ, Rosen N, Rosner M, Spierer A. Intralesional triamcinolone acetonide injection versus incision and curettage for primary chalazia: a prospective, randomized study. *Am J Ophthalmol.* 2011;151(4):714-718.
5. Goawalla A, Lee V. A prospective randomized treatment study comparing three treatment options for chalazia: triamcinolone acetonide injections, incision and curettage and treatment with hot compresses. *Clin Exp Ophthalmol.* 2007;35(8):706-712.
6. Chung CF, Lai JS, Li PS. Subcutaneous extralesional triamcinolone acetonide injection versus conservative management in the treatment of chalazion. *Hong Kong Med J.* 2006;12(4):278-281.
7. Singhania R, Sharma N, Vashisht S, Dewan T. Intralesional triamcinolone acetonide (TA) versus incision and curettage (I & C) for medium and large size chalazia. *Nepal J Ophthalmol.* 2018;10(19):3-10.
8. Wolkow N, Jakobiec FA, Hatton MP. A common procedure with an uncommon pathology: triamcinolone acetonide eyelid injection. *Ophthalmic Plast Reconstr Surg.* 2018;34(3):e72-e73.

Keloid Scar

Keloids are pathogenic scars occurring as the result of an abnormal overgrowth of dense fibrous tissue that develops in areas of prior skin trauma. The tissue elevates above the surface of the surrounding skin, extends beyond the borders of the original wound, does not regress spontaneously, and often recurs after excision. Keloids usually occur during the second and third decades of life, with a higher prevalence in persons with darker pigmented skin. They are most commonly asymptomatic but can present with itching and pain if they become inflamed or enlarged.

Since primary surgical excision may result in worsening of the keloid scar, other therapeutic modalities for keloids and hypertrophic scars may be considered in clinical practice. These include ablative laser, fractional laser, photodynamic therapy, silicone gel application, and cryosurgery.

Intralesional injection of therapeutic agents is the most commonly used treatment. The primary injectable agent for many years has been corticosteroids. Corticosteroids reduce excessive scarring by decreasing collagen synthesis, suppressing vascular endothelial growth factor, and decreasing production of inflammatory mediators and fibroblast proliferation during wound healing. In a study by Huu et al,[1] the optimal dose for treatment of a keloid was determined to be 7.5 mg/1 cm^2 scar. Complications of repeated corticosteroid injections may include skin atrophy, telangiectasia formation, hypopigmentation, and a depressed scar.

Combinations of various therapies may produce an even greater benefit. Triamcinolone used in combination with 5-flurouracil results in improved scar regression and reduced recurrence of keloids.[2,3] Combined injection of intralesional steroids with botulinum toxin type A appears to be superior to either therapy alone.[4] A recent network meta-analysis showed that injection of intralesional botulinum toxin type A combined with corticosteroids was more effective and had fewer side effects. The optimal treatment course was monthly intralesional injections of triamcinolone acetonide 40 mg/mL (0.1 mL/cm^3) mixed with botulinum toxin type A (2.5 IU/cm^3) for a total of three treatments.[5] Combining intralesional platelet-rich plasma with triamcinolone could yield cosmetically better outcomes in keloid treatment with lower incidence of corticosteroid-induced side effects especially atrophy and hypopigmentation.[6] Finally, combination therapy with intralesional cryosurgery followed by injected steroids[7] and surgical excision followed by corticosteroid injections[8,9] have also been shown to be effective.

PATIENT POSITION

- Supine on the examination table.
- Rotate the patient's head away from the side that is being injected. This minimizes anxiety and pain perception.
- The clinician stands on the side of the patient that allows best access to the keloid scar.

ANESTHESIA

- Local anesthesia of the injection site with topical vapocoolant spray.

EQUIPMENT

- Topical vapocoolant spray
- 3-mL syringe
- 25-gauge 1- or 1½-in needle depending on the size of the keloid
- 0.25 to 1 mL of the 40 mg/mL steroid solution (10-40 mg of triamcinolone acetonide)
- (Optional) 0.25 to 1 mL of 5-fluorouracil solution (50 mg/mL)
- (Optional) 0.1 to 1 mL of onabotulinumtoxinA solution (100 U/mL)
- One alcohol prep pad
- Two povidone-iodine or chlorhexidine prep pads
- Sterile gauze pads
- Sterile adhesive bandage

TECHNIQUE

1. Prep the insertion site with alcohol followed by the povidone-iodine or chlorhexidine pads.
2. Achieve good local anesthesia by using topical vapocoolant spray.
3. Position the needle and syringe parallel to the surface of the skin at the edge of the keloid with the tip of the needle directed toward the center of the keloid scar.
4. Using the no-touch technique, quickly introduce the needle at the edge of the keloid (Fig. 8.3).
5. Advance the needle into the lesion.
6. Withdraw the plunger of the syringe to ensure that there is no blood return.
7. Perform a uniform injection of 0.25 to 1 mL of steroid solution (10-40 mg of triamcinolone acetonide—see above for dosing) (and/or optionally, 0.25-1 mL

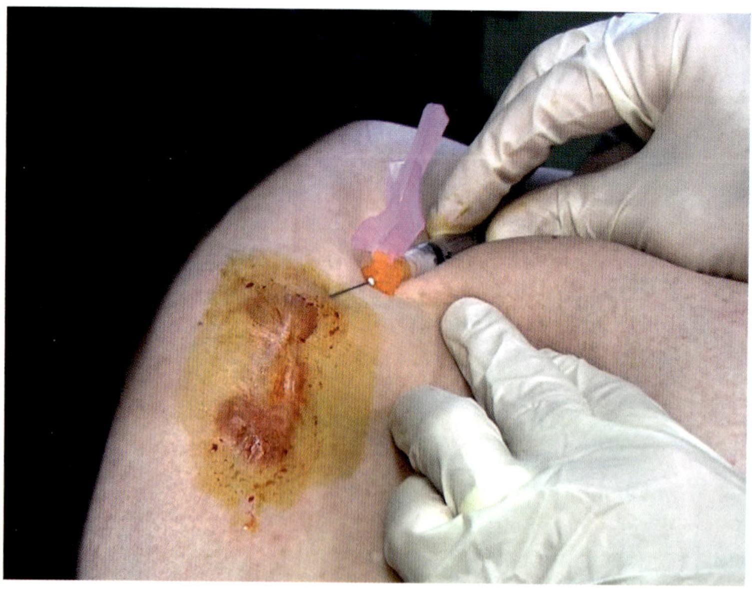

FIGURE 8.3 ● Keloid injection.

[12.5-50 mg] of 5-fluorouracil solution) (and/or optionally, 10-100 units of onabotulinumtoxinA solution—see above for dosing) into the substance of the keloid at a depth that is half the thickness of the keloid.

8. Avoid injection into the subcutaneous fat or surrounding normal skin.
9. Following injection, withdraw the needle.
10. Apply a sterile adhesive bandage.

AFTERCARE

- None needed
- Follow-up examination in 4 to 6 weeks

PEARLS

- If the keloid continues to recur after several injections, more aggressive measures may be used, as noted above.
- Avoid superficial injections as they may increase the likelihood of dermal complications.

Video showing a keloid scar injection can be found in the companion eBook.

REFERENCES

1. Huu ND, Huu SN, Thi XL, et al. Successful treatment of intralesional triamcilonon acetonide injection in keloid patients. *Open Access Maced J Med Sci.* 2019;7(2):275-278.
2. Davison SP, Dayan JH, Clemens MW, Sonni S, Wang A, Crane A. Efficacy of intralesional 5-fluorouracil and triamcinolone in the treatment of keloids. *Aesthet Surg J.* 2009;29(1):40-46.
3. Monteiro RC, Bhat MR, Martis J, Kamath HG. A comparative study of the efficacy of intralesional 5 fluorouracil vs combination of 5 fluorouracil with triamcinolone acetonide in keloids. *Indian J Dermatol.* 2022;67(3):211-215.
4. Gamil HD, Khattab FM, El Fawal MM, Eldeeb SE. Comparison of intralesional triamcinolone acetonide, botulinum toxin type A, and their combination for the treatment of keloid lesions. *J Dermatolog Treat.* 2020;31(5):535-544.
5. Sun P, Lu X, Zhang H, Hu Z. The efficacy of drug injection in the treatment of pathological scar: a network meta-analysis. *Aesthetic Plast Surg.* 2021;45(2):791-805.
6. Hewedy ES, Sabaa BEI, Mohamed WS, Hegab DS. Combined intralesional triamcinolone acetonide and platelet rich plasma versus intralesional triamcinolone acetonide alone in treatment of keloids. *J Dermatolog Treat.* 2022;33(1):150-156.
7. Weshahy AH, Abdel HR. Intralesional cryosurgery and intralesional steroid injection: a good combination therapy for treatment of keloids and hypertrophic scars. *Dermatol Ther.* 2012;25(3):273-276.
8. Hayashi T, Furukawa H, Oyama A, et al. A new uniform protocol of combined corticosteroid injections and ointment application reduces recurrence rates after surgical keloid/hypertrophic scar excision. *Dermatol Surg.* 2012;38(6):893-897.
9. Zhang Y, Wu M, Liu D, et al. Recurrence and complications of peri-operative steroid injection of keloids: a systematic review and meta-analysis. *Aesthetic Plast Surg.* 2024;48(15):2927-2940.

Common Warts

Patients often present to the primary care office for evaluation of common warts. These verrucous structures are the focal dermal expression of human papillomavirus infections. Common warts may be treated with various modalities, including cryosurgery, electrosurgery, laser ablation, cautery, curettage, and injection therapy.

Intradermal injection of antigens—such as Candida albicans, measles-mumps-rubella (MMR), Trichophyton, or tuberculin—at the margin of a wart incites a host immune response mediated by T-helper 1 cytokine activation.[1] This commonly results in spontaneous regression of the treated warts. In addition, an HPV-directed cell-mediated immune response plays a role in the resolution of distant untreated warts. There is a growing body of literature that documents the effectiveness and safety of intralesional and/or perilesional injection therapy with *Candida*[2] and measles-mumps-rubella[3] antigens. A large study yielded a 70% complete response to intralesional injections of *Candida* antigen for children with multiple recalcitrant cutaneous warts.[4] Compared to liquid nitrogen cryotherapy, intralesional injection of *Candida* antigen has a better therapeutic response, needs fewer sessions, and can treat distant warts.[5]

Candida antigen is available as "Candin" (Nielsen BioSciences, Inc., https://nielsenbio.com/candin-hcp/) or the generic (Hollister Stier Allergy. 3525 N. Regal St, Spokane, WA 99207, phone: 509-489-5656, website: http://www.hsallergy.com/).

PATIENT POSITION

- Supine on the examination table.
- Rotate the patient's head away from the side that is being injected. This minimizes anxiety and pain perception.

ANESTHESIA

- Local anesthesia of the skin using topical vapocoolant spray.

EQUIPMENT

- Topical vapocoolant spray
- 3-mL syringe
- 30-gauge 1/2-in needle
- Up to 1 mL of the *Candida* antigen
- Up to 1 mL of 1% lidocaine without epinephrine
- One alcohol prep pad
- Two povidone-iodine or chlorhexidine prep pads
- Sterile gauze pads

- Sterile adhesive bandage
- Nonsterile, clean chucks pad

TECHNIQUE

1. Prepare the injection solution: Mix equal parts of up to 1 mL of *Candida* antigen and up to 1 mL of 1% lidocaine without epinephrine.
2. Prep the insertion site with alcohol followed by the povidone-iodine or chlorhexidine pads.
3. Achieve good local anesthesia by using topical vapocoolant spray.
4. Position the needle and syringe at a 10° angle to the surface of the skin at the edge of the wart with the tip of the needle directed toward the wart.
5. Using the no-touch technique, quickly introduce the needle about 5 mm from the edge of the wart (Fig. 8.4).
6. Advance the needle into the dermis at the edge of the wart. (NOT into the wart itself.)
7. Withdraw the plunger of the syringe to ensure that there is no blood return.
8. Perform an intradermal injection immediately adjacent to the wart using 0.1 mL of the solution per wart. Limit the total amount at any one visit to 1 mL of the *Candida* antigen.
9. Avoid injection into the subcutaneous tissues.
10. Following injection of the solution, withdraw the needle.
11. Apply a sterile adhesive bandage.

AFTERCARE

- None needed.
- Instruct the patient that the following symptoms may occur after injection as the immune system is reacting to the antigen: localized erythema, itching, drying of the wart, lesion turning a black color, peeling of the treated tissue, or simply (and most commonly) spontaneous regression.
- Adverse reactions may also include rash, adenopathy, and persistence of wart(s).
- Consider follow-up examination in 3 weeks.

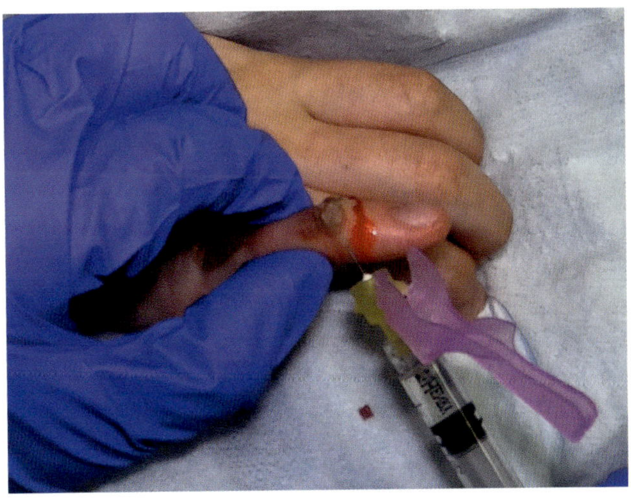

FIGURE 8.4 • Common wart injection using *Candida* antigen.

PEARLS

- *Candida* antigen should not be used after a previous unacceptable adverse reaction such as extreme hypersensitivity or allergy to this antigen or to a similar product.
- Repeat injection in 3 weeks if there is any residual wart.
- Sixty-five to seventy-five percent of warts treated with *Candida* antigen injection resolve after the first injection.[6]
- Fifty percent of the remaining warts respond after a second injection.[6]
- Antigen injection of warts is an "off-label" use of *Candida* and mumps antigens, and there is no J code listed for these antigens. Thus, insurance companies do not provide reimbursement for the antigen used in this procedure. Unfortunately, the injection code does not include this cost, and the antigen itself is more expensive than the payment for the procedure. Therefore, if providing this treatment, consider asking the patient to fill a prescription at a reputable pharmacy, bring the unopened injectable to the office, and then perform the procedure.

A video showing common wart injections can be found in the companion eBook.

REFERENCES

1. Nofal A, Salah E, Nofal E, Yosef A. Intralesional antigen immunotherapy for the treatment of warts: current concepts and future prospects. *Am J Clin Dermatol.* 2013;14(4):253-260.
2. Chang CH, Sung ZY, Huang YC. Efficacy of intralesional *Candida* injection in the treatment of cutaneous warts: a systematic review and meta-analysis. *Acta Derm Venereol.* 2024;104:adv40819.
3. Vania R, Pranata R, Tan ST. Intralesional measles-mumps-rubella is associated with a higher complete response in cutaneous warts: a systematic review and meta-analysis of randomized controlled trial including GRADE qualification. *J Dermatolog Treat.* 2021;32(8):1010-1017.
4. Muñoz Garza FZ, Roé Crespo E, Torres Pradilla M, et al. Intralesional *Candida* antigen immunotherapy for the treatment of recalcitrant and multiple warts in children. *Pediatr Dermatol.* 2015;32(6):797-801.
5. Khozeimeh F, Jabbari Azad F, Mahboubi Oskouei Y, et al. Intralesional immunotherapy compared to cryotherapy in the treatment of warts. *Int J Dermatol.* 2017;56(4):474-478.
6. Phillips R, Ruhl TS, Pfenninger JL, Garber MR. Candida antigen for the treatment of verruca. *Arch Dermatol.* 2000;136:1274-1275.

Granuloma Annulare and Other Thin, Benign, Inflammatory Dermatoses

Granuloma annulare is an example of a *thin* benign inflammatory dermatosis. This is associated with many conditions such as malignancy, trauma, thyroid disease, diabetes mellitus, and HIV infection. In the most common localized form, it presents as skin-colored or erythematous dermal papules and ring-shaped lesions up to 5 cm in diameter (Fig. 8.5). The localized variant has a predilection for the feet, ankles, lower limbs, and wrists and generally self-resolves within 2 years without treatment. However, the generalized form is more chronic and less responsive to therapy.[1,2] Treatment is not evidence-based and is determined by provider preference, expert opinion, and case reports. Potent topical corticosteroids or intralesional corticosteroids are most commonly utilized. There are a myriad of other treatment options, including liquid nitrogen cryosurgery, photodynamic therapy, hydroxychloroquine, dapsone, tacrolimus, pimecrolimus, and imiquimod.[3]

PATIENT POSITION

- Supine on the examination table with the head of the bed elevated 30°.
- The patient's hands are folded in their lap.
- The clinician stands lateral to the patient, on the same side as the affected area.

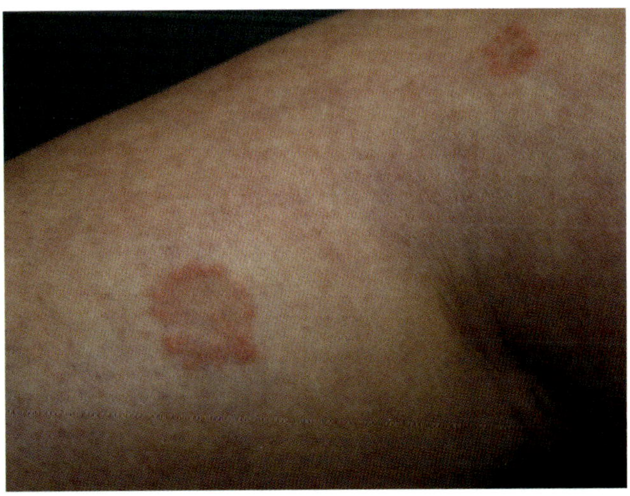

FIGURE 8.5 ● Granuloma annulare lesion.

ANESTHESIA

- Local anesthesia of the injection site with topical vapocoolant spray.

EQUIPMENT

- Topical vapocoolant spray
- 0.5-mL insulin syringe with its attached 8-mm, 31-gauge needle
- Up to 1 mL of the 10 mg/mL steroid solution per lesion (up to 10 mg of triamcinolone acetonide)
- One alcohol prep pad
- Two povidone-iodine or chlorhexidine prep pads
- Sterile gauze pads
- Sterile adhesive bandage

TECHNIQUE

1. Over the lesion, plot out a grid at 1-cm intervals using a ruler and surgical marking pen.
2. Prep the site with alcohol followed by the povidone-iodine or chlorhexidine pads.
3. Achieve good local anesthesia by using Gebauer's Pain Ease Mist topical vapocoolant spray (Fig. 8.6).
4. Position the needle and syringe at about a 20° angle to the surface of the skin at each injection site.
5. Using the no-touch technique, quickly introduce the needle into the skin.
6. Advance the needle into the mid to deep dermis.
7. Withdraw the plunger of the syringe to ensure that there is no blood return.
8. Inject 0.02 to 0.05 mL of the steroid solution (10 mg/mL of triamcinolone acetonide) (Fig. 8.7).
9. Repeat the injections to cover the entire lesion.
10. Following the injections of the corticosteroid solution, withdraw the needle, and apply direct pressure with the gauze pad.

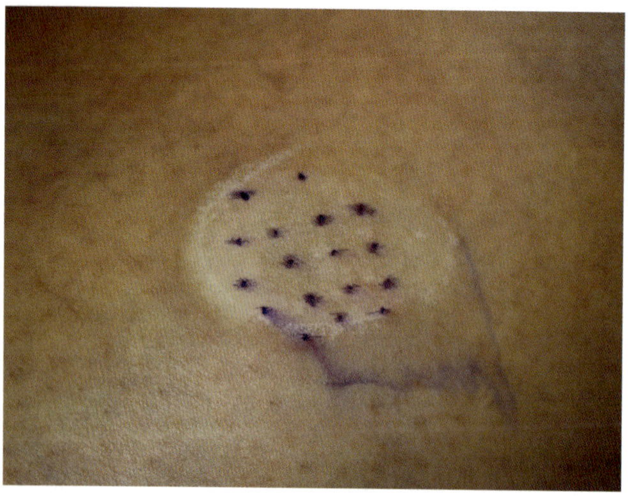

FIGURE 8.6 ● Granuloma annulare lesion with 1-cm grid markings—immediately after Pain Ease Mist topical vapocoolant spray.

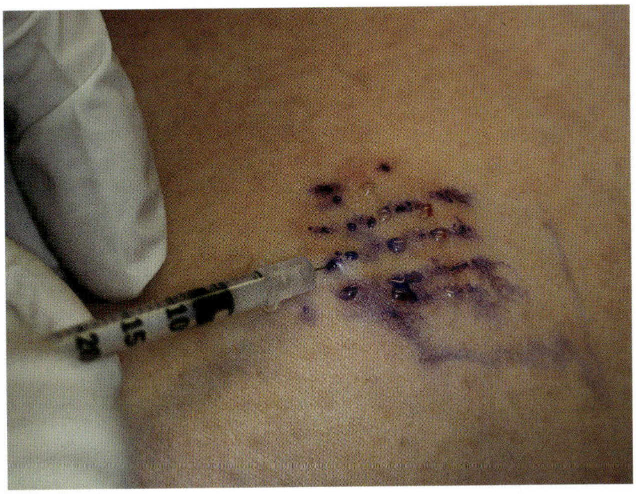

FIGURE 8.7 • Injections of granuloma annulare lesion using an insulin syringe/needle with small volumes of triamcinolone.

11. Apply a sterile adhesive bandage.
12. The injections may be repeated every 4 to 6 weeks until the lesion resolves (Fig. 8.8).

AFTERCARE

- None needed.
- Consider scheduling a follow-up examination in 4 to 6 weeks.

PEARLS

- Avoid injecting into the epidermis or subcutaneous tissues.

A video showing injections for thin, benign, inflammatory dermatoses can be found in the companion eBook.

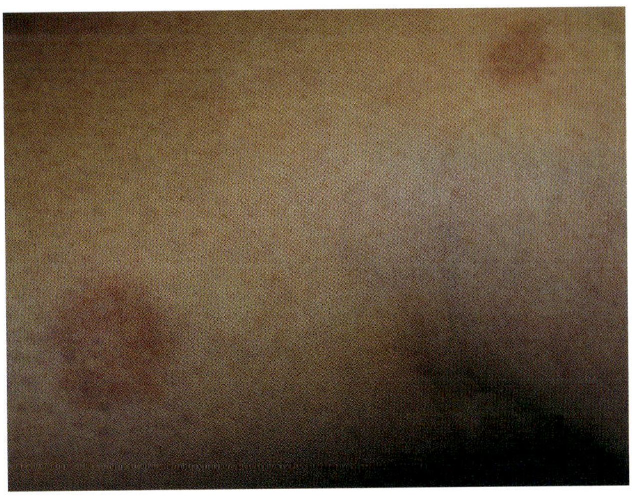

FIGURE 8.8 • Resolving granuloma annulare lesion 7 days after corticosteroid injection.

REFERENCES

1. Wang J, Khachemoune A. Granuloma annulare: a focused review of therapeutic options. *Am J Clin Dermatol.* 2018;19(3):333-344.
2. Joshi TP, Duvic M. Granuloma annulare: an updated review of epidemiology, pathogenesis, and treatment options. *Am J Clin Dermatol.* 2022;23(1):37-50.
3. Thornsberry LA, English JC III. Etiology, diagnosis, and therapeutic management of granuloma annulare: an update. *Am J Clin Dermatol.* 2013;14(4):279-290.

Prurigo Nodularis and Other Thick, Benign, Inflammatory Dermatoses

Prurigo nodularis (PN) is an example of a *thick* benign inflammatory dermatosis. It can occur spontaneously, or as an expression of underlying conditions such as atopic dermatitis, chronic kidney disease, and neurological diseases. There is also a strong association with psychiatric disease. PN is a chronic condition characterized by the presence of generally symmetric, hyperkeratotic, excoriated, hyperpigmented, firm, intensely pruritic nodules. Chronic and repetitive scratching or picking of the nodules causes permanent skin changes, including nodular lichenification, hyperkeratosis, hyperpigmentation, and skin thickening. Unhealed, excoriated lesions are often scaling and crusted. They can involve any part of the body, but generally begin on the arms and legs. PN appears to have a neuropathic origin, with alterations in the dermal and epidermal small diameter nerve fibers.[1] The diagnosis is based on the physical features of the nodules and the presence of itching. A skin biopsy is often performed to exclude other diseases.

PN often has a tremendous impact on the quality of life. Unfortunately, few randomized controlled trials are available to guide therapy.[1] Intralesional steroids are highly effective, and triamcinolone acetonide is commonly used.[2] A total dose of up to 20 mg for adults may need to be repeated monthly for a maximum of 4 months to achieve a good clinical result.[3] More severe or recalcitrant cases may necessitate the use of phototherapy, systemic immunosuppressives, thalidomide, lenalidomide, opioid receptor antagonists, or neurokinin-1 receptor antagonists.[4] Regardless of the intervention, effective management of PN involves consideration of any associated psychological factors.[5]

PATIENT POSITION

- Usually supine on the examination table.
- Rotate the patient's head away from the side that is being injected. This minimizes anxiety and pain perception.
- The clinician stands on the side of the patient that allows best access to the PN lesion.

ANESTHESIA

- Local anesthesia of the injection site with topical vapocoolant spray.

EQUIPMENT

- Topical vapocoolant spray
- 3-mL syringe
- 25-gauge 1-in needle
- 0.25 to 1 mL of the 40 mg/mL steroid solution (10-40 mg of triamcinolone acetonide)
- One alcohol prep pad
- Two povidone-iodine or chlorhexidine prep pads
- Sterile gauze pads
- Sterile adhesive bandage

TECHNIQUE

1. Prep the insertion site with alcohol followed by the povidone-iodine or chlorhexidine pads.
2. Achieve good local anesthesia by using topical vapocoolant spray.
3. Position the needle and syringe at a 10° to 45° angle to the surface of the skin at the edge of the lesion with the tip of the needle directed toward the center of the nodule.
4. Using the no-touch technique, quickly introduce the needle at the edge of the lesion (Fig. 8.9).
5. Advance the needle into the lesion.
6. Withdraw the plunger of the syringe to ensure that there is no blood return.
7. Perform injection(s) of 0.1 mL to a maximum of 1 mL (40 mg/mL of triamcinolone acetonide) into the base of the lesion to uniformly infuse the entire lesion.
8. Avoid injection into the epidermis or subcutaneous tissues.
9. Following the injection of the corticosteroid solution, withdraw the needle.
10. Apply a sterile adhesive bandage.

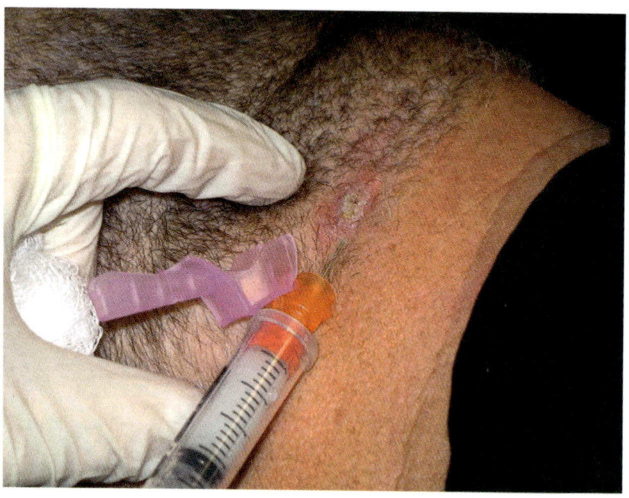

FIGURE 8.9 ● Injection of prurigo nodularis lesion using a 25-gauge needle with triamcinolone.

AFTERCARE

- None needed.
- Schedule a follow-up examination in 4 to 6 weeks.

PEARLS

- Avoid injection into the epidermis or subcutaneous tissues.

REFERENCES

1. Fostini AC, Girolomoni G, Tessari G. Prurigo nodularis: an update on etiopathogenesis and therapy. *J Dermatolog Treat.* 2013;24(6):458-462.
2. Todberg T, Zachariae C, Skov L. Treatment and burden of disease in a cohort of patients with prurigo nodularis: a survey-based study. *Acta Derm Venereol.* 2020;100(8):adv00119.
3. Richards RN. Update on intralesional steroid: focus on dermatoses. *J Cutan Med Surg.* 2010;14(1):19-23.
4. Kowalski EH, Kneiber D, Valdebran M, Patel U, Amber KT. Treatment-resistant prurigo nodularis: challenges and solutions. *Clin Cosmet Investig Dermatol.* 2019;12:163-172.
5. Lotti T, Buggiani G, Prignano F. Prurigo nodularis and lichen simplex chronicus. *Dermatol Ther.* 2008;21(1):42-46.

9

Temporomandibular Joint

James W. McNabb

Patients commonly present to the primary care office for evaluation of jaw pain from temporomandibular joint (TMJ) dysfunction and/or arthritis. Arthrocentesis of the TMJ combined with intra-articular washout and intra-articular injection of pharmacological agents has been used for many years. There is literature support for injecting corticosteroids in pediatric patients with juvenile idiopathic arthritis.[1] However, a recent systematic review of randomized controlled trials in adults shows that intra-articular injections with corticosteroids seem to result in similar findings to other therapeutic drugs, with no significant differences.[2] Furthermore, adverse effects limit their usefulness.[3]

Although not approved by the U.S. Food and Drug Administration, there is an increasing body of evidence that both hyaluronic acid[4,5] and especially platelet-rich plasma intra-articular injections[6,7] are effective in treating the pain of TMJ disorders in the medium and long term.[8] These injections appear significantly more effective than conservative treatments for both pain reduction and improvement of TMJ function. Therefore, injections should be implemented as first-line treatments or should be considered early, if patients do not show a clear benefit from initial conservative treatment.[9]

Ultrasound guidance of the procedure significantly improves localization of TMJ intra-articular injections,[10] especially in the pediatric population.[11,12]

Relevant Anatomy: (Fig. 9.1)

PATIENT POSITION

- Sitting on the examination table.
- The patient's hands are folded in their lap.

LANDMARKS

1. With the patient seated on the examination table, the clinician stands lateral and posterior to the affected jaw.
2. Palpate the TMJ with the mouth in the closed and then the fully open positions.
3. Identify the sulcus that forms with jaw opening and mark that spot with ink.
4. At that site, press firmly on the skin with the retracted tip of a ballpoint pen. This indentation represents the entry point for the needle.
5. After the landmarks are identified, the patient should not move the jaw.
6. The patient must keep his or her mouth open until the completion of the procedure.

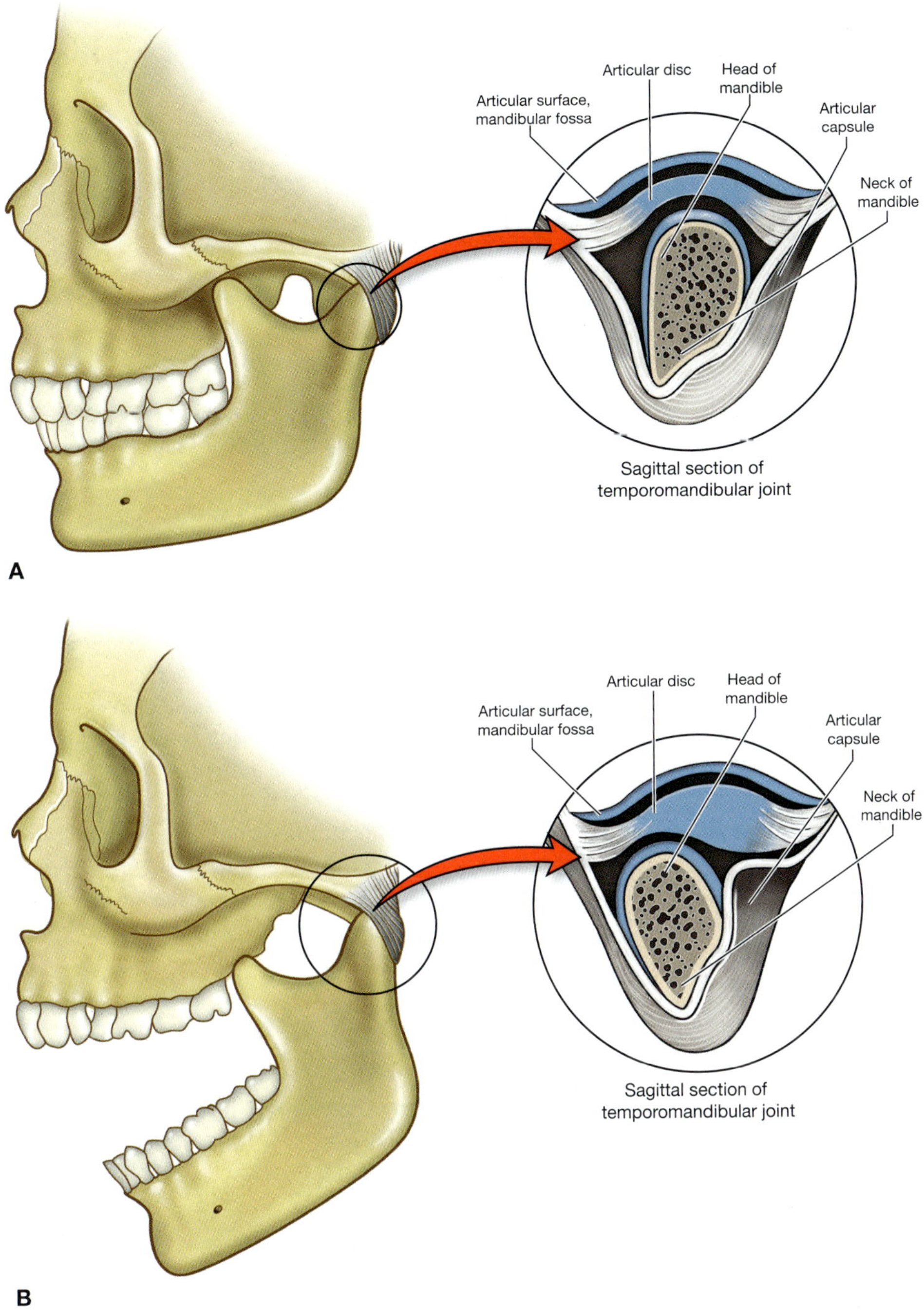

FIGURE 9.1 • Sagittal view of the temporomandibular joint. **A.** Jaw closed. **B.** Jaw open.

ANESTHESIA

- Local anesthesia of the skin using topical vapocoolant spray may be used. Make sure that "overspray" of the vapocoolant chemical does not enter the patient's eyes or external ear canal.

EQUIPMENT

- Topical vapocoolant spray
- 3-mL syringe
- 25-gauge 1-in needle
- 0.5 mL of 1% mepivacaine without epinephrine
- 0.5 mL of the 40 mg/mL steroid solution (20 mg of triamcinolone acetonide)
- One alcohol prep pad
- Two povidone-iodine or chlorhexidine prep pads
- Sterile gauze pads
- Sterile adhesive bandage

TECHNIQUE

1. Prep the insertion site with alcohol followed by the povidone-iodine or chlorhexidine pads.
2. Achieve good local anesthesia by using topical vapocoolant spray.
3. Position the needle and syringe from a posterior approach at a 30° angle to the sagittal plane into the sulcus with the tip of the needle directed anteromedial toward the posterior aspect of the TMJ.
4. Using the no-touch technique, quickly introduce the needle at the insertion site (Fig. 9.2).
5. Advance the needle toward the joint until the needle tip is located in the joint capsule. There will be a decrease in resistance when entering the joint capsule. After entering the joint space, the needle will touch the articular surface or the articular disk. Back up the needle 1 to 2 mm.
6. Withdraw the plunger of the syringe to ensure that there is no blood return.
7. Inject the mepivacaine/corticosteroid solution as a bolus into the TMJ articular capsule. The injected solution should flow smoothly into the space. If increased resistance is encountered, advance or withdraw the needle slightly before attempting further injection.
8. Following injection, withdraw the needle.
9. Apply a sterile adhesive bandage.

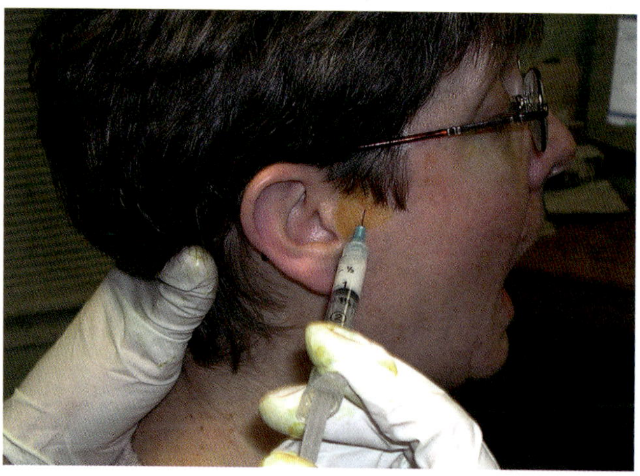

FIGURE 9.2 ● Temporomandibular joint injection.

10. Instruct the patient to move his or her jaw through its full range of motion. This movement distributes the mepivacaine/corticosteroid solution throughout the joint capsule.
11. Reexamine the TMJ in 5 minutes to assess pain relief.

AFTERCARE

- Avoid excessive use of the jaw by avoiding chewing gum, chewing tough foods, and excessive talking over the next 2 weeks.
- Nonsteroidal anti-inflammatory drugs (NSAIDs), ice, and/or physical therapy as indicated.
- Consider follow-up examination in 2 weeks.

PEARLS

- Be aware that there are reports of articular degeneration following corticosteroid joint injections—especially in adult patients.
- Consider ultrasound guidance to enhance both the accuracy and safety of this procedure.

A video showing a TMJ injection can be found in the companion eBook.

REFERENCES

1. Stoll ML, Good J, Sharpe T, et al. Intra-articular corticosteroid injections to the temporomandibular joints are safe and appear to be effective therapy in children with juvenile idiopathic arthritis. *J Oral Maxillofac Surg*. 2012;70(8):1802-1807.
2. Davoudi A, Khaki H, Mohammadi I, et al. Is arthrocentesis of temporomandibular joint with corticosteroids beneficial? A systematic review. *Med Oral Patol Oral Cir Bucal*. 2018;23(3):e367-e375.
3. Isacsson G, Schumann M, Nohlert E, Mejersjö C, Tegelberg Å. Pain relief following a single-dose intra-articular injection of methylprednisolone in the temporomandibular joint arthralgia—a multicentre randomised controlled trial. *J Oral Rehabil*. 2019;46(1):5-13.
4. Manfredini D, Piccotti F, Guarda-Nardini L. Hyaluronic acid in the treatment of TMJ disorders: a systematic review of the literature. *Cranio*. 2010;28(3):166-176.
5. Guarda-Nardini L, Cadorin C, Frizziero A, Ferronato G, Manfredini D. Comparison of 2 hyaluronic acid drugs for the treatment of temporomandibular joint osteoarthritis. *J Oral Maxillofac Surg*. 2012;70(11):2522-2530.
6. Haigler MC, Abdulrehman E, Siddappa S, Kishore R, Padilla M, Enciso R. Use of platelet-rich plasma, platelet-rich growth factor with arthrocentesis or arthroscopy to treat temporomandibular joint osteoarthritis: systematic review with meta-analyses. *J Am Dent Assoc*. 2018;149(11):940-952.e2.
7. Chung PY, Lin MT, Chang HP. Effectiveness of platelet-rich plasma injection in patients with temporomandibular joint osteoarthritis: a systematic review and meta-analysis of randomized controlled trials. *Oral Surg Oral Med Oral Pathol Oral Radiol*. 2019;127(2):106-116.
8. Li F, Wu C, Sun H, Zhou Q. Effect of platelet-rich plasma injections on pain reduction in patients with temporomandibular joint osteoarthrosis: a meta-analysis of randomized controlled trials. *J Oral Facial Pain Headache*. 2020;34(2):149-156.
9. Al-Moraissi EA, Wolford LM, Ellis E III, Neff A. The hierarchy of different treatments for arthrogenous temporomandibular disorders: a network meta-analysis of randomized clinical trials. *J Craniomaxillofac Surg*. 2020;48(1):9-23.
10. Champs B, Corre P, Hamel A, Laffite CD, Le Goff B. US-guided temporomandibular joint injection: validation of an in-plane longitudinal approach. *J Stomatol Oral Maxillofac Surg*. 2019;120(1):67-70.
11. Young CM, Shiels WE II, Coley BD. Ultrasound-guided corticosteroid injection therapy for juvenile idiopathic arthritis: 12-year care experience. *Pediatr Radiol*. 2012;42(12):1481-1489.
12. Habibi S, Ellis J, Strike H, Ramanan AV. Safety and efficacy of US-guided CS injection into temporomandibular joints in children with active JIA. *Rheumatology (Oxford)*. 2012;51(5):874-877.

Suprascapular Nerve

Patients uncommonly present to the primary care office for evaluation of suprascapular neuropathy. It is an underdiagnosed disorder that is the result of nerve entrapment and compression. The suprascapular nerve is vulnerable as it passes through the suprascapular notch and again at the spinoglenoid notch. Entrapment at the former leads to weakness of the supraspinatus and infraspinatus muscles as well as vague unilateral posterior shoulder pain that is described as a deep, dull, aching discomfort that is exacerbated with overhead throwing motions. Entrapment at the latter causes weakness of the infraspinatus muscle and is generally painless. The most common causes of suprascapular neuropathy are acute trauma, inflammatory processes (ie, brachial neuritis), a spinoglenoid notch cyst, and rotator cuff tears and overuse.[1] Spinoglenoid notch cysts and suprascapular notch entrapment respond best to surgical decompression, while overuse and viral etiologies respond best to conservative measures.[2] A nerve block at the suprascapular notch can be used in the conservative management of this condition as well as to treat shoulder pain following surgery,[3] hemiplegic shoulder pain following strokes,[4,5] and pain associated with adhesive capsulitis.[6] Ultrasound-guided suprascapular nerve blocks are more effective and safer than nonguided techniques to treat pain due to suprascapular nerve entrapment.[7]

Relevant Anatomy: (Fig. 9.3)

PATIENT POSITION

- Sitting on an examination stool, with arms resting on the examination table and neck in a neutral position.

LANDMARKS

1. With the patient sitting on an examination stool, the clinician stands posterior to the affected scapula.
2. Find the midpoint between the tip of the acromion and the medial aspect of the spine of the scapula, and mark it with an ink pen.
3. Find the coracoid process, and mark it with an ink pen.
4. Draw a line between these two points, and mark the midposition of this line.
5. At that site, press firmly on the skin with the retracted tip of a ballpoint pen. This indentation represents the entry point for the needle.
6. After the landmarks are identified, the patient should not move.

ANESTHESIA

- Local anesthesia of the skin using topical vapocoolant spray.

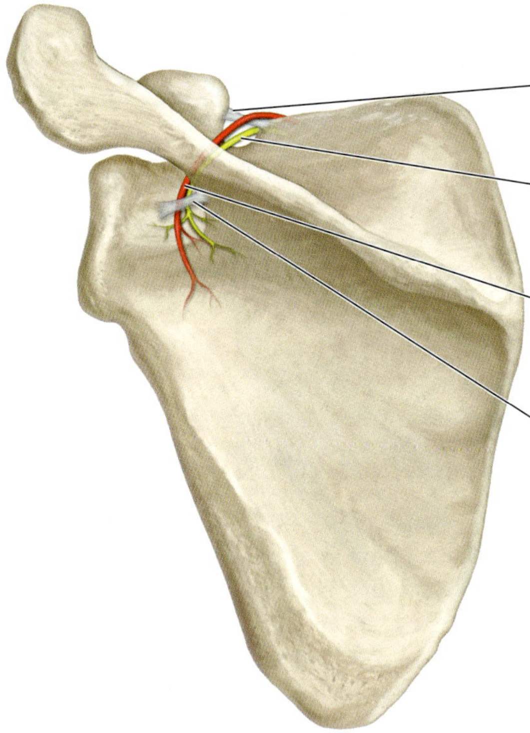

FIGURE 9.3 • Nerves and vessels of left posterior scapular region.

EQUIPMENT

- Topical vapocoolant spray
- 3-mL syringe
- 25-gauge 1½-in needle
- 1 mL of 1% lidocaine without epinephrine
- 1 mL of the 40 mg/mL steroid solution (40 mg of triamcinolone acetonide)
- One alcohol prep pad
- Two povidone-iodine or chlorhexidine prep pads
- Sterile gauze pads
- Sterile adhesive bandage

TECHNIQUE

1. Prep the insertion site with alcohol followed by the povidone-iodine or chlorhexidine pads.
2. Achieve good local anesthesia by using topical vapocoolant spray.
3. Position the needle and syringe perpendicular to the skin with the tip of the needle directed toward the suprascapular notch.
4. Using the no-touch technique, quickly introduce the needle at the insertion site (Fig. 9.4).
5. Advance the needle completely through the supraspinatus muscle and touch the bone of the suprascapular fossa. Back up the needle 1 to 2 mm.
6. Withdraw the plunger of the syringe to ensure that there is no blood return.

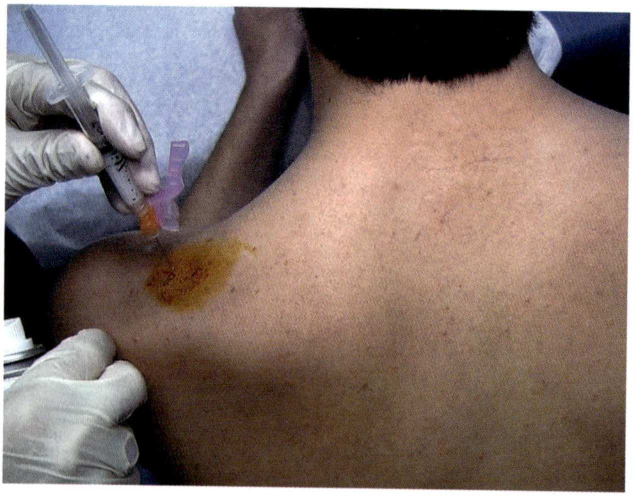

FIGURE 9.4 ● Suprascapular nerve injection.

7. Inject the lidocaine/corticosteroid solution as a bolus into the muscle around the suprascapular nerve. The injected solution should flow smoothly into this area. If increased resistance is encountered, advance or withdraw the needle slightly before attempting further injection.
8. Following injection, withdraw the needle.
9. Apply a sterile adhesive bandage.
10. Instruct the patient to move his or her shoulder through its full range of motion in external rotation and abduction. This movement distributes the lidocaine/corticosteroid solution throughout the suprascapular fossa.
11. Reexamine the shoulder and scapula in 5 minutes to assess pain relief.

AFTERCARE

- Avoid excessive abduction, external rotation, and overhead throwing motions of the shoulder over the next 2 weeks.
- NSAIDs, ice, and/or physical therapy as indicated.
- Consider follow-up examination in 2 weeks.

PEARLS

- Consider ultrasound guidance to enhance both the accuracy and safety of this procedure—particularly to avoid pneumothorax and/or vascular injury (Fig. 9.5).
- Always aspirate before injecting to make sure that the needle tip is not in the suprascapular artery.
- If there is no significant improvement in pain or weakness, and the diagnosis has been confirmed by electromyography, then refer the patient for surgical decompression of the superior or inferior transverse scapular ligaments.

ULTRASOUND-GUIDED PROCEDURE

Please refer to the introductory ultrasound chapter for preprocedure, sterile prep, post-procedure, and documentation information and recommendations.

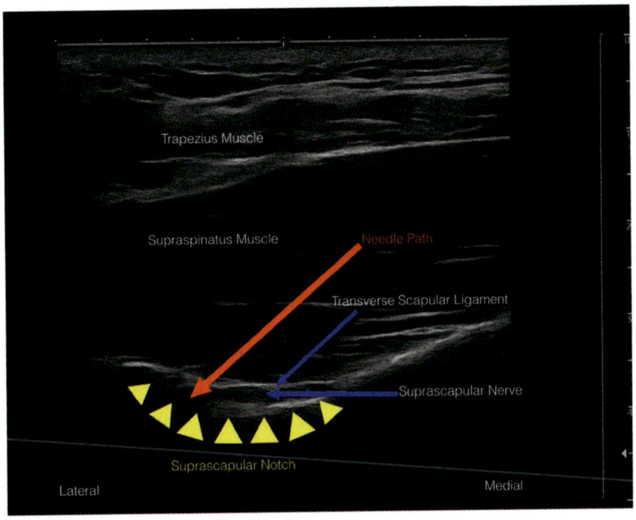

FIGURE 9.5 • Suprascapular nerve at the suprascapular notch ultrasound image.

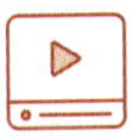
A video showing a landmark-based suprascapular nerve injection can be found in the companion eBook.

REFERENCES

1. Hill LJ, Jelsing EJ, Terry MJ, Strommen JA. Evaluation, treatment, and outcomes of suprascapular neuropathy: a 5-year review. *PM R*. 2014;6(9):774-780. pii:S1934-1482(14)00071-9.
2. Antoniou J, Tae SK, Williams GR, Bird S, Ramsey ML, Iannotti JP. Suprascapular neuropathy. Variability in the diagnosis, treatment, and outcome. *Clin Orthop Relat Res*. 2001;(386):131-138.
3. Jerosch J, Saad M, Greig M, Filler T. Suprascapular nerve block as a method of preemptive pain control in shoulder surgery. *Knee Surg Sports Traumatol Arthrosc*. 2008;16(6):602-607.
4. Picelli A, Bonazza S, Lobba D, et al. Suprascapular nerve block for the treatment of hemiplegic shoulder pain in patients with long-term chronic stroke: a pilot study. *Neurol Sci*. 2017;38(9):1697-1701.
5. Adey-Wakeling Z, Crotty M, Shanahan EM. Suprascapular nerve block for shoulder pain in the first year after stroke: a randomized controlled trial. *Stroke*. 2013;44(11):3136-3141.
6. Jones DS, Chattopadhyay C. Suprascapular nerve block for the treatment of frozen shoulder in primary care: a randomized trial. *Br J Gen Pract*. 1999;49(438):39-41.
7. Aydın T, Şen Eİ, Yardımcı MY, Kesiktaş FN, Öneş K, Paker N. Efficacy of ultrasound-guided suprascapular nerve block treatment in patients with painful hemiplegic shoulder. *Neurol Sci*. 2019;40(5):985-991.

Scapulothoracic Syndrome

Scapulothoracic syndrome is an uncommon problem in general clinical practice. It primarily affects middle-aged persons whose occupations require them to extend their arms for prolonged periods of time. This can also occur as a complication from preexisting shoulder lesions or in disabled patients who are unable to control the scapulothoracic relationship. The abnormal positioning causes bursitis because of altered biomechanics of the scapula and the underlying posterior chest wall. Scapulothoracic syndrome is characterized by pain that may be localized to the medial superior border of the scapula or may radiate to the neck and shoulder. Nonsurgical therapy utilizing scapular stabilization, postural exercises, and/or local corticosteroid injections can be effective for symptoms due to scapular dyskinesis or benign, nonosseous lesions.[1] However, these techniques are less successful than surgical management in patients with anatomic abnormalities.[2] In patients with normal anatomy, this condition can be successfully treated with a local corticosteroid injection at site of maximum tenderness at the medial superior scapular border.[3] Ultrasound guidance improves the accuracy and safety of scapulothoracic bursa injections.[4]

Relevant Anatomy: (Fig. 9.6)

PATIENT POSITION

- Sitting erect on an examination stool, with their ipsilateral hand on the contralateral shoulder.

LANDMARKS

1. With the patient seated on the examination stool, the clinician stands or sits behind the affected scapula.
2. Palpate to determine the area of most intense pain. This is usually along the superior aspect of the medial border of the scapula. Mark this location with an ink pen.
3. At that site, press firmly on the skin with the retracted tip of a ballpoint pen. This indentation represents the entry point for the needle.
4. After the landmarks are identified, the patient should not move.

ANESTHESIA

- Local anesthesia of the skin using topical vapocoolant spray.

EQUIPMENT

- Topical vapocoolant spray
- 3-mL syringe

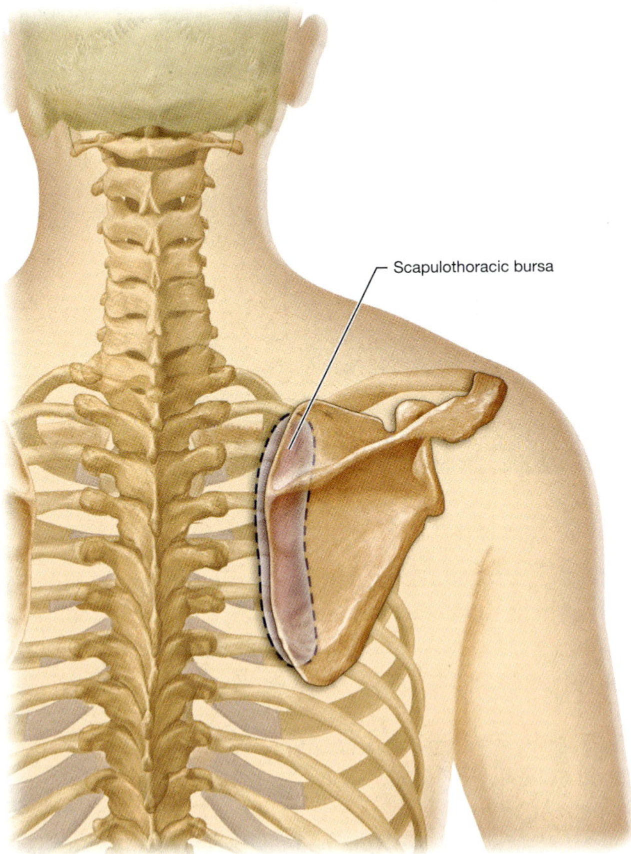

FIGURE 9.6 ● Scapulothoracic bursa.

- 25-gauge 1½-in needle
- 1 mL of 1% lidocaine without epinephrine
- 1 mL of the 40 mg/mL steroid solution (40 mg of triamcinolone acetonide)
- One alcohol prep pad
- Two povidone-iodine or chlorhexidine prep pads
- Sterile gauze pads
- Sterile adhesive bandage

TECHNIQUE

1. Prep the insertion site with alcohol followed by the povidone-iodine or chlorhexidine pads.
2. Achieve good local anesthesia by using topical vapocoolant spray.
3. Position the needle and syringe at a 20° angle to the skin with the tip of the needle directed toward the area of tenderness in the scapulothoracic space.
4. Using the no-touch technique, quickly introduce the needle at the insertion site (Fig. 9.7).
5. Advance the needle into the point of maximal tenderness in a plane parallel to the undersurface of the scapula, not toward the chest wall.
6. Withdraw the plunger of the syringe to ensure that there is no blood return.

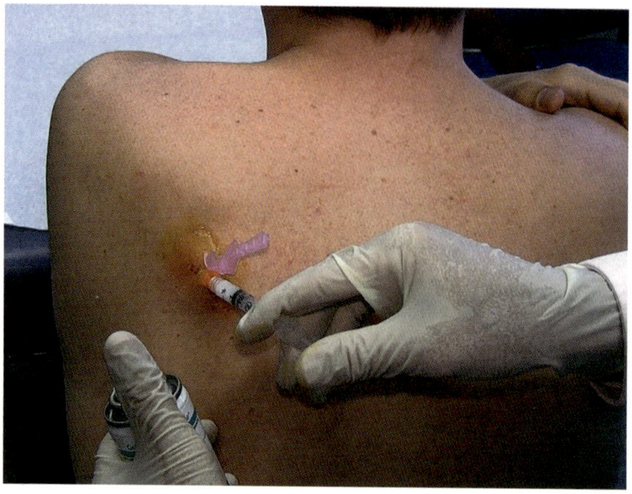

FIGURE 9.7 ● Scapulothoracic bursa injection.

7. Inject half of the lidocaine/corticosteroid solution as a bolus at the point of maximal tenderness and the remainder in the scapulothoracic space. The injected solution should flow smoothly into the space. If increased resistance is encountered, advance or withdraw the needle slightly before attempting further injection.
8. Following injection, withdraw the needle.
9. Apply a sterile adhesive bandage.
10. Instruct the patient to move his or her shoulder through its full range of motion. This movement distributes the lidocaine/corticosteroid solution throughout the area.
11. Reexamine the scapula in 5 minutes to assess pain relief.

AFTERCARE

- Avoid excessive shoulder abduction, protraction, retraction, or pushing, pulling, and overhead throwing motions over the next 2 weeks.
- NSAIDs, ice, and/or physical therapy as indicated.
- Consider follow-up examination in 2 weeks.

PEARLS

- Consider ultrasound guidance to enhance both the accuracy and safety of this procedure (Fig. 9.8).
- Avoid advancing the needle so deeply as to risk the complication of pneumothorax.

ULTRASOUND-GUIDED PROCEDURE

Please refer to the introductory ultrasound chapter for preprocedure, sterile prep, post-procedure, and documentation information and recommendations.

A video showing a landmark-guided scapulothoracic bursa injection can be found in the companion eBook.

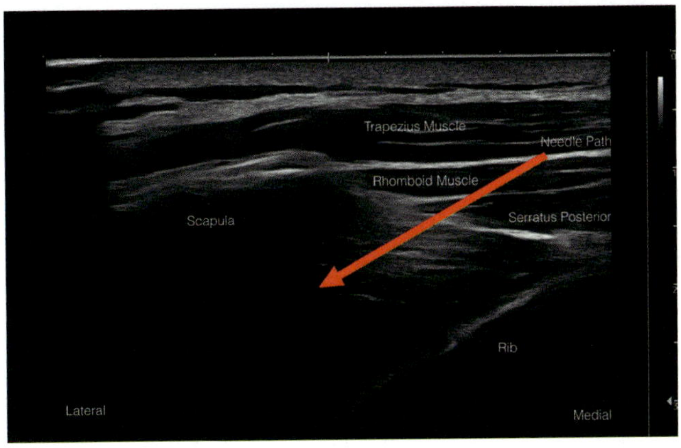

FIGURE 9.8 • Scapulothoracic bursa ultrasound image.

REFERENCES

1. Osias W, Matcuk GR Jr, Skalski MR, et al. Scapulothoracic pathology: review of anatomy, pathophysiology, imaging findings, and an approach to management. *Skeletal Radiol.* 2018;47(2):161-171.
2. Gaskill T, Millett PJ. Snapping scapula syndrome: diagnosis and management. *J Am Acad Orthop Surg.* 2013;21(4):214-224.
3. Boneti C, Arentz C, Klimberg VS. Scapulothoracic bursitis as a significant cause of breast and chest wall pain: underrecognized and undertreated. *Ann Surg Oncol.* 2010;17(Suppl 3):321-324.
4. Walter WR, Burke CJ, Adler RS. Ultrasound-guided therapeutic scapulothoracic interval injections. *J Ultrasound Med.* 2019;38(7):1899-1906.

Sacroiliac Joint

Pain involving the sacroiliac (SI) joint(s) is a common condition seen by primary care physicians.[1] SI joint pain may be caused by acute or repetitive trauma, spondyloarthropathies, degenerative arthritis, pregnancy, and rarely by an infection of the joint. Injection into the SI joint(s) can be both diagnostic and therapeutic. Corticosteroid injections are an effective conservative treatment option for sacroiliitis.[2] These can be safely and effectively performed using landmark-guided techniques because significant extra-articular sources of SI region pain exist.[3,4] However, ultrasound-guided SI joint injections are shown to increase the accuracy[5] and improve the treatment effect of pain relief and function. In addition, ultrasound may improve safety by facilitating the identification and avoidance of critical vessels around or within the SI joints.[6] Other agents including platelet-rich plasma,[7] botulinum toxin injections,[8] and prolotherapy[9] utilizing dextrose show promise for the treatment of SI joint pain.

Relevant Anatomy: (Fig. 9.9)

PATIENT POSITION

- Patient is standing and leaning over an examination table with the forearms supported by the table. The back is held in a position of 45° of forward flexion.

LANDMARKS

1. With the patient standing fully upright, the clinician stands directly behind the patient.
2. Identify tenderness over the SI joint.
3. While continuously palpating the location of the SI joint, have the patient lean forward, to 45° of forward flexion, over the examination table and support their upper body with the forearms.
4. Mark the location of the SI joint with ink.
5. At that site, press firmly on the skin with the retracted tip of a ballpoint pen. This indentation represents the entry point for the needle.

ANESTHESIA

- Local anesthesia of the skin using Pain Ease Mist topical vapocoolant spray.

EQUIPMENT

- Topical vapocoolant spray
- 3-mL syringe
- 25-gauge 2-in needle

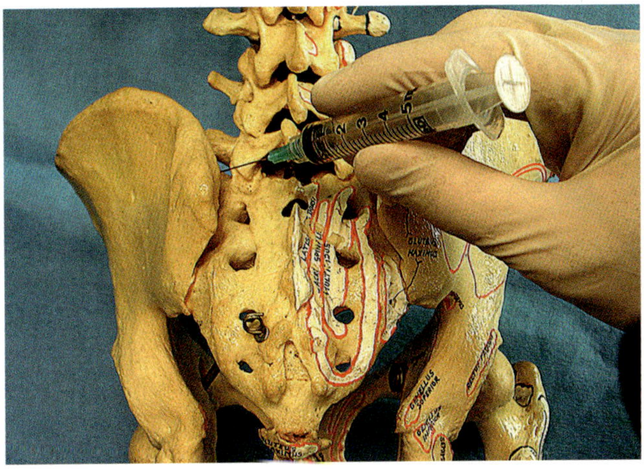

FIGURE 9.9 ● Sacroiliac anatomy—note the angle of insertion.

- 1 mL of 1% mepivacaine without epinephrine
- 1 mL of the 40 mg/mL steroid solution (40 mg of triamcinolone acetonide)
- One alcohol prep pad
- Two povidone-iodine or chlorhexidine prep pads
- Sterile gauze pads
- Sterile adhesive bandage

TECHNIQUE

1. Prep the insertion site with alcohol followed by the povidone-iodine or chlorhexidine pads.
2. Achieve good local anesthesia by using Pain Ease Mist topical vapocoolant spray.
3. Position the 25-gauge 2-in needle at a 30° angle laterally, relative to the sagittal plane, and 15° inferiorly, relative to the axial plane, with the tip of the needle directed toward the SI joint.
4. Using the no-touch technique, quickly introduce the needle at the insertion site (Fig. 9.10).

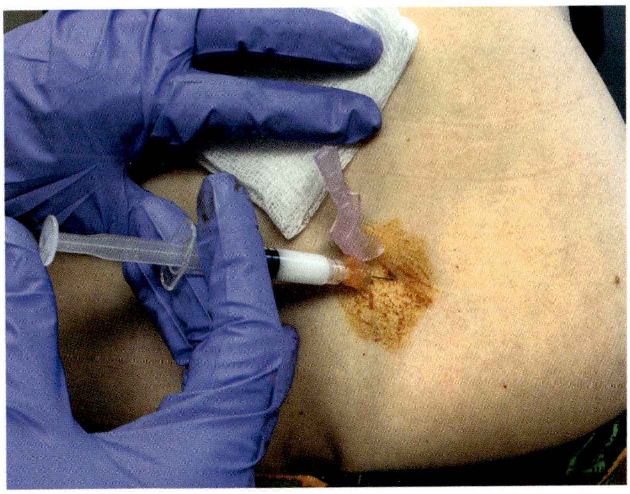

FIGURE 9.10 ● Sacroiliac joint injection.

5. Advance the needle slowly and carefully into the SI joint.
6. Withdraw the plunger of the syringe to ensure that there is no blood return.
7. Inject the mepivacaine/corticosteroid solution as a bolus into the SI joint. The injected solution should flow smoothly into the space. If increased resistance is encountered, advance or withdraw the needle slightly before attempting further injection.
8. Following injection, withdraw the needle.
9. Apply a sterile adhesive bandage.
10. Reexamine the SI joint in 5 minutes to assess pain relief.

AFTERCARE

- NSAIDs, ice, and/or physical therapy as indicated.
- Treatment of the underlying condition.
- Consider follow-up examination in 2 weeks.

PEARLS

- Consider ultrasound guidance to enhance both the accuracy and safety of this procedure (Fig. 9.11).
- Use Pain Ease Mist spray to provide a topical vapocoolant anesthetic effect. That product does not "run" down the skin. Both Ethyl Chloride and Pain Ease Stream Spray products leave a liquid residue that will follow gravity and accumulate in the patients' groin, thus turning this injection into a very uncomfortable experience!

ULTRASOUND-GUIDED PROCEDURE

Please refer to the introductory ultrasound chapter for preprocedure, sterile prep, post-procedure, and documentation information and recommendations.

A video showing a landmark-based sacroiliac joint injection can be found in the companion eBook.

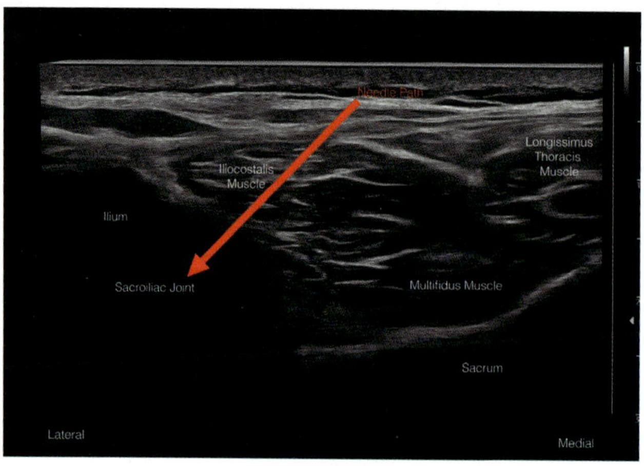

FIGURE 9.11 ● Sacroiliac joint ultrasound image.

REFERENCES

1. Wu L, Varacallo M. Sacroiliac joint injection. *StatPearls [Internet].* StatPearls Publishing; 2020. http://www.ncbi.nlm.nih.gov/books/NBK513245/
2. Hawkins J, Schofferman J. Serial therapeutic sacroiliac joint injections: a practice audit. *Pain Med.* 2009;10(5):850-853.
3. Borowsky CD, Fagen G. Sources of sacroiliac region pain: insights gained from a study comparing standard intra-articular injection with a technique combining intra- and peri-articular injection. *Arch Phys Med Rehabil.* 2008;89(11):2048-2056.
4. Hartung W, Ross CJ, Straub R, et al. Ultrasound-guided sacroiliac joint injection in patients with established sacroiliitis: precise IA injection verified by MRI scanning does not predict clinical outcome. *Rheumatology (Oxford).* 2010;49(8):1479-1482.
5. De Luigi AJ, Saini V, Mathur R, Saini A, Yokel N. Assessing the accuracy of ultrasound-guided needle placement in sacroiliac joint injections. *Am J Phys Med Rehabil.* 2019;98(8):666-670.
6. Jee H, Lee JH, Park KD, Ahn J, Park Y. Ultrasound-guided versus fluoroscopy-guided sacroiliac joint intra-articular injections in the noninflammatory sacroiliac joint dysfunction: a prospective, randomized, single-blinded study. *Arch Phys Med Rehabil.* 2014;95(2):330-337.
7. Mohi Eldin M, Sorour OO, Hassan ASA, Baraka M, Ahmed MF. Percutaneous injection of autologous platelet-rich fibrin versus platelet-rich plasma in sacroiliac joint dysfunction: an applied comparative study. *J Back Musculoskelet Rehabil.* 2019;32(3):511-518.
8. Lee JH, Lee SH, Song SH. Clinical effectiveness of botulinum toxin A compared to a mixture of steroid and local anesthetics as a treatment for sacroiliac joint pain. *Pain Med.* 2010;11(5):692-700.
9. Kim WM, Lee HG, Jeong CW, Kim CM, Yoon MH. A randomized controlled trial of intra-articular prolotherapy versus steroid injection for sacroiliac joint pain. *J Altern Complement Med.* 2010;16(12):1285-1290.

10

Subacromial Space—Posterior Approach

James W. McNabb

The shoulder is the most common site of nonaxial musculoskeletal pain. Subacromial disorders comprise the bulk of these complaints presenting to primary care clinicians. Most of these are treatable by conservative management augmented with injection therapy. These conditions commonly arise from acute trauma, overuse injury, and/or chronic degenerative changes that involve the rotator cuff complex, a group of muscles and tendons that stabilize the shoulder joint. Since the subacromial space is in close proximity to the rotator cuff complex, it allows convenient access to these structures for injection therapies. If the rotator cuff is intact, the subacromial bursa is separate and distinct from the glenohumeral (GH) joint. In patients with full-thickness rotator cuff tears, the subacromial bursa may communicate with the GH joint, which can be noted on advanced imaging such as magnetic resonance imaging. In this case, consider a surgical referral. If surgery is not an option, through a shared decision-making process with the patient, a well-placed subacromial space injection can provide therapy to the rotator cuff, GH joint, and even the proximal aspect of the long head of the biceps tendon.[1,2]

There are three main approaches for performing subacromial space injections: lateral, anterior, and posterior. However, the **posterior approach is generally preferred**. It is the least technical and most patient-friendly approach, whether performing landmark-guided or ultrasound-guided injections. Since patients cannot see the advancing needle, anxiety is diminished. Of the three standard portals, it holds an additional advantage over the others when performing landmark-guided injections. When using the landmark-guided posterior approach, the needle is directed cephalad piercing the deltoid muscle, passing over the supraspinatus muscle/tendon, entering the subacromial space, and ultimately contacting the underside of the acromion. Therefore, accurate placement is confirmed. When utilizing the anterior and lateral approaches without ultrasound guidance, there is a high risk of injecting the corticosteroid into the supraspinatus muscle/tendon, potentially leading to further tendinopathy or even rupture. Dependent on body habitus, the posterior approach typically requires a 25-gauge 2-in needle to accurately inject anesthetic and/or steroid solution into the subacromial space.[3] A large-diameter needle is infrequently used because a significant effusion rarely collects in the subacromial-subdeltoid (SA-SD) bursa.

The medical literature demonstrates that low-volume corticosteroid injections[4] in the subacromial space are effective in the short- to medium-term treatment of rotator cuff disorders[5,6] and for the treatment of adhesive capsulitis.[7,8] On the other hand, a meta-analysis showed that corticosteroid injections provide only small and transient pain relief in patients with rotator cuff tendinosis.[9] In studies of optimal corticosteroid dosing, there was no difference in pain or function between intra-articular injections of 20 or 40 mg of triamcinolone acetonide.[10,11] Safety is also increased since the use of corticosteroid injections in patients with subacromial impingement does not result in an increase in rotator cuff tears.[12] Platelet-rich plasma (PRP) injections are an emerging therapeutic option.[13] Hyaluronic acid viscosupplementation for the treatment of GH osteoarthritis has been studied and shown to be effective at 12 weeks.[14-17] However, this has not been approved by the Food and Drug Administration for use outside of osteoarthritis of the knee. The use of ultrasound improves the accuracy[18] and efficacy of therapeutic injections.[19]

A subacromial injection performed using local anesthetic without steroid can help the clinician differentiate the cause of nonlocalized shoulder pain. The injected anesthetic removes pain from subacromial impingement as a confounding factor and allows the clinician to physically test the integrity of the rotator cuff complex by asking the patient to abduct the shoulder. This is known as the "impingement injection test." Injection of local anesthetic does not cause muscle weakness and therefore does not affect the validity of this test.[20]

Relevant Anatomy: (Figs. 10.1 and 10.2)

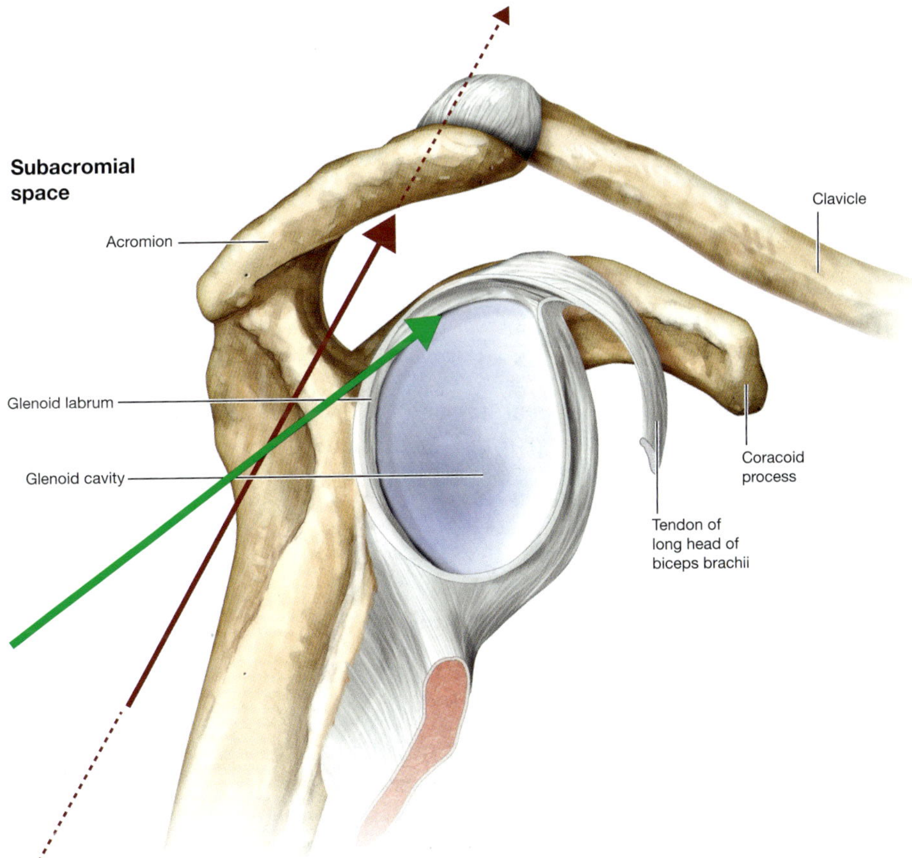

FIGURE 10.1 ● Lateral aspect of right shoulder (*red arrow* indicates path of the needle for landmark-guided injections and the *green arrow* indicates the path of the needle for the ultrasound-guided injections). (Reprinted with permission from Agur AMR, Dalley AF II. *Grant's Atlas of Anatomy*. 16th ed. Wolters Kluwer; 2025.)

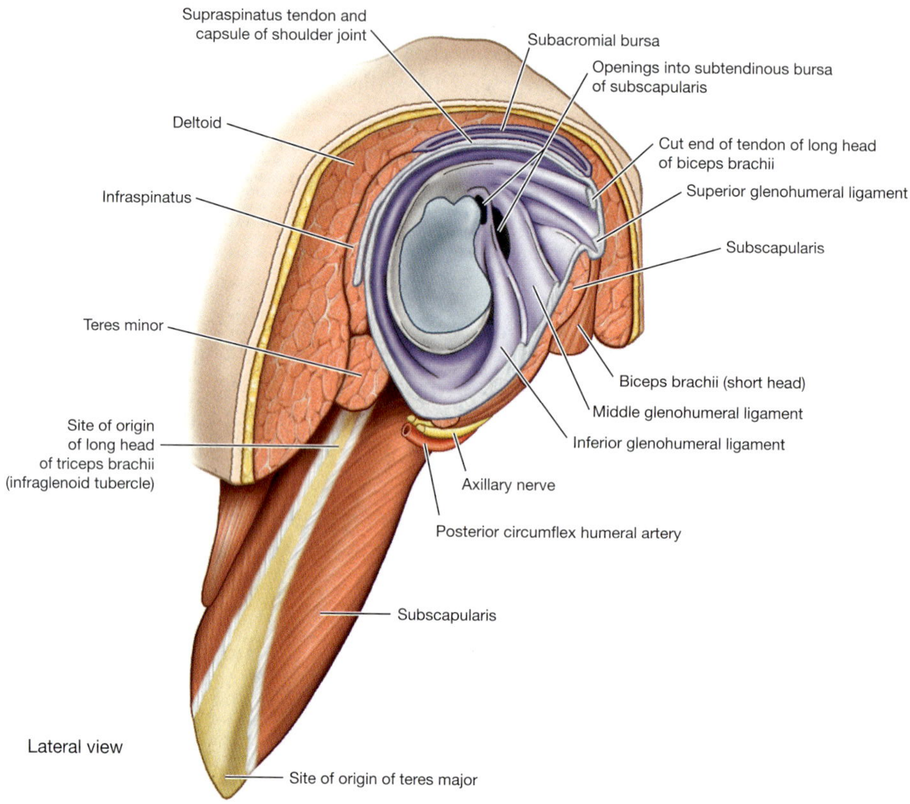

FIGURE 10.2 ● Interior of right shoulder. (Reprinted with permission from Agur AMR, Dalley AF II. *Grant's Atlas of Anatomy*. 16th ed. Wolters Kluwer; 2025.)

LANDMARK-GUIDED PROCEDURE

PATIENT POSITION

- Sitting on the examination table.
- The patient's hands are folded in their lap with fingers interlaced.
- This allows consistent positioning of the shoulder so that the landmarks do not change from the time that they are identified and marked until the time of injection.

PROVIDER POSITION

- The provider stands lateral and posterior to the affected shoulder.

LANDMARKS

1. Find the lateral edge of the acromion and mark it with an ink pen.
2. Palpate the posterior border of the acromion and mark that.
3. Having identified the posterior lateral corner of the acromion, drop a vertical line down from that point and mark a spot 2 cm below the posterior lateral corner.
4. At that site, press firmly with the retracted tip of a ballpoint pen. This indentation represents the entry point for the needle.

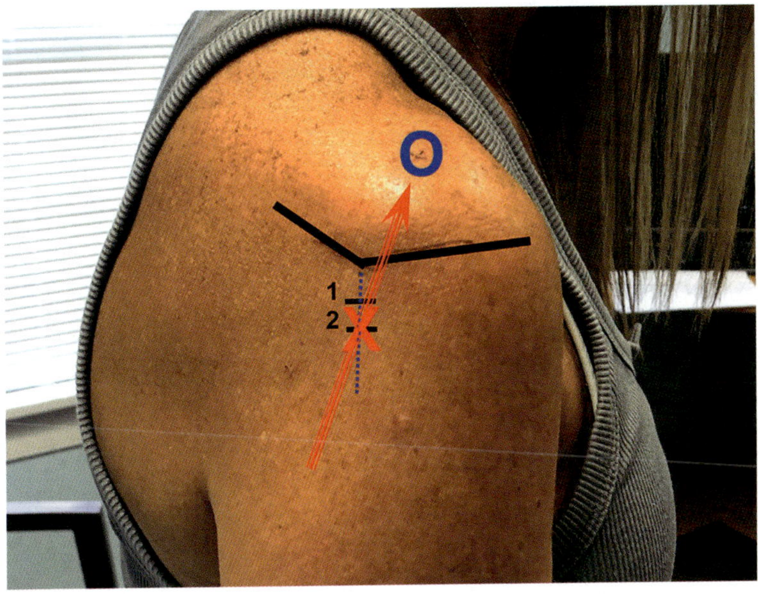

FIGURE 10.3 ● Right shoulder injection landmarks.

5. Next, identify the target site by placing the index finger of the nondominant hand over the superior aspect of the acromion posterior to the acromioclavicular (AC) joint. As you palpate, please realize that the acromion has length and width. The target site is in the center of the acromion. This will be the target for the tip of the needle (Fig. 10.3). If the index finger is at the target site—on top of the acromion—it should be protected from accidental needlestick.
6. After the landmarks are identified, the patient should not move the shoulder or arm.

ANESTHESIA

- The no-touch technique is utilized for the injection to avoid infections. However, tactile skin distraction is administered by firmly stroking the skin **outside** of the injection point immediately before and during the time that the small-diameter needle is quickly introduced into the skin.
- Topical vapocoolant spray or injection of a local anesthetic is unnecessary in almost all patients.

EQUIPMENT

- 3-mL syringe
- 25-gauge 2-in needle (Consider a 3½-in 22-gauge spinal needle in large individuals.)
- 1 mL of 1% mepivacaine without epinephrine
- 0.5 to 1 mL of the 40 mg/mL steroid solution (20-40 mg of triamcinolone acetonide)
- One alcohol prep pad
- Two povidone-iodine or chlorhexidine prep pads
- Sterile gauze pads
- Sterile adhesive bandage

TECHNIQUE

1. Prep the insertion site with alcohol followed by the povidone-iodine or chlorhexidine pads.
2. Position the needle and syringe at about a 30° angle to the skin with the needle tip directed cephalad toward the acromion.
3. Using the no-touch technique, quickly introduce the needle at the insertion site (Fig. 10.4).
4. Direct the needle underneath the acromion and advance it toward the target until the needle tip touches the undersurface of the acromion. Back up the needle 1 to 2 mm.
5. Withdraw the plunger of the syringe to ensure that there is no blood return.
6. Inject the mepivacaine/corticosteroid solution as a bolus into the subacromial space. The injected solution should flow smoothly into the space. Increased resistance may indicate that the injected fluid is entering the supraspinatus muscle or tendon. In that case, advance or withdraw the needle slightly before attempting further injection.
7. Following injection, withdraw the needle.
8. Apply a sterile adhesive bandage.
9. Instruct the patient to move their shoulder through its full range of motion. This movement distributes the mepivacaine/corticosteroid solution throughout the subacromial space.
10. Reexamine the shoulder in 5 minutes to assess pain relief.

AFTERCARE

- Avoid excessive use of the shoulder over the next 2 weeks.
- Consider the use of an arm sling.

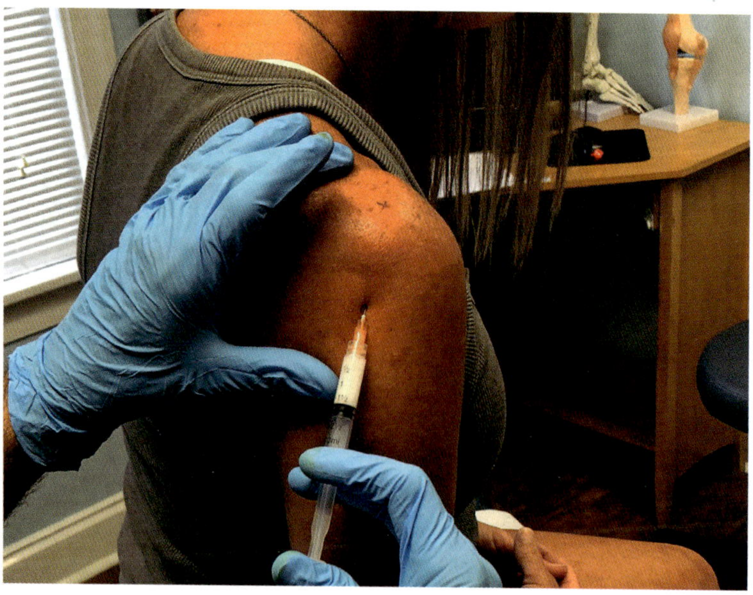

FIGURE 10.4 ● Right shoulder subacromial space injection.

- Nonsteroidal anti-inflammatory drugs (NSAIDs), ice, and/or physical therapy as indicated.
- Consider follow-up examination in 2 weeks.

PEARLS

- The correct identification of the acromion landmarks is more difficult than many primary care providers realize. Make sure to take time and recheck the landmarks before proceeding with the injection.
- When palpating to determine the anatomy of the acromion, use the tips of the index, middle, and ring fingers positioned in a straight line. Firmly, carefully, and methodically move in a distal to proximal direction. Mark the site where fingers contact the lateral and posterior margins of the acromion.
- For most patients, use a long 2-in 25-gauge needle for this injection.
- Ensure that the needle is underneath the acromion before advancing it toward the target finger.
- Always keep the target finger over the acromion to protect it from accidental needlestick.

ULTRASOUND-GUIDED PROCEDURE

Please refer to the introductory ultrasound chapter for preprocedure, sterile prep, post-procedure, and documentation information and recommendations.

PATIENT POSITION

- Lateral decubitus on the examination table with their affected shoulder upward.
- Internally rotate the affected shoulder across the patient's body, maintaining 90° of elbow flexion.
- Place a pillow under their head for comfort.
- Adjust the patient's position as needed for comfort.

PROVIDER/ULTRASOUND POSITION

- The provider sits behind the patient's affected shoulder.
- Adjust the examination table to position the injection site between the provider's umbilicus and axillary level, ensuring optimal ergonomics and visualization of the ultrasound screen, transducer, and needle's approach (Fig. 10.5).
- Position the ultrasound machine on the opposite side of the table from the provider at the level of the patient's shoulders with the screen facing the provider.

LANDMARKS

See the landmarks for the landmark-guided injection procedure.

ANESTHESIA

- Local anesthesia of the skin using topical vapocoolant spray.

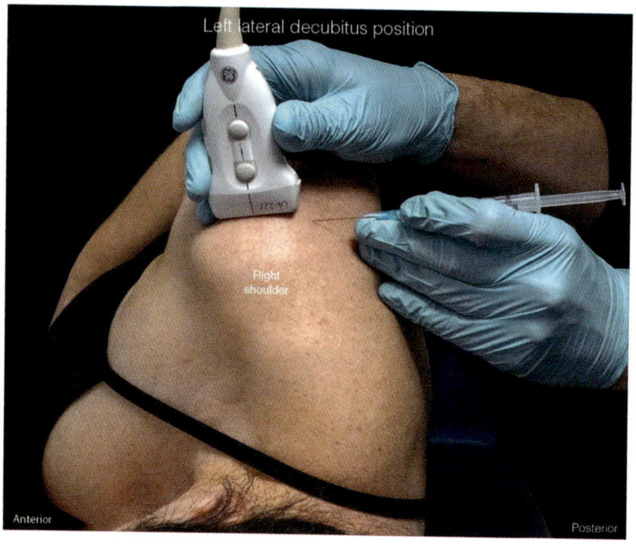

FIGURE 10.5 ● Right shoulder ultrasound-guided subacromial-subdeltoid bursa injection. Left lateral decubitus position, with the affected shoulder uppermost.

EQUIPMENT

- 3-mL syringe
- 25-gauge 2-in needle (adjust needle length based on body habitus)
- 1 mL of 1% mepivacaine without epinephrine
- 0.5 to 1 mL of the 40 mg/mL steroid solution (20-40 mg of triamcinolone acetonide)
- Three chlorhexidine swabs
- 12-4 MHz linear ultrasound transducer and machine
- Sterile ultrasound transducer cover
- Sterile ultrasound gel
- Nonlatex sterile or nonsterile gloves
- Two 4 × 4 sterile gauze pads
- One sterile adhesive bandage

TECHNIQUE

1. For an ultrasound-guided SA-SD bursa injection, position a high-frequency linear 12-4 MHz ultrasound transducer in the axial plane lateral to the acromion with the affected SA-SD bursa centered beneath it.
2. Advance a 25-gauge 2-in needle using an in-plane approach, directing it from posterior to anterior, with an initial needle insertion depth of about 2 cm from the face of the transducer and an initial needle angle of approximately 0° to 5° relative to the skin surface where the transducer is positioned.
3. The target area is the affected SA-SD bursa.
4. Utilize real-time ultrasound guidance throughout the procedure to precisely place the needle within the desired target area and minimize the risk of inadvertently injuring surrounding structures (Fig. 10.6).
5. Upon completion of the procedure, carefully withdraw the needle. Adhere to established postprocedure care protocols and ensure appropriate follow-up as recommended.

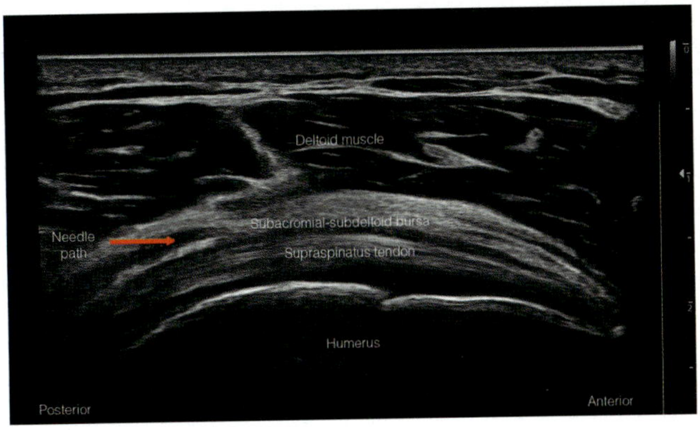

FIGURE 10.6 • Subacromial-subdeltoid ultrasound axial image.

PEARLS

- The SA-SD bursa lies superficial to the supraspinatus and infraspinatus tendons.
- If an effusion is present in the SA-SD bursa, it appears as a hypoechoic or anechoic structure on ultrasound. Without an effusion, the bursa appears hyperechoic on ultrasound.
- The SA-SD bursa can be identified by shoulder rotation, as it lies between the moving rotator cuff tendons and the stationary deltoid.

Videos showing landmark-guided and ultrasound-guided subacromial space injections can be found in the companion eBook.

REFERENCES

1. Gofeld M, Hurdle MF, Agur A. Biceps tendon sheath injection: an anatomical conundrum. *Pain Med.* 2019;20(1):138-142.
2. Pujalte G, Hudspeth LJ, Troyer WD, Shapiro SA. Ultrasound-guided injection of the long head of the biceps tendon sheath with concomitant subacromial bursa injection through the same needlestick. *Clin Anat.* 2023;36(3):400-405.
3. Sardelli M, Burks RT. Distances to the subacromial bursa from 3 different injection sites as measured arthroscopically. *Arthroscopy.* 2008;24(9):992-996.
4. Boonard M, Sumanont S, Arirachakaran A, et al. Short-term outcomes of subacromial injection of combined corticosteroid with low-volume compared to high-volume local anesthetic for rotator cuff impingement syndrome: a randomized controlled non-inferiority trial. *Eur J Orthop Surg Traumatol.* 2018;28(6):1079-1087.
5. Gialanella B, Prometti P. Effects of corticosteroids injection in rotator cuff tears. *Pain Med.* 2011;12(10):1559-1565.
6. Hsieh LF, Kuo YC, Huang YH, Liu Y-F, Hsieh T-L. Comparison of corticosteroid injection, physiotherapy and combined treatment for patients with chronic subacromial bursitis—a randomised controlled trial. *Clin Rehabil.* 2023;37(9):1189-1200.
7. Shin SJ, Lee SY. Efficacies of corticosteroid injection at different sites of the shoulder for the treatment of adhesive capsulitis. *J Shoulder Elbow Surg.* 2013;22(4):521-527.
8. Goyal T, Singh A, Negi P, Kharkwal B. Comparative functional outcomes of patients with adhesive capsulitis receiving intra-articular versus sub-acromial steroid injections: case-control study. *Musculoskelet Surg.* 2019;103(1):31-35.
9. Mohamadi A, Chan JJ, Claessen FM, Ring D, Chen NC. Corticosteroid injections give small and transient pain relief in rotator cuff tendinosis: a meta-analysis. *Clin Orthop Relat Res.* 2017;475(1):232-243.
10. Hong JY, Yoon SH, Moon DJ, Kwack K-S, Joen B, Lee HY. Comparison of high- and low-dose corticosteroid in subacromial injection for periarticular shoulder disorder: a randomized, triple-blind, placebo-controlled trial. *Arch Phys Med Rehabil.* 2011;92(12):1951-1960.
11. Kim KH, Park JW, Kim SJ. High- vs low-dose corticosteroid injection in the treatment of adhesive capsulitis with severe pain: a randomized controlled double-blind study. *Pain Med.* 2018;19(4):735-741.
12. Bhatia M, Singh B, Nicolaou N, Ravikumar KJ. Correlation between rotator cuff tears and repeated subacromial steroid injections: a case-controlled study. *Ann R Coll Surg Engl.* 2009;91(5):414-416.

13. Barman A, Mishra A, Maiti R, Sahoo J, Thakur KB, Sasidharan SK. Can platelet-rich plasma injections provide better pain relief and functional outcomes in persons with common shoulder diseases: a meta-analysis of randomized controlled trials. *Clin Shoulder Elb.* 2022;25(1):73-89.
14. Jiménez I, Marcos-García A, Muratore-Moreno G, Romero-Pérez B, Álvarez-León EE, Medina J. Subacromial sodium hyaluronate injection for the treatment of chronic shoulder pain: a prospective series of eighty patients. *Acta Ortop Mex.* 2018;32(2):70-75.
15. Kim YS, Park JY, Lee CS, Lee S-J. Does hyaluronate injection work in shoulder disease in early stage? A multicenter, randomized, single blind and open comparative clinical study. *J Shoulder Elbow Surg.* 2012;21(6):722-727.
16. Merolla G, Bianchi P, Porcellini G. Ultrasound-guided subacromial injections of sodium hyaluronate for the management of rotator cuff tendinopathy: a prospective comparative study with rehabilitation therapy. *Musculoskelet Surg.* 2013;97(Suppl 1):49-56.
17. Noël E, Hardy P, Hagena FW, et al. Efficacy and safety of Hylan G-F 20 in shoulder osteoarthritis with an intact rotator cuff. Open-label prospective multicenter study. *Joint Bone Spine.* 2009;76(6):670-673.
18. Daley EL, Bajaj S, Bisson LJ, Cole BJ. Improving injection accuracy of the elbow, knee, and shoulder: does injection site and imaging make a difference? A systematic review. *Am J Sports Med.* 2011;39(3):656-662.
19. Messina C, Banfi G, Orlandi D, et al. Ultrasound-guided interventional procedures around the shoulder. *Br J Radiol.* 2016;89(1057):20150372.
20. Farshad M, Jundt-Ecker M, Sutter R, Schubert M, Gerber C. Does subacromial injection of a local anesthetic influence strength in healthy shoulders? A double-blinded, placebo-controlled study. *J Bone Joint Surg Am.* 2012;94(19):1751-1755.

Glenohumeral Joint—Posterior Approach

The GH joint is a relatively common injection site for most primary care providers. It is typically accessed for the treatment of adhesive capsulitis as well as GH osteoarthritis. Both anterior and posterior approaches can be used. However, the **posterior approach to the GH joint is generally preferred** for reasons listed in the previous chapter. This posterior approach to the GH joint also helps avoid confusion with other sources of pain that are located over the anterior aspect of the GH joint (subscapularis tendon and proximal aspect of the long head of the biceps). The same injection site identified in the "Subacromial Space Injection—Posterior Approach" chapter is used for this procedure.

Since the long head of the biceps tendon has its origin within the GH joint capsule, this injection may offer an alternative approach to injecting this structure[1] in select patients.

Intra-articular corticosteroid injections are more effective in pain relief in the short term (8-12 weeks) but not long term. However, they provide greater passive range of motion[2] and overall function.[3] In studies of optimal corticosteroid dosing for adhesive capsulitis, there is no difference in pain or function between intra-articular injections of 20 or 40 mg of triamcinolone acetonide.[4,5] Thus, the smaller 20-mg dose is recommended. Providers should consider corticosteroid injection to treat adhesive capsulitis, especially in the early stages when pain is the predominant presentation.[6]

A small-diameter needle is selected since this technique is used to inject steroid solution into the joint space. A large-diameter needle is infrequently used because a significant effusion rarely collects in the subacromial bursa. There is a growing body of literature supporting injection therapy using PRP[7] and other biologics.[8] The use of ultrasound improves the accuracy[9] and efficacy of therapeutic injections.[10]

Relevant Anatomy: (Figs. 10.7 and 10.8)

PATIENT POSITION

- Sitting on the examination table.
- The patient's hands are folded in their lap with fingers interlaced.
- This allows consistency of positioning of the shoulder so that the landmarks do not change from the time that they are identified and marked until the time of injection.

LANDMARKS

1. With the patient seated on the examination table, the clinician stands lateral and posterior to the affected shoulder.
2. Find the lateral edge of the acromion and mark it with an ink pen.

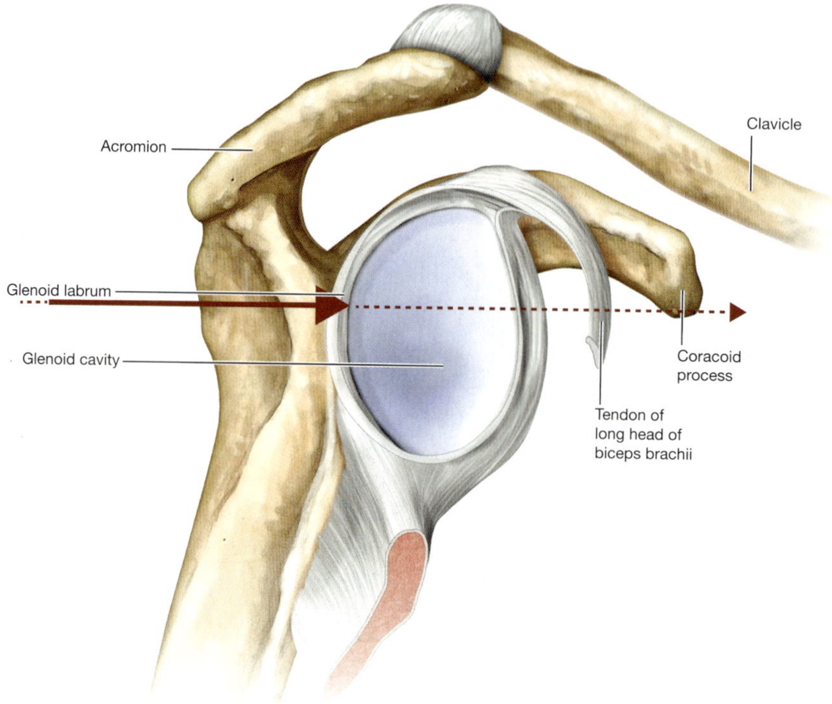

FIGURE 10.7 Lateral aspect of right shoulder (*red arrow* indicates path of the needle). (Reprinted with permission from Agur AMR, Dalley AF II. *Grant's Atlas of Anatomy*. 16th ed. Wolters Kluwer; 2025.)

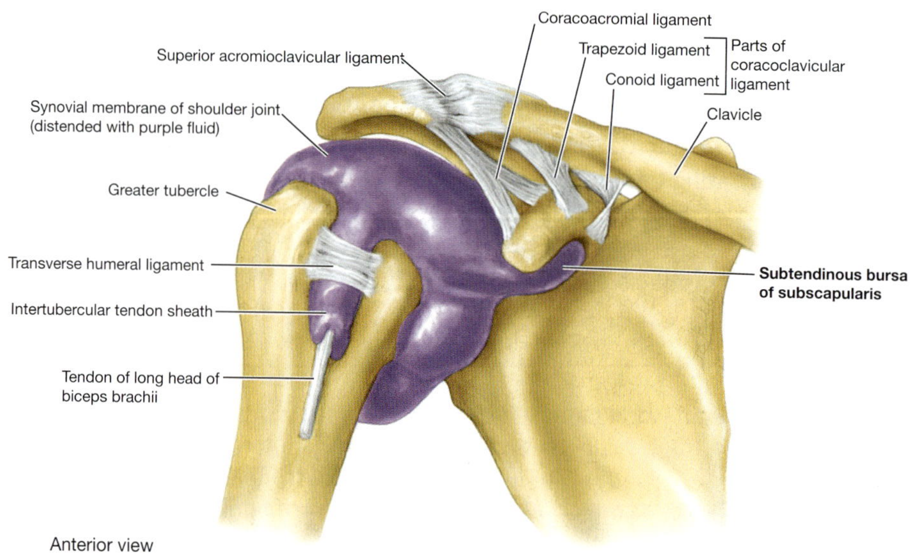

FIGURE 10.8 Right glenohumeral joint capsule. (Reprinted with permission from Agur AMR, Dalley AF II. *Grant's Atlas of Anatomy*. 16th ed. Wolters Kluwer; 2025.)

3. Palpate the posterior border of the acromion and mark that.
4. Having identified the posterior lateral corner of the acromion, drop a vertical line down from that point and mark a spot 2 cm below the posterior lateral corner.
5. At that site, press firmly with the retracted tip of a ballpoint pen. This indentation represents the entry point for the needle.
6. Next, identify the target site by placing the index finger of the nondominant hand over the coracoid process. This will be the target for the tip of the needle.
7. After the landmarks are identified, the patient should not move the shoulder or arm.

ANESTHESIA

- Tactile skin distraction is administered by firmly stroking the skin outside of the injection point as the needle is quickly introduced into the skin. Topical vapocoolant spray or injection of a local anesthetic is unnecessary in almost all patients.

EQUIPMENT

- 3-mL syringe
- 25-gauge 1½-in needle
- 1 mL of 1% mepivacaine without epinephrine
- 0.5 mL of the 40 mg/mL steroid solution (20 mg of triamcinolone acetonide)
- One alcohol prep pad
- Two povidone-iodine or chlorhexidine prep pads
- Sterile gauze pads
- Sterile adhesive bandage

TECHNIQUE

1. Prep the insertion site with alcohol followed by the povidone-iodine or chlorhexidine pads.
2. Position the needle and syringe perpendicular to the skin with the needle tip directed anterior toward the coracoid process.
3. Using the no-touch technique, quickly introduce the needle at the insertion site (Fig. 10.9).
4. Advance the needle toward the target until the needle tip touches the humeral head. Back up the needle 1 to 2 mm.
5. Withdraw the plunger of the syringe to ensure that there is no blood return.
6. Inject the mepivacaine/corticosteroid solution as a bolus into the GH joint. The injected solution should flow smoothly into the joint space. If increased resistance is encountered, advance or withdraw the needle slightly before attempting further injection.
7. Following injection, withdraw the needle.
8. Apply a sterile adhesive bandage.
9. Instruct the patient to move their shoulder through its full range of motion. This movement distributes the mepivacaine/corticosteroid solution throughout the subacromial space.
10. Reexamine the shoulder in 5 minutes to assess pain relief.

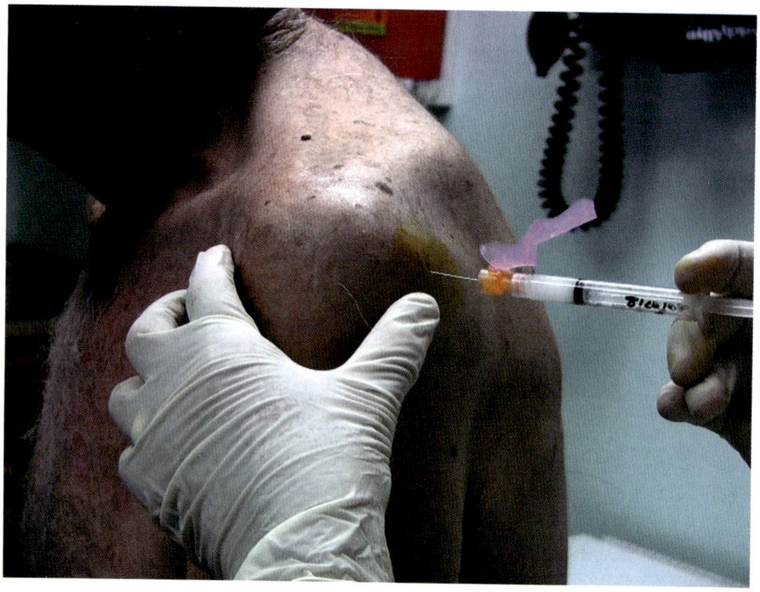

FIGURE 10.9 ● Left shoulder glenohumeral joint injection—posterior approach.

AFTERCARE

- Avoid excessive use of the shoulder over the next 2 weeks.
- Consider the use of an arm sling.
- NSAIDs, ice, and/or physical therapy as indicated.
- Consider follow-up examination in 2 weeks.

PEARLS

- The correct identification of the acromion landmarks is more difficult than many primary care providers realize. Make sure to take time and recheck the landmarks before proceeding with the injection.
- When palpating to determine the anatomy of the acromion, use the tips of the index, middle, and ring fingers positioned in a straight line. Firmly, carefully, and methodically move in a distal to proximal direction. Mark the site where fingers contact the lateral and posterior margins of the acromion.

ULTRASOUND-GUIDED PROCEDURE

Please refer to the introductory ultrasound chapter for preprocedure, sterile prep, post-procedure, and documentation information and recommendations.

PATIENT POSITION

- Lateral decubitus on the examination table with the affected shoulder upward.
- Internally rotate the affected shoulder across the patient's body, maintaining 90° of elbow flexion.

- Place a pillow under their head for comfort.
- Adjust the patient's position as needed for comfort.

PROVIDER/ULTRASOUND POSITION

- The provider stands in front of the patient at the patient's affected shoulder.
- Adjust the table to position the injection site approximately at the provider's umbilicus level, ensuring optimal ergonomics and visualization of the ultrasound screen, transducer, and needle's approach (Fig. 10.10).
- Position the ultrasound machine on the opposite side of the table from the provider at the level of the patient's shoulders with the screen facing the provider.

LANDMARKS

- See the landmarks for the landmark-guided injection procedure.

ANESTHESIA

- Local anesthesia of the skin using topical vapocoolant spray.

EQUIPMENT

- 3-mL syringe
- 22-gauge 3.5-in needle (adjust needle length based on body habitus)

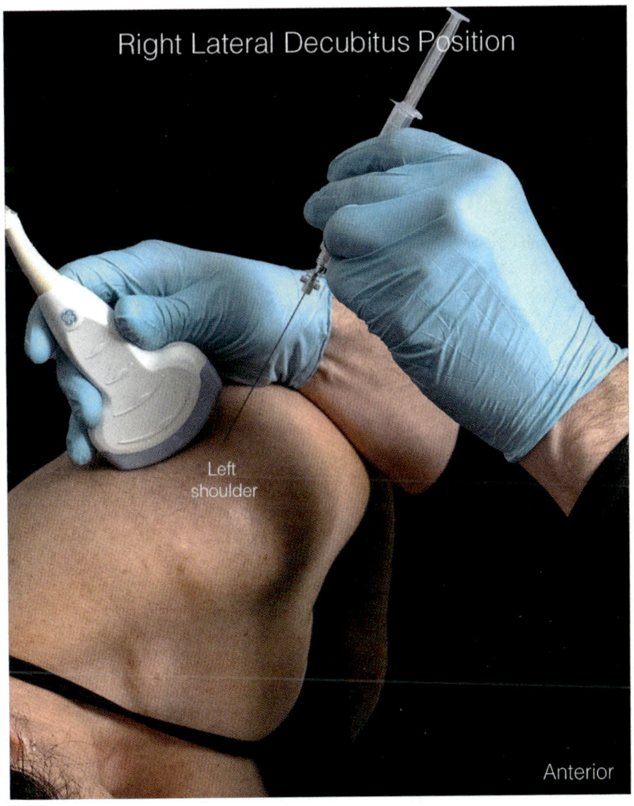

FIGURE 10.10 • Ultrasound-guided left glenohumeral joint injection. Right lateral decubitus position, with the affected shoulder uppermost and the patient's head facing the camera.

- 1 mL of 1% mepivacaine without epinephrine
- 0.5 mL of the 40 mg/mL steroid solution (20 mg of triamcinolone acetonide)
- Three chlorhexidine swabs
- 5-1 MHz curvilinear ultrasound transducer and machine
- Sterile ultrasound transducer cover
- Sterile ultrasound gel
- Nonlatex sterile or nonsterile gloves
- Two 4 × 4 sterile gauze pads
- One sterile adhesive bandage
- Topical vapocoolant spray

TECHNIQUE

1. Position a low-frequency curvilinear 5-1 MHz ultrasound transducer in the axial plane at the posterolateral aspect of the acromion adjacent to the scapular spine with the affected GH joint centered beneath it.
2. Advance a 22-gauge 3.5-in needle using an in-plane approach from a posterolateral to anteromedial direction, with an initial needle angle of approximately 30° to 45° relative to the skin surface where the transducer is positioned.
3. The target area is the affected joint.
4. Utilize real-time ultrasound guidance throughout the procedure to precisely place the needle within the desired target area and minimize the risk of inadvertently injuring surrounding structures (Fig. 10.11).
5. Upon completion of the procedure, carefully withdraw the needle. Adhere to established postprocedure care protocols and ensure appropriate follow-up as recommended.

PEARLS

- "Toe" the curvilinear transducer by pressing the distal edge away while lifting the proximal edge. If an air gap forms, use a sterile ultrasound gel standoff.
- Perform active or passive internal or external shoulder rotation during the preprocedural ultrasound examination to differentiate the joint from surrounding structures.

Videos showing landmark-guided and ultrasound-guided posterior glenohumeral joint injections can be found in the companion eBook.

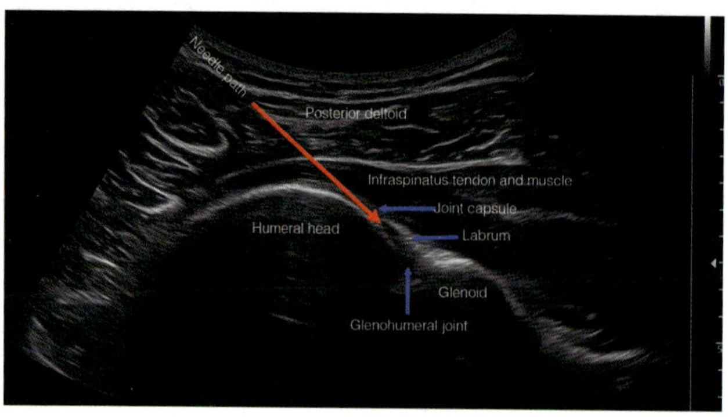

FIGURE 10.11 ● Glenohumeral joint ultrasound axial image.

REFERENCES

1. Gofeld M, Hurdle MF, Agur A. Biceps tendon sheath injection: an anatomical conundrum. *Pain Med.* 2019;20(1):138-142.
2. Wang W, Shi M, Zhou C, et al. Effectiveness of corticosteroid injections in adhesive capsulitis of shoulder: a meta-analysis. *Medicine (Baltimore).* 2017;96(28):e7529.
3. Ranalletta M, Rossi LA, Bongiovanni SL, Tanoira I, Elizondo CM, Maignon GD. Corticosteroid injections accelerate pain relief and recovery of function compared with oral NSAIDs in patients with adhesive capsulitis: a randomized controlled trial. *Am J Sports Med.* 2016;44(2):474-481.
4. Kim KH, Park JW, Kim SJ. High- vs low-dose corticosteroid injection in the treatment of adhesive capsulitis with severe pain: a randomized controlled double-blind study. *Pain Med.* 2018;19(4):735-741.
5. Yoon SH, Lee HY, Lee HJ, Kwack KS. Optimal dose of intra-articular corticosteroids for adhesive capsulitis: a randomized, triple-blind, placebo-controlled trial. *Am J Sports Med.* 2013;41(5):1133-1139.
6. Koh KH. Corticosteroid injection for adhesive capsulitis in primary care: a systematic review of randomised clinical trials. *Singapore Med J.* 2016;57(12):646-657.
7. Barman A, Mukherjee S, Sahoo J, et al. Single intra-articular platelet-rich plasma versus corticosteroid injections in the treatment of adhesive capsulitis of the shoulder: a cohort study. *Am J Phys Med Rehabil.* 2019;98(7):549-557.
8. Carr JB II, Rodeo SA. The role of biologic agents in the management of common shoulder pathologies: current state and future directions. *J Shoulder Elbow Surg.* 2019;28(11):2041-2052.
9. Daley EL, Bajaj S, Bisson LJ, Cole BJ. Improving injection accuracy of the elbow, knee, and shoulder: does injection site and imaging make a difference? A systematic review. *Am J Sports Med.* 2011;39(3):656-662.
10. Messina C, Banfi G, Orlandi D, et al. Ultrasound-guided interventional procedures around the shoulder. *Br J Radiol.* 2016;89(1057):20150372.

Acromioclavicular Joint

The AC joint is an uncommon injection site for most primary care providers. Despite its superficial location, accurate identification and successful injection can be challenging without the aid of imaging.[1] Clinical trials demonstrate the effectiveness of a corticosteroid injection into the AC joint in only a minority of patients.[2] This is most likely a result of inaccurate needle placement due to the small size of the joint.[3] Multiple studies show that this is a difficult injection to perform successfully, with only about 40% of injections actually reaching the intended intra-articular target.[4] Ultrasound guidance greatly improves accuracy to nearly 100%.[5] Ultrasound-guided AC joint intra-articular injections have also been demonstrated to result in better pain and functional status improvement than palpation-guided injections.[6] An emerging therapeutic option is ultrasound-guided prolotherapy using an injection of 15% dextrose solution for the treatment of AC joint moderate to severe acromial enthesopathy and AC joint arthropathy.[7]

Relevant Anatomy: (Fig. 10.12)

PATIENT POSITION

- Sitting or lying supine on the examination table with the head of the bed elevated 45°.
- The patient's hands are folded in their lap with fingers interlaced.

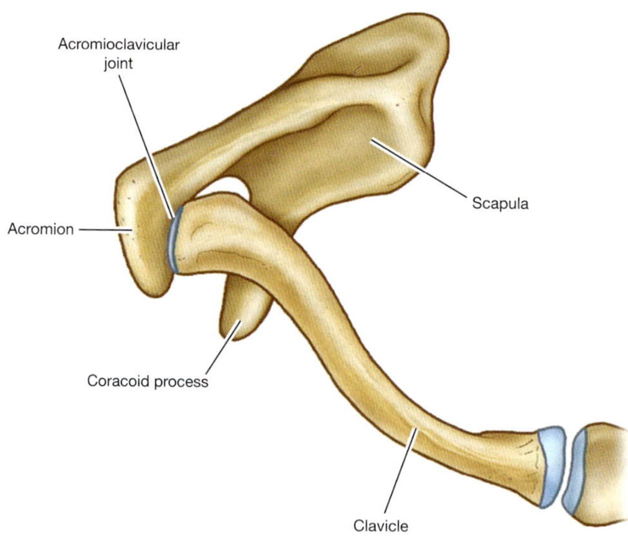

FIGURE 10.12 ● Right acromioclavicular joint.

- This allows consistency of positioning of the shoulder so that the landmarks do not change from the time that they are identified and marked until the time of injection.
- Rotate the patient's head away from the side that is being injected. This minimizes anxiety and pain perception.

LANDMARKS

1. With the patient seated or lying supine on the examination table, the clinician stands lateral and anterior to the affected shoulder.
2. Identify the AC joint. Palpate the clavicle in a medial to lateral direction. At the lateral aspect of the clavicle, there is a small depression that will be tender in the above conditions.
3. The injection point is located directly over the AC joint. At that site, press firmly with the retracted tip of a ballpoint pen. As an alternative, pressure can be placed with the fingernail or a paperclip positioned across the AC joint. This indentation represents the entry point for the needle.
4. Once the landmarks are identified, the patient should not move the chest or shoulder.

ANESTHESIA

- Local anesthesia of the skin using topical vapocoolant spray.

EQUIPMENT

- Topical vapocoolant spray
- 3-mL syringe
- 25-gauge 5/8-in needle
- 0.5 mL of 1% mepivacaine without epinephrine
- 0.5 mL of the 40 mg/mL steroid solution (20 mg of triamcinolone acetonide)
- One alcohol prep pad
- Two povidone-iodine or chlorhexidine prep pads
- Sterile gauze pads
- Sterile adhesive bandage

TECHNIQUE

1. Prep the insertion site with alcohol followed by the povidone-iodine or chlorhexidine pads.
2. Achieve good local anesthesia by using topical vapocoolant spray.
3. Position the needle and syringe perpendicular to the skin with the needle tip directed caudad.
4. Using the no-touch technique, quickly introduce the needle at the insertion site (Fig. 10.13).
5. Advance the needle into the AC joint at an angle 30° medially in the coronal plane.[8] If the needle does not "drop" into the AC joint, then "walk" the needle in the area until it does so.
6. Withdraw the plunger of the syringe to ensure that there is no blood return.
7. Inject the mepivacaine/corticosteroid solution as a bolus into the AC joint. The injected solution should flow smoothly into the joint space. If increased resistance

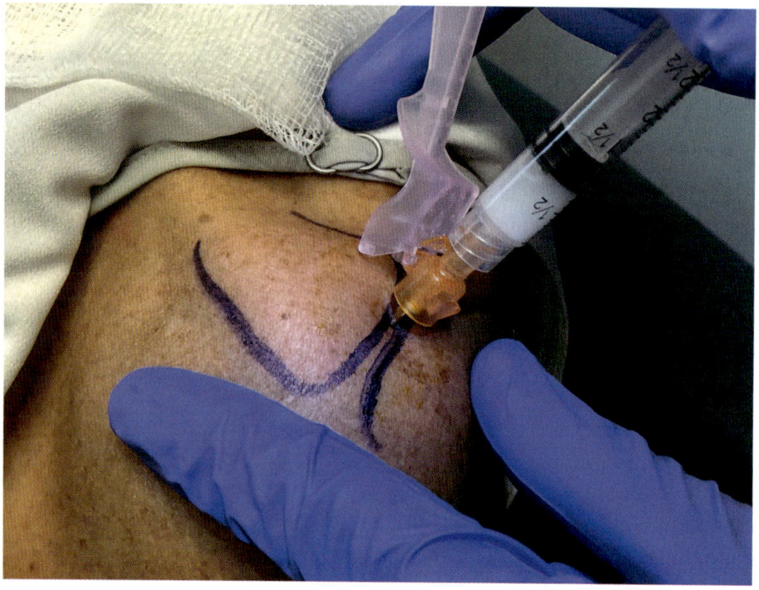

FIGURE 10.13 ● Left acromioclavicular joint injection with landmarks.

is encountered, advance or withdraw the needle slightly before attempting further injection. If the needle will not drop into the joint, then employ the aid of ultrasound imaging, or as a last resort, perform a periarticular injection.

8. Following injection, withdraw the needle.
9. Apply a sterile adhesive bandage.
10. Instruct the patient to move their shoulder through its full range of motion. This movement distributes the mepivacaine/corticosteroid solution throughout the AC joint.
11. Reexamine the shoulder in 5 minutes to assess pain relief.

AFTERCARE

- Avoid excessive use of the shoulder over the next 2 weeks.
- Consider the use of an arm sling.
- NSAIDs, ice, and/or physical therapy as indicated.
- Consider follow-up examination in 2 weeks.

PEARLS

- The AC joint is superficial. Depositing corticosteroid in the subcutaneous tissues can result in the complication of skin atrophy and hypopigmentation. Avoid the development of a subdermal wheal while performing all injections of corticosteroid solutions.
- Perform the "pinch technique" as described in the "Lateral Epicondyle" chapter.

ULTRASOUND-GUIDED PROCEDURE

Please refer to the introductory ultrasound chapter for preprocedure, sterile prep, postprocedure, and documentation information and recommendations.

PATIENT POSITION

- Seated on the examination table.
- Shoulder in the neutral position with the patient's hand supinated in their lap.
- Adjust the patient's position as needed for comfort.

PROVIDER/ULTRASOUND POSITION

- The provider stands behind the patient.
- Adjust the examination table to position the injection site between the provider's umbilicus and axillary level, ensuring optimal ergonomics and visualization of the ultrasound screen, transducer, and needle's approach (Fig. 10.14).
- Position the ultrasound machine on the opposite side of the table from the provider with the screen facing the provider.

LANDMARKS

- See the landmarks for the landmark-guided injection procedure.

ANESTHESIA

- Local anesthesia of the skin using topical vapocoolant spray.

EQUIPMENT

- 3-mL syringe
- 25-gauge 1.5-in needle (adjust needle length based on provider's comfort)
- 0.5 mL of 1% mepivacaine without epinephrine

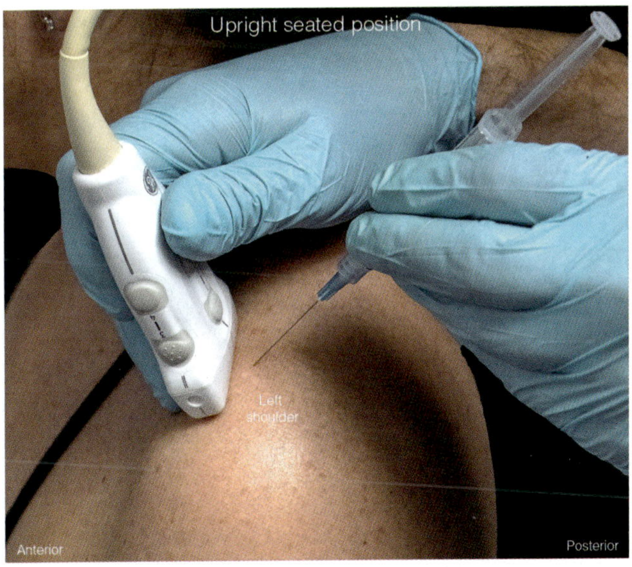

FIGURE 10.14 • Ultrasound-guided left acromioclavicular joint injection. Seated upright on the examination table, with the affected shoulder positioned directly facing the camera.

- 0.5 mL of the 40 mg/mL steroid solution (20 mg of triamcinolone acetonide)
- Three chlorhexidine swabs
- 12-4 MHz linear ultrasound transducer and machine
- Sterile ultrasound transducer cover
- Sterile ultrasound gel
- Nonlatex sterile or nonsterile gloves
- Two 4 × 4 sterile gauze pads
- One sterile adhesive bandage
- Topical vapocoolant spray

TECHNIQUE

1. Position a high-frequency linear 12-4 MHz ultrasound transducer in the coronal plane with the affected AC joint centered beneath it.
2. Advance a 25-gauge 1.5-in needle using an out-of-plane approach, directing it from posterior to anterior, with an initial needle angle of approximately 30° to 45° relative to the skin surface where the transducer is positioned.
3. The target area is the affected joint.
4. Utilize real-time ultrasound guidance throughout the procedure to precisely place the needle within the desired target area and minimize the risk of inadvertently injuring surrounding structures (Fig. 10.15).
5. Upon completion of the procedure, carefully withdraw the needle. Adhere to established postprocedure care protocols and ensure appropriate follow-up as recommended.

PEARLS

- If visualization of the AC joint is challenging, position the transducer in the coronal plane over the acromion, perform a longitudinal scan by sliding the transducer medially to the AC joint.
- During an injection, increased resistance can be felt when the needle tip is inside the joint capsule compared to when positioned inside the joint itself. If increased resistance is encountered, the needle is carefully advanced further while maintaining visualization of the tip in the joint until the resistance decreases.

Videos showing landmark-guided and ultrasound-guided acromioclavicular joint injections can be found in the companion eBook.

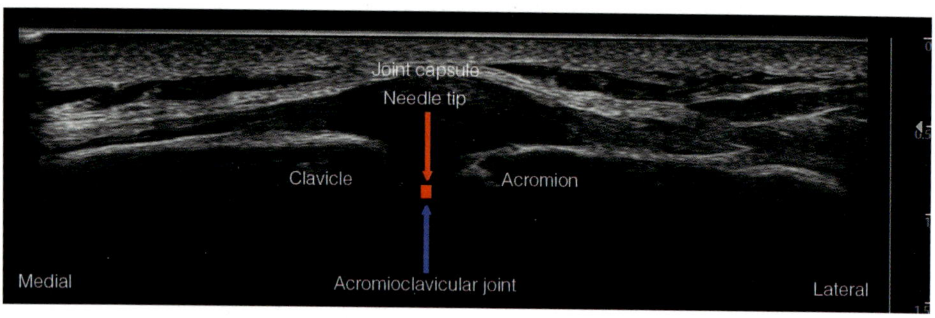

FIGURE 10.15 ● Acromioclavicular joint ultrasound coronal image.

REFERENCES

1. Scillia A, Issa K, McInerney VK, et al. Accuracy of in vivo palpation-guided acromioclavicular joint injection assessed with contrast material and fluoroscopic evaluations. *Skeletal Radiol.* 2015;44(8):1135-1139.
2. van Riet RP, Goehre T, Bell SN. The long term effect of an intra-articular injection of corticosteroids in the acromioclavicular joint. *J Shoulder Elbow Surg.* 2012;21(3):376-379.
3. Javed S, Sadozai Z, Javed A, Din A, Schmitgen G. Should all acromioclavicular joint injections be performed under image guidance? *J Orthop Surg (Hong Kong).* 2017;25(3):2309499017731633.
4. Wasserman BR, Pettrone S, Jazrawi LM, Zuckerman JD, Rokito AS. Accuracy of acromioclavicular joint injections. *Am J Sports Med.* 2013;41(1):149-152.
5. Sabeti-Aschraf M, Lemmerhofer B, Lang S, et al. Ultrasound guidance improves the accuracy of the acromioclavicular joint infiltration: a prospective randomized study. *Knee Surg Sports Traumatol Arthrosc.* 2011;19(2):292-295.
6. Park KD, Kim TK, Lee J, Lee WY, Ahn JK, Park Y. Palpation versus ultrasound-guided acromioclavicular joint intra-articular corticosteroid injections: a retrospective comparative clinical study. *Pain Physician.* 2015;18(4):333-341.
7. Hsieh PC, Chiou HJ, Wang HK, Lai Y-C, Lin Y-H. Ultrasound-guided prolotherapy for acromial enthesopathy and acromioclavicular joint arthropathy: a single-arm prospective study. *J Ultrasound Med.* 2019;38(3):605-612.
8. Crönlein M, Postl L, Beirer M, et al. Analysis of the bony geometry of the acromio-clavicular joint. *Eur J Med Res.* 2018;23(1):50.

Sternoclavicular Joint

The sternoclavicular (SC) joint is a rare injection site for most primary care providers. Successful injection can be difficult because of the small joint space. Physical examination following the use of anesthetic injections can be helpful to confirm the diagnosis of SC arthropathy. High-frequency ultrasound can visualize the anterior SC ligament, interclavicular ligament, and anterior intra-articular structures.[1] The use of ultrasound-guided injections of the SC joint has been shown to be a safe and accurate diagnostic method.[2] Using ultrasound instead of computed tomography scanning avoids potentially harmful radiation, unnecessary expense, and delayed care. Patients who fail to respond to steroid injection therapy might be candidates for resection arthroplasty.

Relevant Anatomy: (Fig. 10.16)

PATIENT POSITION

- Supine on the examination table.
- The patient's hands are folded in their lap with fingers interlaced.
- Rotate the patient's head away from the side that is being injected. This minimizes anxiety and pain perception.

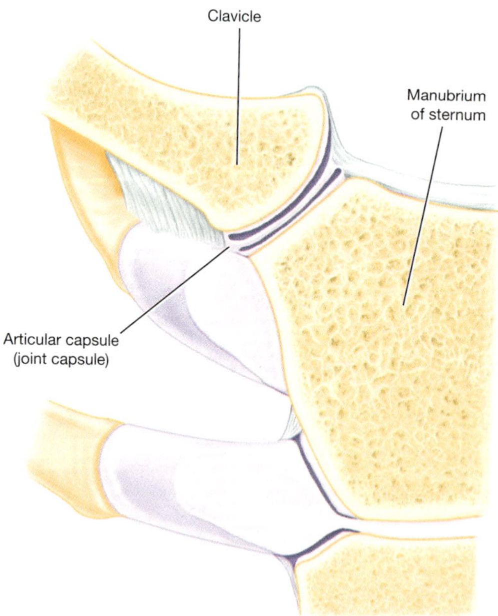

FIGURE 10.16 ● Sternoclavicular joint. (Modified with permission from Gest TR. *Lippincott® Atlas of Anatomy.* 2nd ed. Wolters Kluwer; 2020.)

LANDMARKS

1. With the patient supine on the examination table, the clinician stands to the patient's affected side.
2. Identify the SC joint. Palpate the clavicle in a lateral to medial direction. At the medial aspect of the clavicle, there is a small depression that represents the SC joint. This structure will be tender in patients with pathology.
3. It may be helpful to move the ipsilateral shoulder in order to more easily identify the SC joint.
4. The injection point is located directly over the SC joint. At that site, press firmly with the retracted tip of a ballpoint pen. As an alternative, pressure can be placed with the fingernail or a paperclip positioned across the SC joint. This indentation represents the entry point for the needle.
5. After the landmarks are identified, the patient should not move the chest or shoulder.

ANESTHESIA

- Local anesthesia of the skin using topical vapocoolant spray.

EQUIPMENT

- Topical vapocoolant spray
- 3-mL syringe
- 25-gauge 5/8-in needle
- 0.5 mL of 1% mepivacaine without epinephrine
- 0.5 mL of the 40 mg/mL steroid solution (20 mg of triamcinolone acetonide)
- One alcohol prep pad
- Two povidone-iodine or chlorhexidine prep pads
- Sterile gauze pads
- Sterile adhesive bandage

TECHNIQUE

1. Prep the insertion site with alcohol followed by the povidone-iodine or chlorhexidine pads.
2. Achieve good local anesthesia by using topical vapocoolant spray.
3. Position the needle and syringe perpendicular to the skin with the needle tip directed posteriorly.
4. Using the no-touch technique, quickly introduce the needle at the insertion site (Fig. 10.17).
5. Advance the needle into the SC joint space.
6. Withdraw the plunger of the syringe to ensure that there is no blood return.
7. Inject the mepivacaine/corticosteroid solution as a bolus into the SC joint. The injected solution should flow smoothly into the joint space. If increased resistance is encountered, advance or withdraw the needle slightly before attempting further injection. If the needle will not drop into the joint, then employ the aid of ultrasound imaging, or as a last resort, perform a periarticular injection.
8. Following injection of the mepivacaine/corticosteroid solution, withdraw the needle.
9. Apply a sterile adhesive bandage.

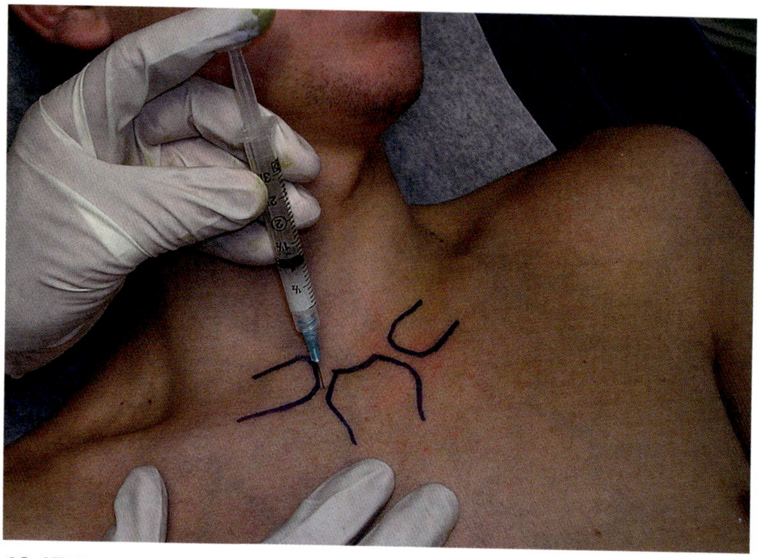

FIGURE 10.17 ● Sternoclavicular joint injection with landmarks.

10. Instruct the patient to move their shoulder through its full range of motion. This movement distributes the mepivacaine/corticosteroid solution throughout the SC joint.
11. Reexamine the SC joint in 5 minutes to assess pain relief.

AFTERCARE

- Avoid excessive use of the shoulder over the next 2 weeks.
- Consider the use of an arm sling.
- NSAIDs, ice, and/or physical therapy as indicated.
- Consider follow-up examination in 2 weeks.

PEARLS

- The SC joint is superficial. Depositing corticosteroid in the subcutaneous tissues can result in the complication of skin atrophy and hypopigmentation. Avoid the development of a subdermal wheal while performing all injections of corticosteroid solutions.
- Perform the "pinch technique" as described in the "Lateral Epicondyle" chapter.

ULTRASOUND-GUIDED PROCEDURE

Please refer to the introductory ultrasound chapter for preprocedure, sterile prep, post-procedure, and documentation information and recommendations.

PATIENT POSITION

- Supine on the examination table.
- Place the affected shoulder in the neutral position.
- Place the patient's neck in extension with a pillow under their neck or shoulders.

- Consider rotating the patient's head toward the affected side.
- Adjust the patient's position as needed for patient comfort.

PROVIDER/ULTRASOUND POSITION

- The provider stands at the contralateral shoulder.
- Adjust the examination table to position the injection site between the provider's umbilicus and axillary level, ensuring optimal ergonomics and visualization of the ultrasound screen, transducer, and needle's approach (Fig. 10.18).
- Position the ultrasound machine on the opposite side of the table from the provider at the level of the patient's head with the screen facing the provider.

LANDMARKS

- See the landmarks for the landmark-guided injection procedure.

ANESTHESIA

- Local anesthesia of the skin using topical vapocoolant spray.

EQUIPMENT

- 3-mL syringe
- 25-gauge 1.5-in needle (adjust needle length based on provider's comfort)
- 0.5 mL of 1% mepivacaine without epinephrine
- 0.5 mL of the 40 mg/mL steroid solution (20 mg of triamcinolone acetonide)
- Three chlorhexidine swabs
- 12-4 MHz linear ultrasound transducer and machine
- Sterile ultrasound transducer cover
- Sterile ultrasound gel
- Nonlatex sterile or nonsterile gloves
- Two 4 × 4 sterile gauze pads

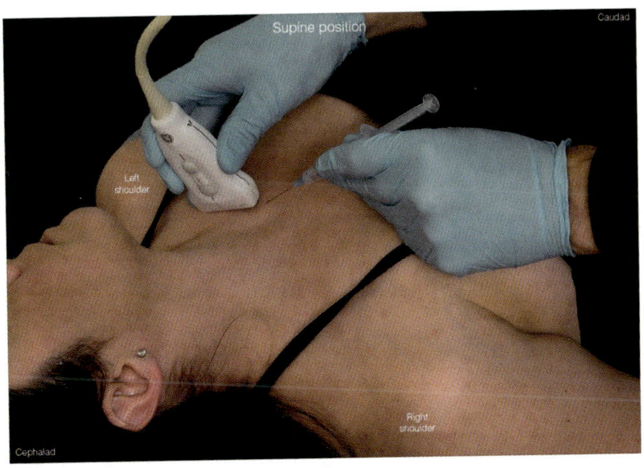

FIGURE 10.18 ● Ultrasound-guided left sternoclavicular joint injection. Supine position with the affected SC joint contralateral to the provider.

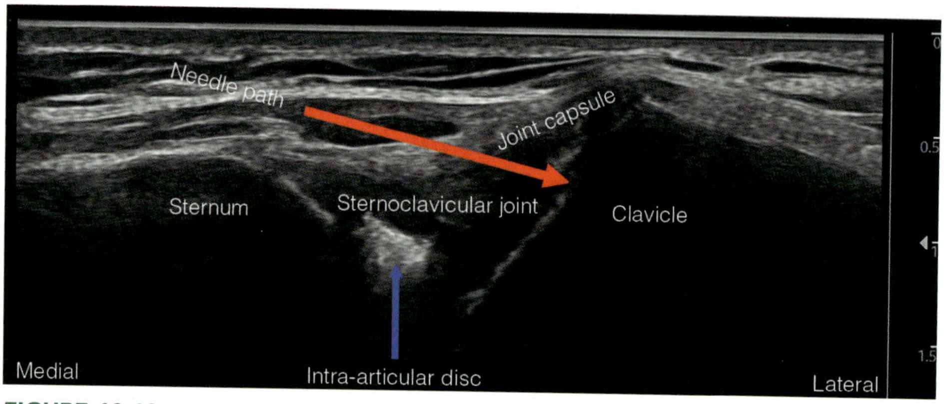

FIGURE 10.19 ● Sternoclavicular joint ultrasound axial oblique image.

- One sterile adhesive bandage
- Topical vapocoolant spray

TECHNIQUE

1. Position a high-frequency linear 12-4 MHz ultrasound transducer in the axial oblique plane with the affected SC joint centered beneath it.
2. Advance a 25-gauge 1.5-in needle using an in-plane approach, directing it from medial to lateral, with an initial needle angle of approximately 15° to 30° relative to the skin surface where the transducer is positioned.
3. The target area is the affected joint.
4. Utilize real-time ultrasound guidance throughout the procedure to precisely place the needle within the desired target area and minimize the risk of inadvertently injuring surrounding structures (Fig. 10.19).
5. Upon completion of the procedure, carefully withdraw the needle. Adhere to established postprocedure care protocols and ensure appropriate follow-up as recommended.

PEARLS

- If the transducer lifts on the sternal end, creating an air gap, use a sterile ultrasound gel standoff to improve image quality.
- The SC joint is surrounded by vital structures. Extreme caution is crucial due to the risk of complications like bleeding, nerve damage, and pneumothorax. Real-time ultrasound guidance with the use of Doppler is essential for safe needle placement.

A video showing ultrasound-guided sternoclavicular joint injection can be found in the companion eBook.

REFERENCES

1. Olivier T, Kasprzak K, Herteleer M, Demondion X, Jacques T, Cotten A. Anatomical study of the sterno-clavicular joint using high-frequency ultrasound. Insights. *Imaging.* 2022;13(1):66.
2. Min KS, Lopez A, Powlan FJ, Pham B, Lause G. Ultrasound-guided sternoclavicular joint injection: technique and case series. *JSES Rev Rep Tech.* 2021;1(4):393-397.

Biceps Tendon—Long Head

Patients occasionally present to the primary care office for evaluation and treatment of pain caused by tendinopathy of the long head of biceps. This is an inflammatory and/or degenerative condition that is much more frequently seen in the long head rather than the short head of the biceps brachii muscle. It develops either from direct acute trauma or chronic overuse with repeated microtears in throwing athletes and nonathletes who use their arms to do repetitive biceps activation, resisted forearm supination, or overhead work. Biceps tendinopathy is frequently diagnosed in association with rotator cuff disease as a component of the impingement syndrome or secondary to intra-articular pathology, such as labral tears. Local tenderness is usually located over the bicipital groove of the humerus. Conservative management of biceps tendon pain usually consists of rest, ice, oral analgesics, physical therapy, or corticosteroid injections.

As demonstrated in the literature, physicians have difficulty correctly identifying the intertubercular groove that contains the tendon of the long head of the biceps. Localization attempts are usually far medial of the tendon's actual location.[1] Consequently, clinicians should exercise caution when relying on clinical palpation to perform a biceps long head tendon sheath injection. Corticosteroid injections are an effective treatment for primary long head biceps tendonitis. When performed under ultrasound guidance, injections to the bicipital groove are more accurate,[2] faster to perform, produce less discomfort, and demonstrate superior clinical outcomes.[3,4]

Relevant Anatomy: (Fig. 10.20)

PATIENT POSITION

- Supine on the examination table with the head of the bed elevated 30°.
- The patient's hands are placed in a position of supination at their side with slight external rotation of the arm.
- Rotate the patient's head away from the side that is being injected. This minimizes anxiety and pain perception.

LANDMARKS

1. With the patient lying supine on the examination table, the clinician stands lateral to the affected arm.
2. Instruct the patient to flex the elbow and contract the biceps muscle.
3. Palpate the course of the long head of the bicipital tendon over the anterior aspect of the upper arm.
4. Determine the location of maximal tenderness, which will most likely be under the edge of the pectoralis major muscle. Mark that spot with an ink pen.

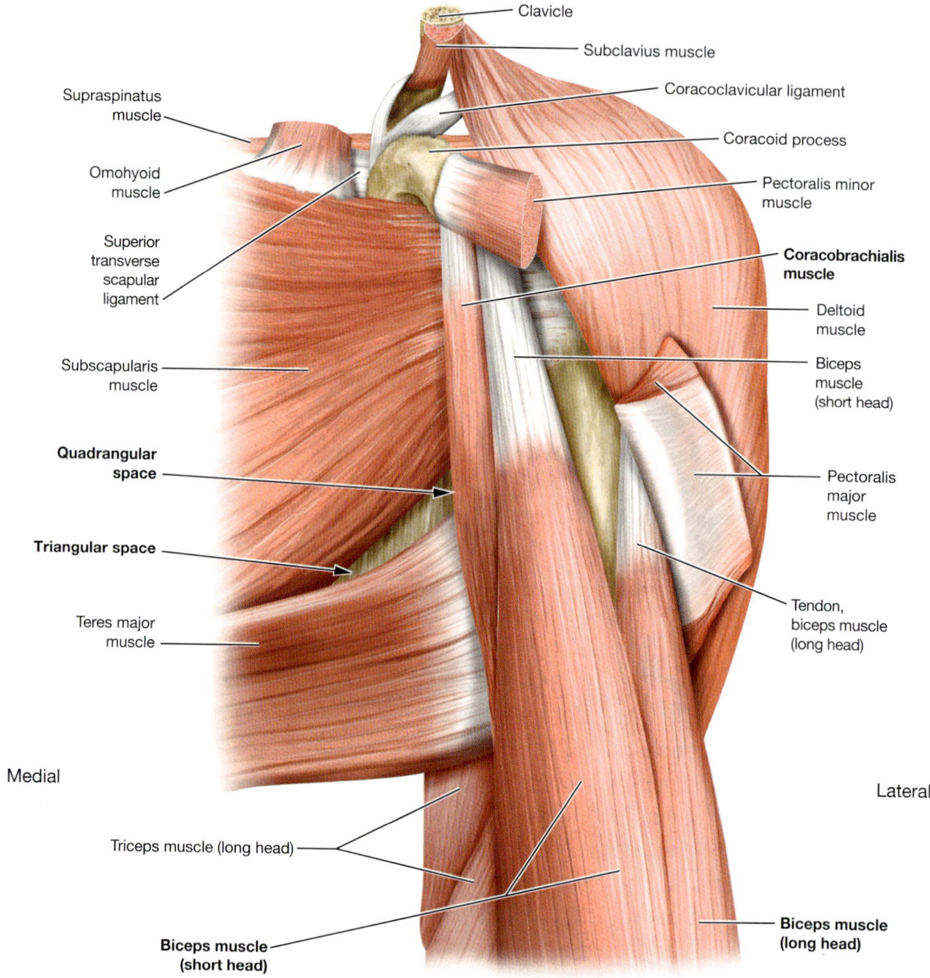

FIGURE 10.20 Muscles of anterior left arm. (Modified with permission from Paulsen F, Waschke J. *Sobotta Atlas of Human Anatomy*. 25th ed. Urban & Fischer; 2022. Copyright © 2022 Elsevier GmbH.)

5. At that site, press firmly on the skin with the retracted tip of a ballpoint pen. This indentation represents the entry point for the needle.
6. After the landmarks are identified, the patient should not move the shoulder or arm.

ANESTHESIA

- Local anesthesia of the skin using topical vapocoolant spray.

EQUIPMENT

- Topical vapocoolant spray
- 3-mL syringe
- 25-gauge 1½-in needle
- 1 mL of 1% lidocaine without epinephrine
- 0.5 to 1 mL of the 40 mg/mL steroid solution (20-40 mg of triamcinolone acetonide)
- One alcohol prep pad

- Two povidone-iodine or chlorhexidine prep pads
- Sterile gauze pads
- Sterile adhesive bandage

TECHNIQUE

1. Prep the insertion site with alcohol followed by the povidone-iodine or chlorhexidine pads.
2. Achieve good local anesthesia by using topical vapocoolant spray.
3. Position the needle and syringe at a 45° angle to the skin with the needle tip directed proximally.
4. Using the no-touch technique, quickly introduce the needle at the insertion site (Fig. 10.21).
5. Advance the needle until the needle tip touches the tendon. (An increase in resistance will be detected.) Back up the needle 1 to 2 mm.
6. Withdraw the plunger of the syringe to ensure that there is no blood return.
7. Inject the lidocaine/corticosteroid solution as a bolus around the bicipital tendon. The injected solution should flow smoothly into the tenosynovial sheath. If increased resistance is encountered, advance or withdraw the needle slightly before attempting further injection.
8. Following injection of the lidocaine/corticosteroid solution, withdraw the needle.
9. Apply a sterile adhesive bandage.
10. Instruct the patient to move their biceps muscle and shoulder through their full range of motion. This movement distributes the lidocaine/corticosteroid solution throughout the tenosynovial sheath.
11. Reexamine the arm in 5 minutes to assess pain relief.

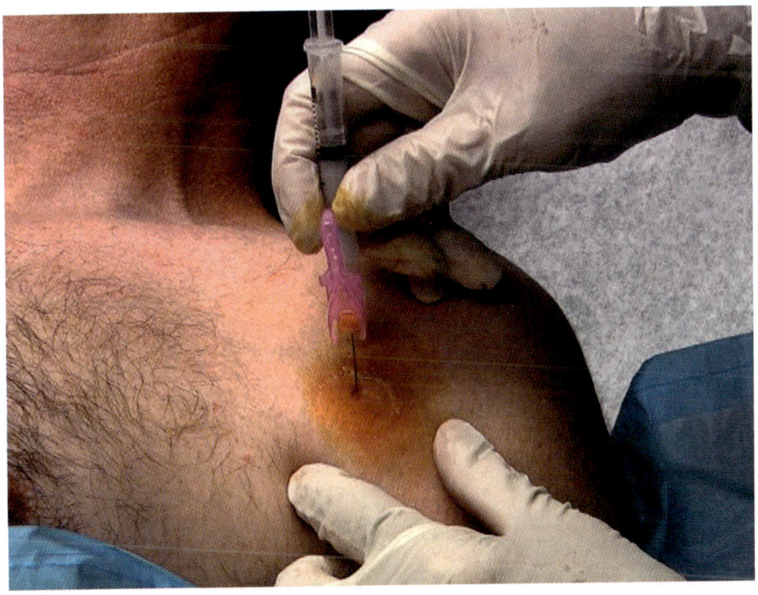

FIGURE 10.21 • Injection of the tendon of the long head of the left biceps brachii muscle.

AFTERCARE

- Avoid all throwing and excessive use of the arm and shoulder over the next 2 weeks.
- NSAIDs, ice, and/or physical therapy as indicated.
- Consider follow-up examination in 2 weeks.

PEARLS

- Failure to recognize or treat this condition may lead to rupture of the tendon of the long head of the biceps brachii.
- Make sure to place the injection around the tendon and not into the substance of the tendon in order to avoid iatrogenic degeneration of the tendon and subsequent rupture.
- For patients with persistent cases of biceps tendinitis, consider the use of ultrasound-guided imaging or even a well-placed subacromial space injection. An SA space injection can often provide deposition of corticosteroid solution to the proximal aspect of the long head of the biceps tendon.[5,6]

ULTRASOUND-GUIDED PROCEDURE

Please refer to the introductory ultrasound chapter for preprocedure, sterile prep, post-procedure, and documentation information and recommendations.

PATIENT POSITION

- Supine on the examination table.
- On the affected side, place the shoulder in external rotation with 30° to 60° of elbow flexion.
- Place a pillow under their head for comfort.
- Adjust the patient's position as needed for comfort.

PROVIDER/ULTRASOUND POSITION

- The provider sits at the patient's affected shoulder.
- Adjust the examination table to position the injection site between the provider's umbilicus and axillary level, ensuring optimal ergonomics and visualization of the ultrasound screen, transducer, and needle's approach (Fig. 10.22).
- Position the ultrasound machine on the opposite side of the table from the provider at the level of the patient's shoulders with the screen facing the provider.

LANDMARKS

- See the landmarks for the landmark-guided injection procedure.

ANESTHESIA

- Local anesthesia of the skin using topical vapocoolant spray.

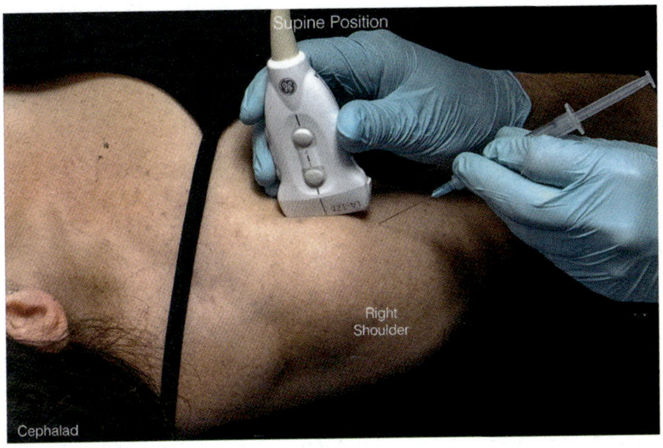

FIGURE 10.22 Ultrasound-guided right long head bicep tendon sheath injection. Supine position with the affected shoulder toward the provider.

EQUIPMENT

- 3-mL syringe
- 25-gauge 1.5-in needle (adjust needle length based on body habitus)
- 1 mL of 1% mepivacaine without epinephrine
- 0.5 to 1 mL of the 40 mg/mL steroid solution (20-40 mg of triamcinolone acetonide)
- Three chlorhexidine swabs
- 12-4 MHz linear ultrasound transducer and machine
- Sterile ultrasound transducer cover
- Sterile ultrasound gel
- Nonlatex sterile or nonsterile gloves
- Two 4 × 4 sterile gauze pads
- One sterile adhesive bandage
- Topical vapocoolant spray

TECHNIQUE

1. Position a high-frequency linear 12-4 MHz ultrasound transducer in the axial plane over the anterior shoulder at the level of the bicipital grove with the affected long head of the bicep tendon centered beneath it.
2. Advance a 25-gauge 1.5-in needle using an in-plane approach, directing it from lateral to medial, with an initial depth of needle insertion about 2 cm from the face of the transducer and an initial needle angle of approximately 15° to 20° relative to the skin surface where the transducer is positioned.
3. The target area is the medial aspect of the bicep tendon sheath.
4. Utilize real-time ultrasound guidance throughout the procedure to precisely place the needle within the desired target area and minimize the risk of inadvertently injuring surrounding structures (Fig. 10.23).
5. Upon completion of the procedure, carefully withdraw the needle. Adhere to established postprocedure care protocols and ensure appropriate follow-up as recommended.

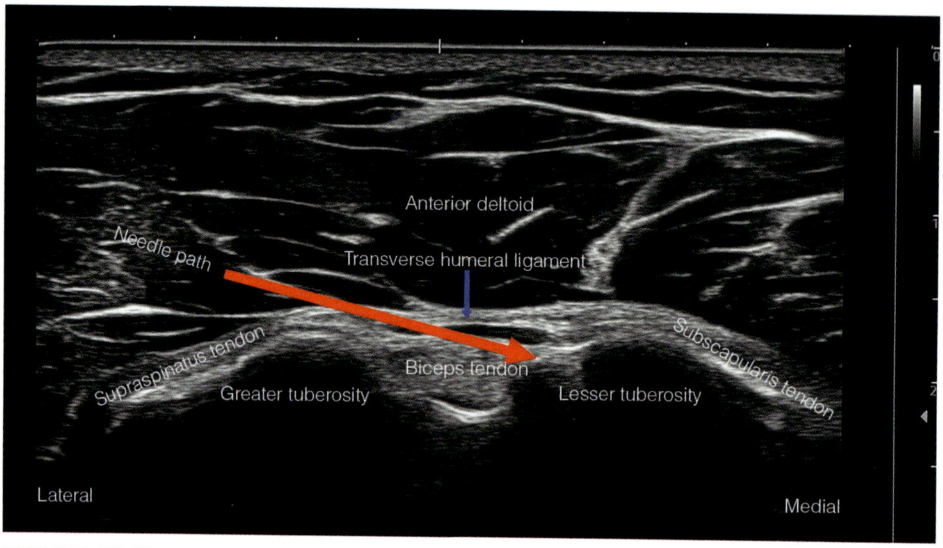

FIGURE 10.23 ● Long head of the bicep tendon within the bicipital groove ultrasound axial image.

PEARLS

- Consider a longer needle (eg, 2-in 25-gauge).
- A "halo sign" (effusion that appears hypo- or anechoic on ultrasound) around the long head of the biceps may indicate tenosynovitis and improves the tendon sheath visualization.
- Utilize power Doppler to identify and avoid the arcuate artery, then target the medial aspect of the sheath toward the lesser tuberosity.

Videos showing landmark-guided and ultrasound-guided biceps tendon: long head injections can be found in the companion eBook.

REFERENCES

1. Gazzillo GP, Finnoff JT, Hall MM, Sayeed YA, Smith J. Accuracy of palpating the long head of the biceps tendon: an ultrasonographic study. *PM R.* 2011;3(11):1035-1040.
2. Hashiuchi T, Sakurai G, Morimoto M, Komei T, Takakura Y, Tanaka Y. Accuracy of the biceps tendon sheath injection: ultrasound guided or unguided injection? A randomized controlled trial. *J Shoulder Elbow Surg.* 2011;20(7):1069-1073.
3. Yiannakopoulos CK, Megaloikonomos PD, Foufa K, Gliatis J. Ultrasound-guided versus palpation-guided corticosteroid injections for tendinosis of the long head of the biceps: a randomized comparative study. *Skeletal Radiol.* 2020;49(4):585-591.
4. Petscavage-Thomas J, Gustas C. Comparison of ultrasound-guided to fluoroscopy-guided biceps tendon sheath therapeutic injection. *J Ultrasound Med.* 2016;35(10):2217-2221.
5. Gofeld M, Hurdle MF, Agur A. Biceps tendon sheath injection: an anatomical conundrum. *Pain Med.* 2019;20(1):138-142.
6. Pujalte G, Hudspeth LJ, Troyer WD, Shapiro SA. Ultrasound-guided injection of the long head of the biceps tendon sheath with concomitant subacromial bursa injection through the same needlestick. *Clin Anat.* 2023;36(3):400-405.

Cubital Tunnel Syndrome

Cubital tunnel syndrome is encountered uncommonly by primary care providers. It develops when the ulnar nerve becomes entrapped in the cubital tunnel posterior to the medial epicondyle. Nonsurgical treatment, aiming to decrease both compression and traction on the ulnar nerve, is successful in most patients with mild nerve dysfunction.[1] Conservative measures usually involve activity modification by the avoidance of predisposing repetitive movements and nighttime application of an elbow (or pediatric knee) splint/brace.[2] The clinician may wish to attempt to provide relief of pain by administration of a corticosteroid injection in carefully selected patients. A single randomized control trial did not demonstrate a positive effect of ultrasound-guided corticosteroid injections compared with placebo.[3] Successful treatment in patients unresponsive to conservative measures, including injection, may require surgical referral for transposition of the ulnar nerve in order to relocate it over the medial epicondyle.

Relevant Anatomy: (Fig. 10.24)

PATIENT POSITION

- Supine on the examination table with the head of the bed elevated 30°.
- Shoulder at 30° of abduction and full external rotation.
- The affected elbow is flexed at 90°.
- The wrist is in a neutral position.
- The elbow is supported with the placement of chucks pads or towels.
- Rotate the patient's head away from the side that is being injected. This minimizes anxiety and pain perception.

LANDMARKS

1. With the patient supine on the examination table, the clinician stands lateral to the affected elbow.
2. Identify and mark the medial epicondyle of the humerus.
3. Identify and mark the course of the ulnar nerve in the ulnar groove posterior to the medial epicondyle.
4. Mark the point of maximal tenderness over the ulnar nerve. This is usually just posterior to the medical epicondyle.
5. At that site, press firmly on the skin with the retracted tip of a ballpoint pen. This indentation represents the entry point for the needle.
6. After the landmarks are identified, the patient should not move the elbow.

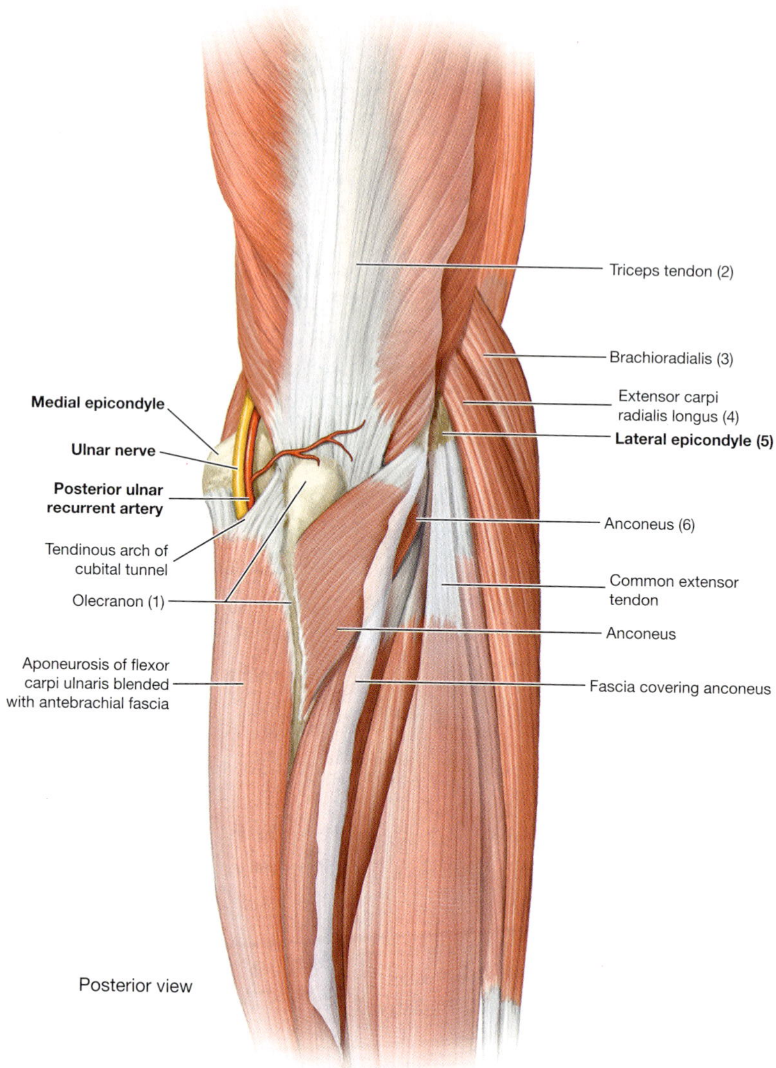

FIGURE 10.24 Posterior aspect of the right elbow.

ANESTHESIA

- Local anesthesia of the skin using topical vapocoolant spray.

EQUIPMENT

- Topical vapocoolant spray
- 3-mL syringe
- 25-gauge 1-in needle

- 1 mL of 1% lidocaine without epinephrine
- 1 mL of the 40 mg/mL steroid solution (40 mg of triamcinolone acetonide)
- One alcohol prep pad
- Two povidone-iodine or chlorhexidine prep pads
- Sterile gauze pads
- Sterile adhesive bandage
- Nonsterile, clean chucks pad

TECHNIQUE

1. Prep the insertion site with alcohol followed by the povidone-iodine or chlorhexidine pads.
2. Achieve good local anesthesia by using topical vapocoolant spray.
3. Position the needle and syringe at a 30° angle to the skin with the tip of the needle directed distally along the ulnar nerve.
4. Using the no-touch technique, quickly introduce the needle at the insertion site (Fig. 10.25).
5. Advance the needle slowly at a shallow angle to a position just along the side of the ulnar nerve.
6. If any pain, paresthesias, or numbness is encountered, withdraw the needle slightly and redirect the needle tip using a slightly different angle.
7. When the needle is placed along the ulnar nerve, withdraw the plunger of the syringe to ensure that there is no blood return.
8. Slowly inject the lidocaine/corticosteroid solution as a bolus around that structure. If increased resistance is encountered, advance or withdraw the needle slightly before attempting further injection.
9. Following injection, withdraw the needle.
10. Apply a sterile adhesive bandage.

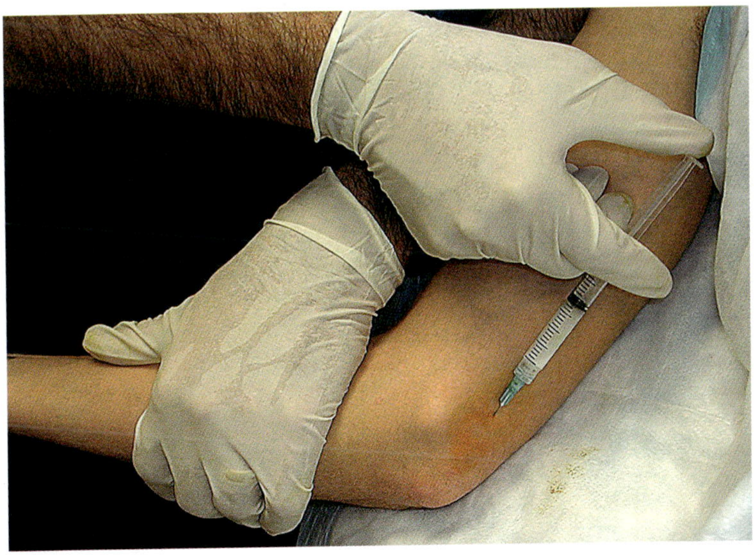

FIGURE 10.25 ● Right cubital tunnel injection.

11. Instruct the patient to move their elbow through its full range of motion. This movement distributes the lidocaine/corticosteroid solution along the course of the ulnar nerve in the cubital tunnel.
12. Reexamine the elbow in 5 minutes to assess pain relief and the development of numbness in the distribution of the ulnar nerve from the local anesthetic.

AFTERCARE

- Avoid further overuse mechanisms of injury.
- Use an elbow extension brace (or pediatric knee brace) while sleeping to avoid excessive elbow flexion.
- NSAIDs, ice, and/or physical therapy as indicated.
- Consider follow-up examination in 2 weeks.

ULTRASOUND-GUIDED PROCEDURE

Please refer to the introductory ultrasound chapter for preprocedure, sterile prep, postprocedure, and documentation information and recommendations.

PATIENT POSITION

- Lateral decubitus on the examination table with the affected elbow resting on a chux pad on the examination table.
- On the affected side, forward flex the shoulder to 90°, supinate the forearm, and flex the elbow to 90°.
- Place a pillow under the patient's head for comfort.
- Adjust the patient's position as needed for optimal comfort and accessibility.

PROVIDER/ULTRASOUND POSITION

- The provider stands on the affected side at the patient's head.
- Adjust the examination table to position the injection site between the provider's umbilicus and axillary level, ensuring optimal ergonomics and visualization of the ultrasound screen, transducer, and needle's approach (Fig. 10.26).
- Position the ultrasound machine at the patient's feet with the screen facing the provider.

LANDMARKS

- See the landmarks for the landmark-guided injection procedure.

ANESTHESIA

- Local anesthesia of the skin using topical vapocoolant spray.

EQUIPMENT

- 3-mL syringe
- 25-gauge 1.5-in needle (adjust needle length as needed)

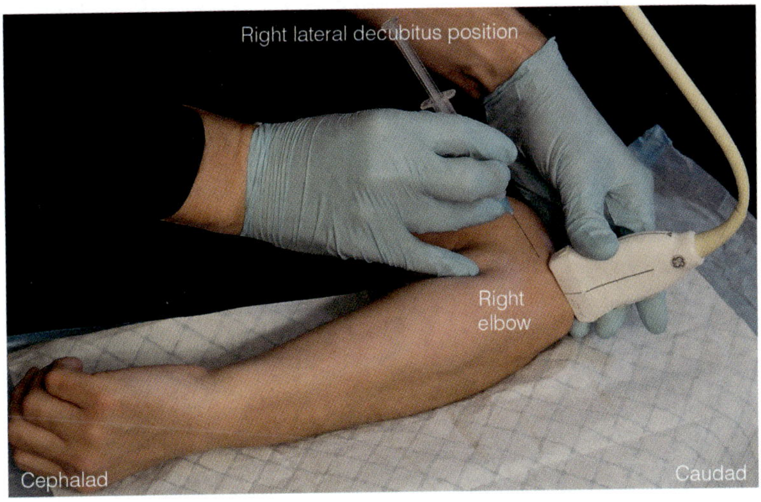

FIGURE 10.26 ● Ultrasound-guided right cubital tunnel injection. Right lateral decubitus position, with the affected elbow ipsilateral to the provider.

- 1 mL of 1% lidocaine without epinephrine
- 1 mL of the 40 mg/mL steroid solution (40 mg of triamcinolone acetonide)
- Three chlorhexidine swabs
- 12-4 MHz linear ultrasound transducer and machine
- Sterile ultrasound transducer cover
- Sterile ultrasound gel
- Nonlatex sterile or nonsterile gloves
- Two 4 × 4 sterile gauze pads
- One sterile adhesive bandage
- Topical vapocoolant spray

TECHNIQUE

1. Position a high-frequency linear 12-4 MHz ultrasound transducer in the axial plane with the ulnar nerve centered beneath it between the medial epicondyle and the olecranon.
2. Advance a 25-gauge 1.5-in needle using an in-plane approach, directing it from anterior to posterior, with an initial needle angle of approximately 5° to 15° relative to the skin surface where the transducer is positioned.
3. The target area is the perineural space of the affected ulnar nerve deep to the Osborne ligament.
4. Utilize real-time ultrasound guidance throughout the procedure to precisely place the needle within the desired target area and minimize the risk of inadvertently injuring surrounding structures (Fig. 10.27).
5. Upon completion of the procedure, carefully withdraw the needle. Adhere to established postprocedure care protocols and ensure appropriate follow-up as recommended.

PEARLS

- The ulnar nerve appears as a hypoechoic or honeycomb, oval-shaped structure within the cubital tunnel.

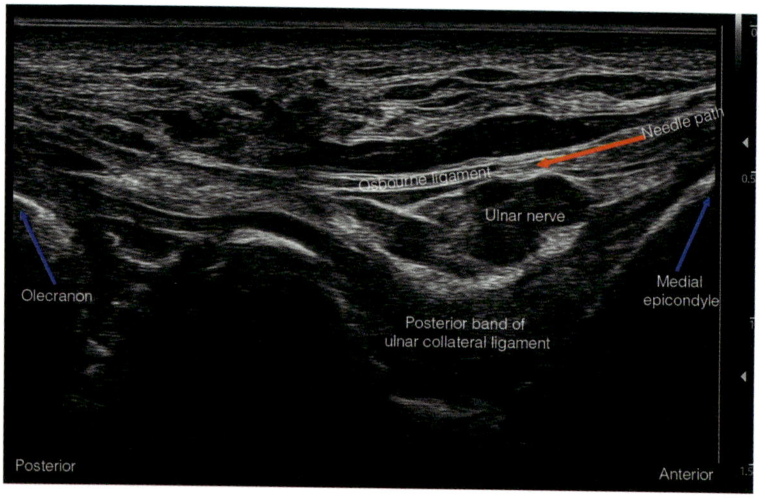

FIGURE 10.27 ● Cubital tunnel ultrasound axial image.

- Advance the needle slowly and with controlled movements, continuously monitoring its position under ultrasound, to avoid intraneural injection.
- This technique distributes the injectate along multiple potential ulnar nerve entrapment sites, including within the cubital tunnel and distally along the nerve.[4]
- Cubital tunnel syndrome can be difficult to differentiate from C8/T1 radiculopathy. Consider a workup for radiculopathy and refer to a specialist as needed before proceeding with injection.

Videos showing landmark-guided and ultrasound-guided cubital tunnel syndrome injections can be found in the companion eBook.

REFERENCES

1. Staples JR, Calfee R. Cubital tunnel syndrome: current concepts. *J Am Acad Orthop Surg.* 2017;25(10):e215-e224.
2. Poenaru D, Ojoga F, Sandulescu M, Cinteza D. Conservative therapy in ulnar neuropathy at the elbow (review). *Exp Ther Med.* 2022;24(2):517.
3. vanVeen KE, Alblas KC, Alons IM, et al. Corticosteroid injection in patients with ulnar neuropathy at the elbow: a randomized, double-blind, placebo-controlled trial. *Muscle Nerve.* 2015;52(3):380-385.
4. Hamscha UM, Tinhofer I, Heber S, Grisold W, Weninger WJ, Meng S. A reliable technique for ultrasound-guided perineural injection in ulnar neuropathy at the elbow. *Muscle Nerve.* 2017;56(2):237-241.

Elbow Joint

Aspiration and injection of the elbow joint is an uncommon procedure in most primary care practices. A tense collection of blood distending the elbow joint commonly develops in association with intra-articular fractures. In that case, significant pain relief may follow aspiration. Arthritis in the elbow with fluid accumulation may occur with gout, rheumatoid arthritis, and osteoarthritis. This may respond to corticosteroid injection, but this aspiration and injection procedure is not described in any clinical trials.

There are two common approaches to the elbow joint. Either the humeroulnar or the radiocapitellar articulations can be accessed. The joint between the humerus and the ulna offers the largest area of joint space and is therefore easier to perform with a landmark-guided approach. Alternatively, with ultrasound guidance, the radiocapitellar articulation approach may be preferred. High-resolution ultrasonography can help clinicians visualize key anatomic structures of the elbow and increase accuracy of periarticular and intra-articular injections.[1,2]

Relevant Anatomy: (Fig. 10.28)

PATIENT POSITION

- Supine on the examination table with the head of the bed elevated 30°.
- The elbow is positioned at 45° of flexion.
- The wrist is in a neutral position.

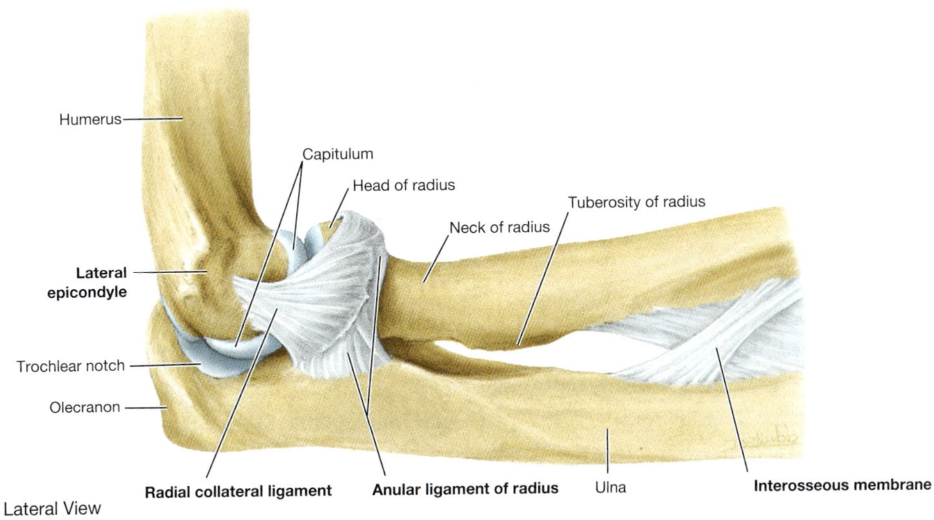

FIGURE 10.28 ● Right lateral elbow joint. (Reprinted with permission from Agur AMR, Dalley AF II. *Grant's Atlas of Anatomy*. 16th ed. Wolters Kluwer; 2025.)

- The elbow is supported with the placement of chucks pads or towels.
- Rotate the patient's head away from the side that is being injected. This minimizes anxiety and pain perception.

LANDMARKS

1. With the patient supine on the examination table, the clinician stands lateral to the affected elbow.
2. (Humeroulnar articulation) This approach may provide the easiest approach to the largest accessible entry point to the elbow joint. Locate the lateral epicondyle. Slide the fingertip over and down the epicondyle until it sits in the sulcus between the epicondyle and the ulna. Mark the deepest point of the sulcus with ink.
3. (Radiocapitellar joint) Alternatively, find the radial head by palpating rotational movement over the lateral aspect of the elbow joint while supinating and pronating the wrist. Find the depression immediately proximal to the radial head and mark it with ink.
4. At the selected site, press firmly on the skin with the retracted tip of a ballpoint pen. This indentation represents the entry point for the needle.
5. After the landmarks are identified, the patient should not move the elbow.

ANESTHESIA

- Local anesthesia of the skin using topical vapocoolant spray.

EQUIPMENT

- Topical vapocoolant spray
- 3-mL syringe
- 10-mL syringe—for optional aspiration
- 25-gauge 1-in needle
- 20-gauge 1-in needle—for optional aspiration
- 0.5 mL of 1% mepivacaine without epinephrine
- 0.5 mL of the 40 mg/mL steroid solution (20 mg of triamcinolone acetonide)
- One alcohol prep pad
- Two povidone-povidone iodine or chlorhexidine prep pads
- Sterile gauze pads
- Sterile adhesive bandage
- Nonsterile, clean chucks pad

TECHNIQUE

1. Prep the selected insertion site with alcohol followed by the povidone-povidone iodine or chlorhexidine pads.
2. Achieve good local anesthesia by using topical vapocoolant spray.
3. Position the needle and syringe perpendicular to the skin with the needle tip directed medially toward the elbow joint.
4. Using the no-touch technique, quickly introduce the needle at the insertion site (Fig. 10.29).

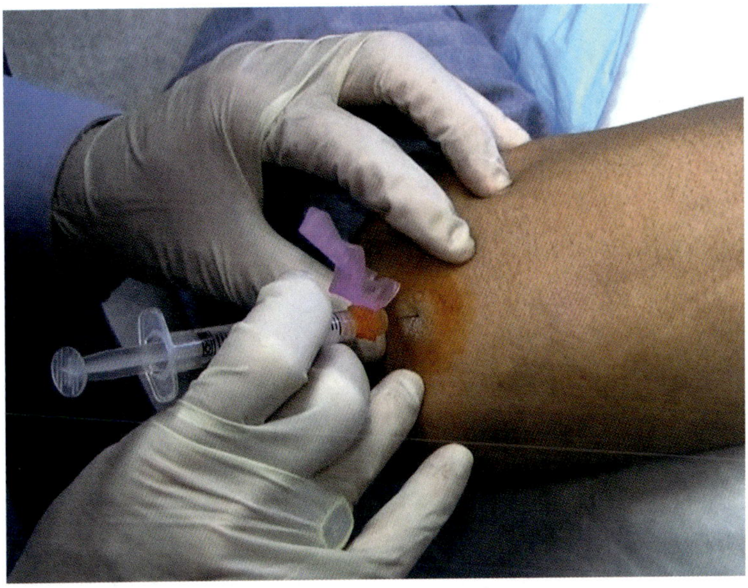

FIGURE 10.29 • Left elbow joint injection.

5. Advance the needle into the elbow joint. This places the needle tip between the humeral lateral condyle and either the ulna or the radial head.
6. If aspirating, withdraw fluid using a 20-gauge 1-in needle with the 10-mL syringe.
7. If injection of corticosteroid is to follow the aspiration, grasp the needle firmly, remove the 10-mL syringe from the 20-gauge needle, and then attach the 3-mL syringe filled with the mepivacaine/corticosteroid mixture.
8. If only injecting the mepivacaine/corticosteroid mixture, use a 25-gauge 1-in needle with the 3-mL syringe.
9. Inject the mepivacaine/corticosteroid solution as a bolus into the elbow joint. The injected solution should flow smoothly into the space. If increased resistance is encountered, advance or withdraw the needle slightly before attempting further injection.
10. Following injection, withdraw the needle.
11. Apply a sterile adhesive bandage.
12. Instruct the patient to move their elbow through its full range of motion. This movement distributes the mepivacaine/corticosteroid solution throughout the elbow joint.
13. Reexamine the elbow in 5 minutes to assess pain relief.

AFTERCARE

- Do not brace or rest the elbow. A study showed a significantly higher rate of synovitis relapse in patients following corticosteroid injection who were rested for 48 hours in an elbow sling versus normal activity without restrictions.[3]
- Consider the use of a neoprene elbow sleeve.
- Avoid vigorous use of the elbow over the next 2 weeks.
- NSAIDs, ice, and/or physical therapy as indicated.
- Consider follow-up examination in 2 weeks.

PEARLS

- The joint space at the radial head may be "opened up" by extending the elbow.
- Since the elbow has a narrow joint space, a 20-gauge needle is used for aspiration instead of the larger diameter, 18-gauge needle.
- If a fracture or infection is suspected, do not inject corticosteroid.

ULTRASOUND-GUIDED PROCEDURE

Please refer to the introductory ultrasound chapter for preprocedure, sterile prep, post-procedure, and documentation information and recommendations.

PATIENT POSITION

- Supine on the examination table.
- On the affected side, internally rotate the shoulder, flex the elbow to 90°, supinate the forearm, and rest the elbow on a chux pad placed on the patient's abdomen.
- Place a pillow under their head for comfort.
- Adjust the patient's position as needed for comfort.

PROVIDER/ULTRASOUND POSITION

- The provider stands slightly distal to the patient's affected elbow.
- Adjust the examination table to position the injection site between the provider's umbilicus and axillary level, ensuring optimal ergonomics and visualization of the ultrasound screen, transducer, and needle's approach (Fig. 10.30).
- Position the ultrasound machine on the same side of the table from the provider at the level of the patient's head with the screen facing the provider.

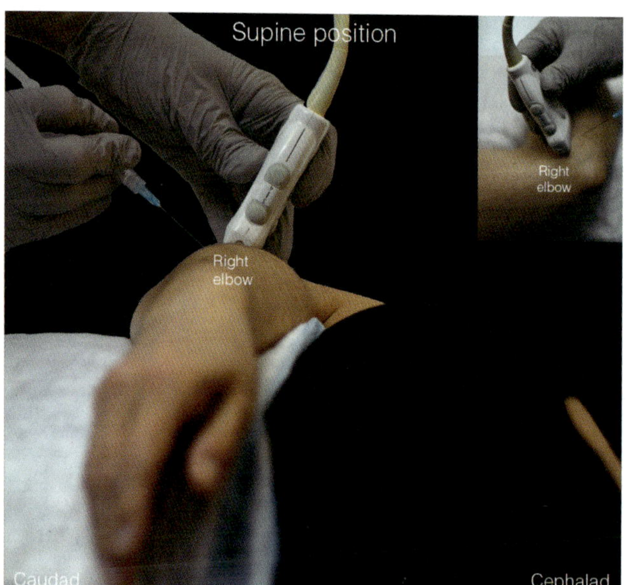

FIGURE 10.30 ● Ultrasound-guided intra-articular right elbow injection. Supine position with the affected elbow flexed and placed across the abdomen. Provider positioned ipsilateral to the affected elbow.

LANDMARKS

- See the landmarks for the landmark-guided injection procedure.

ANESTHESIA

- Local anesthesia of the skin using topical vapocoolant spray.

EQUIPMENT

- 3-mL syringe
- 25-gauge 1.5-in needle (adjust needle length as needed)
- 0.5 mL of 1% mepivacaine without epinephrine
- 0.5 mL of the 40 mg/mL steroid solution (20 mg of triamcinolone acetonide)
- Alternative setup for aspiration
  - 3-mL syringe (anesthesia)
    - 25-gauge 1.5-in needle (adjust needle length as needed)
    - 3 mL of 1% lidocaine without epinephrine
  - 5-mL syringe (aspiration)
    - 18-gauge 1.5-in needle (adjust needle length as needed)
- Three chlorhexidine swabs
- 12-4 MHz linear ultrasound transducer and machine
- Sterile ultrasound transducer cover
- Sterile ultrasound gel
- Nonlatex sterile or nonsterile gloves
- Two 4 × 4 sterile gauze pads
- One sterile adhesive bandage
- Topical vapocoolant spray.

TECHNIQUE

1. Position a high-frequency linear 12-4 MHz ultrasound transducer in the coronal plane with the affected radiocapitellar joint centered beneath it.
2. Advance a 25-gauge 1.5-in needle using an out-of-plane approach, directing it from posterolateral to anteromedial, with an initial needle angle of approximately 5° to 15° relative to the skin surface where the transducer is positioned.
3. The target area is the affected joint.
4. Utilize real-time ultrasound guidance throughout the procedure to precisely place the needle within the desired target area and minimize the risk of inadvertently injuring surrounding structures (Fig. 10.31).
5. For intra-articular steroid injection:
   a. Slowly inject the desired volume of mepivacaine and corticosteroid solution directly into the joint.
6. For situations requiring anesthesia, aspiration, or both:
   a. Utilize a separate 25-gauge 1.5-in needle with a 3-mL syringe to inject 3 mL of 1% lidocaine without epinephrine into the soft tissues overlying the joint.
   b. For aspiration, use an 18-gauge 1.5-in needle with a 5-mL syringe to withdraw the effusion.

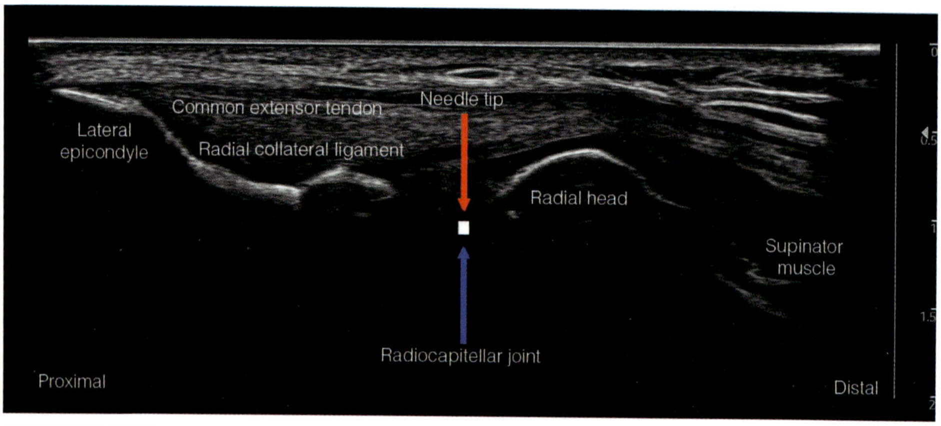

FIGURE 10.31 ● Radiocapitellar joint ultrasound coronal image.

c. If a corticosteroid injection is indicated following aspiration, replace the aspiration syringe with the mepivacaine and corticosteroid solution syringe and reconfirm accurate needle placement using real-time ultrasound guidance before injection.

7. Upon completion of the procedure, carefully withdraw the needle. Adhere to established postprocedure care protocols and ensure appropriate follow-up as recommended.

PEARLS

- The radiocapitellar joint lies deep to the common extensor tendon (CET) and the radial collateral ligament, which should be avoided during the procedure.
- To enhance visualization of the joint, actively supinate and pronate the hand during the preprocedural ultrasound scan. This motion causes the radial head to move, facilitating easier identification of the radiocapitellar joint just proximal to this movement.

Videos showing landmark-guided and ultrasound-guided elbow joint injections can be found in the companion eBook.

REFERENCES

1. Sussman WI, Williams CJ, Mautner K. Ultrasound-guided elbow procedures. *Phys Med Rehabil Clin N Am.* 2016;27(3):573-587.
2. Kim TK, Lee JH, Park KD, Lee SC, Ahn J, Park Y. Ultrasound versus palpation guidance for intra-articular injections in patients with degenerative osteoarthritis of the elbow. *J Clin Ultrasound.* 2013;41(8):479-485.
3. Weitoft T, Forsberg C. Importance of immobilization after intraarticular glucocorticoid treatment for elbow synovitis: a randomized controlled study. *Arthritis Care Res (Hoboken).* 2010;62(5):735-737.

Olecranon Bursa

Olecranon bursitis is a relatively common condition presenting to primary care providers. The subcutaneous olecranon bursa may become inflamed and accumulate fluid when subjected to repeated excessive pressure or friction. The fluid may consist of blood in acute trauma, thick proteinaceous mucoid fluid after repetitive injury, serous fluid in the unusual case of acute gout, or purulent fluid if infected.

In most cases, a conservative treatment regimen can be pursued, following bursal aspirate–based differentiation between septic and nonseptic bursitis.[1] Successful aspiration is usually easily accomplished because the location of the bursa is superficial and readily identified. Injected corticosteroids may be considered in select cases of inflammatory olecranon bursitis such as that encountered with gout or rheumatoid arthritis. However, steroids should not be administered if septic bursitis is suspected. More recent literature has emphasized conservative therapy due to the adverse effects of surgical bursectomy compared with noninvasive management for initial treatment of nonseptic olecranon bursitis.[2] The use of intrabursal doxycycline as a sclerosing agent may be an effective alternative to surgical bursectomy for patients with recurrent disease refractory to conservative management.[3]

Relevant Anatomy: (Fig. 10.32)

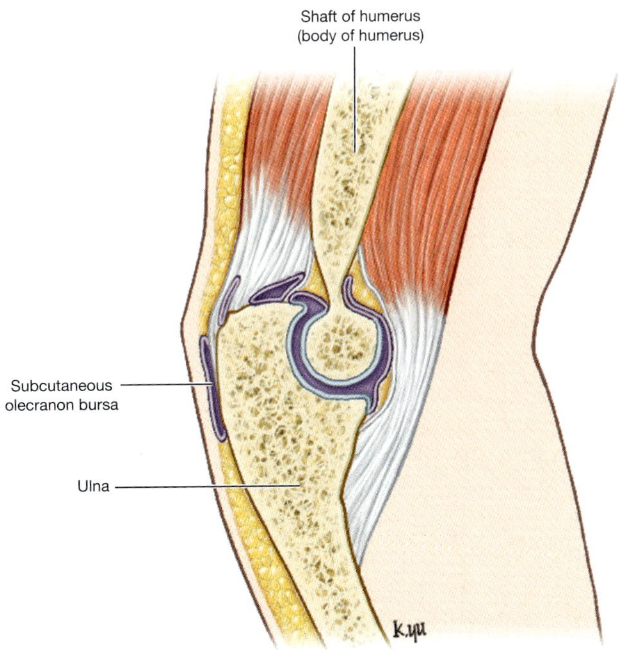

FIGURE 10.32 ● Lateral aspect of left elbow. (Reprinted with permission from Dalley AF II, Agur AMR. *Moore's Clinically Oriented Anatomy*. 9th ed. Wolters Kluwer; 2023.)

PATIENT POSITION

- Supine on the examination table with the head of the bed elevated 30°.
- The affected elbow is maximally flexed.
- The elbow is supported with the placement of chucks pads or towels.
- Rotate the patient's head away from the side that is being injected. This minimizes anxiety and pain perception.

LANDMARKS

1. With the patient supine on the examination table, the clinician stands lateral to the affected elbow.
2. The point of maximal fluctuance is identified.
3. At that site, press firmly on the skin with the retracted tip of a ballpoint pen. This indentation represents the entry point for the needle.
4. After the landmarks are identified, the patient should not move the elbow.

ANESTHESIA

- Local anesthesia of the skin using topical vapocoolant spray.

EQUIPMENT

- Topical vapocoolant spray
- 20-mL syringe—for aspiration
- 3-mL syringe—for optional injection
- 18-gauge 1½-in needle
- 1 mL of 1% lidocaine without epinephrine—for optional injection
- 0.5 mL of the 40 mg/mL steroid solution (20 mg of triamcinolone acetonide)—for optional injection
- One alcohol prep pad
- Two povidone-iodine or chlorhexidine prep pads
- Sterile gauze pads
- Sterile adhesive bandage
- Nonsterile, clean chucks pad

TECHNIQUE

1. Prep the insertion site with alcohol followed by the povidone-iodine or chlorhexidine pads.
2. Achieve good local anesthesia by using topical vapocoolant spray.
3. Grasp the bursa with the thumb and index finger of the nondominant hand and slightly squeeze to stabilize the structure and facilitate stable needle entry.
4. Position the 18-gauge needle and syringe with the needle tip directed toward the center of maximal fluid collection.
5. Using the no-touch technique, quickly introduce the needle at the insertion site (Fig. 10.33).
6. Advance the needle into the center of the bursa.
7. Aspiration should be easily accomplished. Use multiple syringes if the effusion is large.

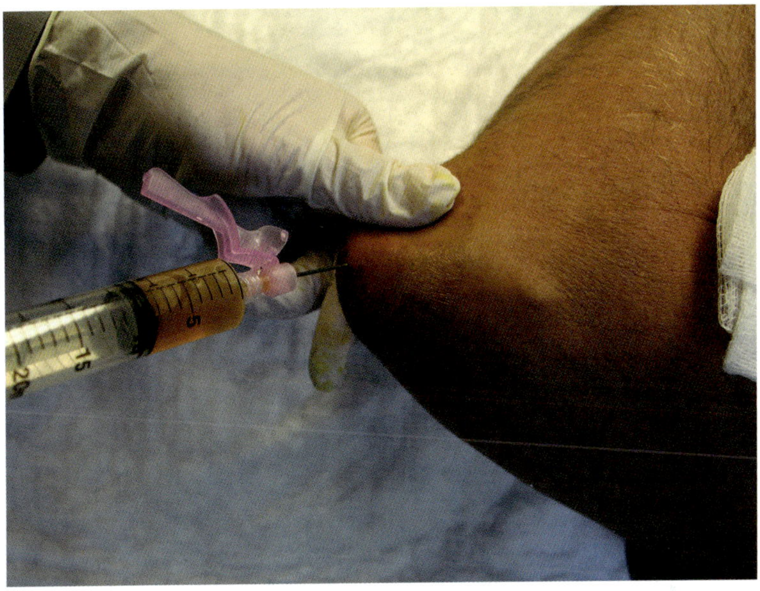

FIGURE 10.33 • Olecranon bursa aspiration.

8. If injection following aspiration is elected, grasp the hub of the needle, remove the large syringe, and then attach the 3-mL syringe filled with the lidocaine/corticosteroid solution.
9. The injected solution should flow smoothly into the space. If increased resistance is encountered, advance or withdraw the needle slightly before attempting further injection.
10. Following complete aspiration, and optional injection, withdraw the needle.
11. Apply a sterile adhesive bandage followed by a compressive elastic bandage.

AFTERCARE

- Avoid excessive use of the elbow over the next 2 weeks.
- Consider the use of a neoprene elbow sleeve or elastic compression bandage.
- NSAIDs, ice, and/or physical therapy as indicated.
- Consider follow-up examination in 2 weeks.

PEARLS

- If the olecranon bursa fluid collection is due to an infection or acute hemorrhagic event, do not follow aspiration with corticosteroid injection.
- Injection of corticosteroid is usually reserved for inflammatory bursitis.

A video showing a landmark-guided olecranon bursa aspiration can be found in the companion eBook.

REFERENCES

1. Baumbach SF, Lobo CM, Badyine I. Prepatellar and olecranon bursitis: literature review and development of a treatment algorithm. *Arch Orthop Trauma Surg.* 2014;134(3):359-370.
2. Nchinda NN, Wolf JM. Clinical management of olecranon bursitis: a review. *J Hand Surg Am.* 2021;46(6):501-506.
3. McDermott D, Wakefield D, Kowalsky M, Sethi P, Vitale MA, Morrey BF. Intrabursal doxycycline sclerotherapy for recurrent olecranon bursitis of the elbow: a case control study. *J Hand Surg Glob Online.* 2024;6(4):504-509.

Lateral Epicondyle

Lateral epicondylitis (aka tennis elbow) is one of the most common soft tissue conditions treated by primary care providers. This is a misnomer and actually involves a noninflammatory tendinosis with collagen disarray—principally involving the CET. It usually is the result of an overuse injury, frequently associated with degenerative microtears to the hypovascular origins of the wrist extensor and supinator muscle groups that originate at the lateral condyle of the distal humerus.

Injection of various therapeutics to treat this condition has been extensively reported in the literature. Although corticosteroid injections have been used for years, it appears that they are beneficial only in the short term.[1,2] Long-term results are no better than placebo and may in fact be worse.[2,3] In addition, corticosteroid injections used in treating this disorder may have both systemic and local adverse effects including well-described skin atrophy[4] and hypopigmentation.[5]

In actuality, there is no injection or physiotherapy intervention that has consistently shown treatment efficacy in the medium to long term in patients diagnosed with lateral epicondylitis.[6-8] In the long term, PRP injections may show greater improvement in pain and function than corticosteroid injections,[9,10] but not all studies are favorable.[11,12] Injections of botulinum toxin have shown promising results.[13,14] Dextrose prolotherapy also shows positive therapeutic effect.[15] More research is needed to determine how to best use orthobiologics and other interventions in the treatment of lateral epicondylitis.[16]

A reduction in the corticosteroid injection rate would be expected following the publication of high-level evidence demonstrating a lack of efficacy; however, this has not been the case.[17,18] The authors suspect that this is due to the positive short-term benefit of corticosteroids on pain.

Relevant Anatomy: (Fig. 10.34)

PATIENT POSITION

- Supine on the examination table with the head of the bed elevated 30°.
- The affected elbow is slightly flexed.
- The wrist is in a neutral to slightly pronated position.
- The elbow is supported with the placement of chucks pads or towels.
- Rotate the patient's head away from the side that is being injected. This minimizes anxiety and pain perception.

LANDMARKS

1. With the patient supine on the examination table, the clinician stands lateral to the affected elbow.
2. Identify and mark the point of maximal tenderness involving the CET, adjacent to the lateral epicondyle.

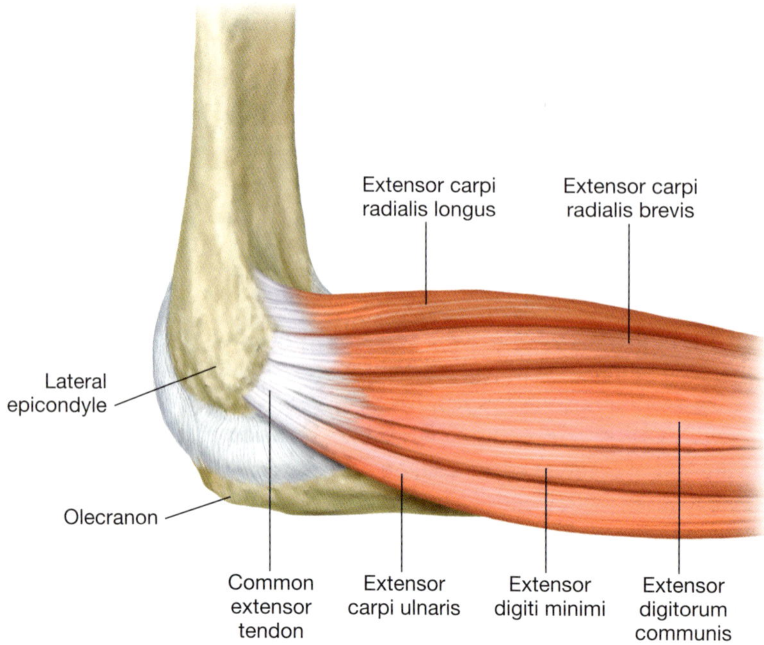

FIGURE 10.34 Lateral view of muscular structures and common extensor tendon of the right elbow.

3. At that site, press firmly on the skin with the retracted tip of a ballpoint pen. This indentation represents the entry point for the needle.
4. After the landmark is identified, the patient should not move the elbow.

ANESTHESIA

- Local anesthesia of the skin using topical vapocoolant spray.

EQUIPMENT

- Topical vapocoolant spray
- 3-mL syringe
- 25-gauge 1-in needle
- 1 mL of 1% lidocaine without epinephrine
- 0.5 to 1 mL of the 40 mg/mL steroid solution (20-40 mg of triamcinolone acetonide)—if desired
- One alcohol prep pad
- Two povidone-iodine or chlorhexidine prep pads
- Sterile gauze pads
- Sterile adhesive bandage
- Nonsterile, clean chucks pad

TECHNIQUE

1. Prep the insertion site with alcohol followed by the povidone-iodine or chlorhexidine pads.
2. Achieve good local anesthesia by using topical vapocoolant spray.

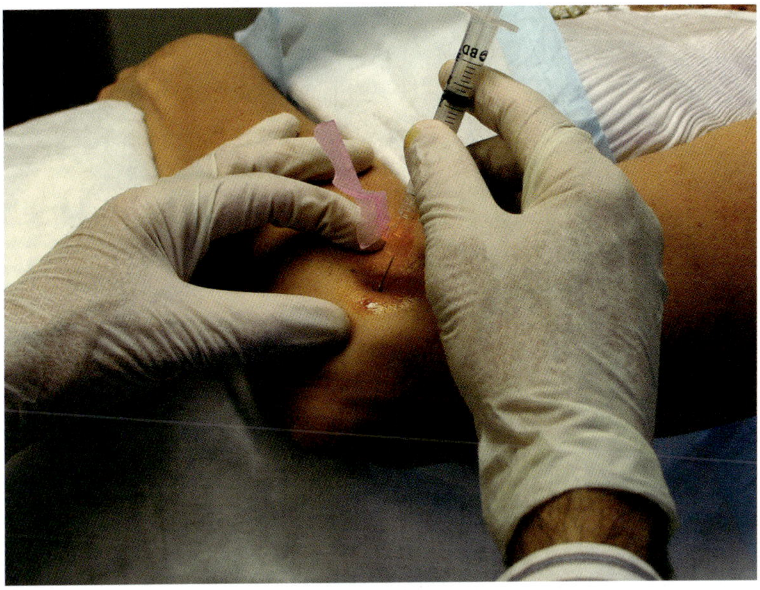

FIGURE 10.35 ● Left elbow lateral epicondyle injection.

3. Position the needle and syringe perpendicular to the skin with the needle tip directed medially toward the lateral epicondyle.
4. Using the no-touch technique, quickly introduce the needle at the insertion site (Fig. 10.35).
5. Advance the needle to the bone of the lateral epicondyle.
6. Withdraw the needle 1 to 2 mm.
7. Perform the "pinch technique" (see description in "Pearls" section—Fig. 10.36).

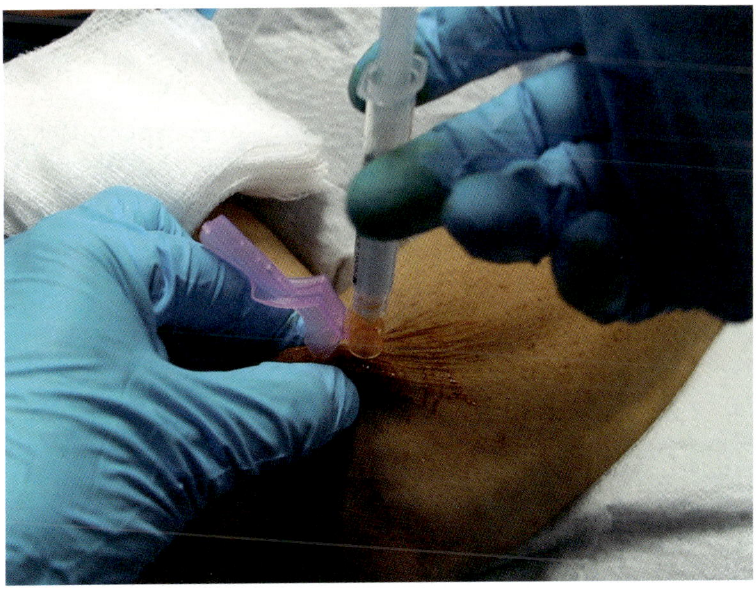

FIGURE 10.36 ● Left elbow—pinch up the tissue to avoid subcutaneous deposition of corticosteroid.

8. Withdraw the plunger of the syringe to ensure that there is no blood return.
9. Inject the lidocaine/corticosteroid or other therapeutic solution steadily into this area. If increased resistance is encountered, advance or withdraw the needle slightly before attempting further injection.
10. Following injection, withdraw the needle.
11. Apply a sterile adhesive bandage.
12. Instruct the patient to move their wrist and elbow through their full range of motion.
13. Reexamine the elbow in 5 minutes to assess pain relief.

AFTERCARE

- Avoid excessive wrist extension and supination over the next 2 weeks.
- Consider the use of a neoprene elbow sleeve or elastic compression bandage.
- Consider the use of a wrist brace to limit wrist extension.
- NSAIDs, ice, heat, and/or physical therapy as indicated.
- Consider follow-up examination in 2 weeks.
- Consider treatment using alternative modalities if initial therapy is not effective.

PEARLS

- Entrapment of branches of the radial nerve in the elbow and forearm can mimic the pain of lateral epicondylitis. Radial tunnel syndrome is most commonly caused by entrapment of the deep radial nerve as it enters the supinator muscle at the arcade of Frohse. Pain in this condition occurs about 4 cm distal to the lateral epicondyle.
- Due to the anatomically superficial location of the lateral epicondyle, especially in thin individuals, an injection of corticosteroid may be inadvertently deposited in the subdermal and subcutaneous tissues rather than beneath the CET. Deposition into these superficial structures commonly leads to the side effects of skin atrophy and hypopigmentation. Avoid the development of an intradermal wheal while performing all injections of corticosteroid solutions.
- In order to prevent this dermal complication, one can use the pinch technique (Fig. 10.36). After insertion, gently grasp the skin on either side of the needle, pinch the soft tissue and push it up the needle toward the syringe. This provides a greater distance between the skin and the actual injection site at the epicondyle, thus minimizing the chance of developing atrophy and hypopigmentation.

ULTRASOUND-GUIDED PROCEDURE

Please refer to the introductory ultrasound chapter for preprocedure, sterile prep, post-procedure, and documentation information and recommendations.

PATIENT POSITION

- Supine on the examination table.
- On the affected side, place the shoulder in internal rotation, flex the elbow to 90°, supinate the forearm, and rest the elbow on a chux pad placed on the patient's abdomen.
- Place a pillow under their head for comfort.
- Adjust the patient's position as needed for comfort.

PROVIDER/ULTRASOUND POSITION

- The provider stands on the opposite side of the table from the patient's affected elbow.
- Adjust the examination table to position the injection site between the provider's umbilicus and axillary level, ensuring optimal ergonomics and visualization of the ultrasound screen, transducer, and needle's approach (Fig. 10.37).
- Position the ultrasound machine on the opposite side of the table from the provider at the level of the patient's affected elbow with the screen facing the provider.

LANDMARKS

- See the landmarks for the landmark-guided injection procedure.

ANESTHESIA

- Local anesthesia of the skin using topical vapocoolant spray.

EQUIPMENT

- 3-mL syringe
- 25-gauge 1.5-in needle (adjust needle length as needed)
- 1 mL of 1% lidocaine without epinephrine
- 0.5 to 1 mL of the 40 mg/mL steroid solution (20-40 mg of triamcinolone acetonide)
- Three chlorhexidine swabs
- 12-4 MHz linear ultrasound transducer and machine
- Sterile ultrasound transducer cover
- Sterile ultrasound gel
- Nonlatex sterile or nonsterile gloves
- Two 4 × 4 sterile gauze pads
- One sterile adhesive bandage
- Topical vapocoolant spray

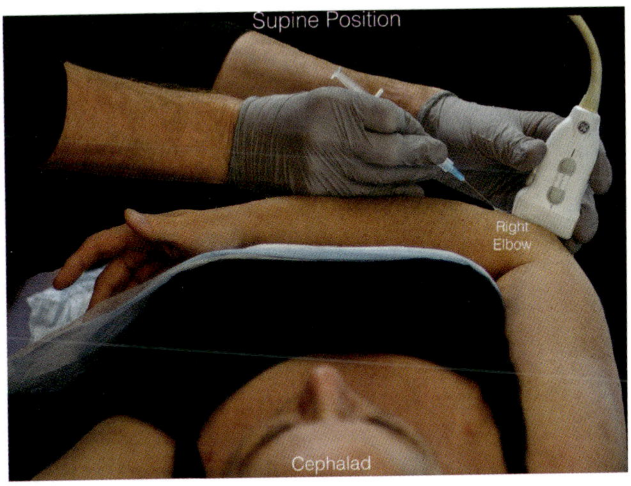

FIGURE 10.37 Ultrasound-guided right lateral epicondylalgia elbow injection. Supine position with the affected elbow flexed across the abdomen. Provider contralateral to the affected elbow.

TECHNIQUE

1. Position a high-frequency linear 12-4 MHz transducer in the coronal plane with the lateral epicondyle centered.
2. Advance a 25-gauge 1.5-in needle using an in-plane approach, directing it from distal to proximal, with an initial needle angle of approximately 15° to 20° relative to the skin surface where the transducer is positioned.
3. Target area:
   a. For corticosteroids: The deep peritendinous space between the CET and radial collateral ligament
   b. For dextrose prolotherapy or PRP: The area of tendinopathy in the tendon (refer to Chapter 4: Orthobiologics)
4. Injectate:
   a. For corticosteroids: Use a 25-gauge 1.5-in needle to inject the solution into the deep peritendinous space.
   b. For dextrose prolotherapy or PRP (refer to Chapter 4: Orthobiologics): Use a 22-gauge 1.5-in needle to inject the solution into the area of tendinopathy in the tendon. Administer a total volume (1-2 mL) of 15% dextrose prolotherapy or PRP in small aliquots (0.5 mL or less).
5. Utilize real-time ultrasound guidance throughout to ensure accurate needle placement and minimize the risk of complications (Fig. 10.38).
6. Upon completion of the procedure, carefully withdraw the needle. Adhere to established postprocedure care protocols and ensure appropriate follow-up as recommended.

PEARLS

- Consider a longer needle (eg, 2-in 25-gauge).
- The CET typically constitutes about 50% of the superficial compact fibrillar structure that inserts onto the lateral epicondyle. The radial collateral ligament is the rest.

Videos showing landmark-guided and ultrasound-guided lateral epicondyle injections can be found in the companion eBook.

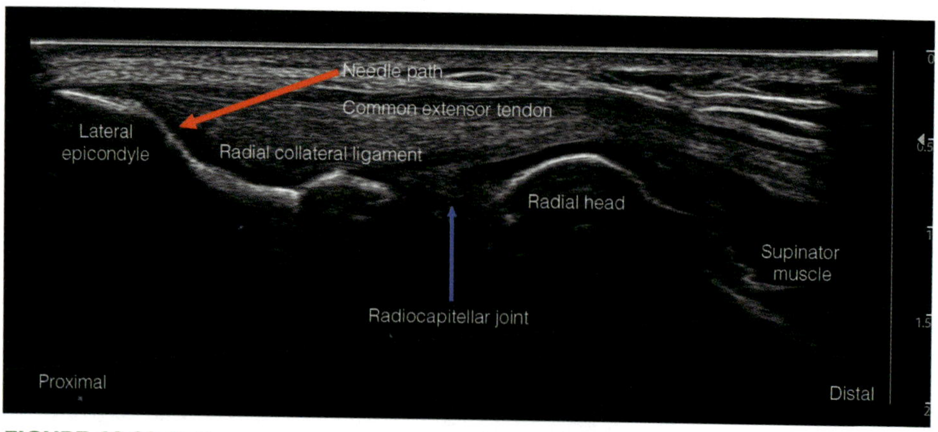

FIGURE 10.38 ● Common extensor tendon ultrasound coronal image.

REFERENCES

1. Krogh TP, Fredberg U, Stengaard-Pedersen K, Christensen R, Jensen P, Ellingsen T. Treatment of lateral epicondylitis with platelet-rich plasma, glucocorticoid, or saline: a randomized, double-blind, placebo-controlled trial. *Am J Sports Med.* 2013;41(3):625-635.
2. Coombes BK, Bisset L, Vicenzino B. Efficacy and safety of corticosteroid injections and other injections for management of tendinopathy: a systematic review of randomised controlled trials. *Lancet.* 2010;376(9754):1751-1767.
3. Coombes BK, Bisset L, Brooks P, Khan A, Vicenzino B. Effect of corticosteroid injection, physiotherapy, or both on clinical outcomes in patients with unilateral lateral epicondylalgia: a randomized controlled trial. *JAMA.* 2013;309(5):461-469.
4. Pace CS, Blanchet NP, Isaacs JE. Soft tissue atrophy related to corticosteroid injection: review of the literature and implications for hand surgeons. *J Hand Surg Am.* 2018;43(6):558-563.
5. Freire V, Bureau NJ. Injectable corticosteroids: take precautions and use caution. *Semin Musculoskelet Radiol.* 2016;20(5):401-408.
6. Gao B, Dwivedi S, DeFroda S, et al. The therapeutic benefits of saline solution injection for lateral epicondylitis: a meta-analysis of randomized controlled trials comparing saline injections with nonsurgical injection therapies. *Arthroscopy.* 2019;35(6):1847-1859.e12.
7. Krogh TP, Bartels EM, Ellingsen T, et al. Comparative effectiveness of injection therapies in lateral epicondylitis: a systematic review and network meta-analysis of randomized controlled trials. *Am J Sports Med.* 2013;41(6):1435-1446.
8. Wolf JM, Ozer K, Scott F, Gordon MJV, Williams AE. Comparison of autologous blood, corticosteroid, and saline injection in the treatment of lateral epicondylitis: a prospective, randomized, controlled multicenter study. *J Hand Surg Am.* 2011;36(8):1269-1272.
9. Li A, Wang H, Yu Z, et al. Platelet-rich plasma vs corticosteroids for elbow epicondylitis: a systematic review and meta-analysis. *Medicine (Baltimore).* 2019;98(51):e18358.
10. Xu Q, Chen J, Cheng L. Comparison of platelet rich plasma and corticosteroids in the management of lateral epicondylitis: a meta-analysis of randomized controlled trials. *Int J Surg.* 2019;67:37-46.
11. Franchini M, Cruciani M, Mengoli C, et al. Efficacy of platelet-rich plasma as conservative treatment in orthopaedics: a systematic review and meta-analysis. *Blood Transfus.* 2018;11; 16(6):502-513.
12. Linnanmäki L, Kanto K, Karjalainen T, Leppänen OV, Lehtinen J. Platelet-rich plasma or autologous blood do not reduce pain or improve function in patients with lateral epicondylitis: a randomized controlled trial. *Clin Orthop Relat Res.* 2020;478(8):1892-1900.
13. Galván Ruiz A, Vergara Díaz G, Rendón Fernández B, Ruiz De CE, Vargas. Effects of ultrasound-guided administration of botulinum toxin (incobotulinumtoxinA) in patients with lateral epicondylitis. *Toxins (Basel).* 2019;11(1):46.
14. Grüner S, Schulz A, Schlüter-Brust K, Lippert-Grüner M. Botulinum toxin for chronic lateral epicondylitis (LE). *Z Orthop Unfall.* 2021;159(5):554-564.
15. Zhu M, Rabago D, Chung VC, Reeves KD, Wong SY-S, Sit RW-S. Effects of hypertonic dextrose injection (prolotherapy) in lateral elbow tendinosis: a systematic review and meta-analysis. *Arch Phys Med Rehabil.* 2022;103(11):2209-2218.
16. Calandruccio JH, Steiner MM. Autologous blood and platelet-rich plasma injections for treatment of lateral epicondylitis. *Orthop Clin North Am.* 2017;48(3):351-357.
17. Fujihara Y, Huetteman HE, Chung TT, Shauver MJ, Chung KC. The effect of impactful articles on clinical practice in the united states: corticosteroid injection for patients with lateral epicondylitis. *Plast Reconstr Surg.* 2018;141(5):1183-1191.
18. Vicenzino B, Britt H, Pollack AJ, Hall M, Bennell KL, Hunter DJ. No abatement of steroid injections for tennis elbow in Australian General Practice: a 15-year observational study with random general practitioner sampling. *PLoS One.* 2017;12(7):e0181631.

Medial Epicondyle

Medial epicondylitis (aka golfer's elbow) is a fairly common soft tissue condition encountered by primary care physicians. Pathophysiologically similar to lateral epicondylitis, this condition also involves a noninflammatory tendinosis with collagen disarray—principally involving the common flexor tendon. It usually is the result of an overuse injury with microtears to the hypovascular origins of the wrist flexor and pronator muscle groups. As with lateral epicondylitis, there is no consistent medical literature that is available to guide treatment with any injectable medication or intervention. A single study suggests short-term improvement only with the use of corticosteroids.[1] Once the acute pain symptoms are alleviated, focus is turned to flexor-pronator mass rehabilitation and injury prevention.[2] A review of the current evidence shows that PRP injections are just as effective as medial epicondyle surgery in relieving pain and restoring function in patients with medial epicondylitis.[3]

Relevant Anatomy: (Fig. 10.39)

PATIENT POSITION

- Supine on the examination table with the head of the bed elevated 30°.
- Shoulder at 30° of abduction and full external rotation.
- The affected elbow is flexed at 90°.
- The wrist is in a neutral position.
- The elbow is supported with the placement of chucks pads or towels.
- Rotate the patient's head away from the side that is being injected. This minimizes anxiety and pain perception.

LANDMARKS

1. With the patient supine on the examination table, the clinician stands lateral to the affected elbow.
2. Identify and mark the point of maximal tenderness involving the common flexor tendon, adjacent to the medial epicondyle.
3. At that site, press firmly on the skin with the retracted tip of a ballpoint pen. This indentation represents the entry point for the needle.
4. After the landmarks are identified, the patient should not move the elbow.

ANESTHESIA

- Local anesthesia of the skin using topical vapocoolant spray.

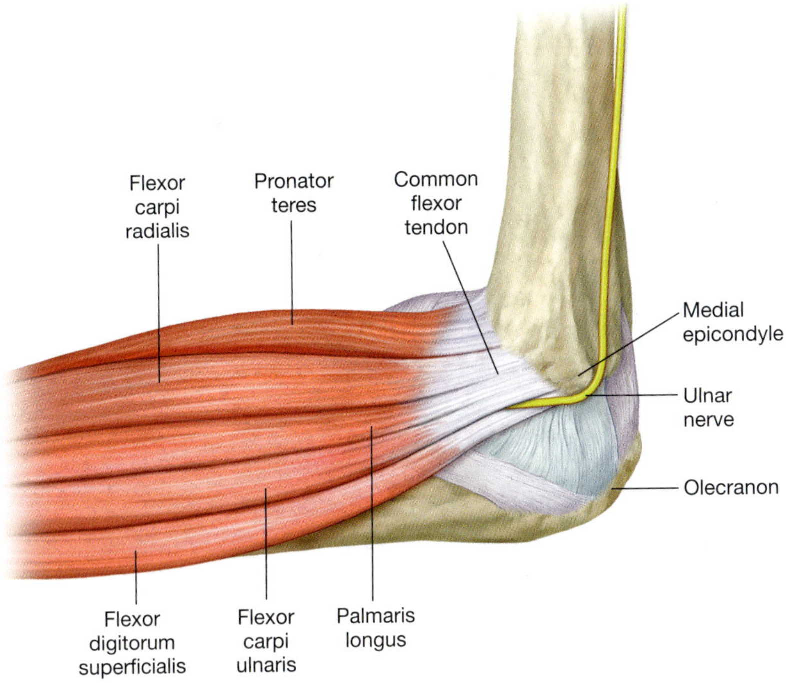

FIGURE 10.39 ● Medial view of muscular structures and common flexor tendon of the right elbow.

EQUIPMENT

- Topical vapocoolant spray
- 3-mL syringe
- 25-gauge 1-in needle
- 1 mL of 1% lidocaine without epinephrine
- 0.5 to 1 mL of the 40 mg/mL steroid solution (20-40 mg of triamcinolone acetonide)
- One alcohol prep pad
- Two povidone-iodine or chlorhexidine prep pads
- Sterile gauze pads
- Sterile adhesive bandage
- Nonsterile, clean chucks pad

TECHNIQUE

1. Prep the insertion site with alcohol followed by the povidone-iodine or chlorhexidine pads.
2. Achieve good local anesthesia by using topical vapocoolant spray.
3. Position the needle and syringe perpendicular to the skin with the needle tip directed laterally toward the medial epicondyle.
4. Using the no-touch technique, quickly introduce the needle at the insertion site (Fig. 10.40).
5. Advance the needle to the bone of the medial epicondyle.
6. Withdraw the needle 1 to 2 mm.

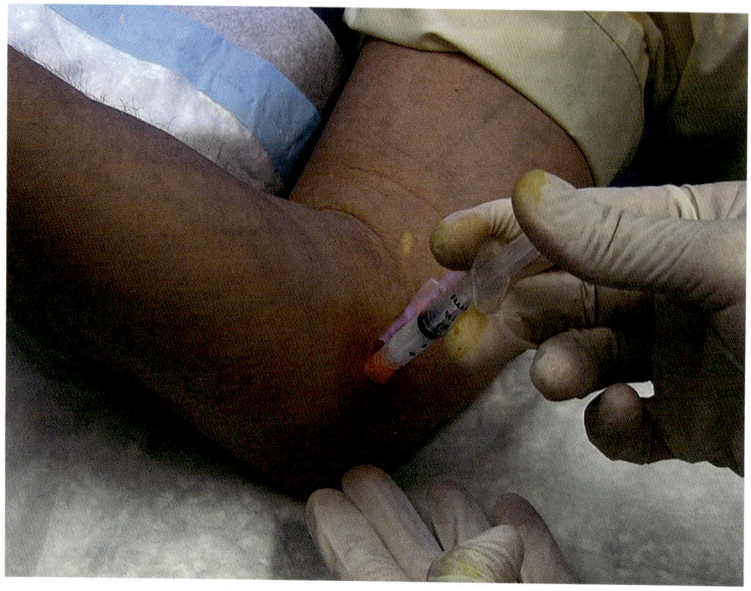

FIGURE 10.40 ● Right elbow medial epicondylitis injection.

7. Withdraw the plunger of the syringe to ensure that there is no blood return.
8. Inject the lidocaine/corticosteroid or other therapeutic solution steadily into this area. If increased resistance is encountered, advance or withdraw the needle slightly before attempting further injection.
9. Following injection, withdraw the needle.
10. Apply a sterile adhesive bandage.
11. Instruct the patient to move their wrist and elbow through their full range of motion.
12. Reexamine the elbow in 5 minutes to assess pain relief.

AFTERCARE

- Avoid excessive wrist flexion or pronation over the next 2 weeks.
- Consider the use of a neoprene elbow sleeve or elastic compression bandage.
- Consider the use of a wrist brace to limit wrist flexion.
- NSAIDs, ice, heat, and/or physical therapy as indicated.
- Consider follow-up examination in 2 weeks.
- Consider treatment using alternative modalities if initial therapy is not effective.

PEARLS

- The ulnar nerve travels in close proximity to this injection. It courses just posterior and inferior to the medial epicondyle. On occasion, the local anesthetic spreading out from a properly placed injection may involve the ulnar nerve. The patient should be warned that transient numbness might occur in the lateral aspect of the hand as well as the ring and little fingers.

ULTRASOUND-GUIDED PROCEDURE

Please refer to the introductory ultrasound chapter for preprocedure, sterile prep, post-procedure, and documentation information and recommendations.

PATIENT POSITION

- Lateral decubitus on the examination table with the affected elbow down.
- On the affected side, place the shoulder in a neutral position, flex the elbow to 90°, supinate the forearm, and rest the elbow on a chux pad placed on the examination table.
- Place a pillow under their head for comfort.
- Adjust the patient's position as needed for comfort.

PROVIDER/ULTRASOUND POSITION

- The provider sits in front of the patient's affected elbow.
- Adjust the examination table to position the injection site between the provider's umbilicus and axillary level, ensuring optimal ergonomics and visualization of the ultrasound screen, transducer, and needle's approach (Fig. 10.41).
- Position the ultrasound machine on the opposite side of the table from the provider at the level of the patient's affected elbow with the screen facing the provider.

LANDMARKS

- See the landmarks for the landmark-guided injection procedure.

ANESTHESIA

- Local anesthesia of the skin using topical vapocoolant spray.

EQUIPMENT

- 3-mL syringe
- 25-gauge 1.5-in needle (adjust needle length as needed)

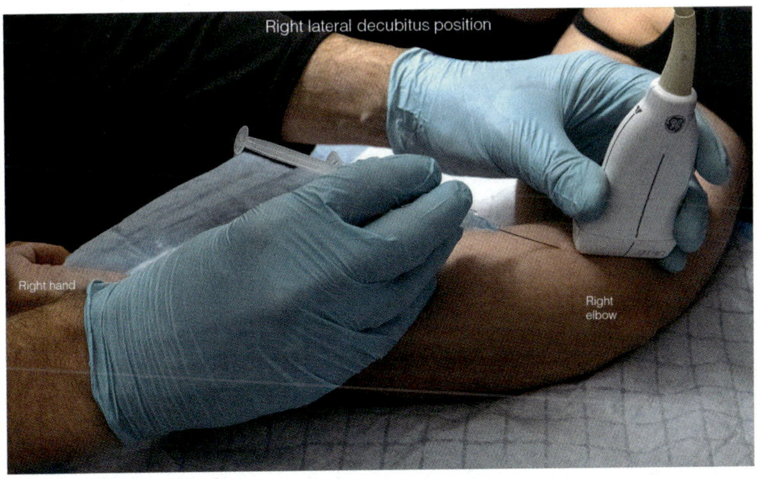

FIGURE 10.41 • Ultrasound-guided right medial epicondylalgia elbow injection. Right lateral decubitus position with the affected elbow flexed and resting on the examination table.

- 1 mL of 1% lidocaine without epinephrine
- 0.5 to 1 mL of the 40 mg/mL steroid solution (20-40 mg of triamcinolone acetonide)
- Three chlorhexidine swabs
- 12-4 MHz linear ultrasound transducer and machine
- Sterile ultrasound transducer cover
- Sterile ultrasound gel
- Nonlatex sterile or nonsterile gloves
- Two 4 × 4 sterile gauze pads
- One sterile adhesive bandage
- Topical vapocoolant spray

TECHNIQUE

1. Position a high-frequency linear 12-4 MHz transducer in the coronal plane with the medial epicondyle centered.
2. Advance a 25-gauge 1.5-in needle using an in-plane approach, directing it from distal to proximal, with an initial needle angle of approximately 15° to 20° relative to the skin surface where the transducer is positioned.
3. Target area:
   a. For corticosteroids: The deep peritendinous space between the common flexor tendon and ulnar collateral ligament.
   b. For dextrose prolotherapy or PRP: The area of tendinopathy in the tendon (refer to Chapter 4: Orthobiologics).
4. Injectate:
   a. For corticosteroids: Use a 25-gauge 1.5-in needle to inject the solution into the deep peritendinous space.
   b. For dextrose prolotherapy or PRP (refer to Chapter 4: Orthobiologics): Use a 22-gauge 1.5-in needle to inject the solution into the area of tendinopathy in the tendon. Administer a total volume (1-2 mL) of 15% dextrose prolotherapy or PRP in small aliquots (0.5 mL or less).
5. Utilize real-time ultrasound guidance throughout to ensure accurate needle placement and minimize the risk of complications (Fig. 10.42).
6. Upon completion of the procedure, carefully withdraw the needle. Adhere to established postprocedure care protocols and ensure appropriate follow-up as recommended.

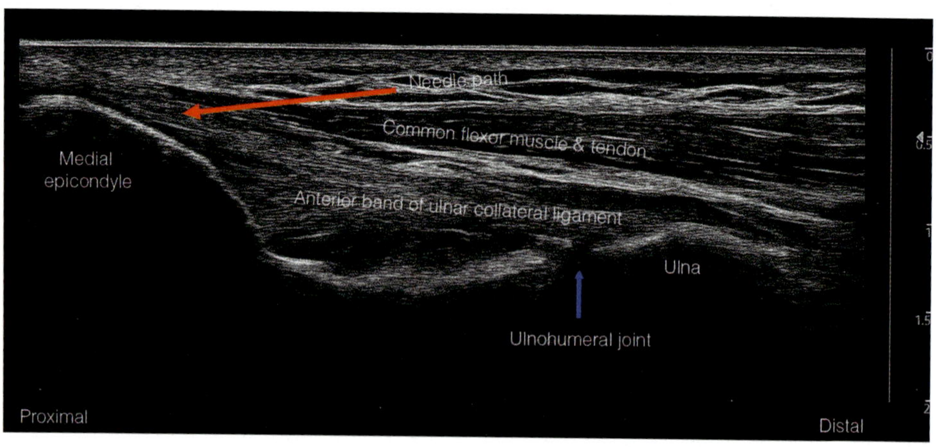

FIGURE 10.42 ● Medial elbow ultrasound coronal image.

PEARLS

- Consider a longer needle (eg, 2-in 25-gauge).
- Exercise caution to avoid inadvertent penetration of the ulnar nerve during needle advancement under ultrasound guidance.

Videos showing landmark-guided and ultrasound-guided medial epicondyle injections can be found in the companion eBook.

REFERENCES

1. Stahl S, Kaufman T. The efficacy of an injection of steroids for medial epicondylitis: a prospective study of sixty elbows. *J Bone Joint Surg Am.* 1997;79(11):1648-1652.
2. Amin NH, Kumar NS, Schickendantz MS. Medial epicondylitis: evaluation and management. *J Am Acad Orthop Surg.* 2015;23(6):348-355.
3. Alzahrani WM. Platelet-rich plasma injections as an alternative to surgery in treating patients with medial epicondylitis: a systematic review. *Cureus.* 2022;14(8):e28378.

Radial Nerve Entrapment

Patients uncommonly present to the primary care office for the treatment of radial nerve entrapment in the forearm. This syndrome is caused by entrapment of the deep branch of the radial nerve (posterior interosseous nerve) as it enters the supinator muscle at the arcade of Frohse. Compression or scarring of the posterior interosseous nerve may cause denervation of the extensor/supinator muscles and numbness or paresthesias involving the distribution of the radial sensory nerve. This can result in pain, weakness, and dysfunction. Pain in this condition occurs about 4 cm distal to the lateral epicondyle.

A nerve block injection utilizing local anesthetic can be given to help confirm diagnosis, and corticosteroid may be added for conservative management.[1] Consider a diagnostic ultrasound-guided injection into the target area with 3 mL of 1% lidocaine without epinephrine. This can help differentiate radial tunnel syndrome from lateral epicondylalgia. Alternative therapies include dry needling[2] and radial nerve hydrodissection. Successful treatment often requires surgical release.

Radial tunnel syndrome can mimic lateral epicondylalgia or C6-C7 radiculopathy. Rule out radiculopathy. If wrist extension weakness is present, refer to a specialist (neurosurgeon, orthopedic spine/hand surgeon).

Relevant Anatomy: (Fig. 10.43)

PATIENT POSITION

- Supine on the examination table with the head of the bed elevated 30°.
- The affected elbow is slightly flexed.
- The wrist is in a neutral to slightly pronated position.
- The elbow is supported with the placement of chucks pads or towels.
- Rotate the patient's head away from the side that is being injected. This minimizes anxiety and pain perception.

LANDMARKS

1. With the patient supine on the examination table, the clinician stands lateral to the affected forearm.
2. Identify the lateral epicondyle.
3. The point of maximal tenderness is usually located about 4 cm distal and anterior to the lateral epicondyle.
4. Identify and mark the point of maximal tenderness.
5. At that site, press firmly on the skin with the retracted tip of a ballpoint pen. This indentation represents the entry point for the needle.
6. After the landmarks are identified, the patient should not move the elbow.

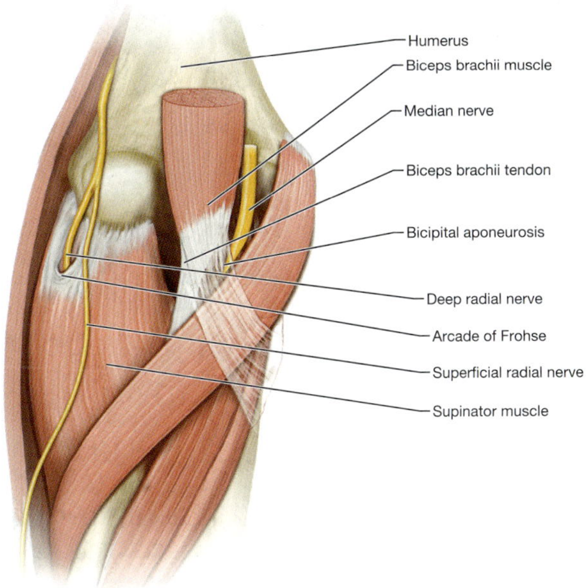

FIGURE 10.43 • Anterior aspect of right elbow. (Modified with permission from Paulsen F, Waschke J. *Sobotta Atlas of Human Anatomy*. 25th ed. Urban & Fischer; 2022. Copyright © 2022 Elsevier GmbH.)

ANESTHESIA

- Local anesthesia of the skin using topical vapocoolant spray.

EQUIPMENT

- Topical vapocoolant spray
- 3-mL syringe
- 25-gauge 1-in needle
- 1 mL of 1% lidocaine without epinephrine
- 1 mL of the 40 mg/mL steroid solution (40 mg of triamcinolone acetonide)
- One alcohol prep pad
- Two povidone-iodine or chlorhexidine prep pads
- Sterile gauze pads
- Sterile adhesive bandage
- Nonsterile, clean chucks pad

TECHNIQUE

1. Prep the insertion site with alcohol followed by the povidone-iodine or chlorhexidine pads.
2. Achieve good local anesthesia by using topical vapocoolant spray.
3. Position the needle and syringe perpendicular to the skin with the needle tip directed posteriorly.
4. Using the no-touch technique, quickly introduce the needle at the insertion site (Fig. 10.44).

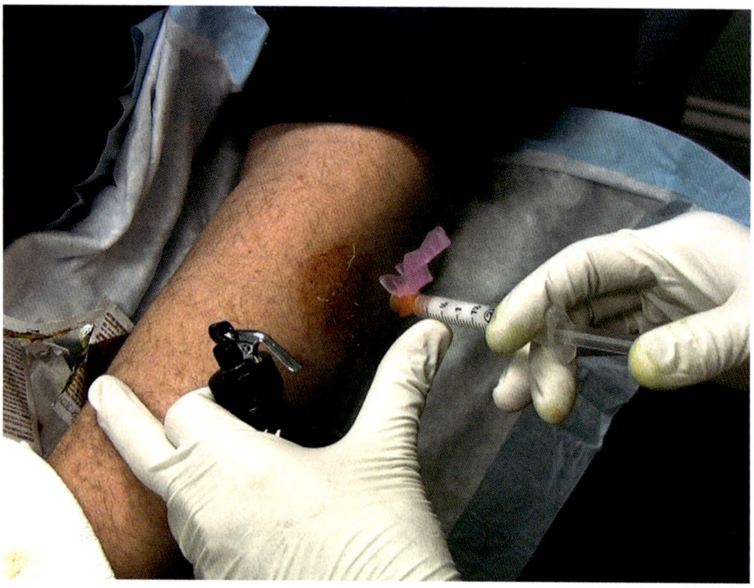

FIGURE 10.44 ● Left arm radial nerve entrapment injection (4 cm distal to the lateral epicondyle).

5. Slowly advance the needle until the needle tip is at the anticipated injection site near the radial nerve.
6. If any pain, paresthesias, or numbness is encountered, withdraw the needle slightly.
7. When the needle is placed along the radial nerve, withdraw the plunger of the syringe to ensure that there is no blood return.
8. Slowly inject the lidocaine/corticosteroid solution as a bolus around the radial nerve.
9. If increased resistance is encountered, advance or withdraw the needle slightly before attempting further injection.
10. Following injection, withdraw the needle.
11. Apply a sterile adhesive bandage.
12. Instruct the patient to move their wrist and elbow through their full range of motion to distribute the lidocaine/corticosteroid solution along the course of the radial nerve.
13. Reexamine the proximal forearm in 5 minutes to assess pain relief and the development of numbness in the distribution of the radial nerve from the local anesthetic.

AFTERCARE

- Avoid excessive wrist extension and supination over the next 2 weeks.
- NSAIDs, ice, and/or physical therapy as indicated.
- Consider follow-up examination in 2 weeks.
- Consider treatment using alternative modalities if initial therapy is not effective.

PEARLS

- Entrapment of branches of the radial nerve in the elbow and forearm can mimic the pain of lateral epicondylitis.

ULTRASOUND-GUIDED PROCEDURE

Please refer to the introductory ultrasound chapter for preprocedure, sterile prep, post-procedure, and documentation information and recommendations.

PATIENT POSITION

- Supine on the examination table.
- On the affected side, place the shoulder in a neutral position and pronate the forearm, resting the ulnar side on a chux pad on the examination table.
- Place a pillow under their head for comfort.
- Adjust the patient's position as needed for comfort.

PROVIDER/ULTRASOUND POSITION

- The provider sits on the affected side.
- Adjust the examination table to position the injection site between the provider's umbilicus and axillary level, ensuring optimal ergonomics and visualization of the ultrasound screen, transducer, and needle's approach (Fig. 10.45).
- Position the ultrasound machine on the opposite side of the table from the provider at the level of the patient's elbow with the screen facing the provider.

LANDMARKS

- See the landmarks for the landmark-guided injection procedure.

ANESTHESIA

- Local anesthesia of the skin using topical vapocoolant spray.

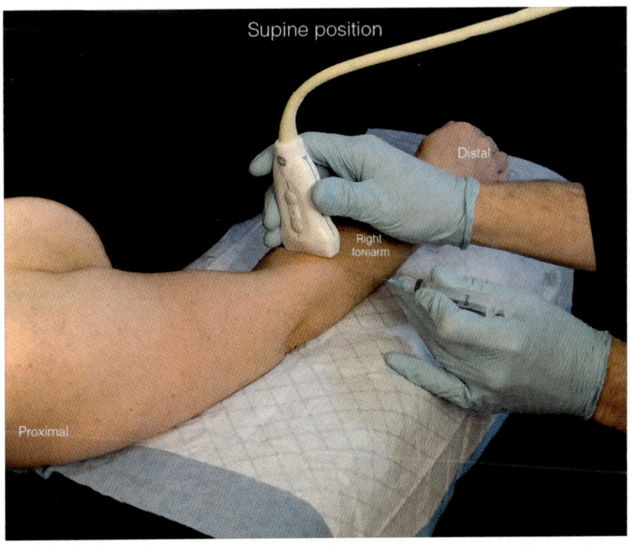

FIGURE 10.45 • Ultrasound-guided right radial tunnel injection. Supine position with the affected forearm resting on the examination table. Provider is on the ipsilateral side.

EQUIPMENT

- 5-mL syringe
- 25-gauge 1.5-in needle (adjust needle length as needed)
- 4 mL of 1% lidocaine without epinephrine
- 1 mL of the 40 mg/mL steroid solution (40 mg of triamcinolone acetonide)
- Three chlorhexidine swabs
- 12-4 MHz linear ultrasound transducer and machine
- Sterile ultrasound transducer cover
- Sterile ultrasound gel
- Nonlatex sterile or nonsterile gloves
- Two 4 × 4 sterile gauze pads
- One sterile adhesive bandage
- Topical vapocoolant spray

TECHNIQUE

1. Position a high-frequency linear 12-4 MHz ultrasound transducer in the axial plane with the radial nerve centered beneath it as it enters the supinator muscle.
2. Prior to the procedure, activate power Doppler imaging to precisely localize the leash of Henry. This visualization is essential for preventing inadvertent injury to the neurovascular bundle.
3. Advance a 25-gauge 1.5-in needle using an in-plane approach, directing it from posterior to anterior, with an initial depth of needle insertion at approximately 2 cm from the face of the transducer and an initial needle angle of approximately 0° to 5° relative to the skin surface where the transducer is positioned.
4. The target area is the perineural space of the deep branch of the radial nerve, distal to the leash of Henry and to the arcade of Frohse.
5. Utilize real-time ultrasound guidance throughout the procedure to precisely place the needle within the desired target area and minimize the risk of inadvertently injuring surrounding structures (Fig. 10.46).
6. Upon completion of the procedure, carefully withdraw the needle. Adhere to established postprocedure care protocols and ensure appropriate follow-up as recommended.

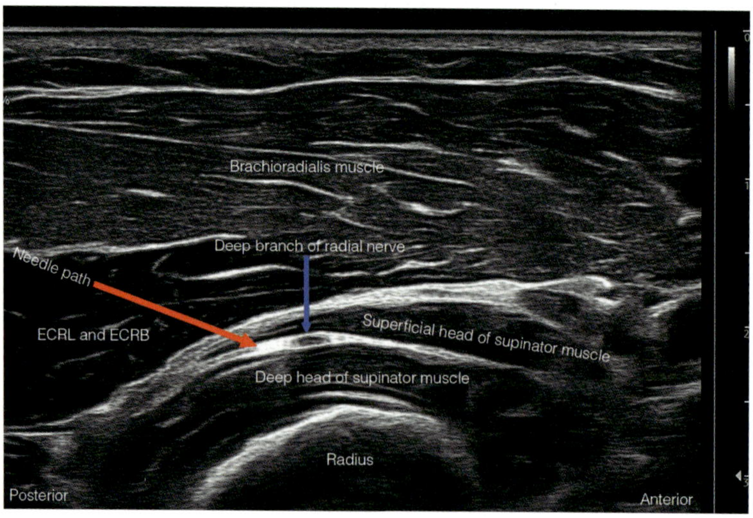

FIGURE 10.46 Radial tunnel ultrasound axial image. ECRB, extensor carpi radialis brevis tendon; ECRL, extensor carpi radialis longus tendon.

PEARLS

- Consider using a longer needle (eg, 2-in 25-gauge).
- Ultrasound-guided radial tunnel injection is an advanced technique requiring caution. Advance the needle slowly and with controlled movements, continuously monitoring its position under ultrasound, to avoid neurovascular structures.

Videos showing landmark-guided and ultrasound-guided radial nerve entrapment injections can be found in the companion eBook.

REFERENCES

1. Carter GT, Weiss MD. Diagnosis and treatment of work-related proximal median and radial nerve entrapment. *Phys Med Rehabil Clin N Am.* 2015;26(3):539-549.
2. Anandkumar S. Effect of dry needling on radial tunnel syndrome: a case report. *Physiother Theory Pract.* 2019;35(4):373-382.

Intersection Syndrome

Injection of corticosteroids for the treatment of intersection syndrome is a rare procedure for primary care providers. This is a painful condition that affects the dorsum of the forearm 4 cm proximal to the wrist joint from Lister tubercle[1] at the intersection of the abductor pollicis longus (APL) and extensor pollicis brevis (EPB) muscles at the point where they crossover (intersect) the extensor carpi radialis longus (ECRL) and the extensor carpi radialis brevis (ECRB) tendons. The mechanism of injury usually involves repetitive resisted wrist extension that occurs in rowers and certain industrial workers. Patients typically describe pain, local swelling, and a rubbing/squeaking sensation when they extend their wrist repeatedly.

Conservative treatment includes rest, activity modification, bracing, and NSAIDs. Alternatively, patients may be treated with a corticosteroid injection or ultrasound-guided saline hydrodissection.[2]

Relevant Anatomy: (Fig. 10.47)

PATIENT POSITION

- Supine on the examination table with the head of the bed elevated 30°.
- The affected wrist is held in a neutral position. The thumb is directed superiorly midway between supination and pronation.
- The wrist is supported with the placement of chucks pads or towels.
- Rotate the patient's head away from the side that is being injected. This minimizes anxiety and pain perception.

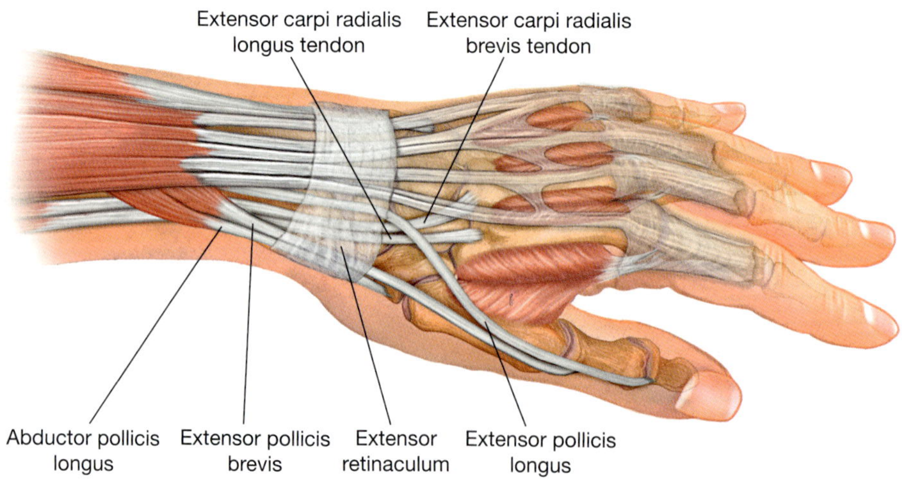

FIGURE 10.47 ● Anatomy of muscles and tendons involved with intersection syndrome.

LANDMARKS

1. With the patient supine on the examination table, the clinician stands lateral to the affected wrist.
2. Identify the maximal point of tenderness located over the dorsal-radial aspect of the forearm 4 cm proximal to the wrist joint from Lister tubercle[3] at the intersection of the APL and EPB muscles at the point where they crossover (intersect) the ECRL and the ECRB tendons.
3. Often, the anatomy is more easily identified by asking the patient to repetitively make very small circular motions with the thumb or perform wrist extensions. The area where these structures intersect can be located by finding the maximal area of pain or palpating for crepitus.
4. At that site, press firmly on the skin with the retracted tip of a ballpoint pen. This indentation represents the target point for the needle.
5. Mark a point 1 cm distal to that spot.
6. At that site, press firmly on the skin with the retracted tip of a ballpoint pen. This indentation represents the entry point for the needle.
7. After the landmarks are identified, the patient should not move the wrist or thumb.

ANESTHESIA

- Local anesthesia of the skin using topical vapocoolant spray.

EQUIPMENT

- Topical vapocoolant spray
- 3-mL syringe
- 25-gauge 1-in needle
- 0.5 mL of 1% lidocaine without epinephrine
- 0.25 mL of the 40 mg/mL steroid solution (10 mg of triamcinolone acetonide)
- One alcohol prep pad
- Two povidone-iodine or chlorhexidine prep pads
- Sterile gauze pads
- Sterile adhesive bandage
- Nonsterile, clean chucks pad

TECHNIQUE

1. Prep the insertion site with alcohol followed by the povidone-iodine or chlorhexidine pads.
2. Achieve good local anesthesia by using topical vapocoolant spray.
3. Position the needle and syringe 1 cm distal to the marked target site—at a 45° angle to the skin with the needle tip directed proximally.
4. Using the no-touch technique, quickly introduce the needle at the insertion site (Fig. 10.48).
5. Advance the needle toward the target that is located about 1 cm deep to the skin.
6. Withdraw the plunger of the syringe to ensure that there is no blood return.
7. Slowly inject the lidocaine/corticosteroid solution as a bolus into the tendon sheath.
8. Following injection, withdraw the needle.
9. Apply a sterile adhesive bandage.

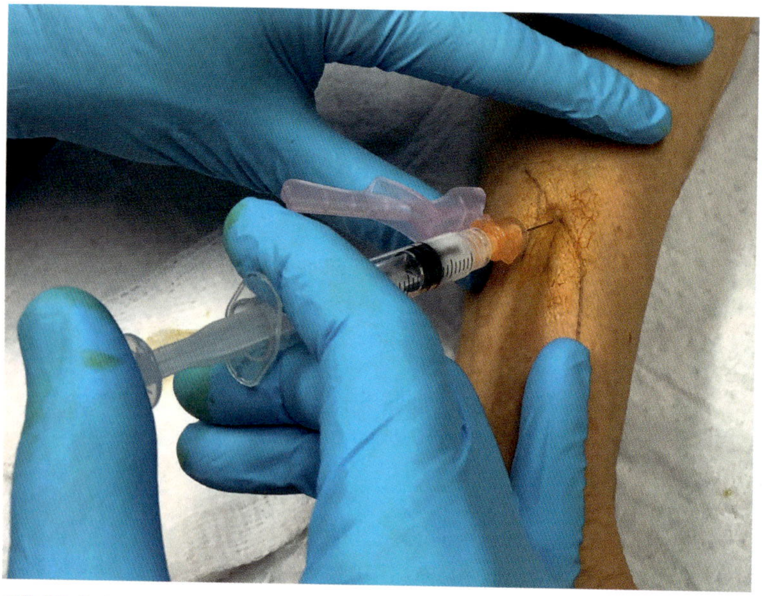

FIGURE 10.48 ● Intersection syndrome injection.

10. Instruct the patient to move their thumb and wrist through its full range of motion. This movement distributes the lidocaine/corticosteroid solution throughout the tenosynovial sheath.
11. Reexamine the hand and wrist in 5 minutes to assess pain relief.

AFTERCARE

- Ensure no excessive wrist or thumb extension/abduction over the next 2 weeks by the application of a wrist and thumb spica splint.
- NSAIDs, ice, heat, and/or physical therapy as indicated.
- Consider follow-up examination in 2 weeks.

PEARLS

- Care should be taken to differentiate this condition from the more common de Quervain tenosynovitis.
- Ultrasound guidance may offer a significant advantage over landmark-based technique.

ULTRASOUND-GUIDED PROCEDURE

Please refer to the introductory ultrasound chapter for preprocedure, sterile prep, post-procedure, and documentation information and recommendations.

PATIENT POSITION

- Supine on the examination table.
- On the affected side, place the shoulder in a neutral position, pronate the forearm, and rest the ulnar aspect of the forearm on a chux pad placed on the examination table.

- Place a pillow under their head for comfort.
- Adjust the patient's position as needed for comfort.

PROVIDER/ULTRASOUND POSITION

- The provider sits on the affected side.
- Adjust the examination table to position the injection site between the provider's umbilicus and axillary level, ensuring optimal ergonomics and visualization of the ultrasound screen, transducer, and needle's approach (Fig. 10.49).
- Position the ultrasound machine on the opposite side of the table from the provider at the level of the contralateral forearm with the screen facing the provider.

LANDMARKS

- See the landmarks for the landmark-guided injection procedure.

ANESTHESIA

- Local anesthesia of the skin using topical vapocoolant spray.

EQUIPMENT

- 3-mL syringe
- 25-gauge 1.5-in needle (adjust needle length as needed)
- 0.5 mL of 1% lidocaine without epinephrine
- 0.25 mL of the 40 mg/mL steroid solution (10 mg of triamcinolone acetonide)
- Three chlorhexidine swabs
- 12-4 MHz linear ultrasound transducer and machine
- Sterile ultrasound transducer cover
- Sterile ultrasound gel

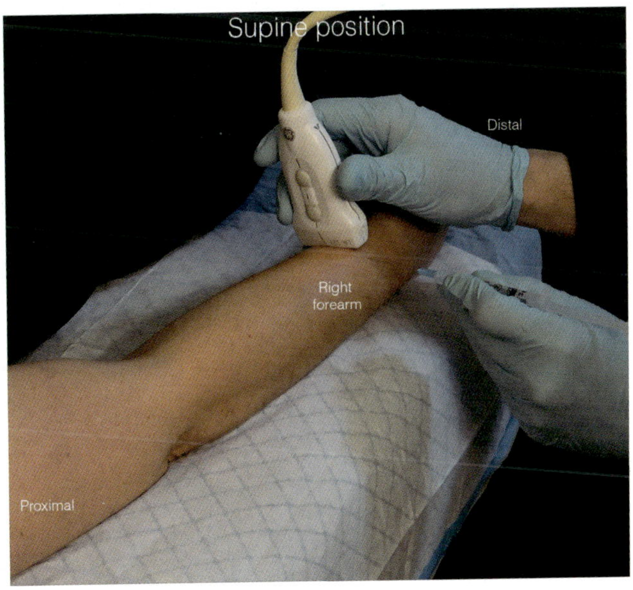

FIGURE 10.49 • Ultrasound-guided right intersection syndrome injection. Supine position with the affected forearm resting on the examination table. Provider on the ipsilateral side.

- Nonlatex sterile or nonsterile gloves
- Two 4 × 4 sterile gauze pads
- One sterile adhesive bandage
- Topical vapocoolant spray

TECHNIQUE

1. Position a high-frequency linear 12-4 MHz ultrasound transducer in the axial plane centered over the point where the first dorsal compartment of the wrist (EPB and APL tendons) crosses over the second dorsal compartment of the wrist (ECRB and longus tendons), approximately 5 to 8 cm proximal to the radial styloid on the affected side.
2. Advance a 25-gauge 1.5-in needle using an in-plane approach, directing it from posterior to anterior, with an initial depth of needle insertion about 0.5 cm from the face of the transducer and an initial needle angle of approximately 0° to 5° relative to the skin surface where the transducer is positioned.
3. The target area is the fascial plane between the first and second dorsal compartments of the wrist.
4. Utilize real-time ultrasound guidance throughout the procedure to precisely place the needle within the desired target area and minimize the risk of inadvertently injuring surrounding structures (Fig. 10.50).
5. Upon completion of the procedure, carefully withdraw the needle. Adhere to established postprocedure care protocols and ensure appropriate follow-up as recommended.

PEARLS

- Dynamically slide the transducer distally and proximally to optimize visualization of the intersection as the first crosses the second dorsal compartment.
- Ensure that the needle tip is placed within the fascial plane between the tendon sheaths and not within the tendons themselves.

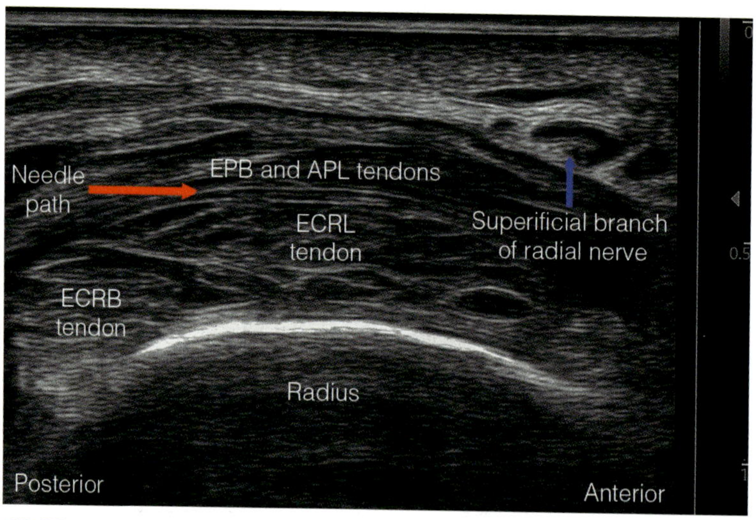

FIGURE 10.50 ● Proximal intersection syndrome ultrasound axial image. This image demonstrates the key anatomical feature of proximal intersection syndrome: the crossing point of the first dorsal compartment (extensor pollicis brevis [EPB] and abductor pollicis longus [APL]) tendons over the second dorsal compartment (extensor carpi radialis brevis [ECRB] and extensor carpi radialis longus [ECRL]) tendons at the wrist.

- Proximal intersection syndrome can cause pain, swelling, crepitus, and tenderness, which may radiate distally, mimicking de Quervain tenosynovitis. If diagnosis is uncertain, consider a diagnostic injection of 1 mL of 1% lidocaine without epinephrine into the fascial plane between the two compartments. Pain relief after injection supports the diagnosis of proximal intersection syndrome.
- Identify and avoid the superficial branch of the radial nerve.

A video showing ultrasound-guided intersection syndrome injection can be found in the companion eBook.

REFERENCES

1. Lee RP, Hatem SF, Recht MP. Extended MRI findings of intersection syndrome. *Skeletal Radiol.* 2009;38(2):157-163.
2. Skinner TM. Intersection syndrome: the subtle squeak of an overused wrist. *J Am Board Fam Med.* 2017;30(4):547-551.
3. Lee RP, Hatem SF, Recht MP. Extended MRI findings of intersection syndrome. *Skeletal Radiol.* 2009;38(2):157-163.

de Quervain Tenosynovitis

Patients with de Quervain tenosynovitis fairly commonly present to primary care providers. This condition represents a stenosing tenosynovitis of the first dorsal compartment over the radial aspect of the wrist. The EPB and APL tendons run parallel and share a common tendon sheath that occupies the first dorsal compartment of the wrist. Overuse movements that involve repetitive extension and abduction of the thumb generally cause this condition. It is commonly encountered during pregnancy—particularly in the postpartum period.

Studies show that a local injection of corticosteroid leads to a high rate of improvement both in the short and long term with few side effects.[1-3] This injection followed by 3 to 4 weeks of immobilization should be considered as first-line treatment.[4] Injections of PRP are also effective.[5] Ultrasound studies show a 28% to 52% incidence of a tendon sheath septum isolating the EPB from the APL.[6,7] The presence of these subcompartments plays a role in recurrence rates.[5,8] The use of ultrasound has been shown to detect the septum, improve injection accuracy by enabling injection into each subcompartment, and improve clinical outcomes.[9,10]

Relevant Anatomy: (Fig. 10.51)

PATIENT POSITION

- Supine on the examination table with the head of the bed elevated 30°.
- The affected wrist is held in a neutral position. The thumb is directed superiorly midway between supination and pronation.
- The wrist is supported with the placement of chucks pads or towels.
- Rotate the patient's head away from the side that is being injected. This minimizes anxiety and pain perception.

LANDMARKS

1. The clinician stands lateral to the affected wrist.
2. Identify tenderness located in the sheath that contains the APL and the EPB tendons.
3. The injection point is located directly between these two tendons. Often, the anatomy is more easily identified by asking the patient to make very small circular motions with their thumb. The space between the APL and EPB tendons may be marked with an indentation made by the examiner's fingernail placed longitudinally between the tendons. This indentation represents the entry point for the needle.
4. After the landmarks are identified, the patient should not move the wrist or thumb.

ANESTHESIA

- Local anesthesia of the skin using topical vapocoolant spray.

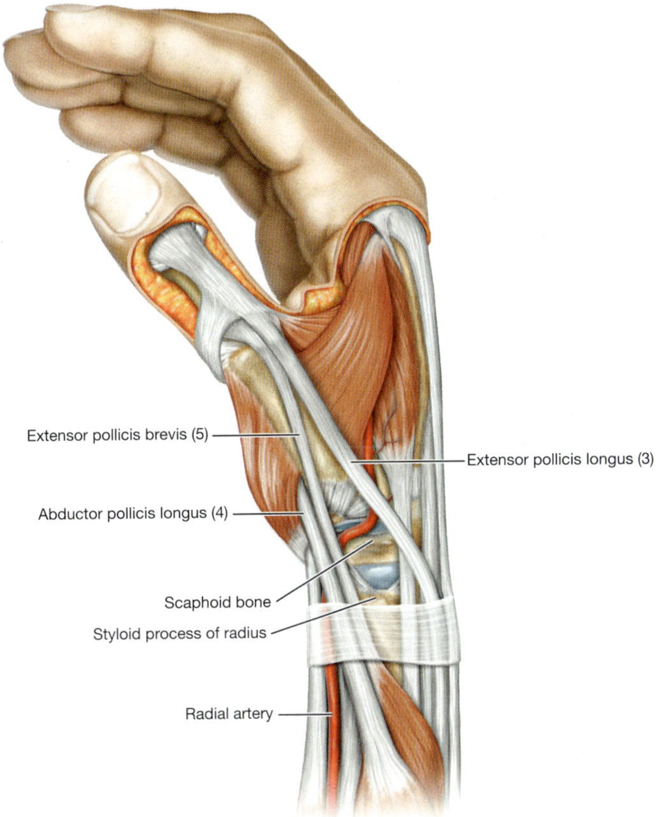

FIGURE 10.51 • Right hand anatomy. (Reprinted with permission from Agur AMR, Dalley AF II. *Grant's Atlas of Anatomy*. 16th ed. Wolters Kluwer; 2025.)

EQUIPMENT

- Topical vapocoolant spray
- 3-mL syringe
- 25-gauge 5/8-in needle
- 0.5 mL of 1% lidocaine without epinephrine
- 0.25 mL of the 40 mg/mL steroid solution (10 mg of triamcinolone acetonide)
- One alcohol prep pad
- Two povidone-iodine or chlorhexidine prep pads
- Sterile gauze pads
- Sterile adhesive bandage
- Nonsterile, clean chucks pad

TECHNIQUE

1. Prep the insertion site with alcohol followed by the povidone-iodine or chlorhexidine pads.
2. Achieve good local anesthesia by using topical vapocoolant spray.
3. Position the needle and syringe at a 30° angle to the skin with the needle tip directed proximally.

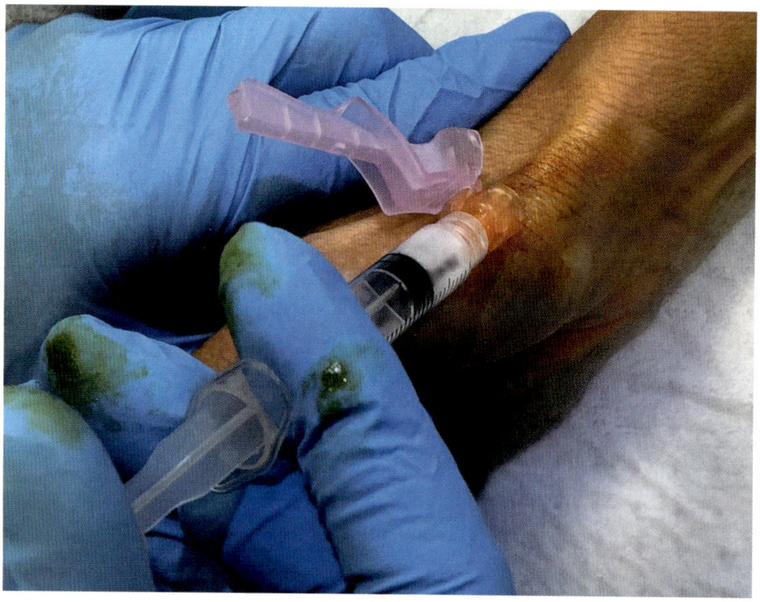

FIGURE 10.52 ● de Quervain tenosynovitis injection.

4. Using the no-touch technique, quickly introduce the needle at the insertion site (Fig. 10.52).
5. Advance the needle toward the convergence of the APL and the EPB tendons until the needle tip is located between the tendons in the tendon sheath.
6. Withdraw the plunger of the syringe to ensure that there is no blood return.
7. Slowly inject the lidocaine/corticosteroid solution as a bolus into the tendon sheath. A small bulge in the shape of a sausage often develops in the tendon sheath.
8. Following injection, withdraw the needle.
9. Apply a sterile adhesive bandage.
10. Instruct the patient to move their thumb through its full range of motion. This movement distributes the lidocaine/corticosteroid solution throughout the tenosynovial sheath.
11. Reexamine the hand and wrist in 5 minutes to assess pain relief.

AFTERCARE

- Ensure no excessive wrist flexion or pronation over the next 2 weeks by the application of a wrist and thumb spica splint.
- NSAIDs, ice, heat, and/or physical therapy as indicated.
- Consider follow-up examination in 2 weeks.

PEARLS

- Care should be taken to differentiate this condition from a painful thumb carpometacarpal joint (CMCJ) and the rare intersection syndrome.
- Due to the anatomically superficial location of the first dorsal compartment, especially in thin individuals, corticosteroid may be inadvertently deposited in the subcutaneous tissues rather than the tendon sheath, leading to skin atrophy and hypopigmentation.

The de Quervain injection is notorious for the development of these complications. Avoid the development of an intradermal wheal while performing all injections of corticosteroid solutions.

ULTRASOUND-GUIDED PROCEDURE

Please refer to the introductory ultrasound chapter for preprocedure, sterile prep, post-procedure, and documentation information and recommendations.

PATIENT POSITION

- Supine on the examination table.
- On the affected side, place the shoulder in a neutral position, pronate the forearm, and rest the ulnar aspect of the forearm on a chux pad placed on the examination table.
- The affected thumb is in a relaxed or flexed position.
- To improve access to the first dorsal compartment, place a rolled-up chux pad under the ulnar side of the wrist to ulnar deviate the wrist during the procedure.
- Place a pillow under their head for comfort.
- Adjust the patient's position as needed for comfort.

PROVIDER/ULTRASOUND POSITION

- The provider sits on the affected side.
- Adjust the examination table to position the injection site between the provider's umbilicus and axillary level, ensuring optimal ergonomics and visualization of the ultrasound screen, transducer, and needle's approach (Fig. 10.53).
- Position the ultrasound machine on the same side of the table from the provider at the level of the shoulders with the screen facing the provider.

EQUIPMENT

- 3-mL syringe
- 25-gauge 1.5-in needle (adjust needle length as needed)
- 0.5 mL of 1% lidocaine without epinephrine

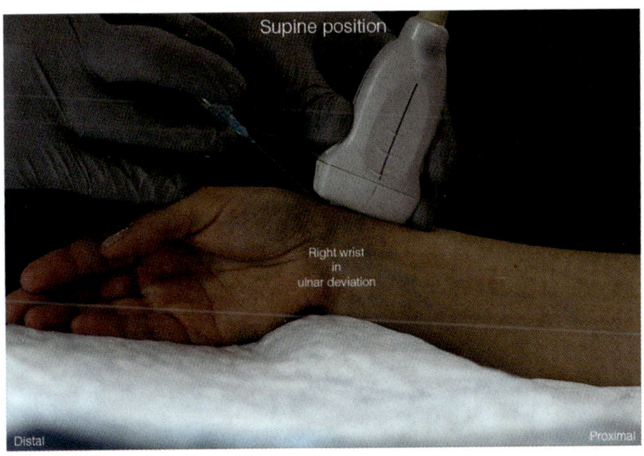

FIGURE 10.53 Ultrasound-guided right de Quervain tenosynovitis injection. Supine position with the affected arm resting on the examination table in ulnar deviation. Provider positioned ipsilaterally distal to the injection site.

- 0.25 mL of the 40 mg/mL steroid solution (10 mg of triamcinolone acetonide)
- Three chlorhexidine swabs
- 12-4 MHz linear ultrasound transducer and machine
- Sterile ultrasound transducer cover
- Sterile ultrasound gel
- Nonlatex sterile or nonsterile gloves
- Two 4 × 4 sterile gauze pads
- One sterile adhesive bandage
- Topical vapocoolant spray

LANDMARKS

- See the landmarks for the landmark-guided injection procedure.

ANESTHESIA

- Local anesthesia of the skin using topical vapocoolant spray.

TECHNIQUE

1. Position a high-frequency linear 12-4 MHz ultrasound transducer in the coronal plane with the first dorsal compartment of the wrist (EPB and APL tendons) in long axis and the radial styloid centered beneath it.
2. Advance a 25-gauge 1.5-in needle using an in-plane approach, directing it from distal to proximal, with an initial needle angle of approximately 20° to 30° relative to the skin surface where the transducer is positioned.
3. The target area is inside the tendon sheath of the first dorsal compartment.
4. Utilize real-time ultrasound guidance throughout the procedure to precisely place the needle within the desired target area and minimize the risk of inadvertently injuring surrounding structures (Fig. 10.54).
5. Upon completion of the procedure, carefully withdraw the needle. Adhere to established postprocedure care protocols and ensure appropriate follow-up as recommended.

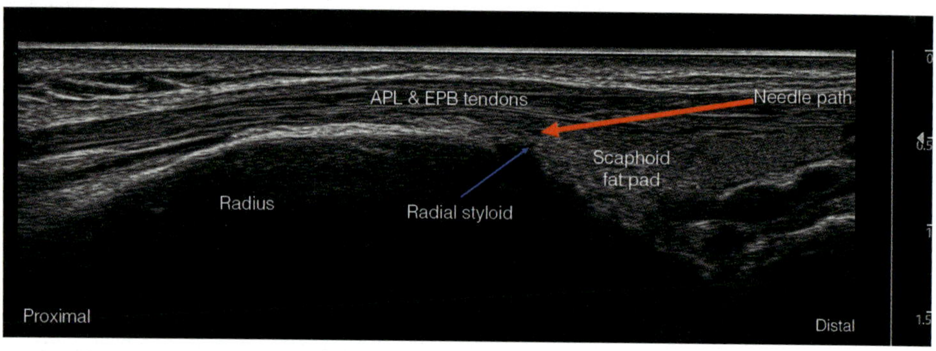

FIGURE 10.54 First dorsal compartment ultrasound coronal image. The first dorsal compartment of the wrist contains the extensor pollicis brevis (EPB) and abductor pollicis longus (APL) tendons.

PEARLS

- If the proximal edge of the transducer lifts off the skin, creating an air gap, use a sterile ultrasound gel standoff to fill the gap and enhance image quality.
- Ensure that the needle tip is placed within the tendon sheath and not within the tendon themselves or superficial soft tissue.
- de Quervain tenosynovitis pain may radiate proximally, potentially mimicking proximal intersection syndrome. If diagnosis is uncertain, consider a diagnostic injection of 1 mL of 1% lidocaine without epinephrine into the first dorsal compartment tendon sheath. Pain relief after injection supports the diagnosis of de Quervain tenosynovitis.

Videos showing landmark-guided and ultrasound-guided de Quervain injections can be found in the companion eBook.

REFERENCES

1. Peters-Veluthamaningal C, van der Windt DAWM, Winters JC, Meyboom-de JB. Corticosteroid injection for de Quervain's tenosynovitis. *Cochrane Database Syst Rev.* 2009;2009(3):CD005616.
2. Cavaleri R, Schabrun SM, Te M, Chipchase LS. Hand therapy versus corticosteroid injections in the treatment of de Quervain's disease: a systematic review and meta-analysis. *J Hand Ther.* 2016;29(1):3-11.
3. Abi-Rafeh J, Kazan R, Safran T, Thibaudeau S. Conservative management of de Quervain's stenosing tenosynovitis: review and presentation of treatment algorithm. *Plast Reconstr Surg.* 2020;146(1):105-126.
4. Challoumas D, Ramasubbu R, Rooney E, Seymour-Jackson E, Putti A, Millar NL. Management of de Quervain tenosynovitis: a systematic review and network meta-analysis. *JAMA Netw Open.* 2023;6(10):e2337001.
5. Hidajat NN, Magetsari RMSN, Steven G, Budiman J, Prasetiyo GT. Platelet-rich plasma for de Quervain's tenosynovitis: a systematic review and meta-analysis. *World J Orthop.* 2024;15(9):858-869.
6. Mirzanli C, Ozturk K, Esenyel CZ, Ayanoglu S, Imren Y, Aliustaoglu S. Accuracy of intrasheath injection techniques for de Quervain's disease: a cadaveric study. *J Hand Surg Eur Vol.* 2012;37(2):155-160.
7. McDermott JD, Ilyas AM, Nazarian LN, Leinberry CF. Ultrasound-guided injections for de Quervain's tenosynovitis. *Clin Orthop Relat Res.* 2012;470(7):1925-1931.
8. De Keating-Hart E, Touchais S, Kerjean Y, Ardouin L, Le Goff B. Presence of an intracompartmental septum detected by ultrasound is associated with the failure of ultrasound-guided steroid injection in de Quervain's syndrome. *J Hand Surg Eur Vol.* 2016;41(2):212-219.
9. Kume K, Amano K, Yamada S, Amano K, Kuwaba N, Ohta H. In de Quervain's with a separate EPB compartment, ultrasound-guided steroid injection is more effective than a clinical injection technique: a prospective open-label study. *J Hand Surg Eur Vol.* 2012;37(6):523-527.
10. Kang JW, Park JW, Lee SH, et al. Ultrasound-guided injection for De Quervain's disease: accuracy and its influenceable anatomical variances in first extensor compartment of fresh cadaver wrists. *J Orthop Sci.* 2017;22(2):270-274.

Carpal Tunnel Syndrome—Preferred Flexor Carpi Radialis Approach

Carpal tunnel syndrome is a very common condition encountered in primary care. It represents a compressive injury to the median nerve as it traverses the carpal tunnel in the wrist. This usually occurs as a result of an overuse injury following repetitive handgrip movements or compression of the contents of the carpal tunnel from various disease or physical processes. Predisposing factors may include previous injury, pregnancy, diabetes, hypothyroidism, rheumatoid arthritis, or amyloidosis. Injection therapy of the carpal tunnel is an effective, but underutilized, treatment option by primary care providers.

In the traditional approach, the needle is inserted 1 cm proximal to the wrist crease and 1 cm ulnar to the palmaris longus tendon, then directed radially and distally at a 30° angle to the coronal plane. With the preferred, landmark-guided, flexor carpi radialis (FCR) approach, the needle is inserted 1 cm proximal to the wrist crease, at the ulnar border of the FCR tendon (or through it), then advanced in an ulnar direction and distally at a 20° angle to the coronal plane.

The preferred, landmark-guided FCR approach is safer and more effective than the traditional approach. Anatomic studies of cadavers have demonstrated a higher risk of ulnar artery and median nerve injury due to the close proximity of those structures as well as median nerve swelling and/or flattening around the distal wrist crease when using the traditional approach.[1–3] The preferred FCR approach gives the highest accuracy rate and is also the safest injection site.[4] Ultrasound guidance further increases the safety[1] and efficacy of this procedure.[5,6]

A single local injection of corticosteroid at or proximal to the carpal tunnel is a remarkably safe procedure.[7] Injection of corticosteroid is more effective than standard conservative therapy[8] and results in long-lasting improvement in at least half of treated patients.[9–12] A second corticosteroid injection appears at least as effective as the first.[13] Favorable prognostic factors include patients with shorter duration of symptoms, no prior injection,[14] electrodiagnostically mild disease,[15] lower symptom severity scores, and lower median nerve ultrasonographic cross-sectional areas at the pisiform bone.[16]

Objective measurable changes following corticosteroid injections include decreased swelling of the median nerve,[17] improvement in distal motor latency of the median nerve,[18] improvement in sonoelasticity of the intracarpal tunnel contents,[19] and decreased vascularity of the median nerve at the distal wrist crease.[20]

Promising alternative therapies of mild to moderate idiopathic carpal tunnel syndrome include nerve hydrodissection[21,22] as well as injections of PRP[23,24] and dextrose.[25]

Relevant Anatomy: (Figs. 10.55 and 10.56)

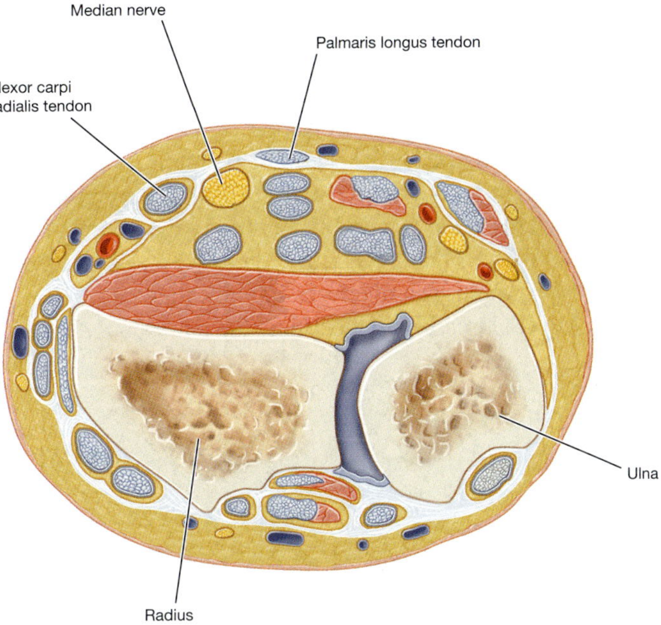

FIGURE 10.55 ● Right wrist cross section at the level of the distal radioulnar joint. (Modified with permission from Gest TR. *Lippincott® Atlas of Anatomy*. 2nd ed. Wolters Kluwer; 2020.)

PATIENT POSITION

- Supine on the examination table with the head of the bed elevated at an angle of 30°.
- The elbow is slightly flexed with the wrist in supination.
- The wrist is then positioned in slight hyperextension with the placement of chucks pads or towels underneath the supinated wrist.
- Rotate the patient's head away from the side that is being injected. This minimizes anxiety and pain perception.

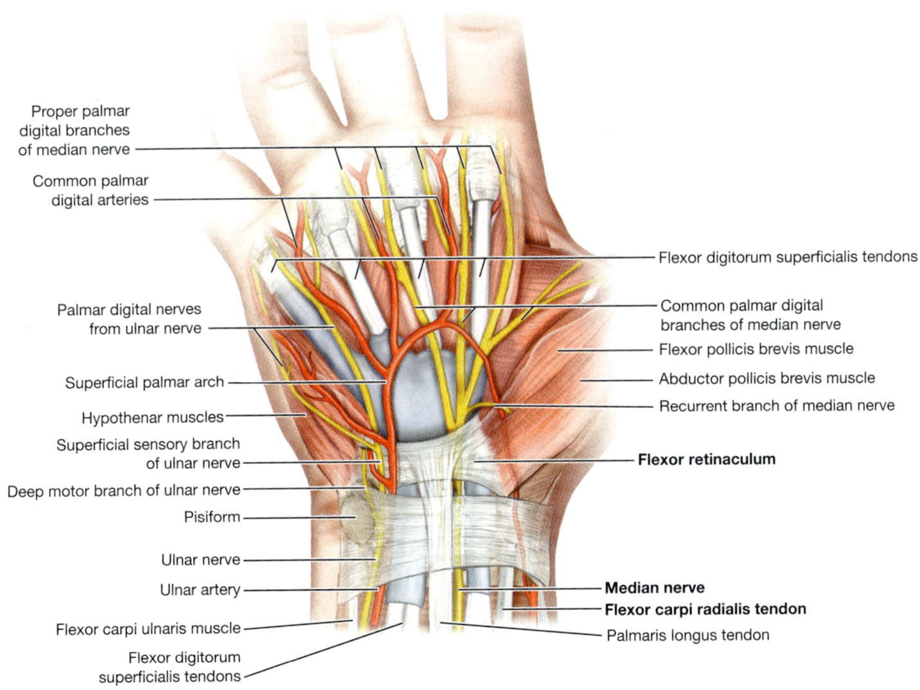

FIGURE 10.56 ● Right wrist—volar aspect.

LANDMARKS

1. With the patient supine on the examination table, the clinician stands lateral to the affected wrist.
2. Identify and mark the distal palmar crease as shown in Figure 10.57.
3. Identify and mark the course of the palmaris longus and FCR tendons (Fig. 10.58).
4. Mark a point 1 cm proximal to the distal palmar crease on the ulnar border of the FCR tendon. This is the entry point for the needle.
5. At both the entry point and the target site, press firmly on the skin with the retracted tip of a ballpoint pen to create skin indentations.
6. After the landmarks are identified, the patient should not move the wrist.

ANESTHESIA

- Local anesthesia of the skin using topical vapocoolant spray.

EQUIPMENT

- Topical vapocoolant spray
- 3-mL syringe
- 25-gauge 1-in needle
- 1 mL of 1% lidocaine without epinephrine
- 0.5 to 1 mL of the 40 mg/mL steroid solution (20-40 mg of triamcinolone acetonide)
- One alcohol prep pad
- Two povidone-iodine or chlorhexidine prep pads
- Sterile gauze pads
- Sterile adhesive bandage
- Nonsterile, clean chucks pad

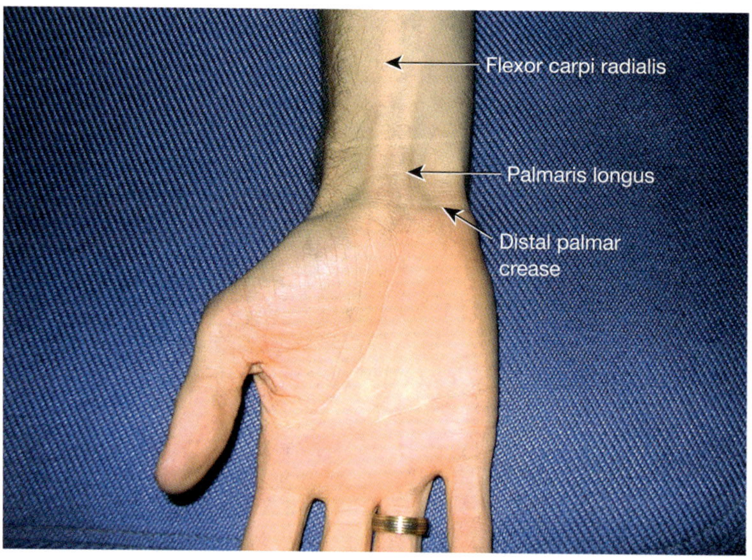

FIGURE 10.57 ● Right hand carpal tunnel injection surface anatomy.

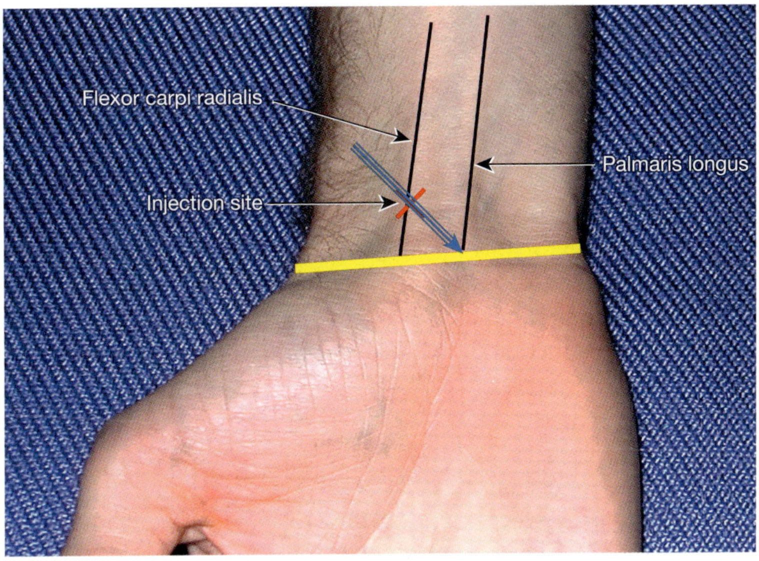

FIGURE 10.58 ● Right hand carpal tunnel injection surface landmarks identified.

TECHNIQUE

1. Prep the insertion site with alcohol followed by the povidone-iodine or chlorhexidine pads.
2. Achieve good local anesthesia by using topical vapocoolant spray.
3. Position the needle and syringe at a 20° angle to the skin with the needle tip directed in an ulnar and distal direction.
4. Using the no-touch technique, quickly introduce the needle at the insertion site (Fig. 10.59).
5. Very slowly advance the needle approximately 1.5 cm.

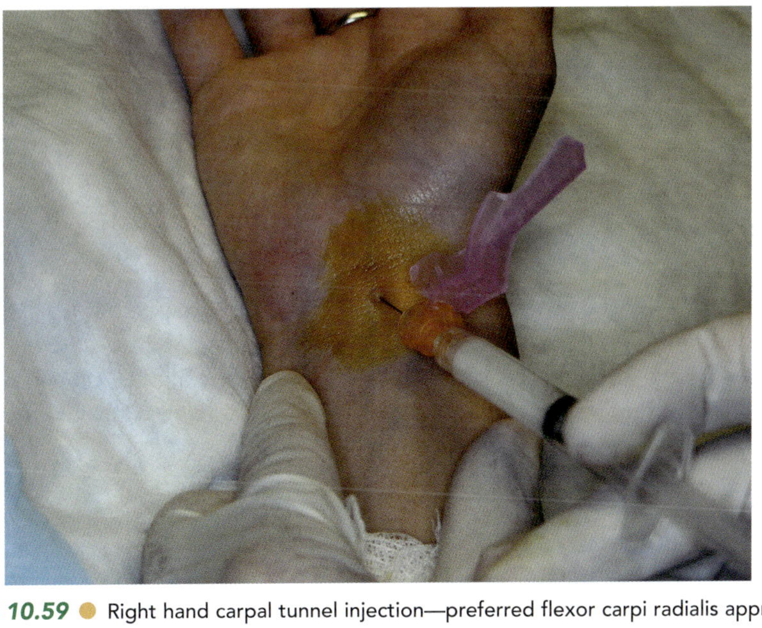

FIGURE 10.59 ● Right hand carpal tunnel injection—preferred flexor carpi radialis approach.

6. If any pain, paresthesias, or numbness is encountered, withdraw the needle 1 to 2 mm.
7. Withdraw the plunger of the syringe to ensure that there is no blood return.
8. Slowly inject the lidocaine/corticosteroid solution as a bolus around the median nerve.
9. If increased resistance is encountered, withdraw the needle slightly before attempting further injection.
10. Following injection, withdraw the needle.
11. Apply a sterile adhesive bandage.
12. Reexamine the hand in 5 minutes to assess pain relief and/or the development of numbness in the distribution of the median nerve from the local anesthetic.

AFTERCARE

- Avoid further overuse mechanisms of injury.
- Use a carpal tunnel wrist brace while sleeping to avoid wrist flexion and extension.
- NSAIDs, ice, and/or physical therapy as indicated.
- Consider follow-up examination in 2 weeks.

PEARLS

- The preferred, landmark-guided FCR approach illustrated here is easy to perform and has few side effects.
- This injection places the steroid solution just proximal to the carpal tunnel. Injections into the carpal tunnel itself may damage the median nerve.
- Warn the patients that the median nerve may be contacted when using this approach.
- Ask them to calmly report any pain or electrical shock sensation without jerking their arm away. If this occurs, simply withdraw the needle 1 to 2 mL before injecting.
- Alternatively, ultrasound guidance of the procedure may be done to increase safety and accuracy of this injection.

ULTRASOUND-GUIDED PROCEDURE

Please refer to the introductory ultrasound chapter for preprocedure, sterile prep, post-procedure, and documentation information and recommendations.

PATIENT POSITION

- Lateral decubitus on the examination table with the affected wrist down.
- On the affected side, keep the shoulder in a neutral position, flex the elbow to 90°, supinate the forearm, and place the forearm on a chux pad on the examination table.
- Patient's fingers are in a relaxed position.
- Improve access to the injection site by extending the affected wrist over the edge of the bed to fully extend the wrist.
- Place a pillow under their head for comfort.
- Adjust the patient's position as needed for comfort.

PROVIDER/ULTRASOUND POSITION

- The provider sits in front of the patient approximately at their waist.
- Adjust the examination table to position the injection site between the provider's umbilicus and axillary level, ensuring optimal ergonomics and visualization of the ultrasound screen, transducer, and needle's approach (Fig. 10.60).
- Position the ultrasound machine on the same side of the table from the provider at the level of the patient's head with the screen facing the provider.

LANDMARKS

- See the landmarks for the landmark-guided injection procedure.

EQUIPMENT

- 5-mL syringe
- 25-gauge 1.5-in needle (adjust needle length as needed)
- 4 mL of 1% lidocaine without epinephrine
- 0.5 to 1 mL of the 40 mg/mL steroid solution (20-40 mg of triamcinolone acetonide)
- Three chlorhexidine swabs
- 12-4 MHz linear ultrasound transducer and machine
- Sterile ultrasound transducer cover
- Sterile ultrasound gel
- Nonlatex sterile or nonsterile gloves
- Two 4 × 4 sterile gauze pads
- One sterile adhesive bandage
- Topical vapocoolant spray

ANESTHESIA

- Topical vapocoolant spray.

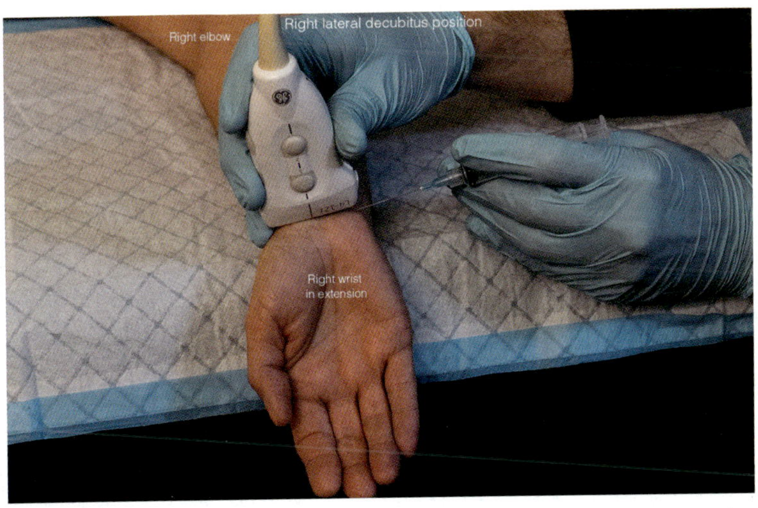

FIGURE 10.60 ● Ultrasound-guided right carpal tunnel injection. Right lateral decubitus position with the affected wrist extended over the edge of the examination table. Provider positioned ipsilaterally on the ulnar aspect of the wrist.

TECHNIQUE

1. Position a high-frequency linear 12-4 MHz ultrasound transducer in the axial plane with the median nerve centered beneath it, located deep to the flexor retinaculum that forms the roof of the carpal tunnel between the pisiform and scaphoid tubercle.
2. Prior to the procedure, identify the ulnar nerve and activate power Doppler imaging to precisely localize the ulnar and radial arteries. This visualization is essential for preventing inadvertent injury to the neurovascular bundle.
3. Advance a 25-gauge 1.5-in needle using an in-plane approach, directing it from ulnar to radial, with an initial needle angle of approximately 0° to 5° relative to the skin surface where the transducer is positioned. It is critical to maintain the needle trajectory superficial to the ulnar artery and nerve and away from the radial artery throughout the procedure.
4. The target area is the perineural space surrounding the median nerve within the carpal tunnel.
5. Utilize real-time ultrasound guidance throughout the procedure to precisely place the needle within the desired target area and minimize the risk of inadvertently injuring surrounding structures (Fig. 10.61).
6. Upon completion of the procedure, carefully withdraw the needle. Adhere to established postprocedure care protocols and ensure appropriate follow-up as recommended.

PEARLS

- The carpal tunnel is anatomically complex. Ultrasound-guided injection requires meticulous technique due to the presence of numerous neurovascular structures.
- Advance the needle slowly and with controlled movements, continuously monitoring its position under ultrasound, to avoid neurovascular structures.
- Differentiate carpal tunnel syndrome from C5 to C8 radiculopathy. Consider workup for radiculopathy or severe carpal tunnel syndrome. Refer to a specialist (neurosurgeon, orthopedic spine/hand surgeon) as needed before proceeding with injection.

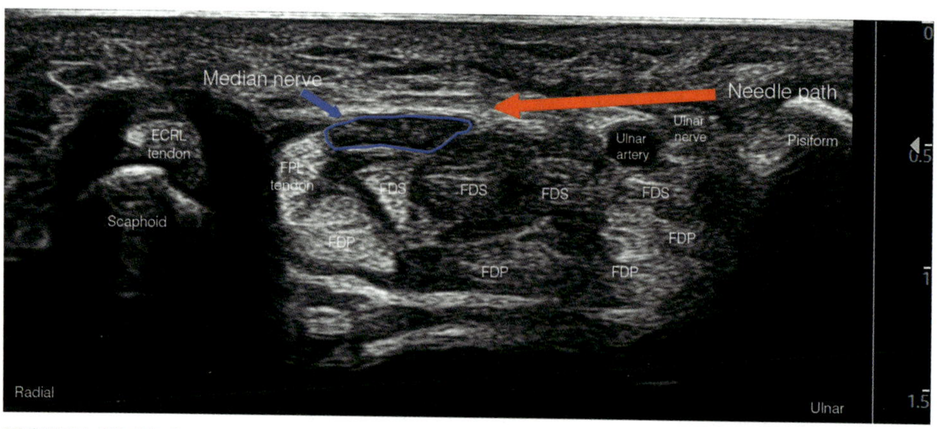

FIGURE 10.61 ● Carpal tunnel ultrasound axial image depicting the extensor carpi radialis longus (ECRL), flexor pollicis longus (FPL), flexor digitorum superficialis (FDS), and flexor digitorum profundus (FDP) tendons within the carpal tunnel.

Videos showing landmark-guided and ultrasound-guided carpal tunnel syndrome injections can be found in the companion eBook.

REFERENCES

1. Kim DH, Jang JE, Park BK. Anatomical basis of ulnar approach in carpal tunnel injection. *Pain Physician.* 2013;16(3):E191-E198.
2. Dubert T, Racasan O. A reliable technique for avoiding the median nerve during carpal tunnel injections. *Joint Bone Spine.* 2006;73(1):77-79.
3. MacLennan A, Schimizzi A, Meier KM. Comparison of needle position proximity to the median nerve in 2 carpal tunnel injection methods: a cadaveric study. *J Hand Surg Am.* 2009;34(5):875-879.
4. Ozturk K, Esenyel CZ, Sonmez M, Esenyel M, Kahraman S, Senel B. Comparison of carpal tunnel injection techniques: a cadaver study. *Scand J Plast Reconstr Surg Hand Surg.* 2008;42(6):300-304.
5. Babaei-Ghazani A, Roomizadeh P, Forogh B, et al. Ultrasound-guided versus landmark-guided local corticosteroid injection for carpal tunnel syndrome: a systematic review and meta-analysis of randomized controlled trials. *Arch Phys Med Rehabil.* 2018;99(4):766-775.
6. Chen PC, Wang LY, Pong YP, Hsin Y-J, Liaw M-Y, Chiang C-W. Effectiveness of ultrasound-guided vs direct approach corticosteroid injections for carpal tunnel syndrome: a double-blind randomized controlled trial. *J Rehabil Med.* 2018;50(2):200-208.
7. Kaile E, Bland JDP. Safety of corticosteroid injection for carpal tunnel syndrome. *J Hand Surg Eur.* 2018;43(3):296-302.
8. Chesterton LS, Blagojevic-Bucknall M, Burton C, et al. The clinical and cost-effectiveness of corticosteroid injection versus night splints for carpal tunnel syndrome (INSTINCTS trial): an open-label, parallel group, randomised controlled trial. *Lancet.* 2018;392(10156):1423-1433.
9. Ashworth NL, Bland JDP, Chapman KM, Tardif G, Albarqouni L, Nagendran A. Local corticosteroid injection versus placebo for carpal tunnel syndrome. *Cochrane Database Syst Rev.* 2023;2(2):CD015148.
10. Ly-Pen D, Andréu JL, Millán I, de Blas G, Sánchez-Olaso A. Comparison of surgical decompression and local steroid injection in the treatment of carpal tunnel syndrome: 2-year clinical results from a randomized trial. *Rheumatology (Oxford).* 2012;51(8):1447-1454.
11. Peters-Veluthamaningal C, Winters JC, Groenier KH, Meyboom-de B, Jong. Randomised controlled trial of local corticosteroid injections for carpal tunnel syndrome in general practice. *BMC Fam Pract.* 2010;11:54.
12. Dammers JW, Roos Y, Veering MM, Vermeulen M. Injection with methylprednisolone in patients with the carpal tunnel syndrome: a randomised double blind trial testing three different doses. *J Neurol.* 2006;253(5):574-577.
13. Ashworth NL, Bland JD. Effectiveness of second corticosteroid injections for carpal tunnel syndrome. *Muscle Nerve.* 2013;48(1):122-126.
14. Jerosch-Herold C, Shepstone L, Houghton J, Wilson ECF, Blake J. Prognostic factors for response to treatment by corticosteroid injection or surgery in carpal tunnel syndrome (palms study): a prospective multicenter cohort study. *Muscle Nerve.* 2019;60(1):32-40.
15. Visser LH, Ngo Q, Groeneweg SJ, Brekelmans G. Long term effect of local corticosteroid injection for carpal tunnel syndrome: a relation with electrodiagnostic severity. *Clin Neurophysiol.* 2012;123(4):838-841.
16. Meys V, Thissen S, Rozeman S, Beekman R. Prognostic factors in carpal tunnel syndrome treated with a corticosteroid injection. *Muscle Nerve.* 2011;44(5):763-768.
17. Lee YS, Choi E. Ultrasonographic changes after steroid injection in carpal tunnel syndrome. *Skeletal Radiol.* 2017;46(11):1521-1530.
18. Milo R, Kalichman L, Volchek L, Reitblat T. Local corticosteroid treatment for carpal tunnel syndrome: a 6-month clinical and electrophysiological follow-up study. *J Back Musculoskelet Rehabil.* 2009;22(2):59-64.
19. Miyamoto H, Siedentopf C, Kastlunger M, et al. Intracarpal tunnel contents: evaluation of the effects of corticosteroid injection with sonoelastography. *Radiology.* 2014;270(3):809-815.
20. Cartwright MS, White DL, Demar S, et al. Median nerve changes following steroid injection for carpal tunnel syndrome. *Muscle Nerve.* 2011;44(1):25-29.
21. Wu YT, Chen SR, Li TY, et al. Nerve hydrodissection for carpal tunnel syndrome: a prospective, randomized, double-blind, controlled trial. *Muscle Nerve.* 2019;59(2):174-180.
22. Neo EJR, Shan NT, Tay SS. Hydrodissection for carpal tunnel syndrome: a systematic review. *Am J Phys Med Rehabil.* 2022;101(6):530-539.
23. Senna MK, Shaat RM, Ali AAA. Platelet-rich plasma in treatment of patients with idiopathic carpal tunnel syndrome. *Clin Rheumatol.* 2019;38(12):3643-3654.
24. Dong C, Sun Y, Qi Y, et al. Effect of platelet-rich plasma injection on mild or moderate carpal tunnel syndrome: an updated systematic review and meta-analysis of randomized controlled trials. *Biomed Res Int.* 2020;2020:5089378.
25. Oh MW, Park JI, Shim GY, Kong HH. Comparative efficacy of 5% dextrose and corticosteroid injections in carpal tunnel syndrome: a systematic review and meta-analysis. *Arch Phys Med Rehabil.* 2025;106(2):300-310.

Carpal Tunnel Syndrome—Traditional Approach

Carpal tunnel syndrome is a very common condition encountered in primary care. It represents a compressive injury to the median nerve as it traverses the carpal tunnel in the wrist. This usually occurs as a result of an overuse injury following repetitive handgrip movements or compression of the contents of the carpal tunnel from various disease or physical processes. Predisposing factors may include previous injury, pregnancy, diabetes, hypothyroidism, rheumatoid arthritis, or amyloidosis. Injection therapy of the carpal tunnel is an effective, but underutilized, treatment option by primary care providers.

This traditional technique is the most commonly performed landmark-guided approach to injection of the carpal tunnel. Compared to the preferred FCR approach, it is a bit more awkward to perform. It is less effective, and there is also a higher risk for direct needle injury to the ulnar artery and median nerve.

Please read the details concerning carpal tunnel injection that are presented in the preceding chapter.

Relevant Anatomy: (Figs. 10.55 and 10.56 in previous chapter)

PATIENT POSITION

- Supine on the examination table with the head of the bed elevated 30°.
- The elbow is slightly flexed with the wrist in supination.
- The wrist is then positioned in slight hyperextension with the placement of chucks pads or towels underneath the supinated wrist.
- Rotate the patient's head away from the side that is being injected. This minimizes anxiety and pain perception.

LANDMARKS

1. With the patient supine on the examination table, the clinician stands lateral to the affected wrist.
2. Identify and mark the distal palmar crease as shown in Figure 10.62.
3. Identify and mark the intersection of the palmaris longus tendon with the distal palmar crease (Fig. 10.62).
4. Mark a spot 1 cm proximal and 1 cm ulnar to this intersection.
5. At that site, press firmly with the retracted tip of a ballpoint pen. This indentation represents the entry point for the needle.
6. After the landmarks are identified, the patient should not move the wrist.

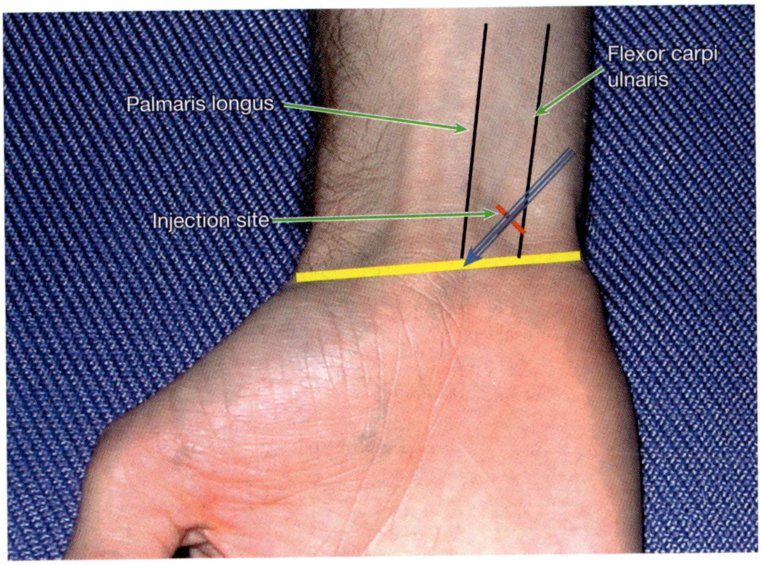

FIGURE 10.62 • Right hand carpal tunnel injection landmarks.

ANESTHESIA

- Local anesthesia of the skin using topical vapocoolant spray.

EQUIPMENT

- Topical vapocoolant spray
- 3-mL syringe
- 25-gauge 1-in needle
- 1 mL of 1% lidocaine without epinephrine
- 0.5 to 1 mL of the 40 mg/mL steroid solution (20-40 mg of triamcinolone acetonide)
- One alcohol prep pad
- Two povidone-iodine or chlorhexidine prep pads
- Sterile gauze pads
- Sterile adhesive bandage
- Nonsterile, clean chucks pad

TECHNIQUE

1. Prep the insertion site with alcohol followed by the povidone-iodine or chlorhexidine pads.
2. Achieve good local anesthesia by using topical vapocoolant spray.
3. Position the needle and syringe at a 30° angle to the skin of the wrist with the needle tip directed toward the base of the thumb.
4. Using the no-touch technique, quickly introduce the needle at the insertion site (Fig. 10.63).
5. Very slowly advance the needle approximately 1 cm toward the base of the thumb.
6. If any pain, paresthesias, or numbness is encountered, withdraw the needle 1 to 2 mm.

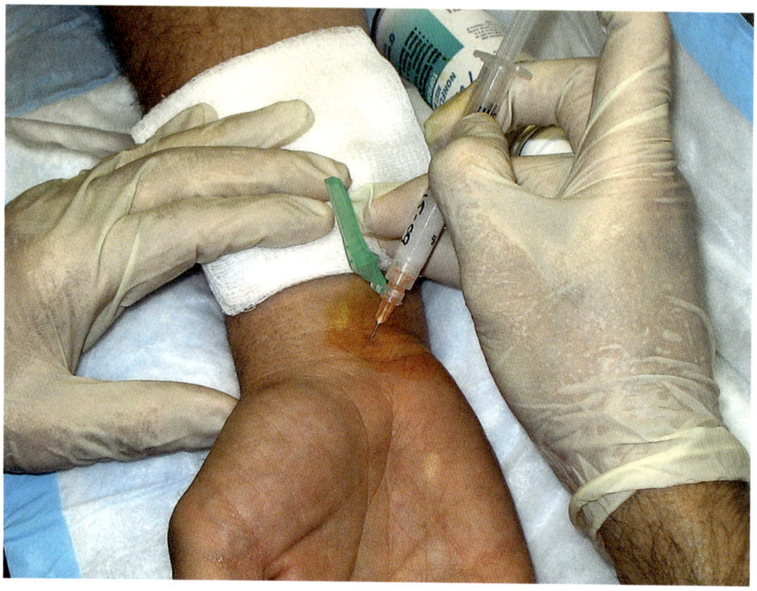

FIGURE 10.63 ● Right hand carpal tunnel injection—traditional approach.

7. Withdraw the plunger of the syringe to ensure that there is no blood return.
8. Slowly inject the lidocaine/corticosteroid solution as a bolus around the median nerve.
9. If increased resistance is encountered, withdraw the needle slightly before attempting further injection.
10. Following injection, withdraw the needle.
11. Apply a sterile adhesive bandage.
12. Reexamine the hand in 5 minutes to assess pain relief and/or the development of numbness in the distribution of the median nerve from the local anesthetic.

AFTERCARE

- Avoid further overuse mechanisms of injury.
- Use a carpal tunnel wrist brace while sleeping to avoid wrist flexion and extension.
- NSAIDs, ice, and/or physical therapy as indicated.
- Consider follow-up examination in 2 weeks.

PEARLS

- The approach illustrated here is easy to perform and has few side effects.
- However, the possibility of direct needle injury to the median nerve is greater with the traditional technique because the nerve is "fixed" in position by the carpal tunnel.
- Warn the patients that the median nerve may be contacted when using this approach.
- Ask them to calmly report any pain or electrical shock sensation without jerking their arm away. If this occurs, simply withdraw the needle 1 to 2 mL before injecting.
- Alternatively, ultrasound guidance of the procedure may be done to increase safety and accuracy of this injection.

A video showing a landmark-guided carpal tunnel injection can be found in the companion eBook.

REFERENCES

Please consult references listed in the preceding chapter, Carpal Tunnel Syndrome: Preferred Flexor Carpi Radialis Approach.

Wrist Joint

Injection of the wrist joint is a relatively uncommon procedure in primary care. Pain and swelling in the wrist may be the result of trauma, osteoarthritis, an infectious etiology, or an inflammatory disorder such as rheumatoid arthritis. A significant number of patients with rheumatoid arthritis on long-term treatment including biologics complain of wrist pain due to synovial proliferation and arthropathic changes. Multiple repeated corticosteroid injections may be safely used to control pain, improve function, and prevent or delay surgery, including synovectomy or joint arthroplasty.[1] Occasionally, one may encounter a small effusion of synovial fluid to remove. The success rates of corticosteroid injections can be significantly improved with use of ultrasound guidance.[2–4]

Relevant Anatomy: (Fig. 10.64)

PATIENT POSITION

- Supine on the examination table with the head of the bed elevated 30°.
- The elbow is slightly flexed with neutral positioning of the wrist in pronation.
- The wrist is supported with the placement of chucks pads or towels.
- Rotate the patient's head away from the side that is being injected. This minimizes anxiety and pain perception.

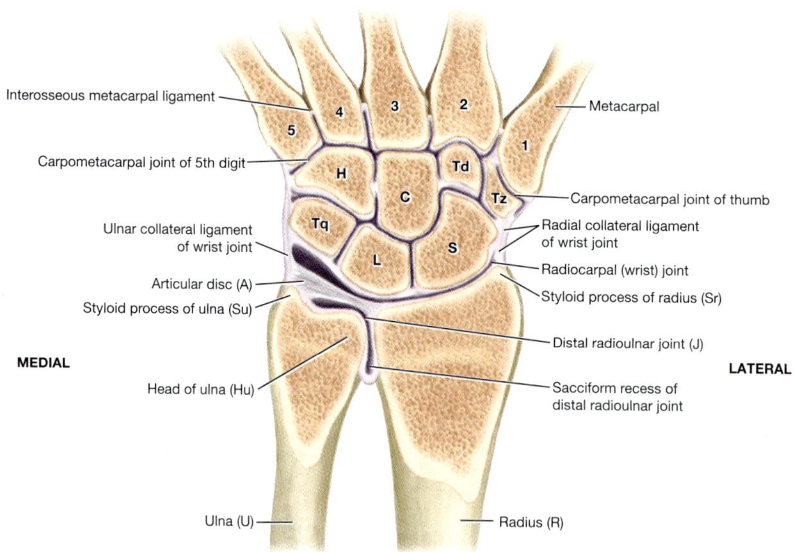

FIGURE 10.64 ● Coronal section of the wrist. (Modified with permission from Gest TR. *Lippincott® Atlas of Anatomy*. 2nd ed. Wolters Kluwer; 2020.)

LANDMARKS

1. With the patient supine on the examination table, the clinician stands lateral to the affected wrist.
2. Identify and mark the area of maximal tenderness and/or swelling over the dorsal aspect of the wrist joint.
3. At that site, press firmly on the skin with the retracted tip of a ballpoint pen. This indentation represents the entry point for the needle.
4. After the landmarks are identified, the patient should not move the wrist.

ANESTHESIA

- Local anesthesia of the skin using topical vapocoolant spray.

EQUIPMENT

- Topical vapocoolant spray
- 3-mL syringe
- 5-mL syringe—for optional aspiration
- 25-gauge 5/8-in or 1-in needle—for injection
- 20-gauge 1-in needle—for optional aspiration
- 0.5 mL of 1% mepivacaine without epinephrine
- 0.25 to 0.5 mL of the 40 mg/mL steroid solution (10-20 mg of triamcinolone acetonide)
- One alcohol prep pad
- Two povidone-iodine or chlorhexidine prep pads
- Sterile gauze pads
- Sterile adhesive bandage
- Nonsterile, clean chucks pad

TECHNIQUE

1. Prep the insertion site with alcohol followed by the povidone-iodine or chlorhexidine pads.
2. Achieve good local anesthesia by using topical vapocoolant spray.
3. Position the needle and syringe perpendicular to the skin with the needle tip directed posteriorly.
4. Using the no-touch technique, quickly introduce the needle at the insertion site (Fig. 10.65).
5. Advance the needle down into the wrist joint.
6. If aspirating, withdraw the fluid using a 20-gauge 1-in needle with the 5-mL syringe and then inject through the same syringe.
7. If only injecting, use a 25-gauge 5/8-in or 1-in needle with the 3-mL syringe.
8. If injection following aspiration is elected, remove the large syringe from the 20-gauge needle and then attach the 3-mL syringe filled with the mepivacaine/corticosteroid solution.
9. Inject the mepivacaine/corticosteroid solution as a bolus into the wrist joint. The injected solution should flow smoothly into the space. If increased resistance is encountered, advance or withdraw the needle slightly before attempting further injection.
10. Following injection, withdraw the needle.

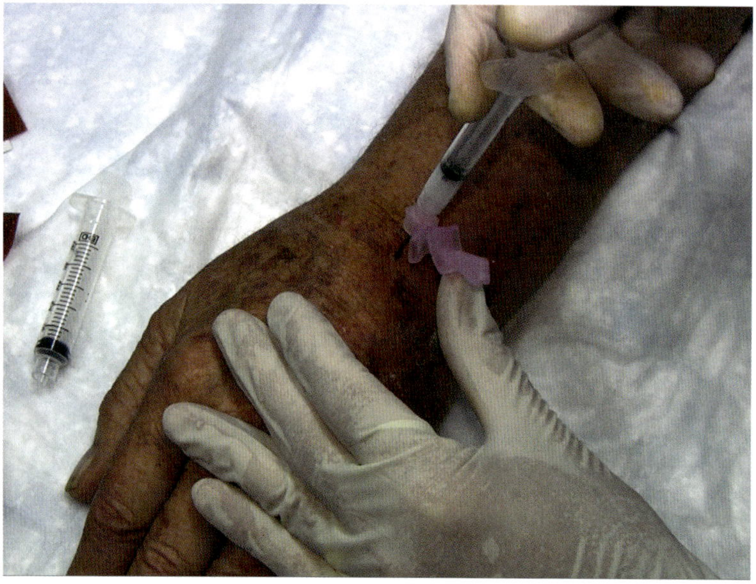

FIGURE 10.65 ● Right dorsal wrist joint injection.

11. Apply a sterile adhesive bandage.
12. Instruct the patient to move their wrist through its full range of motion. This movement distributes the mepivacaine/corticosteroid solution throughout the joint.
13. Reexamine the wrist in 5 minutes to assess pain relief.

AFTERCARE

- Consider the use of a wrist brace.
- Avoid excessive use of the wrist over the next 2 weeks.
- NSAIDs, ice, and/or physical therapy as indicated.
- Consider follow-up examination in 2 weeks.

PEARLS

- There are septa that create multiple partitions within the wrist joint complex. Increasing degrees of synovitis also inhibit flow to all wrist compartments. Therefore, a single injection into a standard injection site in the proximal part of the wrist cannot be assumed to distribute and treat the entire joint.[5] Successful administration of corticosteroid involves pinpoint precision and may require multiple injections during the same office visit.
- Work on the dorsal aspect of the wrist. The volar aspect contains the radial artery, median nerve, ulnar artery, and thicker musculature. These must all be avoided.
- Ultrasound guidance will improve accuracy, efficacy, and safety.

ULTRASOUND-GUIDED PROCEDURE

Please refer to the introductory ultrasound chapter for preprocedure, sterile prep, post-procedure, and documentation information and recommendations.

PATIENT POSITION

- Supine on the examination table.
- On the affected side, place the shoulder in a neutral position, extend the elbow to comfort, pronate the forearm, and rest the ventral aspect of the wrist on a chux pad.
- Wrist flexion can enhance joint space visualization. Place a rolled chux pad under the wrist to achieve approximately 20° to 30° of flexion.
- Place a pillow under their head for comfort.
- Adjust the patient's position as needed for comfort.

PROVIDER/ULTRASOUND POSITION

- The provider sits on the affected side of the table just distal to the patient's fingers.
- Adjust the examination table to position the injection site between the provider's umbilicus and axillary level, ensuring optimal ergonomics and visualization of the ultrasound screen, transducer, and needle's approach (Fig. 10.66).
- Position the ultrasound machine on the same side of the table from the provider at the level of the patient's shoulder with the screen facing the provider.

LANDMARKS

- See the landmarks for the landmark-guided injection procedure.

ANESTHESIA

- Local anesthesia of the skin using topical vapocoolant spray.

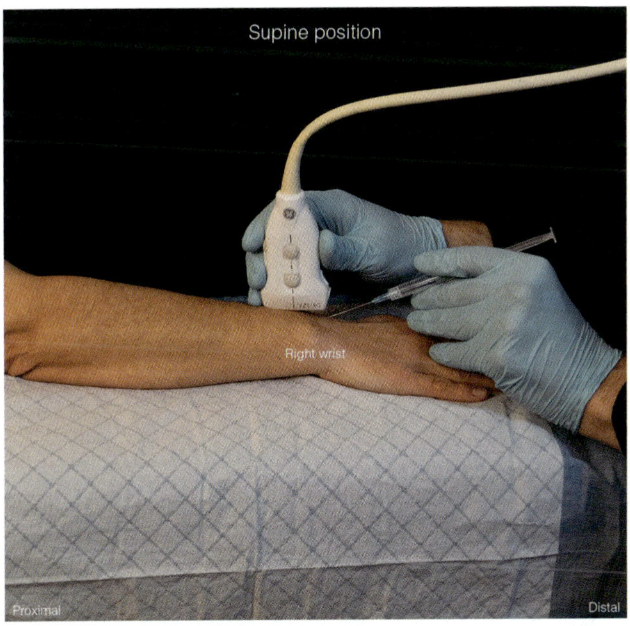

FIGURE 10.66 ● Ultrasound-guided right wrist injection. Supine position with the affected wrist pronated and resting on the examination table. Provider positioned ipsilaterally distal to the injection site.

EQUIPMENT

- 3-mL syringe
- 25-gauge 1.5-in needle (adjust needle length as needed)
- 0.5 mL of 1% mepivacaine without epinephrine
- 0.5 mL of the 40 mg/mL steroid solution (20 mg of triamcinolone acetonide)
- Alternative setup for aspiration
  - 3-mL syringe (anesthesia)
    - 25-gauge 1.5-in needle (adjust needle length as needed)
    - 3 mL of 1% lidocaine without epinephrine
  - 5-mL syringe (aspiration)
    - 18-gauge 1.5-in needle (adjust needle length as needed)
- Three chlorhexidine swabs
- 12-4 MHz linear ultrasound transducer and machine
- Sterile ultrasound transducer cover
- Sterile ultrasound gel
- Nonlatex sterile or nonsterile gloves
- Two 4 × 4 sterile gauze pads
- One sterile adhesive bandage
- Topical vapocoolant spray

TECHNIQUE

1. Position a high-frequency linear 12-4 MHz ultrasound transducer in the sagittal plane on the dorsal aspect of the wrist with the affected joint centered beneath it.
2. Advance a 25-gauge 1.5-in needle using an in-plane approach, directing it from distal to proximal, with an initial needle angle of approximately 20° to 30° relative to the skin surface where the transducer is positioned.
3. The target area is the contiguous synovial joint connecting the distal radius, triangular fibrocartilage disc, and the scaphoid, lunate, and triquetrum carpal bones.
4. Utilize real-time ultrasound guidance throughout the procedure to precisely place the needle within the desired target area and minimize the risk of inadvertently injuring surrounding structures (Fig. 10.67).
5. For intra-articular steroid injection:
   a. Slowly inject the desired volume of mepivacaine and corticosteroid solution directly into the joint.

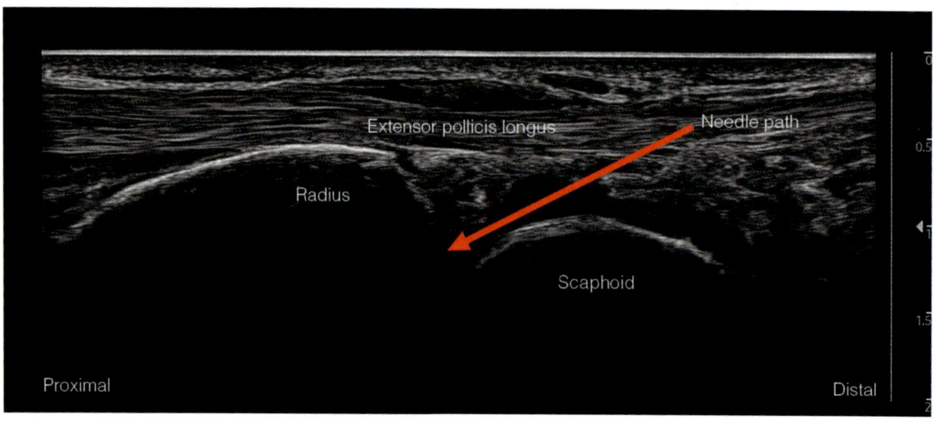

FIGURE 10.67 Radiocarpal joint ultrasound sagittal image.

6. For situations requiring anesthesia, aspiration, or both:
   a. Utilize a separate 25-gauge 1.5-in needle with a 3-mL syringe to inject 3 mL of 1% lidocaine without epinephrine into the soft tissues overlying the joint.
   b. For aspiration, use an 18-gauge 1.5-in needle with a 5-mL syringe to withdraw the effusion.
   c. If a corticosteroid injection is indicated following aspiration, replace the aspiration syringe with the mepivacaine and corticosteroid solution syringe and reconfirm accurate needle placement using real-time ultrasound guidance before injection.
7. Upon completion of the procedure, carefully withdraw the needle. Adhere to established postprocedure care protocols and ensure appropriate follow-up as recommended.

PEARLS

- If the wrist joint is challenging to locate, palpate Lister tubercle on the dorsal aspect of the radius. With the wrist in pronation and flexion, position the 12-4 MHz linear transducer in an axial plane over Lister tubercle. Identify the extensor pollicis longus tendon in the third dorsal compartment (located to the ulnar side of Lister tubercle). Rotate to a sagittal plane to visualize the extensor pollicis longus tendon in long axis. Slide the transducer distally to locate the radioscaphoid joint, which is congruent with the other wrist joints.
- Observe for distention of the joint capsule during injection to confirm intra-articular placement.
- Exercise caution to avoid inadvertent injury of the extensor tendons during needle advancement.

Videos showing landmark-guided and ultrasound-guided wrist joint injections can be found in the companion eBook.

REFERENCES

1. Fukui A, Yamada H, Yoshii T. Effect of intraarticular triamcinolone acetonide injection for wrist pain in rheumatoid arthritis patients: a statistical investigation. *J Hand Surg Asian Pac*. 2016;21(2):239-245.
2. Smith J, Brault JS, Rizzo M, Sayeed YA, Finnoff JT. Accuracy of sonographically guided and palpation guided scaphotrapeziotrapezoid joint injections. *J Ultrasound Med*. 2011;30(11):1509-1515.
3. Shen PC, Lin TY, Wu WT, Özçakar L, Chang K-V. Comparison of ultrasound- vs. landmark-guided injections for musculoskeletal pain: an umbrella review. *J Rehabil Med*. 2024;56:jrm40679.
4. Ali AH, Qenawy OK, Saleh WR, Ali AM, Abdul Monem ES, Omar NN. Radio-carpal wrist MR arthrography: comparison of ultrasound with fluoroscopy and palpation-guided injections. *Skeletal Radiol*. 2022;51(4):765-775.
5. Boesen M, Jensen KE, Torp-Pedersen S, Cimmino MA, Danneskiold-Samsøe B, Bliddal H. Intra-articular distribution pattern after ultrasound-guided injections in wrist joints of patients with rheumatoid arthritis. *Eur J Radiol*. 2009;69(2):331-338.

Dorsal Wrist Ganglion Cyst

Patients commonly present to primary care providers with dorsal wrist ganglion cysts. These are simple cysts containing clear mucinous, gelatinous fluid that originate from the wrist joint or tendon sheaths. They are seen over the dorsum of the wrist, usually between the extensor carpi radialis brevis and extensor digitorum communis, at the level of the scapholunate ligament. Although most prevalent in the wrists, ganglion cysts may also occur in other joints including the feet. Those located over the dorsal surface of the wrist joint can be easily treated with needle aspiration and expression of the cyst contents.

The very few studies reported in the medical literature suggest a poor response rate to traditional single aspiration attempts[1] with success in only 27% reported by Richman[2] and 42% by Dias.[3] Aspiration combined with corticosteroid injection gave only a 38.5% success rate.[4] In a study by Zubowicz,[5] up to three separate aspirations yielded 85% resolution. The author (JWM) suspects that the reason for the poor overall response rate is due to incomplete evacuation of the contents of the ganglion cyst with an aspiration attempt. Therefore, the author developed a technique that combines aspiration with a large-bore needle followed by firm compression of the cyst with the wrist in a flexed position "Mash technique." Corticosteroid is not injected. Since employing this technique for more than 25 years, the author is aware of only two patients who have failed this conservative treatment. Both were young women with chronic (>6 months), large dorsal wrist ganglion cysts greater than 1 cm in diameter (anecdotal and unpublished).

Ganglion cysts involving the volar surface of the wrist are usually intimately associated with the radial artery. Aspiration should never be attempted without ultrasound guidance with color flow Doppler monitoring and are best managed by orthopedic surgical referral.

Ultrasound-guided imaging for aspiration of dorsal wrist ganglion cysts is not necessary due to their obvious presentation.

Relevant Anatomy: (Fig. 10.68)

PATIENT POSITION

- Supine on the examination table with the head of the bed elevated 30°.
- For ganglion cysts over the dorsal aspect, the wrist is held in pronation and slight flexion.
- The wrist is supported with the placement of chucks pads or towels.
- Rotate the patient's head away from the side that is being injected. This minimizes anxiety and pain perception.

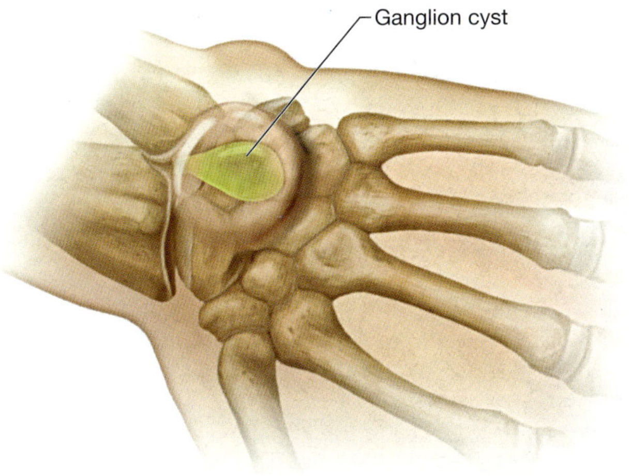

FIGURE 10.68 • Dorsal wrist ganglion cyst.

LANDMARKS

1. With the patient supine on the examination table, the clinician stands lateral to the affected wrist.
2. Position the wrist in flexion.
3. Identify the cystic structure over the dorsal aspect of the wrist joint.
4. The injection point is located directly over the cyst.
5. At that site, press firmly on the skin with the retracted tip of a ballpoint pen. This indentation represents the entry point for the needle.
6. After the landmarks are identified, the patient should not move the wrist.

ANESTHESIA

- Local anesthesia of the skin using topical vapocoolant spray.

EQUIPMENT

- Topical vapocoolant spray
- 3-mL syringe
- 18-gauge 1½ in needle
- One alcohol prep pad
- Two povidone-iodine or chlorhexidine prep pads
- Sterile gauze pads
- Sterile adhesive bandage
- Nonsterile, clean chucks pad

TECHNIQUE

1. Prep the insertion site with alcohol followed by the povidone-iodine or chlorhexidine pads.
2. Achieve good local anesthesia by using topical vapocoolant spray.
3. Position the needle and syringe perpendicular to the skin with the needle tip directed toward the palm.

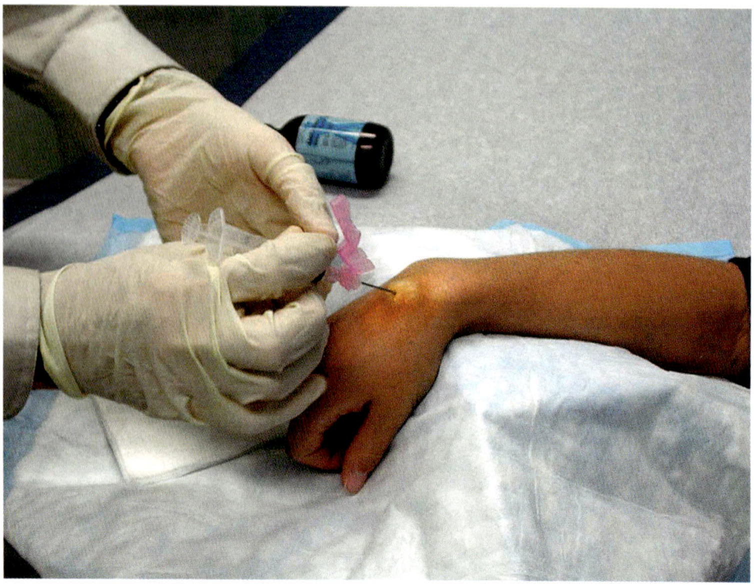

FIGURE 10.69 ● Right wrist dorsal ganglion cyst aspiration.

4. Using the no-touch technique, quickly introduce the needle at the insertion site (Fig. 10.69).
5. Advance the needle quickly but carefully into the cyst.
6. Apply suction with the syringe and withdraw the expected small amount of a clear gel.
7. Following aspiration, withdraw the needle.
8. With gloved fingers, apply very firm pressure to the tissues surrounding the punctured cyst "Mash technique." Do not contact the injection site with nonsterile gloves. Remove all extruded clear gel with sterile gauze pads (Fig. 10.70).
9. Apply a sterile adhesive bandage.

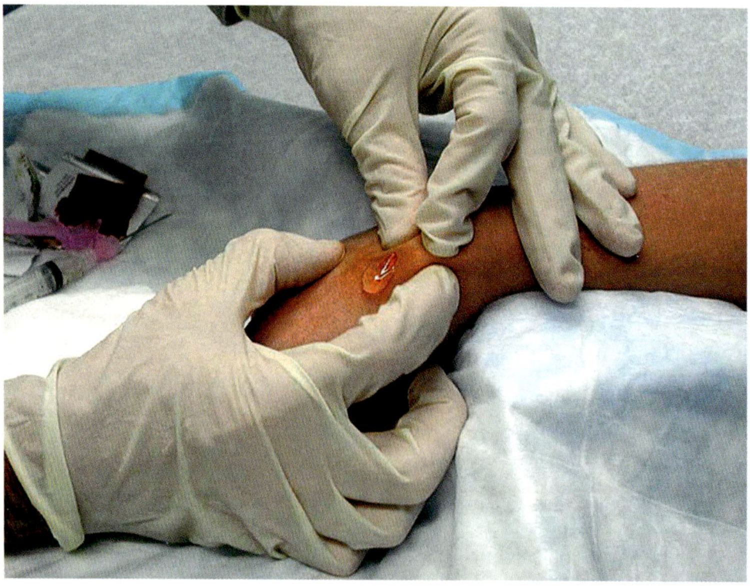

FIGURE 10.70 ● Expression of fluid remaining following aspiration of a ganglion cyst with direct pressure applied to the surrounding tissues "Mash technique."

AFTERCARE

- Consider immobilizing the wrist with a splint for 2 weeks.
- Consider follow-up examination in 2 weeks.

PEARLS

- Use extreme caution when treating ganglion cysts over the volar aspect of the wrist. These commonly involve the area immediately adjacent to the radial artery. An accidental injury of this artery with an 18-gauge needle can result in disastrous consequences.
- Initial treatment of a symptomatic ganglion cyst usually requires only cyst aspiration with manual extrusion of remaining contents.
- Treatment success may improve with wrist immobilization for 3 weeks.[1]
- Even with proficient technique, ganglion cysts frequently recur and may require surgical referral for definitive management.

REFERENCES

1. Horvath A, Zsidai B, Konaporshi S, et al. Treatment of primary dorsal wrist ganglion—a systematic review. *J Wrist Surg.* 2022;12(2):177-190.
2. Richman JA, Gelberman RH, Engber WD, Salamon PB, Bean DJ. Ganglions of the wrist and digits: results of treatment by aspiration and cyst wall puncture. *J Hand Surg.* 1987;12:1041-1043.
3. Dias JJ, Dhukaram V, Kumar P. The natural history of untreated dorsal wrist ganglia and patient reported outcome 6 years after intervention. *J Hand Surg Eur.* 2007;32(5):502-508.
4. Limpaphayom N, Wilairatana V. Randomized controlled trial between surgery and aspiration combined with methylprednisolone acetate injection plus wrist immobilization in the treatment of dorsal carpal ganglion. *J Med Assoc Thai.* 2004;87(12):1513-1517.
5. Zubowicz VN. Management of ganglion cysts of the hand by simple aspiration. *J Hand Surg Am.* 1987;12A(4):618.

Thumb Carpometacarpal Joint

The CMCJ of the thumb is a relatively common injection site for most primary care providers. This joint articulates the trapezium and the first metacarpal bone of the thumb. It is the most common site of osteoarthritis in the hand. The diagnosis of thumb carpometacarpal osteoarthritis is based on symptoms of localized pain, tenderness, and instability on physical examination as well as radiographic findings.

Review of the medical literature supports the use of corticosteroid injections for short-term[1,2] and perhaps medium- and even long-term treatment.[3,4] Improvement is noted in pain, grip strength, and overall hand function. The therapeutic effect may be more beneficial in mild rather than moderate or severe osteoarthritis.[5,6] Hyaluronic acid viscosupplements may play a future role in this condition.[7,8] Autologous fat transplantation is an interesting alternative, especially in early-stage osteoarthritis of this joint.[9] Thumb carpometacarpal injection accuracy can be significantly improved with ultrasound.[10] Those with persistent and recalcitrant symptoms may benefit from surgical intervention.

Relevant Anatomy: (Fig. 10.71)

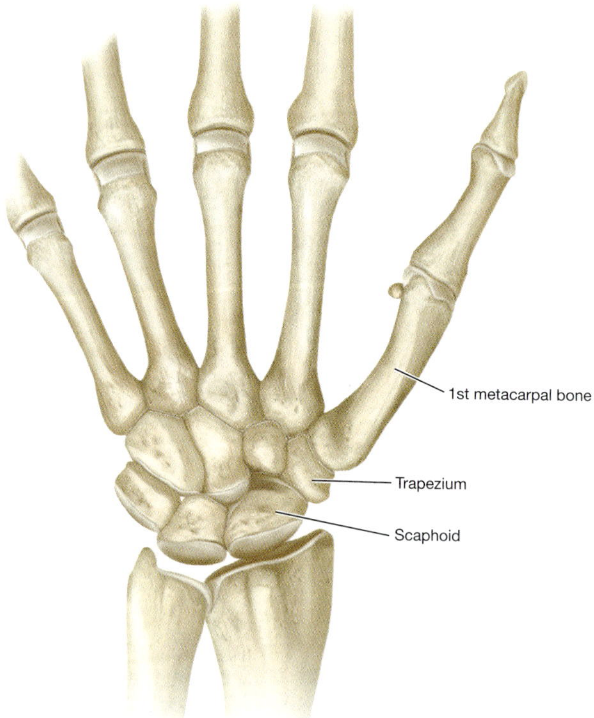

FIGURE 10.71 ● Dorsal aspect of the left hand.

PATIENT POSITION

- Supine on the examination table with the head of the bed elevated 30°.
- The affected wrist is held in pronation.
- The wrist is supported with the placement of chucks pads or towels.
- Rotate the patient's head away from the side that is being injected. This minimizes anxiety and pain perception.

LANDMARKS

1. With the patient supine on the examination table, the clinician stands lateral to the affected hand.
2. Locate the CMCJ by palpating the thumb metacarpal bone in a distal to proximal direction. At the proximal aspect of the first metacarpal, there will be tenderness as the examiner's finger passes over, then drops into the CMCJ. This is located between the first metacarpal and the trapezium bone. The patient will report tenderness in this joint.
3. Mark the injection point directly over the CMCJ.
4. At that site, press firmly on the skin with the retracted tip of a ballpoint pen. This indentation represents the entry point for the needle.
5. After the landmarks are identified, the patient should not move the hand or thumb.

ANESTHESIA

- Local anesthesia of the skin using topical vapocoolant spray.

EQUIPMENT

- Topical vapocoolant spray
- 3-mL syringe
- 25-gauge 5/8 in needle
- 0.25 mL of 1% mepivacaine without epinephrine
- 0.25 mL of the 40 mg/mL steroid solution (10 mg of triamcinolone acetonide)
- One alcohol prep pad
- Two povidone-iodine or chlorhexidine prep pads
- Sterile gauze pads
- Sterile adhesive bandage
- Nonsterile, clean chucks pad

TECHNIQUE

1. Prep the insertion site with alcohol followed by the povidone-iodine or chlorhexidine pads.
2. Achieve good local anesthesia by using topical vapocoolant spray.
3. Position the needle and syringe perpendicular to the skin with the needle tip directed posteriorly toward the first CMCJ.
4. Using the no-touch technique, quickly introduce the needle at the insertion site (Fig. 10.72).
5. Advance the needle in a palmar direction down into the joint.

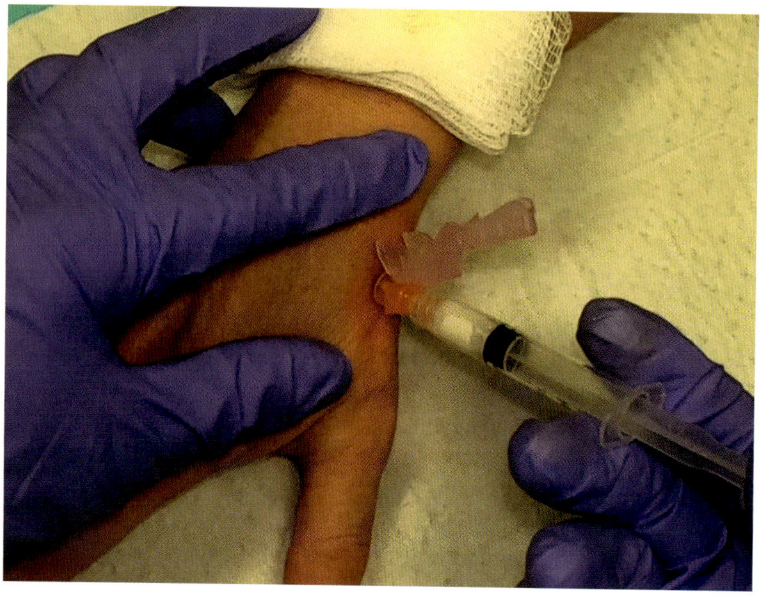

FIGURE 10.72 ● Left hand—thumb carpometacarpal joint injection.

6. Withdraw the plunger of the syringe to ensure that there is no blood return.
7. Inject the mepivacaine/corticosteroid solution as a bolus into the joint. The injected solution should flow smoothly into the space. If increased resistance is encountered, advance or withdraw the needle slightly before attempting further injection.
8. Following injection, withdraw the needle.
9. Apply a sterile adhesive bandage.
10. Instruct the patient to move their thumb through its full range of motion. This movement distributes the mepivacaine/corticosteroid solution throughout the CMCJ.
11. Reexamine the CMCJ in 5 minutes to assess pain relief.

AFTERCARE

- Avoid excessive use of the thumb over the next 2 weeks.
- Consider the use of a thumb spica splint.
- NSAIDs, ice, and/or physical therapy as indicated.
- Consider follow-up examination in 2 weeks.

PEARLS

- Care should be taken to differentiate this condition from de Quervain tenosynovitis.
- Applying traction to the thumb in a distal direction may help "open up" the joint to accommodate the needle.

ULTRASOUND-GUIDED PROCEDURE

Please refer to the introductory ultrasound chapter for preprocedure, sterile prep, post-procedure, and documentation information and recommendations.

PATIENT POSITION

- Supine on the examination table.
- On the affected side, place the shoulder in a neutral position, extend the elbow to comfort, pronate the forearm, and rest the ulnar aspect of the forearm on a chux pad placed on the examination table.
- Ulnar deviation of the wrist can enhance visualization. Place a rolled chux pad under the ulnar aspect of the wrist to achieve approximately 15° to 20° of ulnar deviation. The thumb should be in a relaxed, or flexed, position.
- Place a pillow under their head for comfort.
- Adjust the patient's position as needed for comfort.

PROVIDER/ULTRASOUND POSITION

- The provider sits on the same side of the table as the affected CMCJ.
- Adjust the examination table to position the injection site between the provider's umbilicus and axillary level, ensuring optimal ergonomics and visualization of the ultrasound screen, transducer, and needle's approach (Fig. 10.73).
- Position the ultrasound machine on the opposite side of the table from the provider at the level of the patient's wrist with the screen facing the provider.

LANDMARKS

- See the landmarks for the landmark-guided injection procedure.

ANESTHESIA

- Local anesthesia of the skin using topical vapocoolant spray.

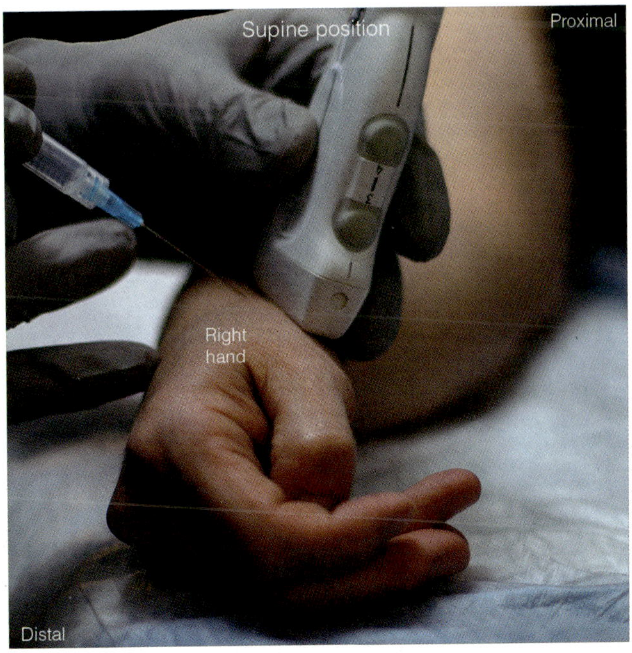

FIGURE 10.73 Ultrasound-guided right carpometacarpal joint injection. Supine position with the ulnar aspect of the wrist resting on the table in ulnar deviation. Provider positioned ipsilaterally at the injection site.

EQUIPMENT

- 3-mL syringe
- 25-gauge 1.5-in needle (adjust needle length as needed)
- 0.5 mL of 1% mepivacaine without epinephrine
- 0.25 to 0.5 mL of the 40 mg/mL steroid solution (10-20 mg of triamcinolone acetonide)
- Three chlorhexidine swabs
- 12-4 MHz linear ultrasound transducer and machine
- Sterile ultrasound transducer cover
- Sterile ultrasound gel
- Nonlatex sterile or nonsterile gloves
- Two 4 × 4 sterile gauze pads
- One sterile adhesive bandage
- Topical vapocoolant spray

TECHNIQUE

1. Position a high-frequency linear 12-4 MHz ultrasound transducer in the coronal plane over the apex of the anatomical snuff box with the CMCJ centered beneath it.
2. Advance a 25-gauge 1.5-in needle using an out-of-plane approach, directing it from dorsolateral to ventromedial, with an initial needle angle of approximately 15° to 30° relative to the skin surface where the transducer is positioned.
3. The target area is the affected CMCJ.
4. Utilize real-time ultrasound guidance throughout the procedure to precisely place the needle within the desired target area and minimize the risk of inadvertently injuring surrounding structures (Fig. 10.74).
5. Upon completion of the procedure, carefully withdraw the needle. Adhere to established postprocedure care protocols and ensure appropriate follow-up as recommended.

PEARLS

- If identifying the CMCJ is challenging, palpate the distal aspect of the anatomical snuffbox while the patient flexes and extends the thumb. The first metacarpal will move under the provider's fingers. The trapezium will remain stationary. If palpating over the scaphotrapezial joint, neither bone will move with thumb flexion/extension.
- Observe for distention of the joint capsule during injection to confirm intra-articular placement.

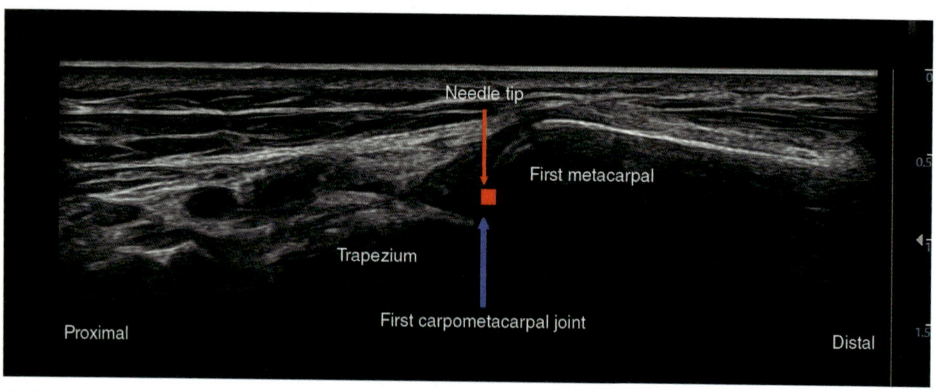

FIGURE 10.74 ● Carpometacarpal joint ultrasound coronal image.

Videos showing landmark-guided and ultrasound-guided thumb carpometacarpal joint injections can be found in the companion eBook.

REFERENCES

1. Maarse W, Watts AC, Bain GI. Medium-term outcome following intra-articular corticosteroid injection in first CMC joint arthritis using fluoroscopy. *Hand Surg.* 2009;14(2-3):99-104.
2. Joshi R. Intraarticular corticosteroid injection for first carpometacarpal osteoarthritis. *J Rheumatol.* 2005;32(7):1305-1306.
3. Swindells MG, Logan AJ, Armstrong DJ, Chan P, Burke FD, Lindau TR. The benefit of radiologically-guided steroid injections for trapeziometacarpal osteoarthritis. *Ann R Coll Surg Engl.* 2010;92(8):680-684.
4. Bahadir C, Onal B, Dayan VY, Gürer N. Comparison of therapeutic effects of sodium hyaluronate and corticosteroid injections on trapeziometacarpal joint osteoarthritis. *Clin Rheumatol.* 2009;28(5):529-533.
5. Meenagh GK, Patton J, Kynes C, Wright GD. A randomised controlled trial of intra-articular corticosteroid injection of the carpometacarpal joint of the thumb in osteoarthritis. *Ann Rheum Dis.* 2004;63(10):1260-1263.
6. Day CS, Gelberman R, Patel AA, Vogt MT, Ditsios K, Boyer MI. Basal joint osteoarthritis of the thumb: a prospective trial of steroid injection and splinting. *J Hand Surg Am.* 2004;29(2):247-251.
7. Bahadir C, Onal B, Dayan VY, Gürer N. Comparison of therapeutic effects of sodium hyaluronate and corticosteroid injections on trapeziometacarpal joint osteoarthritis. *Clin Rheumatol.* 2009;28(5):529-533.
8. Koh SH, Lee SC, Lee WY, Kim J, Park Y. Ultrasound-guided intra-articular injection of hyaluronic acid and ketorolac for osteoarthritis of the carpometacarpal joint of the thumb: a retrospective comparative study. *Medicine (Baltimore).* 2019;98(19):e15506.
9. Herold C, Rennekampff HO, Groddeck R, Allert S. Autologous fat transfer for thumb carpometacarpal joint osteoarthritis: a prospective study. *Plast Reconstr Surg.* 2017;140(2):327-335.
10. To P, McClary KN, Sinclair MK, Stout BA. The accuracy of common hand injections with and without ultrasound: an anatomical study. *Hand (N Y).* 2017;12(6):591-596.

Metacarpophalangeal Joint

Metacarpophalangeal joints (MCPJs) of the hand are uncommon injection sites for most primary care providers. An MCPJ may become inflamed with osteoarthritis, septic arthritis, and inflammatory arthritis—particularly rheumatoid. Ultrasound-guided intra-articular injections of corticosteroid have shown effectiveness in the short and medium term.[1–3]

A small-diameter needle is employed since this technique is generally only used to inject steroid solution into the MCPJ. There should not be a significant joint effusion to remove.

Relevant Anatomy: (Fig. 10.75)

PATIENT POSITION

- Supine on the examination table with the head of the bed elevated 30°.
- The affected wrist is held in a neutral position. The wrist is pronated, and the patient is asked to make a loose fist.

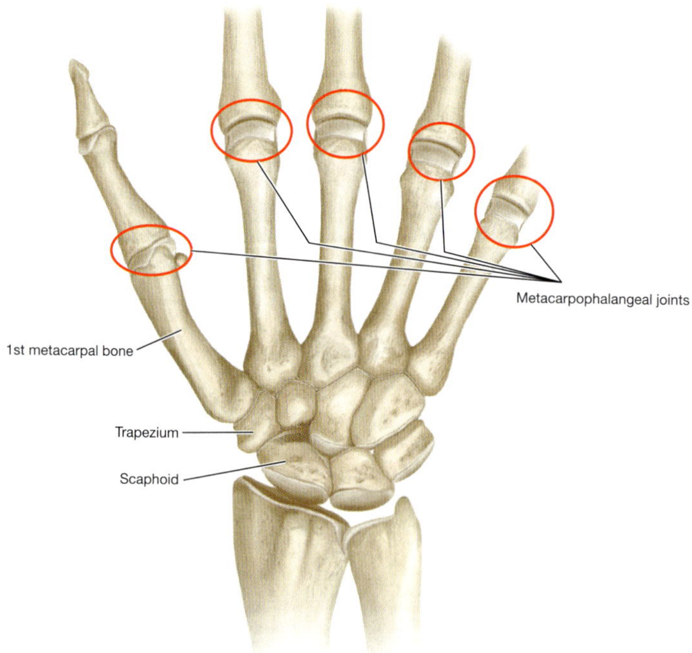

FIGURE 10.75 Dorsal aspect of the right hand.

- The hand is supported with the placement of chucks pads or towels.
- Rotate the patient's head away from the side that is being injected. This minimizes anxiety and pain perception.

LANDMARKS

1. With the patient supine on the examination table, the clinician stands lateral to the affected hand.
2. Locate the affected MCPJ.
3. The point of entry is located directly over the MCPJ, just radial or ulnar to the extensor tendon.
4. At that site, press firmly on the skin with the retracted tip of a ballpoint pen. This indentation represents the entry point for the needle.
5. After the landmarks are identified, the patient should not move the hand or fingers.

ANESTHESIA

- Local anesthesia of the skin using topical vapocoolant spray.

EQUIPMENT

- Topical vapocoolant spray
- 3-mL syringe
- 25-gauge 5/8-in needle
- 0.25 mL of 1% mepivacaine without epinephrine
- 0.25 mL of the 40 mg/mL steroid solution (10 mg of triamcinolone acetonide)
- One alcohol prep pad
- Two povidone-iodine or chlorhexidine prep pads
- Sterile gauze pads
- Sterile adhesive bandage
- Nonsterile, clean chucks pad

TECHNIQUE

1. Prep the insertion site with alcohol followed by the povidone-iodine or chlorhexidine pads.
2. Achieve good local anesthesia by using topical vapocoolant spray.
3. Position the needle and syringe perpendicular to the skin with the needle tip directed in a palmar direction toward the MCPJ.
4. Using the no-touch technique, quickly introduce the needle at the insertion site (Fig. 10.76).
5. Advance the needle down into the joint.
6. Withdraw the plunger of the syringe to ensure that there is no blood return.
7. Inject the mepivacaine/corticosteroid solution as a bolus into the joint. The injected solution should flow smoothly into the joint space. If increased resistance is encountered, advance or withdraw the needle slightly before attempting further injection.
8. Following injection, withdraw the needle.
9. Apply a sterile adhesive bandage.

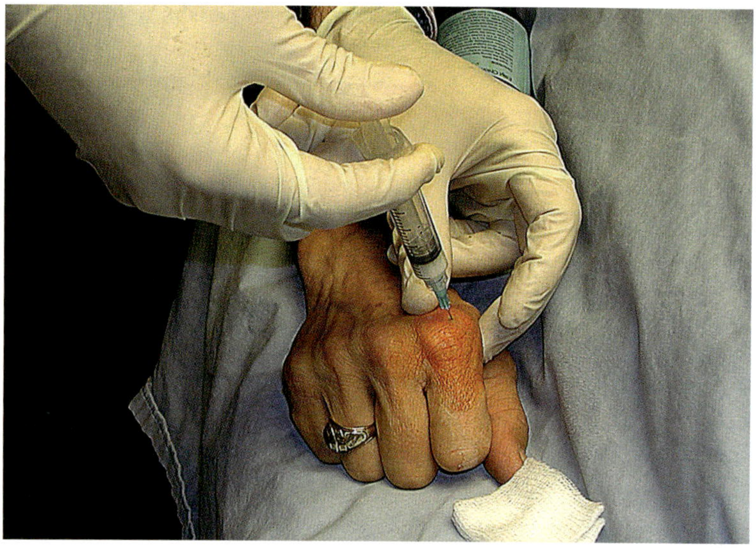

FIGURE 10.76 ● Metacarpophalangeal joint injection.

10. Instruct the patient to move their MCPJ through its full range of motion. This movement distributes the mepivacaine/corticosteroid solution throughout the joint.
11. Reexamine the MCPJ in 5 minutes to assess pain relief.

AFTERCARE

- Avoid excessive use of the affected hand and finger over the next 2 weeks.
- Consider the use of a volar wrist splint.
- NSAIDs, ice, and/or physical therapy as indicated.
- Consider follow-up examination in 2 weeks.

PEARLS

- Approach the MCPJ dorsally but avoid inserting the needle through the extensor tendon.
- Applying traction to the affected finger in a distal direction may help "open up" the joint to accommodate the needle.
- Avoid the development of a subdermal wheal during injection. This indicates the deposition of steroid solution that may cause localized skin atrophy and hypopigmentation.

ULTRASOUND-GUIDED PROCEDURE

Please refer to the introductory ultrasound chapter for preprocedure, sterile prep, post-procedure, and documentation information and recommendations.

PATIENT POSITION

- Supine on the examination table.
- On the affected side, place the shoulder in a neutral position, extend the elbow to comfort, pronate the forearm, and rest the palm on a chux pad placed on the examination table.

- MCPJ flexion can enhance joint space visualization. Place a rolled chux pad under the palmar aspect of the MCPJ to achieve approximately 5° to 10° of flexion of the affected finger.
- Place a pillow under their head for comfort.
- Adjust the patient's position as needed for comfort.

PROVIDER/ULTRASOUND POSITION

- The provider sits on the same side of the table as the affected MCPJ.
- Adjust the examination table to position the injection site between the provider's umbilicus and axillary level, ensuring optimal ergonomics and visualization of the ultrasound screen, transducer, and needle's approach (Fig. 10.77).
- Position the ultrasound machine on the opposite side of the table from the provider at the level of the patient's hand with the screen facing the provider.

LANDMARKS

- See the landmarks for the landmark-guided injection procedure.

ANESTHESIA

- Local anesthesia of the skin using topical vapocoolant spray.

EQUIPMENT

- 3-mL syringe
- 25-gauge 1.5-in needle (adjust needle length as needed)
- 0.25 mL of 1% mepivacaine without epinephrine
- 0.25 mL of the 40 mg/mL steroid solution (10 mg of triamcinolone acetonide)

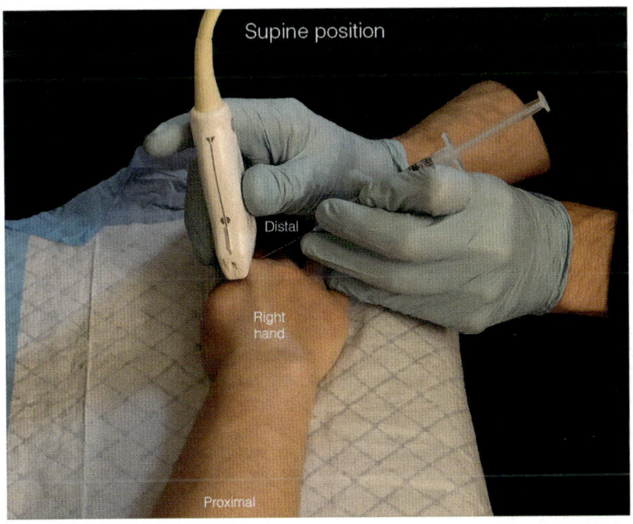

FIGURE 10.77 ● Ultrasound-guided right metacarpophalangeal joint injection. Supine position with affected wrist pronated and resting on examination table. Provider positioned ipsilaterally at the injection site.

- Three chlorhexidine swabs
- 12-4 MHz linear ultrasound transducer and machine
- Sterile ultrasound transducer cover
- Sterile ultrasound gel
- Nonlatex sterile or nonsterile gloves
- Two 4 × 4 sterile gauze pads
- One sterile adhesive bandage
- Topical vapocoolant spray

TECHNIQUE

1. Position a high-frequency linear 12-4 MHz ultrasound transducer in the sagittal plane with the dorsal aspect of the affected MCPJ centered beneath it.
2. Advance a 25-gauge 1.5-in needle using an out-of-plane approach, directing it from dorsomedial to ventrolateral, with an initial needle angle of approximately 30° to 45° relative to the skin surface where the transducer is positioned.
3. The target is the affected MCPJ.
4. Utilize real-time ultrasound guidance throughout the procedure to precisely place the needle within the desired target area and minimize the risk of inadvertently injuring surrounding structures (Fig. 10.78).
5. Upon completion of the procedure, carefully withdraw the needle. Adhere to established postprocedure care protocols and ensure appropriate follow-up as recommended.

PEARLS

- Observe for distention of the joint capsule during injection to confirm intra-articular placement.
- Due to the small size of the MCPJ, precise needle placement is crucial for successful intra-articular injection.

Videos showing landmark-guided and ultrasound-guided metacarpophalangeal joint injections can be found in the companion eBook.

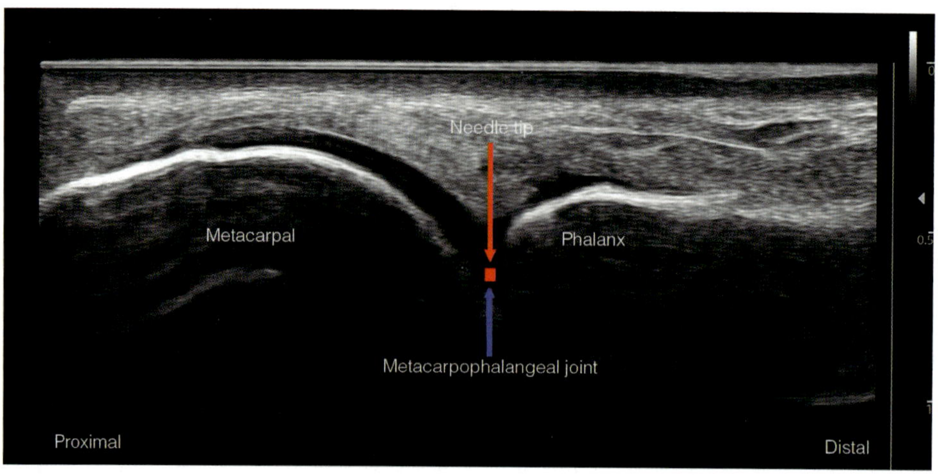

FIGURE 10.78 ● Metacarpophalangeal joint ultrasound sagittal image.

REFERENCES

1. Urits I, Smoots D, Anantuni L, et al. Injection techniques for common chronic pain conditions of the hand: a comprehensive review. *Pain Ther.* 2020;9(1):129-142.
2. Wang S, Wang X, Liu Y, Sun X, Tang Y. Ultrasound-guided intra-articular triamcinolone acetonide injection for treating refractory small joints arthritis of rheumatoid arthritis patients. *Medicine (Baltimore).* 2019;98(33):e16714.
3. Furtado RNV, Machado FS, Luz KRD, et al. Intra-articular injection with triamcinolone hexacetonide in patients with rheumatoid arthritis: prospective assessment of goniometry and joint inflammation parameters. *Rev Bras Reumatol Engl Ed.* 2017;57(2):115-121.

Trigger Finger

Stenosing tenosynovitis, or trigger finger, is the term given for tendinosis of the flexor tendons of the digits. This tendinopathy with nodule formation usually occurs as a result of repetitive compression injuries. It is more common in patients with diabetes and rheumatoid arthritis. In this disorder, the nodule forms where the flexor tendon passes over the metacarpal head of a finger or the thumb. Ultrasound studies show associated thickening of the first annular (A1) pulley and the volar plate.[1] With flexion of the digit, the nodule passes over the proximal edge of the thickened A1 pulley of the tendon sheath and becomes entrapped.

Trigger finger corticosteroid injection is a procedure that can easily be performed by primary care providers. A discrete injection at the site of the palpable, painful nodule offers an effective nonsurgical first-line treatment of this condition.[2,3] A study by Dala-Ali et al[4] showed 66% success rate with a single injection. Dardas further demonstrated 39% long-term response to second and third injections.[5] Ultrasound-guided extrasheath injection at the level of A1 pulley is as effective as an intrasheath administration.[6] However, ultrasound-guided injections are more effective than landmark-based procedures.[7] Schultz showed a greater treatment response in patients with mild to moderate symptoms versus those with moderate to severe disease.[8] Prognostic indicators for recurrence include younger age, insulin-dependent diabetes mellitus,[9] involvement of multiple digits, and a history of other tendinopathies of the upper extremity.[10]

Corticosteroid injection is a viable first-line option for patients presenting with mild to moderate triggering. Initial and repeat injections of trigger fingers should be considered in patients who prefer nonsurgical treatment. For more severe triggering or in patients with poor prognostic indicators, the success of steroid injection is lower and an early referral for surgery should be considered.

Relevant Anatomy: (Fig. 10.79)

PATIENT POSITION

- Supine on the examination table with the head of the bed elevated 30°.
- The affected wrist is held in a neutral position and fully supinated.
- The hand is supported with the placement of chucks pads or towels.
- Rotate the patient's head away from the side that is being injected. This minimizes anxiety and pain perception.

LANDMARKS

1. With the patient supine on the examination table, the clinician stands anterior to the affected hand.
2. Identify and mark the tender nodule located in the finger's flexor tendon and its sheath. This should be located over the metatarsal heads.

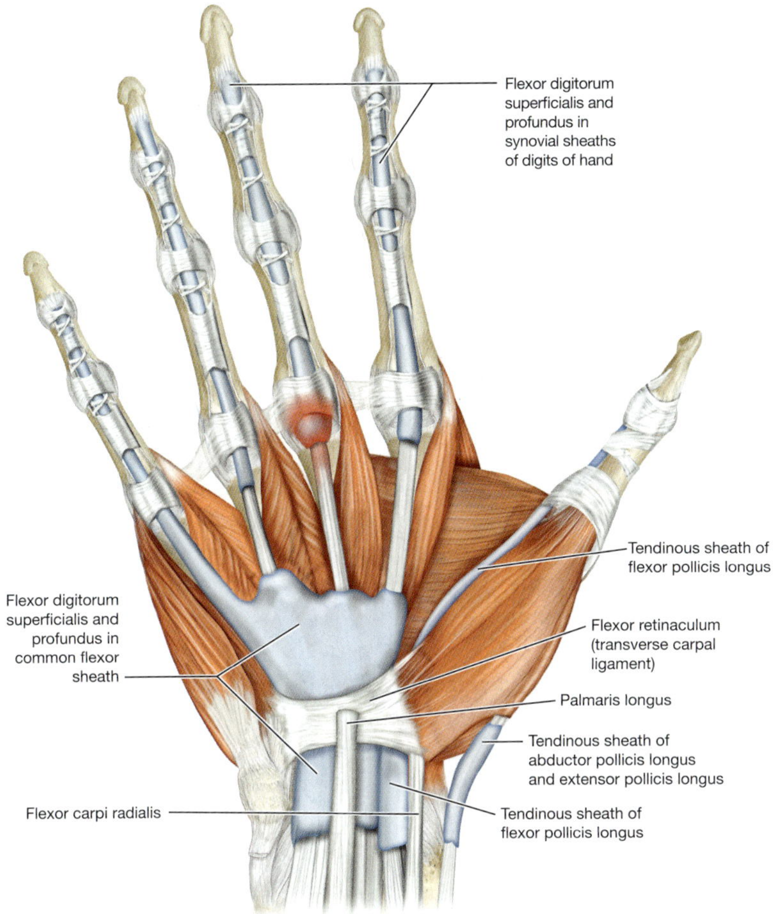

FIGURE 10.79 • Tendinous (synovial) sheaths of long flexor tendons of the digits. An inflamed nodule is shown in the flexor tendon of the long finger.

3. Mark a point 1 cm distal to the nodule.
4. At that site, press firmly on the skin with the retracted tip of a ballpoint pen. This indentation represents the entry point for the needle.
5. After the landmarks are identified, the patient should not move the hand or the fingers.

ANESTHESIA

- Local anesthesia of the skin using topical vapocoolant spray.

EQUIPMENT

- Topical vapocoolant spray
- 3-mL syringe
- 25-gauge 5/8-in needle
- 0.5 mL of 1% lidocaine without epinephrine
- 0.5 mL of the 40 mg/mL steroid solution (20 mg of triamcinolone acetonide)[11]
- One alcohol prep pad

- Two povidone-iodine or chlorhexidine prep pads
- Sterile gauze pads
- Sterile adhesive bandage
- Nonsterile, clean chucks pad

TECHNIQUE

1. Prep the insertion site with alcohol followed by the povidone-iodine or chlorhexidine pads.
2. Achieve good local anesthesia by using topical vapocoolant spray.
3. Position the needle and syringe at a 45° angle to the skin with the needle tip directed proximally at the nodule.
4. Using the no-touch technique, quickly introduce the needle at the insertion site (Fig. 10.80).
5. Advance the needle until the needle tip is located at the tendon nodule. Back up the needle 1 mm.
6. Withdraw the plunger of the syringe to ensure that there is no blood return.
7. Slowly inject the lidocaine/corticosteroid solution around the nodule into the tendon sheath. A subtle bulge in the shape of a sausage may develop in the tendon sheath.
8. If increased resistance is encountered, advance or withdraw the needle slightly before attempting further injection.
9. Following injection, withdraw the needle.
10. Apply a sterile adhesive bandage.
11. Instruct the patient to move their finger through its full range of motion. This movement distributes the lidocaine/corticosteroid solution throughout the tenosynovial sheath.
12. Reexamine the hand in 5 minutes to assess pain relief.

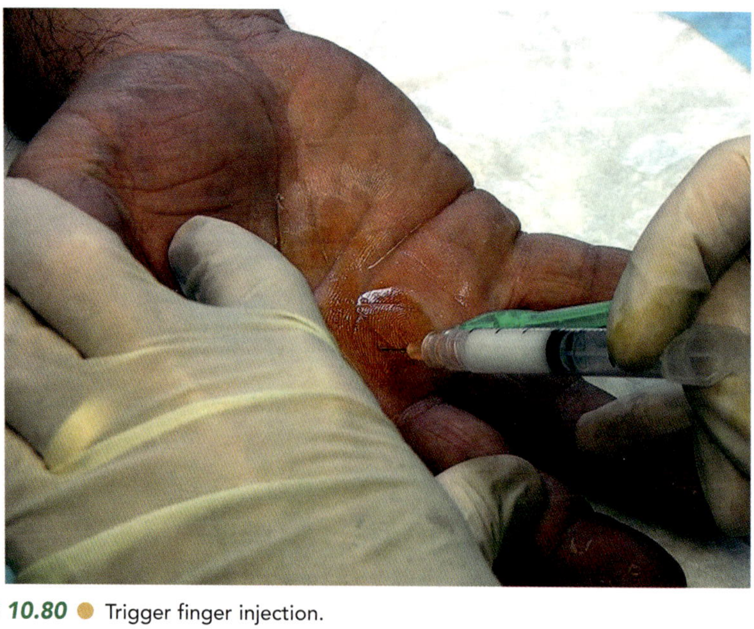

FIGURE 10.80 ● Trigger finger injection.

AFTERCARE

- Avoid excessive repetitive handgrip activities over the next 2 weeks.
- NSAIDs, ice, heat, and/or physical therapy as indicated.
- Consider follow-up examination in 2 weeks.

PEARLS

- The flexor tendon nodule may be approached from either a distal or a proximal direction. It, however, is easier and safer to perform this injection in a distal to proximal direction.

ULTRASOUND-GUIDED PROCEDURE

Please refer to the introductory ultrasound chapter for preprocedure, sterile prep, post-procedure, and documentation information and recommendations.

PATIENT POSITION

- Supine on the examination table.
- On the affected side, place the shoulder in a neutral position, extend the elbow to comfort, supinate the forearm, and rest the dorsal aspect of the hand on a chux pad on the examination table.
- Place a rolled-up chux pad under the dorsal aspect of the MCPJ to achieve approximately 10° to 15° of MCPJ extension, which can improve visualization and access to the tendon sheath deep to the A1 pulley.
- Place a pillow under their head for comfort.
- Adjust the patient's position as needed for comfort.

PROVIDER/ULTRASOUND POSITION

- The provider sits on the same side as the affected trigger finger, slightly distal to the fingers.
- To minimize patient finger movement during the procedure, consider gently resting the provider's transducer hand and wrist on the patient's fingers. This can help stabilize the patient's hand and facilitate a smoother procedure.
- Adjust the examination table to position the injection site between the provider's umbilicus and axillary level, ensuring optimal ergonomics and visualization of the ultrasound screen, transducer, and needle's approach (Fig. 10.81).
- Position the ultrasound machine on the same side of the table from the provider at the level of the patient's shoulder with the screen facing the provider.

LANDMARKS

- See the landmarks for the landmark-guided injection procedure.

ANESTHESIA

- Local anesthesia of the skin using topical vapocoolant spray.

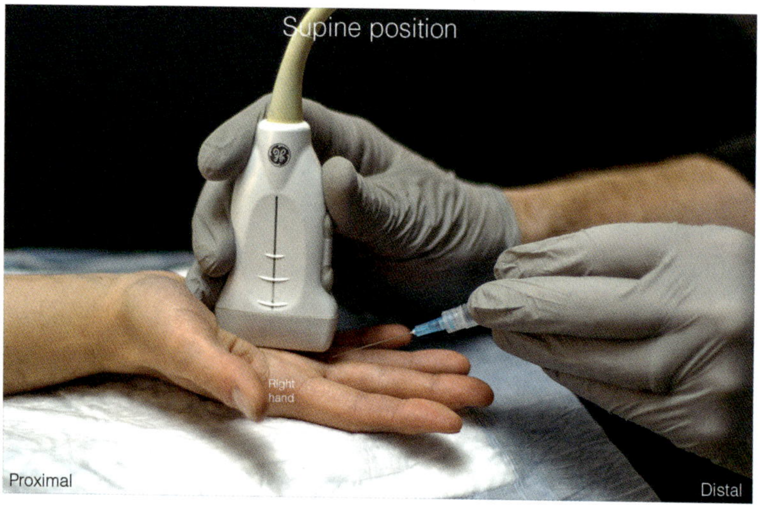

FIGURE 10.81 Ultrasound-guided right trigger finger injection. Supine position with the affected hand resting on the examination table in supination. Provider positioned ipsilaterally distal to the injection site.

EQUIPMENT

- 3-mL syringe
- 25-gauge 1.5-in needle (adjust needle length as needed)
- 0.5 mL of 1% lidocaine without epinephrine
- 0.5 mL of the 40 mg/mL steroid solution (20 mg of triamcinolone acetonide)
- Three chlorhexidine swabs
- 12-4 MHz linear ultrasound transducer and machine
- Sterile ultrasound transducer cover
- Sterile ultrasound gel
- Nonlatex sterile or nonsterile gloves
- Two 4×4 sterile gauze pads
- One sterile adhesive bandage
- Topical vapocoolant spray

TECHNIQUE

1. Position a high-frequency linear 12-4 MHz ultrasound transducer on the volar aspect in the sagittal plane of the affected finger, aligning with the flexor tendon and centering the A1 pulley or MCPJ beneath it.
2. Advance a 25-gauge 1.5-in needle using an in-plane approach, directing it from distal to proximal, with an initial needle angle of approximately 15° to 30° relative to the skin surface where the transducer is positioned.
3. The target area is the flexor tendon sheath deep to the A1 pulley.
4. Utilize real-time ultrasound guidance throughout the procedure to precisely place the needle within the desired target area and minimize the risk of inadvertently injuring surrounding structures (Fig. 10.82).
5. Upon completion of the procedure, carefully withdraw the needle. Adhere to established postprocedure care protocols and ensure appropriate follow-up as recommended.

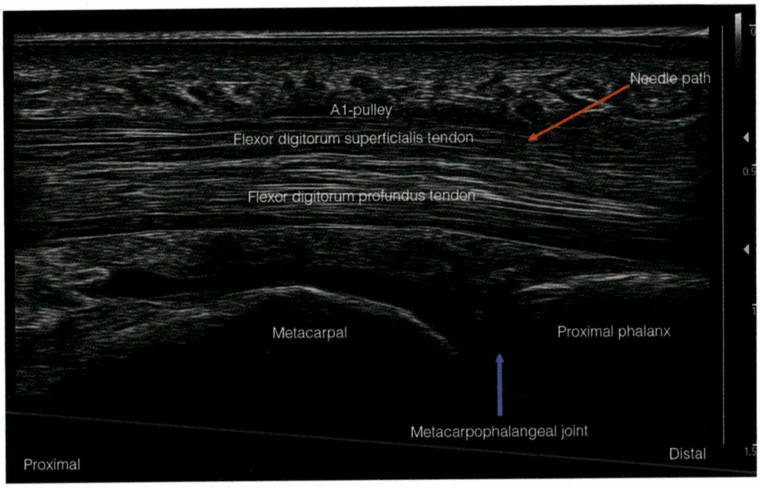

FIGURE 10.82 • A1 pulley and metacarpophalangeal joint ultrasound sagittal image.

PEARLS

- Identify the A1 pulley in the preprocedure evaluation by palpating the area under the distal palmar crease. Often, the provider can also feel the finger triggering in this region.
- Exercise caution to avoid inadvertent injection into the flexor tendon itself during needle advancement.

Videos showing landmark-guided and ultrasound-guided trigger finger injections can be found in the companion eBook.

REFERENCES

1. Tanaka Y, Gotani H, Yano K, Sasaki K. Sonographic evaluation of effects of the volar plate on trigger finger. *J Orthop Sci.* 2015;20(6):999-1004.
2. Ma S, Wang C, Li J, Zhang Z, Yu Y, Lv F. Efficacy of corticosteroid injection for treatment of trigger finger: a meta-analysis of randomized controlled trials. *J Invest Surg.* 2019;32(5):433-441.
3. Peters-Veluthamaningal C, van der Windt DA, Winters JC, Meyboom-de B, Jong. Corticosteroid injection for trigger finger in adults. *Cochrane Database Syst Rev.* 2009;2009(1):CD005617.
4. Dala-Ali BM, Nakhdjevani A, Lloyd MA, Schreuder FB. The efficacy of steroid injection in the treatment of trigger finger. *Clin Orthop Surg.* 2012;4(4):263-268.
5. Dardas AZ, VandenBerg J, Shen T, Gelberman RH, Calfee RP. Long-term effectiveness of repeat corticosteroid injections for trigger finger. *J Hand Surg Am.* 2017;42(4):227-235.
6. Mardani-Kivi M, Karimi-Mobarakeh M, Babaei Jandaghi A, Keyhani S, Saheb-Ekhtiari K, Hashemi-Motlagh K. Intra-sheath versus extra-sheath ultrasound guided corticosteroid injection for trigger finger: a triple blinded randomized clinical trial. *Phys Sportsmed.* 2018;46(1):93-97.
7. Tunçez M, Turan K, Aydın ÖD, Çetin Tunçez H. Ultrasound guided versus blinded injection in trigger finger treatment: a prospective controlled study. *J Orthop Surg Res.* 2023;18(1):459.
8. Shultz KJ, Kittinger JL, Czerwinski WL, Weber RA. Outcomes of corticosteroid treatment for trigger finger by stage. *Plast Reconstr Surg.* 2018;142(4):983-990.
9. Chang CJ, Chang SP, Kao LT, Tai T-W, Jou I-M. A meta-analysis of corticosteroid injection for trigger digits among patients with diabetes. *Orthopedics.* 2018;41(1):e8-e14.
10. Rozental TD, Zurakowski D, Blazar PE. Trigger finger: prognostic indicators of recurrence following corticosteroid injection. *J Bone Joint Surg Am.* 2008;90(8):1665-1672.
11. Kosiyatrakul A, Loketkrawee W, Luenam S. Different dosages of triamcinolone acetonide injection for the treatment of trigger finger and thumb: a randomized controlled trial. *J Hand Surg Asian Pac.* 2018;23(2):163-169.

Digital Mucous Cyst

Patients frequently present to their primary care providers with digital mucous cysts (aka digital myxoid cysts). These cysts, which have either a ganglion or myxomatous origin,[1] are located over the dorsal aspect of terminal digits adjacent to the fingernail. They contain clear mucinous fluid. Typically, there is underlying osteoarthritis of the distal interphalangeal joint. It is believed that a dorsal osteophyte weakens the joint capsule and allows the fluid to track distally. This pedicle terminates at the proximal nailfold where the fluid accumulates as a cystic structure. Over time, the cyst enlarges, exerts pressure on the nail matrix, and produces an indention in the fingernail.[1]

Digital mucous cysts can be treated similarly to ganglion cysts with repeated needle drainage. Unfortunately, the recurrence rate is high.[2] In a recent review, surgery yielded the highest cure rate among all treatment modalities (95%) compared to sclerotherapy (77%), liquid nitrogen cryotherapy (72%), corticosteroid injection (61%), and drainage of cyst contents (39%).[3] If recurrent, they may be managed with surgical excision of the cyst that includes a rotation advancement skin flap,[4] or osteophyte excision and joint débridement.[5]

Relevant Anatomy: (Figs. 10.83 and 10.84)

PATIENT POSITION

- Supine on the examination table with the head of the bed elevated 30°.
- The wrist is held in pronation.
- The hand is supported with the placement of chucks pads or towels.
- Rotate the patient's head away from the side that is being injected. This minimizes anxiety and pain perception.

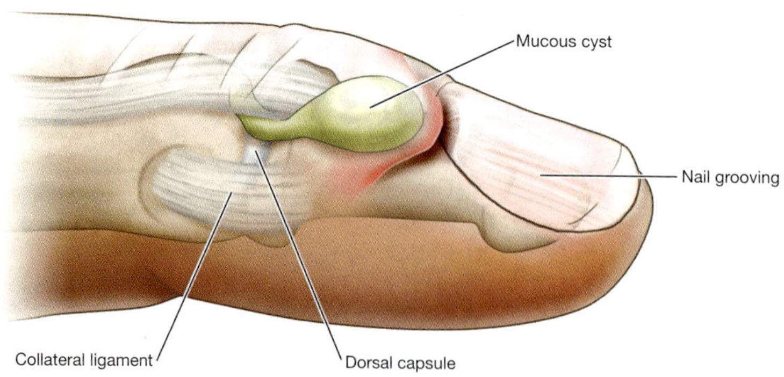

FIGURE 10.83 ● Digital mucous cyst.

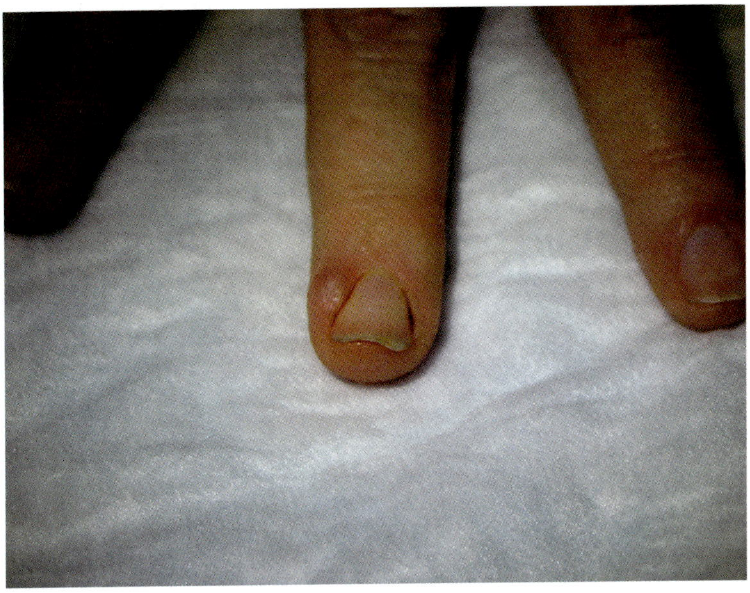

FIGURE 10.84 • Digital mucous cyst.

LANDMARKS

1. With the patient supine on the examination table, the clinician stands lateral to the affected hand.
2. Identify the cystic structure over the dorsal aspect of the finger, just proximal to the nailfold.
3. The injection point is located directly over the cyst.
4. The patient should not move the hand.

ANESTHESIA

- Digital block anesthesia of the finger using injected 1% lidocaine.

EQUIPMENT

- Topical vapocoolant spray
- 3-mL syringe
- 18-gauge 1½-in needle
- One alcohol prep pad
- Two povidone-iodine or chlorhexidine prep pads
- Sterile gauze pads
- Sterile adhesive bandage
- Nonsterile, clean chucks pad

TECHNIQUE

1. Achieve good digital block anesthesia.
2. Prep the insertion site with alcohol followed by the povidone-iodine or chlorhexidine pads.

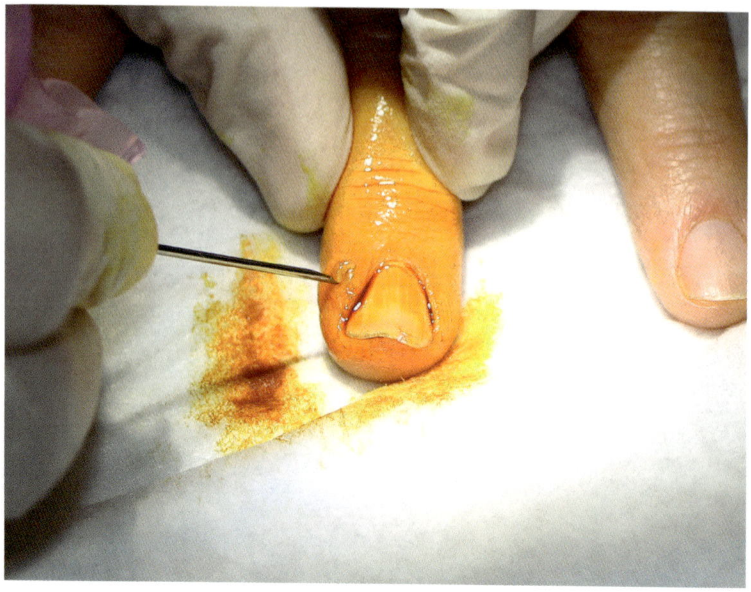

FIGURE 10.85 ● Digital mucous cyst aspiration.

3. Position the needle and syringe perpendicular to the skin with the needle tip directed to the center of the cyst.
4. Using the no-touch technique, quickly introduce the needle at the insertion site (Fig. 10.85).
5. Advance the needle quickly but carefully into the cyst.
6. Apply suction with the syringe and withdraw the expected small amount of a clear gel.
7. Following aspiration, withdraw the needle.
8. With either the shaft of the sterile needle or gloved fingers, apply firm pressure to the tissues surrounding the punctured cyst. Remove all extruded clear gel with sterile gauze pads (Fig. 10.86).
9. Injection of steroid solution is often not helpful.
10. Apply a sterile adhesive bandage.

AFTERCARE

- Consider follow-up examination in 2 weeks.

PEARLS

- Initial treatment of a symptomatic digital mucous cyst usually requires only cyst aspiration with manual extrusion of remaining contents.
- Cysts that recur despite repeated aspirations/needling have not been found to respond to injections of corticosteroid.
- Even with proficient technique, digital mucous cysts frequently recur and may require early surgical treatment.

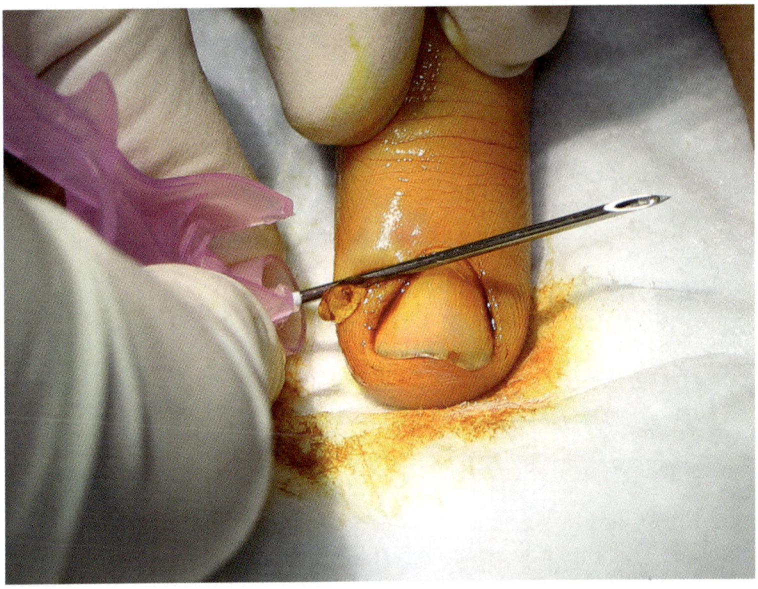

FIGURE 10.86 • Expression of fluid remaining following aspiration of a ganglion cyst with direct pressure to the surrounding tissues.

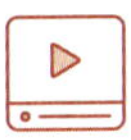

A video showing a landmark-guided digital mucous cyst needle drainage can be found in the companion eBook.

REFERENCES

1. Lin YC, Wu YH, Scher RK. Nail changes and association of osteoarthritis in digital myxoid cyst. *Dermatol Surg*. 2008;34(3):364-369.
2. Epstein E. A simple technique for managing digital mucous cysts. *Arch Dermatol*. 1979;115(11):1315-1316.
3. Jabbour S, Kechichian E, Haber R, Tomb R. Management of digital mucous cysts: a systematic review and treatment algorithm. *Int J Dermatol*. 2017;56(7):701-708.
4. Johnson SM, Treon K, Thomas S, Cox QG. A reliable surgical treatment for digital mucous cysts. *J Hand Surg Eur Vol*. 2014;39(8):856-860.
5. Fan Z, Chang L, Su X, Yang B, Zhu Z. Treatment of mucous cyst of the distal interphalangeal joint with osteophyte excision and joint debridement. *Front Surg*. 2022;8:767098.

11

Hip Joint—Preferred Lateral Approach

James W. McNabb

Hip joint pain from arthritis or capsulitis is a common condition seen in primary care medical practice. This often occurs as a result of osteoarthrosis, posttraumatic arthritis, and rheumatoid arthritis. Patients typically represent the middle-aged and older populations. Septic arthritis in children is fortunately now a rare occurrence following the development of the *Haemophilus influenzae* and pneumococcal vaccines. Diagnostic injections using anesthetic (mepivacaine) and therapeutic injections into and around the hip have become an important part of the treatment algorithm for hip pain.

The selection of therapeutic agent and clinical circumstances are of utmost importance. In the case of diagnostic injections, mepivacaine can be used alone. Although corticosteroids have been used for many years, it appears that there may be substantial risk involved. Four main adverse joint findings have been structurally observed in patients after intra-articular corticosteroid injections: accelerated osteoarthritis progression, subchondral insufficiency fracture, complications of osteonecrosis, and rapid joint destruction, including bone loss.[1,2] Considering these potential risks, it may be preferable to reserve corticosteroid injections for use in patients who present with severe pain,[3] those pending total hip arthroplasty,[4] or patients with malignant hip pain.[5] Promising treatment options for patients with osteoarthritis of the hip include tanezumab,[6,7] platelet-rich plasma (PRP),[8,9] and hyaluronic acid (HA).[10] More research is needed to identify the treatment efficacy and safety of these and other therapeutic options.

Because of the joint's perceived inaccessibility, fear of vascular puncture, and the remote risk of avascular necrosis of the head of the femur, primary care providers rarely perform aspiration and corticosteroid injections of the hip joint. In fact, access to this joint is straightforward. Anterior and lateral approaches have been described. The landmark-guided anterior approach has success rates of 60% to 93%.[11,12] The lateral approach also has good success rates of about 80%.[1,13] However, the anterior approach is associated with significantly more risk to the femoral artery and femoral nerve than the lateral approach.[1,3] For this reason, the landmark-guided lateral approach is preferred in the setting where image guidance is not available. When ultrasound guidance is available, the anterior approach is favored. In both cases, the use of ultrasound to guide needle placement significantly improves the safety and success rates of hip injections.[14,15] Guidance is particularly important in obese patients, patients with advanced osteoarthritis with little to no joint space, and those with flexion deformity.[16]

Relevant Anatomy: (Fig. 11.1)

PATIENT POSITION

- Lying on the examination table in the lateral decubitus position on the unaffected hip.

LANDMARKS

1. With the patient lying on the examination table in the lateral decubitus position on the unaffected hip, the clinician stands posterior to the affected hip.
2. Identify the trochanter of the femur.
3. Mark a point 1 cm proximal to the tip of the greater trochanter.
4. At that site, press firmly on the skin with the retracted tip of a ballpoint pen. This indentation represents the entry point for the needle.
5. After the landmarks are identified, the patient should not move the hip.

ANESTHESIA

- Local anesthesia of the skin using topical vapocoolant spray.

EQUIPMENT

- Topical vapocoolant spray
- 20-mL syringe—for aspiration

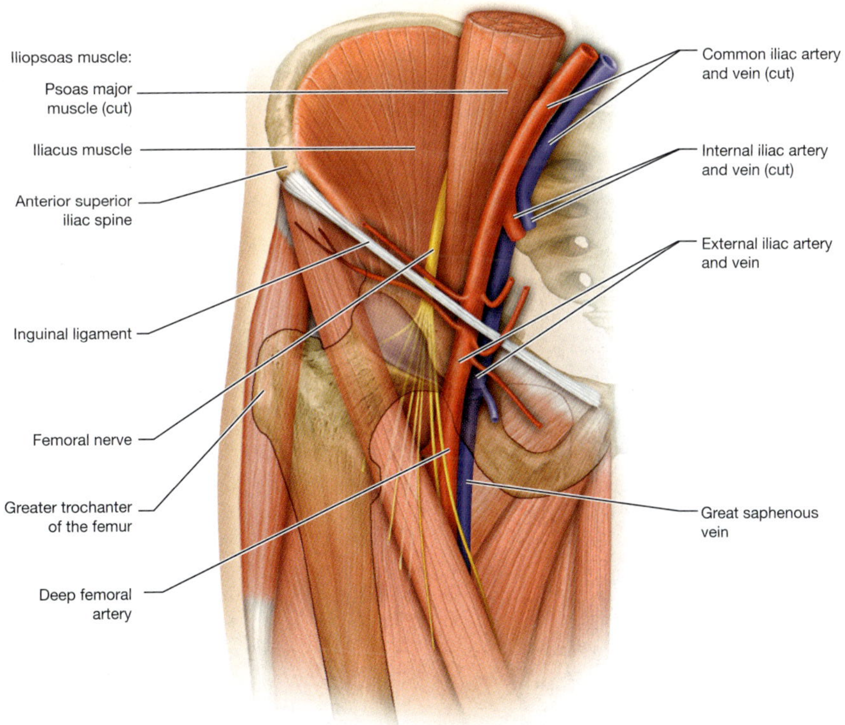

FIGURE 11.1 • Right lateral hip and femoral triangle. (Modified with permission from Gest TR. *Lippincott® Atlas of Anatomy*. 2nd ed. Wolters Kluwer; 2020.)

- 3-mL syringe—for the injection of corticosteroid/local anesthetic mixture
- 25-gauge 2-in needle in thin individuals. Otherwise, use a 25-gauge 3½-in spinal needle (for injections only)
- 20-gauge 2-in needle in thin individuals. Otherwise, use a 20-gauge 3½-in spinal needle (for aspirations and injections)
- 1 mL of 1% mepivacaine without epinephrine
- 1 mL of the steroid solution (40 mg of triamcinolone acetonide)
- One alcohol prep pad
- Two povidone-iodine or chlorhexidine prep pads
- Sterile gauze pads
- Sterile adhesive bandage
- Nonsterile, clean chucks pad

TECHNIQUE

1. (Optional) Use an ultrasound to image the hip joint using an adjacent but separate acoustic window. This allows imaging separate from the injection site so that there is no contamination from the ultrasound gel. Alternatively, the entire site may be prepped in an aseptic manner and sterile ultrasound gel utilized.
2. Prep the insertion site with alcohol followed by the povidone-iodine or chlorhexidine pads.
3. Achieve good local anesthesia by using topical vapocoolant spray.
4. Position the needle and syringe perpendicular to the skin with the tip of the needle directed medially toward the hip joint.
5. Using the no-touch technique, quickly introduce the needle at the insertion site (Fig. 11.2).
6. Advance the needle toward the hip joint until the needle tip contacts the femoral neck/head. Back up the needle 1 to 2 mm.
7. Withdraw the plunger of the syringe to ensure that there is no blood return.

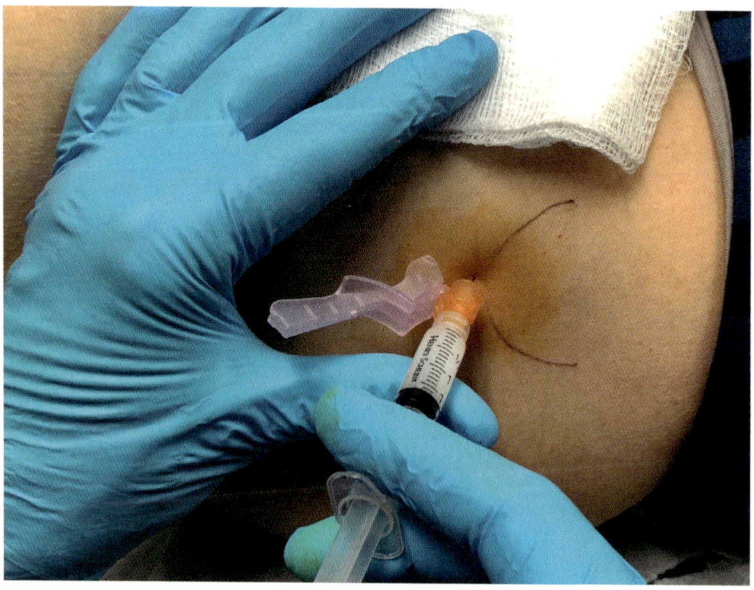

FIGURE 11.2 ● Hip joint injection—preferred lateral approach.

8. Inject the mepivacaine/corticosteroid solution as a bolus into the hip joint capsule. The injected solution should flow smoothly into the space. If increased resistance is encountered, advance or withdraw the needle slightly before attempting further injection.
9. Following injection, withdraw the needle.
10. Apply a sterile adhesive bandage.
11. Instruct the patient to move their hip through its full range of motion. This movement distributes the mepivacaine/corticosteroid solution throughout the hip joint capsule.
12. Reexamine the hip in 5 minutes to assess pain relief.

AFTERCARE

- Avoid excessive weight bearing and hip movement over the next 2 weeks.
- Nonsteroidal anti-inflammatory drugs (NSAIDs) and/or physical therapy as indicated.
- Consider follow-up examination in 2 weeks.

PEARLS

- Imaging guidance is particularly important in obese patients, patients with advanced osteoarthritis with little to no joint space, and those with flexion deformity.[14]

ULTRASOUND-GUIDED PROCEDURE

Please refer to the details of the ultrasound-guided, anterior-approach, hip joint injection procedure in the next chapter.

Videos showing landmark-guided and ultrasound-guided hip joint injections can be found in the companion eBook.

REFERENCES

1. Kompel AJ, Roemer FW, Murakami AM, Diaz LE, Crema MD, Guermazi A. Intra-articular corticosteroid injections in the hip and knee: perhaps not as safe as we thought? *Radiology*. 2019;293(3):656-663.
2. Simeone FJ, Vicentini JRT, Bredella MA, Chang CY. Are patients more likely to have hip osteoarthritis progression and femoral head collapse after hip steroid/anesthetic injections? A retrospective observational study. *Skeletal Radiol*. 2019;48(9):1417-1426.
3. van Middelkoop M, Arden NK, Atchia I, et al. The OA Trial Bank: meta-analysis of individual patient data from knee and hip osteoarthritis trials show that patients with severe pain exhibit greater benefit from intra-articular glucocorticoids. *Osteoarthr Cartil*. 2016;24(7):1143-1152.
4. Pereira LC, Kerr J, Jolles BM. Intra-articular steroid injection for osteoarthritis of the hip prior to total hip arthroplasty: is it safe? A systematic review. *Bone Joint J*. 2016;98-B(8):1027-1035.
5. Rakesh N, Magram YC, Shah JM, Gulati A. Localized corticosteroid injections for malignant joint pain in the oncologic population: a case series. *A A Pract*. 2019;13(1):27-30.
6. Schnitzer TJ, Easton R, Pang S, et al. Effect of tanezumab on joint pain, physical function, and patient global assessment of osteoarthritis among patients with osteoarthritis of the hip or knee: a randomized clinical trial. *JAMA*. 2019;322(1):37-48.
7. Conaghan PG, Abraham L, Viktrup L, Cislo P. Impact of tanezumab on health status, non-work activities and work productivity in adults with moderate-to-severe osteoarthritis. *BMC Musculoskelet Disord*. 2022;23(1):106.
8. De Luigi AJ, Blatz D, Karam C, Gustin Z, Gordon AH. Use of platelet-rich plasma for the treatment of acetabular labral tear of the hip: a pilot study. *Am J Phys Med Rehabil*. 2019;98(11):1010-1017.
9. Sambe HG, Yasir M, Man RK, et al. Comparing intra-articular platelet-rich plasma with hyaluronic acid for the treatment of hip osteoarthritis: a systematic review and meta-analysis. *Cureus*. 2023;15(10):e47919.

10. Clementi D, D'Ambrosi R, Bertocco P, et al. Efficacy of a single intra-articular injection of ultra-high molecular weight hyaluronic acid for hip osteoarthritis: a randomized controlled study. *Eur J Orthop Surg Traumatol*. 2018;28(5):915-922.
11. Leopold SS, Battista V, Oliverio JA. Safety and efficacy of intraarticular hip injection using anatomic landmarks. *Clin Orthop Relat Res*. 2001;(391):192-197.
12. Mei-Dan O, McConkey MO, Petersen B, McCarty E, Moreira B, Young DA. The anterior approach for a non-image-guided intra-articular hip injection. *Arthroscopy*. 2013;29(6):1025-1033.
13. Ziv YB, Kardosh R, Debi R, Backstein D, Safir O, Kosashvili Y. An inexpensive and accurate method for hip injections without the use of imaging. *J Clin Rheumatol*. 2009;15(3):103-105.
14. Gilliland CA, Salazar LD, Borchers JR. Ultrasound versus anatomic guidance for intra-articular and peri-articular injection: a systematic review. *Phys Sportsmed*. 2011;39(3):121-131.
15. Lynch TS, Oshlag BL, Bottiglieri TS, Desai NN. Ultrasound-guided hip injections. *J Am Acad Orthop Surg*. 2019;27(10):e451-e461.
16. Kurup H, Ward P. Do we need radiological guidance for hip joint injections? *Acta Orthop Belg*. 2010;76(2):205-207.

Hip Joint—Anterior Approach

Hip joint pain from arthritis or capsulitis is a common condition seen in primary care medical practice. This often occurs as a result of osteoarthrosis, posttraumatic arthritis, and rheumatoid arthritis. Patients typically represent the middle-aged and older populations. Septic arthritis in children is fortunately now a rare occurrence following the development of the *H influenzae* and pneumococcal vaccines. Diagnostic injections using anesthetic (mepivacaine) and therapeutic injections into and around the hip have become an important part of the treatment algorithm for hip pain.

Because of the joint's perceived inaccessibility, fear of vascular puncture, and the remote risk of avascular necrosis of the head of the femur, primary care providers rarely perform aspiration and corticosteroid injections of the hip joint. In fact, access to this joint is straightforward. Anterior and lateral approaches have been described. The landmark-guided anterior approach has success rates of 60% to 93%.[1,2] The lateral approach also has good success rates of about 80%.[1,3] However, the anterior approach is associated with significantly more risk to the femoral artery and femoral nerve than the lateral approach.[1,3] For this reason, the lateral approach is preferred in the setting where image guidance is not available. When ultrasound guidance is available, the anterior approach is favored. In both cases, the use of ultrasound to guide needle placement significantly improves the safety and success rates of hip injections.[4,5] Guidance is particularly important in obese patients, patients with advanced osteoarthritis with little to no joint space, and those with flexion deformity.[6]

Please read additional details concerning hip joint injection that are presented in the preceding chapter.

Relevant Anatomy: (Fig. 11.3)

PATIENT POSITION

- Supine on the examination table with the head of the bed slightly elevated.

LANDMARKS

1. With the patient supine on the examination table, the clinician stands lateral to the affected hip.
2. Over the anterior aspect of the hip, identify the point at the intersection of two perpendicular lines. The first is distal and sagittal from the anterior superior iliac spine, and the second line is transverse from the proximal tip of the greater trochanter. This point will be located about 3 cm lateral to the femoral artery. Mark that spot, which is directly over the hip joint.
3. (Optional) Use ultrasound to image the hip joint.

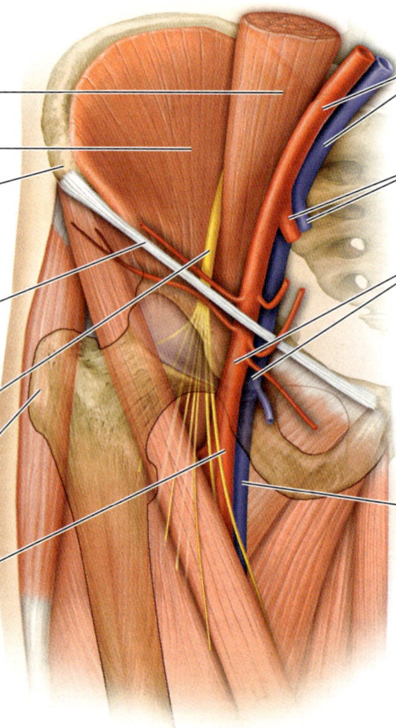

FIGURE 11.3 Right anterior hip and femoral triangle. (Modified with permission from Gest TR. *Lippincott® Atlas of Anatomy*. 2nd ed. Wolters Kluwer; 2020.)

4. At that site, press firmly on the skin with the retracted tip of a ballpoint pen. This indentation represents the entry point for the needle.
5. After the landmarks are identified, the patient should not move the hip.

ANESTHESIA

- Local anesthesia of the skin using topical vapocoolant spray.

EQUIPMENT

- Topical vapocoolant spray
- 20-mL syringe—for aspiration
- 3-mL syringe—for the injection of corticosteroid/local anesthetic mixture
- 25-gauge 1½-in needle in thin individuals. Otherwise, use a 25-gauge 3½-in needle (for injections only)
- 20-gauge 1½-in needle in thin individuals. Otherwise, use a 20-gauge 3½-in needle (for aspirations and injections)
- 1 mL of 1% mepivacaine without epinephrine
- 1 mL of the steroid solution (40 mg of triamcinolone acetonide)
- One alcohol prep pad
- Two povidone-iodine or chlorhexidine prep pads
- Sterile gauze pads
- Sterile adhesive bandage
- Nonsterile, clean chucks pad

TECHNIQUE

1. Prep the insertion site with alcohol followed by the povidone-iodine or chlorhexidine pads.
2. Achieve good local anesthesia by using topical vapocoolant spray.
3. Position the needle and syringe perpendicular to the skin with the tip of the needle directed posteriorly toward the hip joint.
4. Using the no-touch technique, quickly introduce the needle at the insertion site (Fig. 11.4).
5. Advance the needle toward the hip joint until the needle tip contacts the junction of the femoral neck and femoral head. Back up the needle 1 to 2 mm.
6. Withdraw the plunger of the syringe to ensure that there is no blood return.
7. Inject the mepivacaine/corticosteroid solution as a bolus into the hip joint capsule. The injected solution should flow smoothly into the space. If increased resistance is encountered, advance or withdraw the needle slightly before attempting further injection.
8. Following injection, withdraw the needle.
9. Apply a sterile adhesive bandage.
10. Instruct the patient to move their hip through its full range of motion. This movement distributes the mepivacaine/corticosteroid solution throughout the hip joint capsule.
11. Reexamine the hip in 5 minutes to assess pain relief.

AFTERCARE

- Avoid excessive weight bearing and hip movement over the next 2 weeks.
- NSAIDs and/or physical therapy as indicated.
- Consider follow-up examination in 2 weeks.

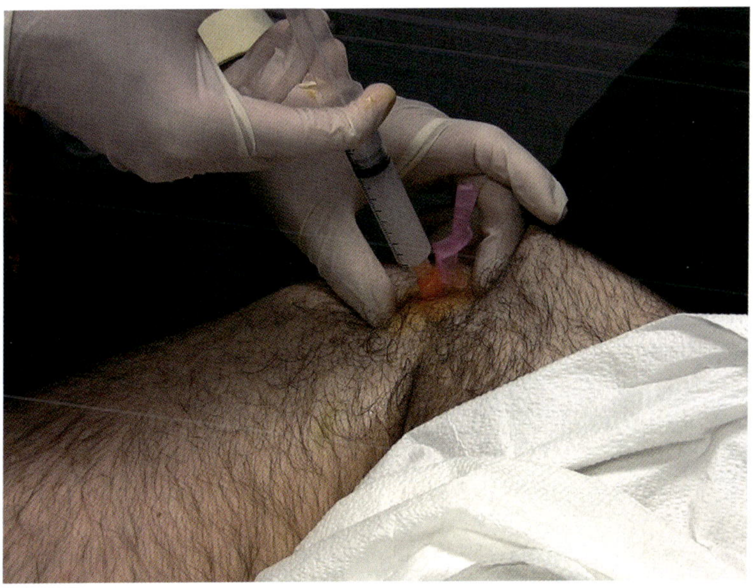

FIGURE 11.4 ● Hip joint injection—anterior approach.

PEARLS

- Ultrasound guidance is particularly important in obese patients, patients with advanced osteoarthritis with little to no joint space, and those with flexion deformity.[6]

ULTRASOUND-GUIDED PROCEDURE

Please refer to the introductory ultrasound chapter for preprocedure, sterile prep, postprocedure, and documentation information and recommendations.

PATIENT POSITION

- Supine on the examination table.
- On the affected side, place the hip in a neutral position resting on the examination table.
- Place a pillow under their head for comfort.
- Adjust the patient's position as needed for comfort.

PROVIDER/ULTRASOUND POSITION

- The provider stands on the same side of the table as the affected hip.
- Adjust the examination table to position the injection site between the provider's umbilicus and axillary level, ensuring optimal ergonomics and visualization of the ultrasound screen, transducer, and needle's approach (Fig. 11.5).
- Position the ultrasound machine on the opposite side of the table from the provider at the level of the patient's shoulder with the screen facing the provider.

LANDMARKS

- See the landmarks for the landmark-guided injection procedure.

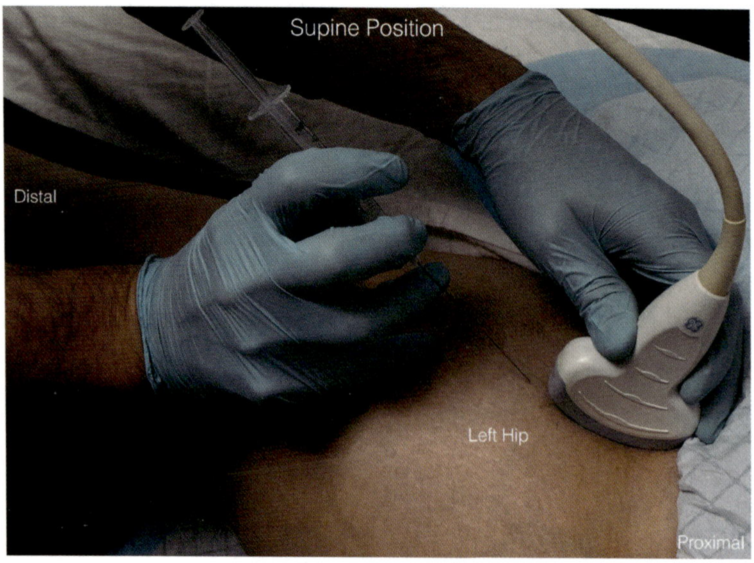

FIGURE 11.5 ● Ultrasound-guided left hip injection. Supine position with the affected hip resting on the examination table. Feet positioned to the left of the image. Provider positioned ipsilaterally and distal to the injection site.

ANESTHESIA

- Local anesthesia of the skin using topical vapocoolant spray.

EQUIPMENT

- 3-mL syringe
- 22-gauge 3.5-in needle (adjust needle length as needed)
- 1 mL of 1% mepivacaine without epinephrine
- 1 mL of 40 mg/mL of triamcinolone acetonide
- Alternative setup for aspiration
  - 5-mL syringe (anesthesia)
    - 22-gauge 3.5-in needle (adjust needle length as needed)
    - 5 mL of 1% lidocaine without epinephrine
  - 10-mL syringe (aspiration)
    - 18-gauge 3.5-in needle (adjust needle length as needed)
- Three chlorhexidine swabs
- 5-1 MHz curvilinear ultrasound transducer and machine
- Sterile ultrasound transducer cover
- Sterile ultrasound gel
- Nonlatex sterile or nonsterile gloves
- Two 4 × 4 sterile gauze pads
- One sterile adhesive bandage
- Topical vapocoolant spray

TECHNIQUE

1. Position a low-frequency curvilinear 5-1 MHz ultrasound transducer in the sagittal-oblique plane in long axis with the femoral head-neck junction centered beneath it.
2. Prior to the procedure, activate power Doppler imaging to precisely localize the lateral circumflex femoral artery. This visualization is essential for preventing inadvertent injury to the neurovascular bundle.
3. Advance a 22-gauge 3.5-in needle using an in-plane approach, directing it from distal to proximal, with an initial needle angle of approximately 30° to 45° relative to the skin surface where the transducer is positioned.
4. The target area is the anterior joint recess of the capsule at the head-neck junction.
5. Utilize real-time ultrasound guidance throughout the procedure to precisely place the needle within the desired target area and minimize the risk of inadvertently injuring surrounding structures (Fig. 11.6).
6. For intra-articular steroid injection:
   a. Slowly inject the desired volume of mepivacaine and corticosteroid solution directly into the joint.
7. For situations requiring anesthesia, aspiration, or both:
   a. Utilize a separate 22-gauge 3.5-in needle with a 5-mL syringe to inject 5 mL of 1% lidocaine without epinephrine into the soft tissues overlying the joint.
   b. For aspiration, use an 18-gauge 3.5-in needle with a 10-mL syringe to withdraw the effusion.
   c. If a steroid injection is indicated following aspiration, replace the aspiration syringe with the mepivacaine and corticosteroid solution syringe and reconfirm accurate needle placement using real-time ultrasound guidance before injection.
8. Upon completion of the procedure, carefully withdraw the needle. Adhere to established postprocedure care protocols and ensure appropriate follow-up as recommended.

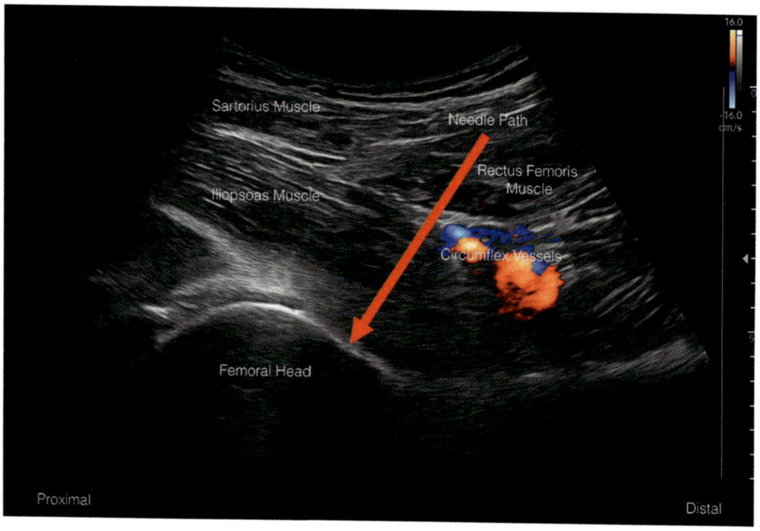

FIGURE 11.6 ● Femoroacetabular joint sagittal-oblique ultrasound with power Doppler.

PEARLS

- Needle visualization is generally better in the first half of the curvilinear transducer, closer to the insertion site.
- "Toe" the transducer to improve visualization. If an air gap forms, use a sterile gel standoff.
- If the hip is challenging to locate, use a sagittal-oblique plane between the greater trochanter and pubic symphysis and perform a dynamic short-axis sliding distally and proximally while passively rotating the hip during the preprocedural examination to identify movement of the femoral head at the acetabulum.
- Utilize power Doppler to identify and avoid the circumflex vessels along the femoral neck.
- Advance the needle slowly and with controlled movements, continuously monitoring its position under ultrasound.
- Observe for distention of the joint capsule during injection to confirm intra-articular placement.
- Be mindful of the potential risk of osteonecrosis with repeated intra-articular corticosteroid injections.

REFERENCES

1. Leopold SS, Battista V, Oliverio JA. Safety and efficacy of intraarticular hip injection using anatomic landmarks. *Clin Orthop Relat Res.* 2001;391:192-197.
2. Mei-Dan O, McConkey MO, Petersen B, McCarty E, Moreira B, Young DA. The anterior approach for a non-image-guided intra-articular hip injection. *Arthroscopy.* 2013;29(6):1025-1033.
3. Ziv YB, Kardosh R, Debi R, Backstein D, Safir O, Kosashvili Y. An inexpensive and accurate method for hip injections without the use of imaging. *J Clin Rheumatol.* 2009;15(3):103-105.
4. Gilliland CA, Salazar LD, Borchers JR. Ultrasound versus anatomic guidance for intra-articular and periarticular injection: a systematic review. *Phys Sportsmed.* 2011;39(3):121-131.
5. Lynch TS, Oshlag BL, Bottiglieri TS, Desai NN. Ultrasound-guided hip injections. *J Am Acad Orthop Surg.* 2019;27(10):e451-e461.
6. Kurup H, Ward P. Do we need radiological guidance for hip joint injections? *Acta Orthop Belg.* 2010;76(2):205-207.

Piriformis Syndrome

Piriformis syndrome is an often overlooked disorder attributed to 6% to 8% of patients presenting with low back and leg pain. It is presumed to be a compression neuropathy that occurs when an abnormally tight piriformis muscle compresses the underlying sciatic nerve. Piriformis syndrome may occur following trauma, vigorous physical activity, developmental abnormalities, tumor, or after total hip arthroplasty. There is a common pathological end pathway involving hypertrophy, spasm, contracture, inflammation, and scarring of the piriformis muscle, leading to impingement of the sciatic nerve. The diagnosis may be made by excluding other causes of sciatica, palpating an abnormally tight and tender piriformis muscle, and the demonstration of a positive figure-four test. Treatment consists of stretching, physical therapy, local corticosteroid injection,[1,2] botulinum toxin injection,[3,4] or hydrodissection.[5] Dry needling treatment is also a viable option.[6-8] Ultrasound guidance improves injection success rates.[1,9] Recalcitrant lesions may require surgical release.

Relevant Anatomy: (Fig. 11.7)

PATIENT POSITION

- Standing up with the back in forward flexion and hands/arms supported by the examination table.
- Alternatively, this injection may be performed with the patient lying in the lateral decubitus position on the examination table.

LANDMARKS

1. With the patient standing up with the back in forward flexion and hands/arms supported by the examination table, the clinician stands directly behind the patient.
2. Locate the S2 median sacral crest and the lateral aspect of the femoral trochanter.
3. Identify the point of maximal tenderness over the piriformis muscle. This will be one-third to one-half of the distance from the sacral crest.
4. At that site, press firmly on the skin with the retracted tip of a ballpoint pen. This indentation represents the entry point for the needle.
5. After the landmarks are identified, the patient should not move.

ANESTHESIA

- Local anesthesia of the skin with a topical vapocoolant spray may be used, but it is not necessary in most patients.

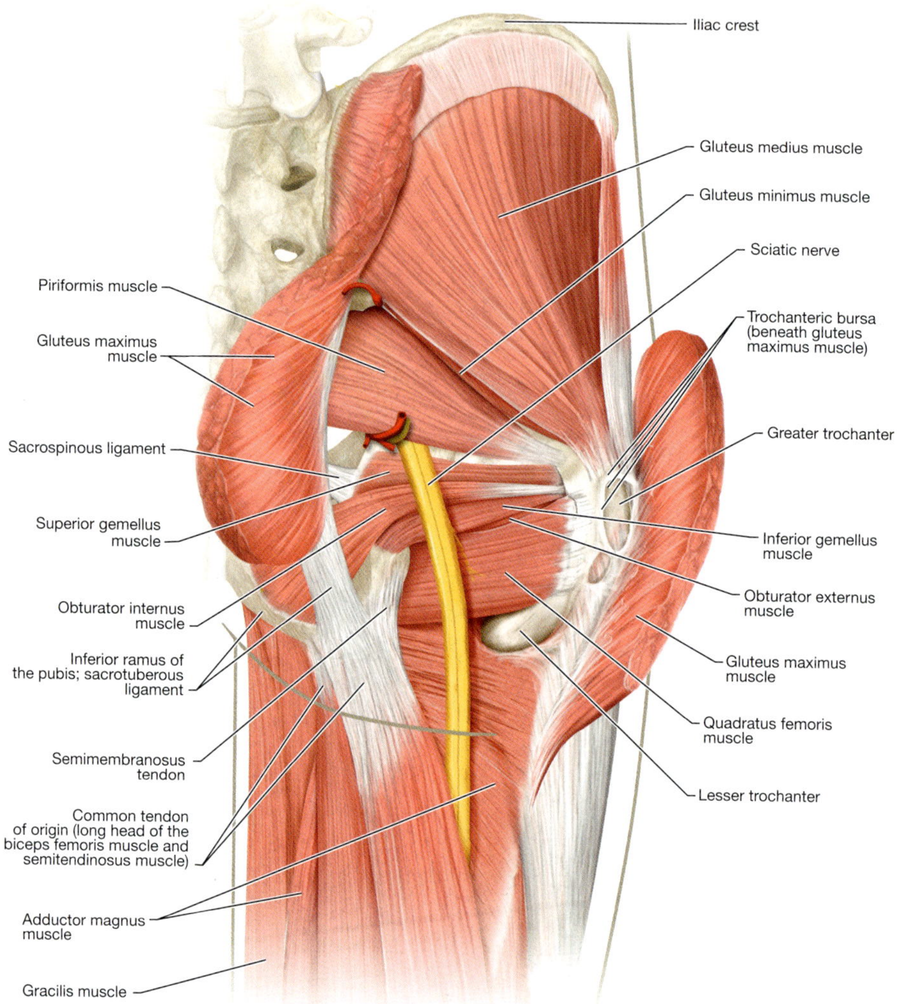

FIGURE 11.7 Middle and deep gluteal muscles and sciatic nerve. (Modified with permission from Gest TR. *Lippincott® Atlas of Anatomy*. 2nd ed. Wolters Kluwer; 2020.)

EQUIPMENT

- Topical vapocoolant spray
- 3-mL syringe
- 25-gauge 2-in needle
- 1 mL of 1% lidocaine without epinephrine
- 1 mL of the steroid solution (40 mg of triamcinolone acetonide)
- One alcohol prep pad
- Two povidone-iodine or chlorhexidine prep pads
- Sterile gauze pads
- Sterile adhesive bandage

TECHNIQUE

1. Prep the insertion site with alcohol followed by the povidone-iodine or chlorhexidine pads.
2. Achieve good local anesthesia by using a topical vapocoolant spray.
3. Position the needle and syringe perpendicular to the skin with the tip of the needle directed anteriorly.
4. Using the no-touch technique, quickly introduce the needle at the insertion site (Fig. 11.8).
5. Advance the needle until you feel that there is an increase in resistance in the muscle due to spasm and/or fibrosis. If the patient experiences sudden shooting pain down the leg, the sciatic nerve has been contacted. Back up the needle a few millimeters until there is no pain.
6. Withdraw the plunger of the syringe to ensure that there is no blood return.
7. Inject the lidocaine/corticosteroid solution into the soft tissues. The injected solution should flow smoothly. If increased resistance is encountered, advance or withdraw the needle slightly before attempting further injection.
8. Following injection, withdraw the needle.
9. Apply a sterile adhesive bandage.
10. Instruct the patient to move their hip through its full range of motion. This movement distributes the lidocaine/corticosteroid solution throughout the course of the piriformis muscle.
11. Reexamine the piriformis muscle in 5 minutes to assess pain relief.

AFTERCARE

- Avoid excessive use of the affected hip over the next 2 weeks.
- NSAIDs, ice, and/or physical therapy as indicated.
- Consider follow-up examination in 2 weeks.

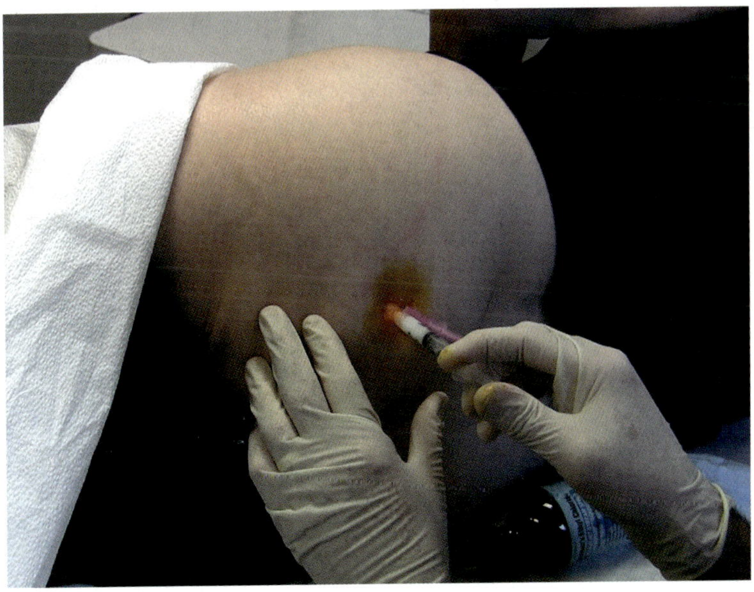

FIGURE 11.8 ● Piriformis muscle injection.

ULTRASOUND-GUIDED PROCEDURE

Please refer to the introductory ultrasound chapter for preprocedure, sterile prep, postprocedure, and documentation information and recommendations.

PATIENT POSITION

- Prone position on the examination table.
- On the affected side, place the hip in a neutral position with slight internal rotation while resting on the examination table with the patient's feet off the end of the examination table.
- Place a pillow under their head for comfort.
- Adjust the patient's position as needed for comfort.

PROVIDER/ULTRASOUND POSITION

- The provider stands on the same side of the table as the affected piriformis muscle.
- Adjust the examination table to position the injection site between the provider's umbilicus and axillary level, ensuring optimal ergonomics and visualization of the ultrasound screen, transducer, and needle's approach (Fig. 11.9).
- Position the ultrasound machine on the opposite side of the table from the provider at the level of the patient's hip with the screen facing the provider.

LANDMARKS

- See the landmarks for the landmark-guided injection procedure.

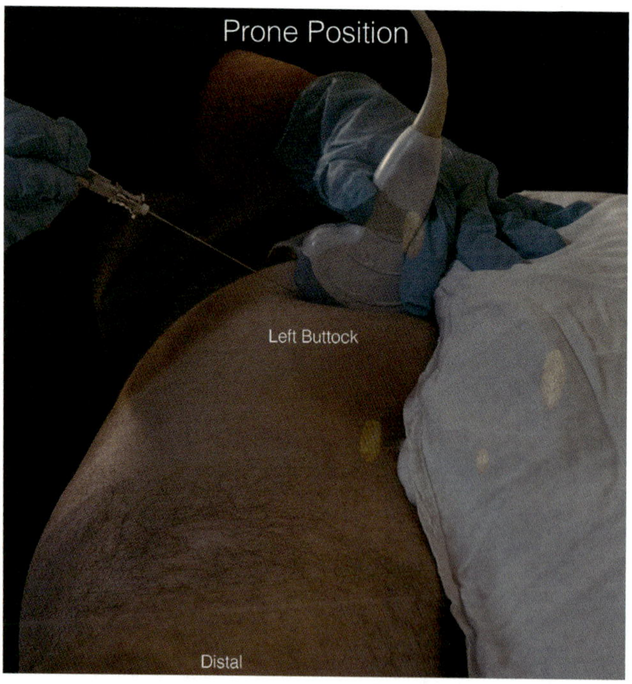

FIGURE 11.9 ● Ultrasound-guided left piriformis muscle injection. Prone position with the affected hip resting on the examination table. Feet positioned at the bottom of the image. Provider positioned ipsilaterally at the injection site.

ANESTHESIA

- Local anesthesia of the skin using topical vapocoolant spray.

EQUIPMENT

- 3-mL syringe
- 22-gauge 3.5-in needle (adjust needle length as needed)
- 1 mL of 1% lidocaine without epinephrine
- 1 mL of 40 mg/mL triamcinolone acetonide
- Three chlorhexidine swabs
- 5-1 MHz curvilinear ultrasound transducer and machine
- Sterile ultrasound transducer cover
- Sterile ultrasound gel
- Nonlatex sterile or nonsterile gloves
- Two 4 × 4 sterile gauze pads
- One sterile adhesive bandage
- Topical vapocoolant spray

TECHNIQUE

1. Position a low-frequency curvilinear 5-1 MHz ultrasound transducer in the axial plane over the posterior hip with the piriformis muscle centered beneath it.
2. Advance a 22-gauge 3.5-in needle using an in-plane approach, directing it from lateral to medial, with an initial needle angle of approximately 30° to 45° relative to the skin surface where the transducer is positioned.
3. The target is to place the needle tip within the affected piriformis muscle.
4. Utilize real-time ultrasound guidance throughout the procedure to precisely place the needle within the desired target area and minimize the risk of inadvertently injuring surrounding structures (Fig. 11.10).
5. Upon completion of the procedure, carefully withdraw the needle. Adhere to established postprocedure care protocols and ensure appropriate follow-up as recommended.

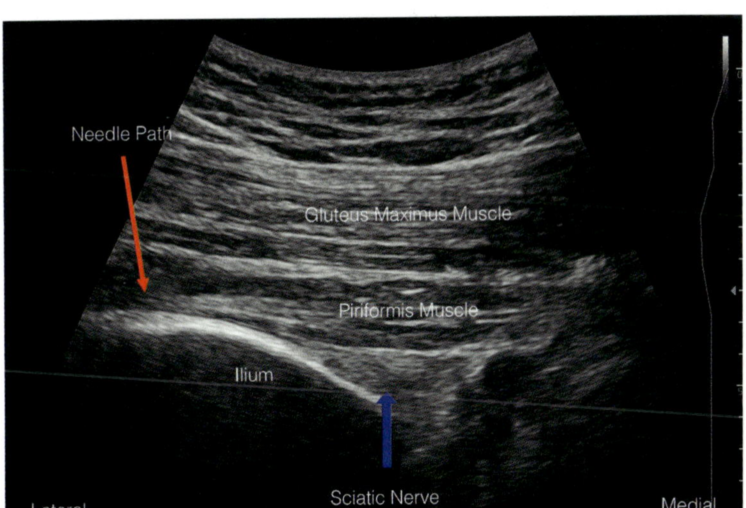

FIGURE 11.10 • Piriformis muscle axial ultrasound image.

PEARLS

- "Toe" the curvilinear transducer to improve visualization. If an air gap forms, use a sterile gel standoff.
- If the piriformis muscle is difficult to visualize, place the transducer in an axial plane between the greater trochanter and midsacrum. Perform short-axis sliding distally and proximally with passive hip rotation during the preprocedural examination. The piriformis can be seen moving between the sacrum and greater trochanter.
- Identify and avoid the sciatic nerve and vasculature, which typically lies deep to the medial aspect of the piriformis muscle.

Videos showing landmark-guided and ultrasound-guided piriformis muscle injections can be found in the companion eBook.

REFERENCES

1. Terlemez R, Erçalık T. Effect of piriformis injection on neuropathic pain. *Agri.* 2019;31(4):178-182.
2. Hilal FM, Bashawyah A, Allam AE, et al. Efficacy of botulinum toxin, local anesthetics, and corticosteroids in patients with piriformis syndrome: a systematic review and meta-analysis. *Pain Physician.* 2022;25(5):325-337.
3. Waseem Z, Boulias C, Gordon A, Ismail F, Sheean G, Furlan AD. Botulinum toxin injections for low-back pain and sciatica. *Cochrane Database Syst Rev.* 2011;(1):CD008257.
4. Koh MM, Tan YL. Use of botulinum neurotoxin in the treatment of piriformis syndrome: a systematic review. *J Clin Orthop Trauma.* 2022;31:101951.
5. Burke CJ, Walter WR, Adler RS. Targeted ultrasound-guided perineural hydrodissection of the sciatic nerve for the treatment of piriformis syndrome. *Ultrasound Q.* 2019;35(2):125-129.
6. Guner D, Ozcete ZA. Evaluation of the efficacy of ultrasound-guided dry needling therapy and exercise in piriformis muscle syndrome. *Cureus.* 2023;15(8):e43804.
7. Tabatabaiee A, Takamjani IE, Sarrafzadeh J, Salehi R, Ahmadi M. Ultrasound-guided dry needling decreases pain in patients with piriformis syndrome. *Muscle Nerve.* 2019;60(5):558-565.
8. Bağcıer F, Tufanoğlu FH. A new treatment modality in piriformis syndrome: ultrasound guided dry needling treatment. *Agri.* 2020;32(3):175-176.
9. Chang KV, Wu WT, Lew HL, Özçakar L. Ultrasound imaging and guided injection for the lateral and posterior hip. *Am J Phys Med Rehabil.* 2018;97(4):285-291.

Hamstring Tendon and Ischial Bursa

Patients occasionally present to the primary care office for the evaluation and treatment of pain over the buttock and posterior thigh upon extension of the hip and flexion of the lower leg. The semimembranosus, semitendinosus, and biceps femoris muscles/ tendons span between the ischial tuberosity to the proximal aspect of the tibia and fibula. Hamstring injuries almost always occur at the proximal myotendinous junction. Acute injury or chronic overuse may cause tendonitis, tendinopathy, or disruption of the hamstring tendons. The biceps femoris is most commonly injured. The main presenting complaint is pain in the lower gluteal or ischial region that usually radiates along the hamstrings in the posterior thigh. The pain increases with direct palpation over the ischial tuberosity and proximal tendons, passive stretching, and resistance to contraction. Proximal hamstring tendinopathy pain and dysfunction are often long-standing and limit athletic and daily activities. Imaging with either ultrasound or magnetic resonance imaging (MRI) may be required to delineate the anatomic pathology and extent of injury.

In chronic tendinopathy, treatment is often lengthy and difficult. Physical therapy is the cornerstone of treatment. Zissen showed that 50% of patients receiving corticosteroid injections had symptomatic improvement lasting longer than 1 month and 24% of patients had symptom relief for more than 6 months.[1] Ultrasound guidance improves the accuracy and efficacy of this injection.[2] Intratendinous injections of PRP[3,4] and percutaneous needle fenestration[5] may improve pain and function. When refractory to conservative management, hamstring injuries may be treated with surgical débridement and reattachment.[6]

Relevant Anatomy: (Fig. 11.11)

PATIENT POSITION

- Lying prone on the examination table.
- The hip will be in a position of extension.

LANDMARKS

1. With the patient lying supine on the examination table, the clinician stands lateral to the opposite hip.
2. Locate the ischial tuberosity and firmly palpate the pubic bone laterally until meeting the origin of the hamstring tendons.
3. Determine the site of maximal tenderness over the ischial tuberosity and tendons and mark it with an ink pen.

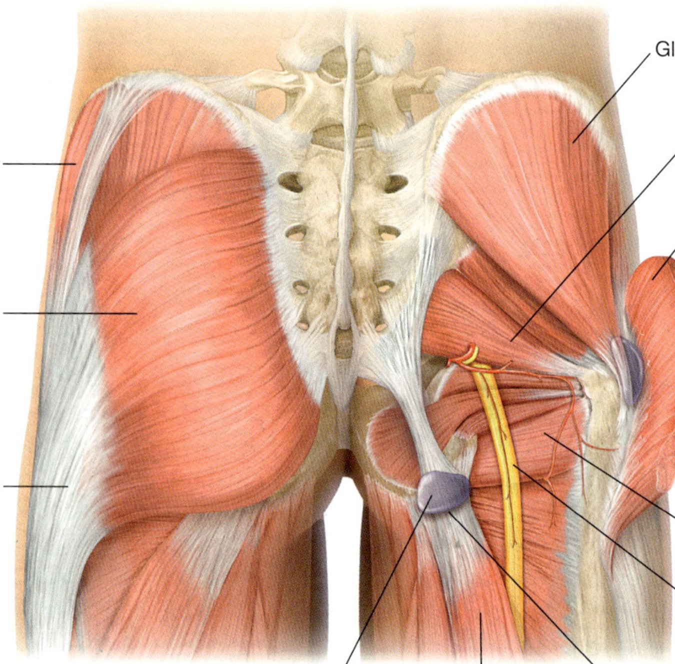

FIGURE 11.11 ● Ischial bursa.

4. At that site, press firmly on the skin with the retracted tip of a ballpoint pen. This indentation represents the entry point for the needle.
5. After the landmarks are identified, the patient should not move the hip.

ANESTHESIA

- Local anesthesia of the skin using a topical vapocoolant spray.

EQUIPMENT

- Topical vapocoolant spray
- 3-mL syringe
- 25-gauge 2-in needle
- 1 mL of 1% lidocaine without epinephrine
- 1 mL of the steroid solution (40 mg of triamcinolone acetonide)
- One alcohol prep pad
- Two povidone-iodine or chlorhexidine prep pads
- Sterile gauze pads
- Sterile adhesive bandage

TECHNIQUE

1. Prep the insertion site with alcohol followed by the povidone-iodine or chlorhexidine pads.
2. Achieve good local anesthesia by using a topical vapocoolant spray.

3. Position the needle and syringe perpendicular to the skin with the tip of the needle directed anteriorly.
4. Using the no-touch technique, quickly introduce the needle at the insertion site (Fig. 11.12).
5. Advance the needle so that it is positioned at the junction of the ischial tuberosity and tendons, but not in the substance of the tendons.
6. Withdraw the plunger of the syringe to ensure that there is no blood return.
7. Inject the lidocaine/corticosteroid solution as a bolus around the adductor tendon(s). The injected solution should flow smoothly into the space. If increased resistance is encountered, advance or withdraw the needle slightly before attempting further injection.
8. Following injection, withdraw the needle.
9. Apply a sterile adhesive bandage.
10. Instruct the patient to massage the area and move their hip through its full range of motion. This movement distributes the lidocaine/corticosteroid solution along the hamstring tendons.
11. Reexamine the affected area in 5 minutes to assess pain relief.

AFTERCARE

- Avoid excessive use of the hip and thigh—hip extension and lower leg flexion (especially running/sprinting) over the next 2 weeks.
- Begin a program of physical therapy.
- NSAIDs, ice, and heat as indicated.
- Consider follow-up examination in 2 weeks.

ULTRASOUND-GUIDED PROCEDURE

Please refer to the introductory ultrasound chapter for preprocedure, sterile prep, post-procedure, and documentation information and recommendations.

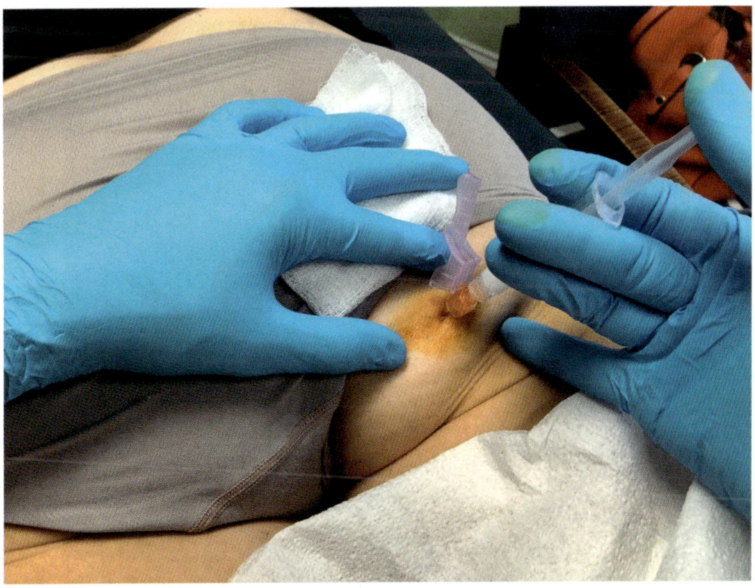

FIGURE 11.12 • Hamstring tendon origin and ischial bursa injection.

PATIENT POSITION

- Prone on the examination table.
- On the affected side, place the hip in a neutral or 30° flexed position resting on the examination table with the patient's feet off the end of the table.
- If desired, place a small bolster under the hips to achieve approximately 30° of flexion.
- Place a pillow under their head for comfort.
- Adjust the patient's position as needed to ensure comfort.

PROVIDER/ULTRASOUND POSITION

- The provider stands on the same side of the table as the affected hamstring tendon.
- Adjust the examination table to position the injection site between the provider's umbilicus and axillary level, ensuring optimal ergonomics and visualization of the ultrasound screen, transducer, and needle's approach (Fig. 11.13).
- Place the ultrasound machine on the opposite side of the table from the provider at the level of the patient's head with the screen facing the provider.

LANDMARKS

- See the landmarks for the landmark-guided injection procedure.

ANESTHESIA

- Local anesthesia of the skin using topical vapocoolant spray.

EQUIPMENT

- 3-mL syringe
- 22-gauge 3.5-in needle (adjust needle length as needed)

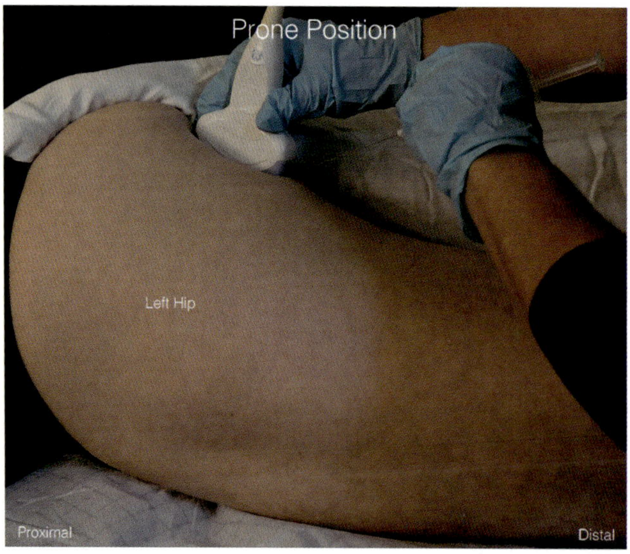

FIGURE 11.13 ● Ultrasound-guided hamstring injection. Prone position with the affected hip resting on the examination table. Feet positioned to the right of the image. Provider positioned ipsilaterally distal to the injection site.

- 1 mL of 1% lidocaine without epinephrine
- 1 mL of 40 mg/mL triamcinolone acetonide
- Three chlorhexidine swabs
- 5-1 MHz curvilinear ultrasound transducer and machine
- Sterile ultrasound transducer cover
- Sterile ultrasound gel
- Nonlatex sterile or nonsterile gloves
- Two 4 × 4 sterile gauze pads
- One sterile adhesive bandage
- Topical vapocoolant spray

TECHNIQUE

1. Position a low-frequency curvilinear 5-1 MHz ultrasound transducer in the sagittal plane over the hamstring tendon in long axis with the ischial tuberosity centered beneath it.
2. Advance a 22-gauge 3.5-in needle using an in-plane approach, directing it from distal to proximal, with an initial needle angle of approximately 30° to 45° relative to the skin surface where the transducer is positioned.
3. Target area:
   a. For corticosteroids: The superficial peritendinous space
   b. For dextrose prolotherapy or PRP: The tendon itself (refer to Chapter 4: Orthobiologics)
4. Injectate:
   a. For corticosteroids: Use a 22-gauge 3.5-in needle to inject the solution into the superficial peritendinous space.
   b. For dextrose prolotherapy or PRP (refer to Chapter 4: Orthobiologics): Use a 22-gauge 3.5-in needle to inject the solution into the tendon itself. Administer a total volume (1-2 mL) of 15% dextrose prolotherapy or PRP in small aliquots (0.5 mL or less).
5. Utilize real-time ultrasound guidance throughout to ensure accurate needle placement and minimize the risk of complications (Fig. 11.14).

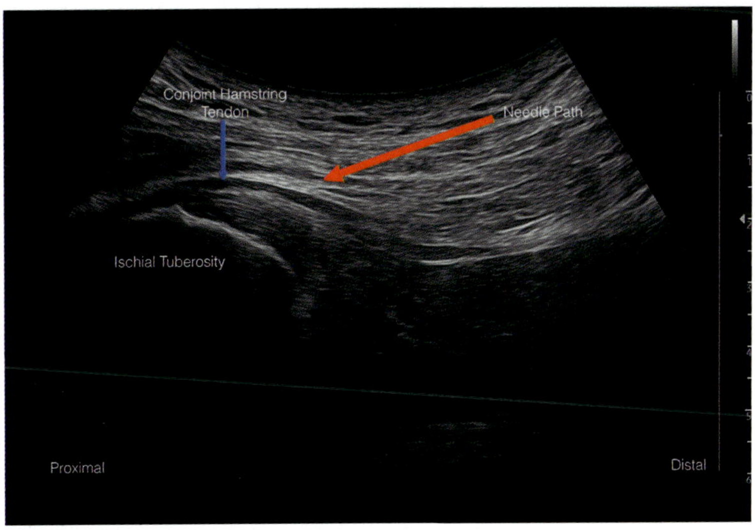

FIGURE 11.14 • Hamstring tendon sagittal ultrasound image.

6. Upon completion of the procedure, carefully withdraw the needle. Adhere to established postprocedure care protocols and ensure appropriate follow-up as recommended.

PEARLS

- "Toe" the curvilinear transducer to improve visualization. If an air gap forms, use a sterile gel standoff.
- If identifying the hamstring tendons is challenging, position the transducer in a sagittal plane over the ischial tuberosity. Instruct the patient to actively flex the hamstring against resistance during the examination. The semitendinosus and biceps femoris form the conjoint tendon and insert on the ischial tuberosity posteriorly. The semimembranosus tendon inserts separately on the lateral aspect of the ischial tuberosity.
- Exercise caution by carefully identifying and avoiding the sciatic nerve, which typically lies deep and lateral.
- Ultrasound-guided peritendinous injections are safe and effective for pain relief.[1] However, the overall risk of tendon rupture warrants careful consideration and patient counseling.

Videos showing landmark-guided and ultrasound-guided hamstring tendon and ischial bursa injections can be found in the companion eBook.

REFERENCES

1. Zissen MH, Wallace G, Stevens KJ, et al. High hamstring tendinopathy: MRI and ultrasound imaging and therapeutic efficacy of percutaneous corticosteroid injection. *AJR Am J Roentgenol.* 2010;195(4):993-998.
2. Chang KV, Wu WT, Lew HL, Özçakar L. Ultrasound imaging and guided injection for the lateral and posterior hip. *Am J Phys Med Rehabil.* 2018;97(4):285-291.
3. Davenport KL, Campos JS, Nguyen J, et al. Ultrasound-guided intratendinous injections with platelet-rich plasma or autologous whole blood for treatment of proximal hamstring tendinopathy: a double-blind randomized controlled trial. *J Ultrasound Med.* 2015;34(8):1455-1463.
4. Wetzel RJ, Patel RM, Terry MA. Platelet-rich plasma as an effective treatment for proximal hamstring injuries. *Orthopedics.* 2013;36(1):e64-e70.
5. Jacobson JA, Rubin J, Yablon CM, et al. Ultrasound-guided fenestration of tendons about the hip and pelvis: clinical outcomes. *J Ultrasound Med.* 2015;34(11):2029-2035.
6. Startzman AN, Fowler O, Carreira D. Proximal hamstring tendinosis and partial ruptures. *Orthopedics.* 2017;40(4):e574-e582.

Meralgia Paresthetica

Patients occasionally present to their primary care provider with burning pain, numbness, or paresthesias over the lateral aspect of the thigh. Meralgia paresthetica is most commonly caused by a compression neuropathy of the lateral femoral cutaneous nerve (LFCN) (a pure sensory nerve) as it passes through a tunnel formed by the lateral attachment of the inguinal ligament and the anterior superior iliac spine (Fig. 11.16). It is more common in patients with diabetes and those who are obese. Percussion of the nerve over this tunnel just anterior to the anterior iliac spine or extending the thigh posteriorly may reproduce or worsen the symptoms. Conservative management includes relieving chronic pressure over the nerve, weight loss, and antineuropathic medications. Corticosteroid injections at the site of nerve compression demonstrate high success rates when guided by ultrasound.[1,2] Other treatment options include ultrasound-guided hydrodissection of the nerve—without or with 5% dextrose,[3,4] and surgical decompression[5] or nerve transection.

Relevant Anatomy: (Figs. 11.15 and 11.16)

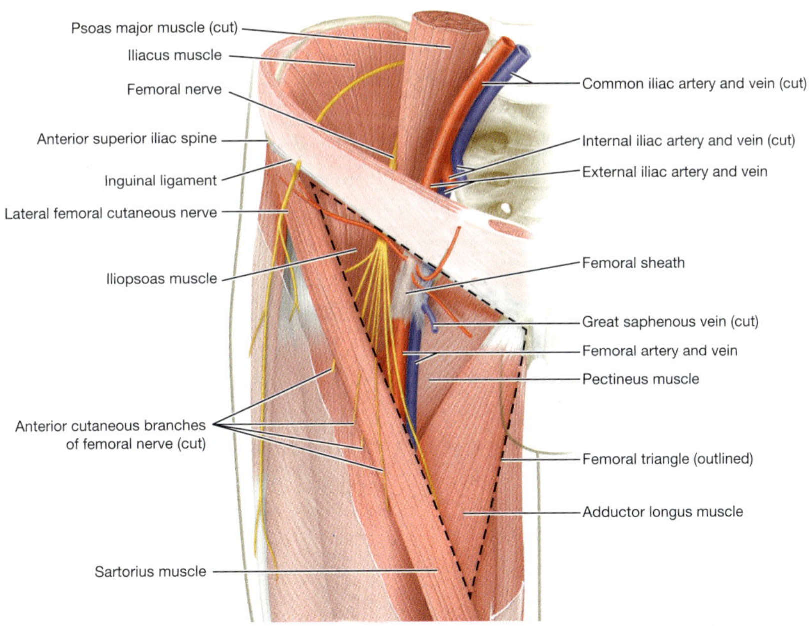

FIGURE 11.15 ● Anterior right hip neurovascular structures. (Modified with permission from Gest TR. *Lippincott® Atlas of Anatomy*. 2nd ed. Wolters Kluwer; 2020.)

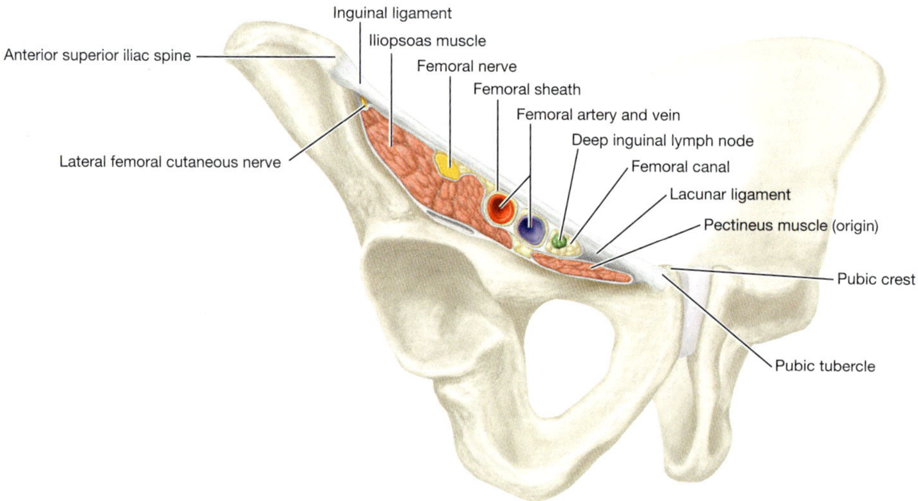

FIGURE 11.16 ● Section through the right femoral sheath. (Reprinted with permission from Gest TR. *Lippincott® Atlas of Anatomy*. 2nd ed. Wolters Kluwer; 2020.)

PATIENT POSITION

- Lying supine on the examination table.
- Rotate the patient's head away from the side that is being injected. This minimizes anxiety and pain perception.

LANDMARKS

1. With the patient supine on the examination table, the clinician stands lateral to the affected hip.
2. Find the anterior superior iliac spine and the pubic bone.
3. Firmly palpate the inguinal ligament that connects these two structures.
4. The LFCN of the thigh traverses the inguinal ligament about 2 cm inferior and medial to the anterior superior iliac spine under the inguinal ligament. Tap over this area or press firmly until discomfort is elicited. Mark that spot with ink.
5. At that site, press firmly on the skin with the retracted tip of a ballpoint pen. This indentation represents the entry point for the needle.
6. After the landmarks are identified, the patient should not move the hip or leg.

ANESTHESIA

- Local anesthesia of the skin with a topical vapocoolant spray may be used, but it is not necessary in most patients.

EQUIPMENT

- Topical vapocoolant spray
- 3-mL syringe
- 25-gauge 1½-in needle
- 2 mL of 1% lidocaine without epinephrine
- 1 mL of the steroid solution (40 mg of triamcinolone acetonide)

- One alcohol prep pad
- Two povidone-iodine or chlorhexidine prep pads
- Sterile gauze pads
- Sterile adhesive bandage

TECHNIQUE

1. Prep the insertion site with alcohol followed by the povidone-iodine or chlorhexidine pads.
2. Achieve good local anesthesia by using a topical vapocoolant spray.
3. Position the needle and syringe perpendicular to the skin with the tip of the needle directed posteriorly.
4. Using the no-touch technique, quickly introduce the needle at the insertion site (Fig. 11.17).
5. Advance the needle 2 to 3 cm until the needle tip is located under the inguinal ligament.
6. Withdraw the plunger to ensure that there is no blood return.
7. Inject the lidocaine/corticosteroid solution as a bolus into the area. The injected solution should flow smoothly into the space. If increased resistance is encountered, advance or withdraw the needle slightly before attempting further injection.
8. Following injection, withdraw the needle.
9. Apply a sterile adhesive bandage.
10. Instruct the patient to move their hip through its full range of motion. This movement distributes the lidocaine/corticosteroid solution throughout the area.

AFTERCARE

- Treatment is directed at relieving the compression and usually consists of avoiding tight belts, wearing looser clothing, and/or losing weight.
- Consider follow-up examination in 2 weeks.

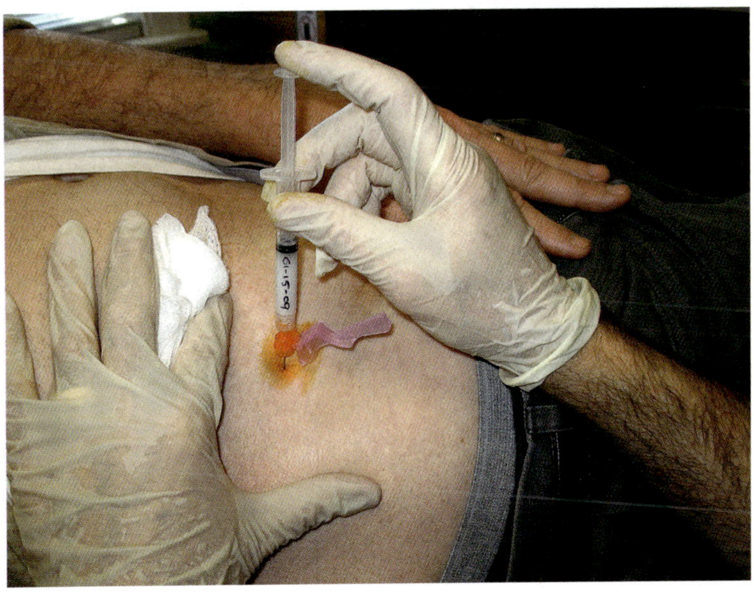

FIGURE 11.17 ● Meralgia paresthetica injection.

ULTRASOUND-GUIDED PROCEDURE

Please refer to the introductory ultrasound chapter for preprocedure, sterile prep, postprocedure, and documentation information and recommendations.

PATIENT POSITION

- Supine on the examination table.
- On the affected side, place the hip in a neutral position resting on the examination table.
- Place a pillow under their head for comfort.
- Adjust the patient's position as needed to ensure comfort.

PROVIDER/ULTRASOUND POSITION

- The provider stands on the same side of the table as the affected LFCN.
- Adjust the examination table to position the injection site between the provider's umbilicus and axillary level, ensuring optimal ergonomics and visualization of the ultrasound screen, transducer, and needle's approach (Fig. 11.18).
- Position the ultrasound machine on the opposite side of the table at the level of the patient's hip with the screen facing the provider.

LANDMARKS

- See the landmarks for the landmark-guided injection procedure.

ANESTHESIA

- Local anesthesia of the skin using topical vapocoolant spray.

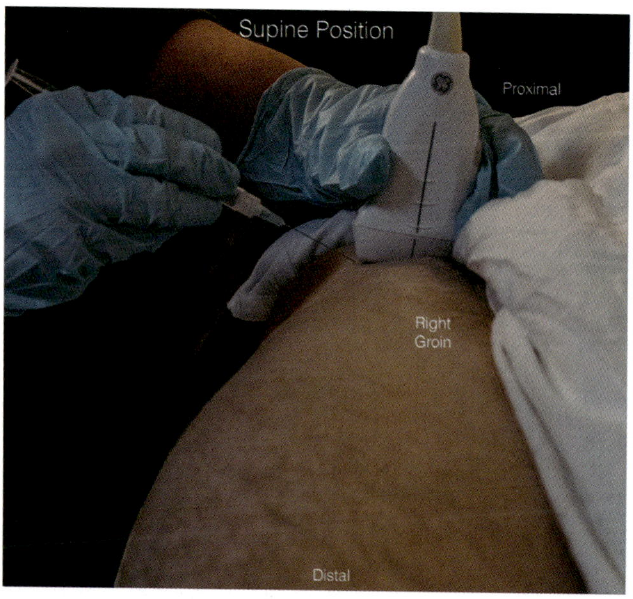

FIGURE 11.18 Ultrasound-guided perineural right lateral femoral cutaneous nerve injection. Supine position with the affected hip resting on the examination table. Feet positioned at the bottom of the image. Provider positioned ipsilaterally at the injection site.

EQUIPMENT

- 3-mL syringe
- 25-gauge 1.5-in needle (adjust needle length as needed)
- 2 mL of 1% lidocaine without epinephrine
- 1 mL of 40 mg/mL triamcinolone acetonide
- Three chlorhexidine swabs
- 12-4 MHz linear ultrasound transducer and machine
- Sterile ultrasound transducer cover
- Sterile ultrasound gel
- Nonlatex sterile or nonsterile gloves
- Two 4 × 4 sterile gauze pads
- One sterile adhesive bandage
- Topical vapocoolant spray

TECHNIQUE

1. Position a high-frequency linear 12-4 MHz ultrasound transducer in the axial plane approximately 1 to 2 cm distal to the anterior superior iliac spine with the LFCN centered in short axis in the space between the sartorius and tensor fasciae latae muscles on the affected side.
2. Advance a 25-gauge 1.5-in needle using an in-plane approach, with an initial needle angle of approximately 15° to 30° relative to the skin surface where the transducer is positioned.
3. The target area is the perineural space surrounding the LFCN.
4. Utilize real-time ultrasound guidance throughout the procedure to precisely place the needle within the desired target area and minimize the risk of inadvertently injuring surrounding structures (Fig. 11.19).
5. Upon completion of the procedure, carefully withdraw the needle. Adhere to established postprocedure care protocols and ensure appropriate follow-up as recommended.

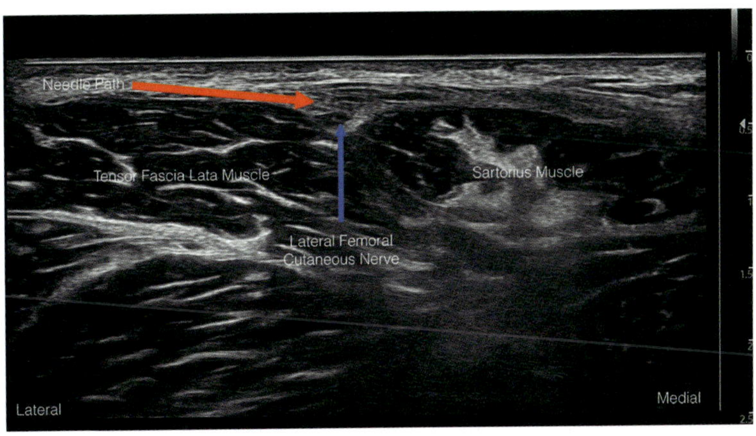

FIGURE 11.19 • Lateral femoral cutaneous nerve axial ultrasound image.

PEARLS

- Consider a longer needle (eg, 2 in, 25 gauge).
- Meralgia paresthetica can mimic L2 or L3 radiculopathy. Consider a workup for radiculopathy. Refer to a specialist (neurosurgeon or orthopedic spine specialist) as appropriate.
- Ultrasound-guided LFCN perineural injection is an advanced technique that requires careful attention to the proximity of neurovascular structures throughout the procedure.
- The LFCN exhibits variable anatomy, piercing or passing deep to the inguinal ligament; sonographic identification is facilitated by initially locating the LFCN in the hypoechoic intermuscular space between the tensor fasciae latae and sartorius muscles.

A video showing ultrasound-guided LFCN injection for the treatment of meralgia paresthetica can be found in the companion eBook.

REFERENCES

1. Hurdle MF, Weingarten TN, Crisostomo RA, Psimos C, Smith J. Ultrasound-guided blockade of the lateral femoral cutaneous nerve: technical description and review of 10 cases. *Arch Phys Med Rehabil.* 2007;88(10):1362-1364.
2. Tagliafico A, Serafini G, Lacelli F, Perrone N, Valsania V, Martinoli C. Ultrasound-guided treatment of meralgia paresthetica (lateral femoral cutaneous neuropathy): technical description and results of treatment in 20 consecutive patients. *J Ultrasound Med.* 2011;30(10):1341-1346.
3. Mulvaney SW. Ultrasound-guided percutaneous neuroplasty of the lateral femoral cutaneous nerve for the treatment of meralgia paresthetica: a case report and description of a new ultrasound-guided technique. *Curr Sports Med Rep.* 2011;10(2):99-104.
4. Xu H, Shi X, Zhu J, Li G, Bai L. A randomized double-blind trial of 5% dextrose versus corticosteroid hydrodissection for meralgia paresthetica. *Pain Physician.* 2024;27(8):E835-E842.
5. Siu TL, Chandran KN. Neurolysis for meralgia paresthetica: an operative series of 45 cases. *Surg Neurol.* 2005;63(1):19-23.

Greater Trochanteric Pain Syndrome

Greater trochanteric pain syndrome is a term used to describe pain involving the lateral aspect of the hip. This common regional pain syndrome includes pain from trochanteric bursitis but also often mimics pain from other sources including myofascial pain, degenerative joint disease, sciatica, and spinal pathology. There is overlap of symptoms due to gluteus medius and minimus disorders including acute inflammation, tendinosis, and tendon tears. The prevalence is higher in women and patients with coexisting low back pain, osteoarthritis, iliotibial band (ITB) tenderness, and obesity. Symptoms include persistent pain over the lateral hip that may radiate along the lateral aspect of the thigh to the knee and occasionally to the buttock. Physical examination reveals point tenderness in the posterolateral area of the greater trochanter.[1]

Conservative therapy includes stretching, therapeutic exercise, and physical modalities focused on the low back/pelvic core and sacroiliac joints. Local corticosteroid injections into the area of maximal tenderness have demonstrated effectiveness and safety.[2-4] Alternative therapies include injections of PRP,[5] percutaneous needle tendon fenestration,[6] and dry needling.[7] Landmark-based injection is generally the method of choice. Ultrasound guidance should be reserved for extreme obesity or injection failure.[8] Recalcitrant cases may be treated with shockwave therapy[2,9] or require surgical referral to consider ITB release, subgluteal bursectomy, or trochanteric reduction osteotomy.

Relevant Anatomy: (Fig. 11.20)

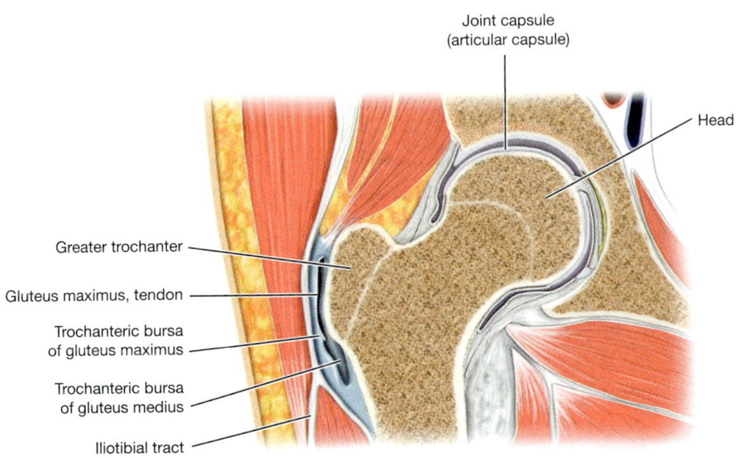

FIGURE 11.20 ● Right anterior hip joint and trochanteric structures.

PATIENT POSITION

- Lying on the examination table in the lateral decubitus position on the unaffected hip.

LANDMARKS

1. With the patient lying on the examination table in the lateral decubitus position on the unaffected hip, the clinician stands behind the patient.
2. Identify and mark the area(s) of maximal tenderness over the greater trochanter.
3. At that area, press firmly on the skin with the retracted tip of a ballpoint pen. This indentation(s) represents the entry point(s) for the needle.
4. After the landmarks are identified, the patient should not move the hip.

ANESTHESIA

- Local anesthesia of the skin with topical vapocoolant spray may be used.

EQUIPMENT

- Topical vapocoolant spray
- 5-mL syringe
- 25-gauge 2-in needle
- 3 mL of 1% lidocaine without epinephrine
- 1 mL of the steroid solution (40 mg of triamcinolone acetonide)
- One alcohol prep pad
- Two povidone-iodine or chlorhexidine prep pads
- Sterile gauze pads
- Sterile adhesive bandage

TECHNIQUE

1. Prep the insertion site(s) with alcohol followed by the povidone-iodine or chlorhexidine pads.
2. Achieve good local anesthesia by using topical vapocoolant spray.
3. Position the needle and syringe perpendicular to the skin with the tip of the needle directed medially.
4. Using the no-touch technique, quickly introduce the needle at the insertion site(s) (Fig. 11.21).
5. Advance the needle toward the femoral trochanter until the needle tip touches the bone. Back up the needle 1 to 2 mm.
6. Withdraw the plunger of the syringe to ensure that there is no blood return.
7. Inject the steroid solution as a bolus steadily in the area of the trochanteric bursa. The injected solution should flow smoothly into the space. If increased resistance is encountered, advance or withdraw the needle slightly before attempting further injection.
8. Repeat the injection at other adjacent painful areas if needed.
9. Following injection(s), withdraw the needle.
10. Apply a sterile adhesive bandage(s).

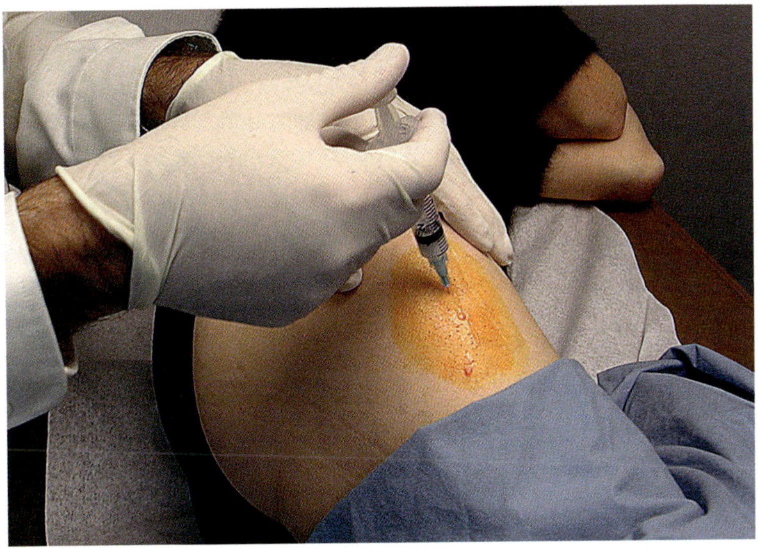

FIGURE 11.21 • Greater trochanteric pain syndrome injection.

11. Instruct the patient to massage the area and move their hip through its full range of motion. This movement distributes the steroid solution throughout the trochanteric bursa.
12. Reexamine the area of the trochanteric bursa in 5 minutes to confirm pain relief.

AFTERCARE

- Avoid excessive hip movement over the next 2 weeks.
- NSAIDs, ice, heat, and/or physical therapy as indicated.
- Consider follow-up examination in 2 weeks.

PEARLS

- Consider fanning this injection to disperse the corticosteroid solution over a wider area.

ULTRASOUND-GUIDED PROCEDURE

Please refer to the introductory ultrasound chapter for preprocedure, sterile prep, post-procedure, and documentation information and recommendations.

PATIENT POSITION

- Lateral decubitus on the examination table with the affected hip upward.
- Place the hips in 15° to 20° of flexion resting on the examination table.
- Place a pillow under their head for comfort.
- Adjust the patient's position as needed to ensure comfort.

PROVIDER/ULTRASOUND POSITION

- The provider stands behind the patient at the level of the affected hip.
- Adjust the examination table to position the injection site between the provider's umbilicus and axillary level, ensuring optimal ergonomics and visualization of the ultrasound screen, transducer, and needle's approach (Fig. 11.22).
- Place the ultrasound machine on the opposite side of the table at the level of the patient's knees with the screen facing the provider.

LANDMARKS

- See the landmarks for the landmark-guided injection procedure.

ANESTHESIA

- Local anesthesia of the skin using topical vapocoolant spray.

EQUIPMENT

- 3-mL syringe
- 22-gauge 3.5-in needle (adjust needle length as needed)
- 3 mL of 1% lidocaine without epinephrine
- 1 mL of 40 mg/mL triamcinolone acetonide
- Three chlorhexidine swabs
- 5-1 MHz curvilinear ultrasound transducer and machine
- Sterile ultrasound transducer cover
- Sterile ultrasound gel
- Nonlatex sterile or nonsterile gloves
- Two 4 × 4 sterile gauze pads
- One sterile adhesive bandage
- Topical vapocoolant spray

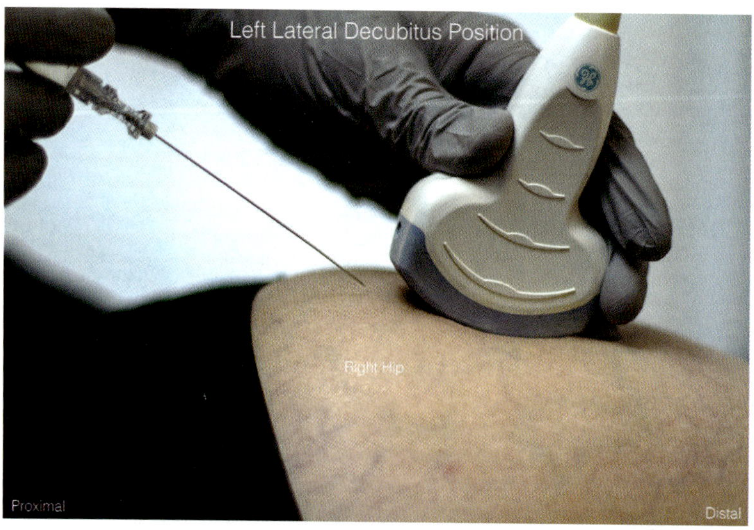

FIGURE 11.22 ● Ultrasound-guided right gluteus medius or minimus tendon injection. Left lateral decubitus position with affected hip uppermost. Feet positioned to the right of the image. Provider positioned ipsilaterally proximal to the injection site.

TECHNIQUE

1. Position a low-frequency curvilinear 5-1 MHz ultrasound transducer in the coronal plane over the greater trochanter with the gluteus medius and minimus tendons centered beneath it.
2. Advance a 22-gauge 3.5-in needle using an in-plane approach, directing it from proximal to distal, with an initial needle angle of approximately 30° to 45° relative to the skin surface where the transducer is positioned.
3. Target area:
   a. For corticosteroids: The deep peritendinous space or into a bursa
   b. For dextrose prolotherapy or PRP: The area of tendinopathy in the tendon (refer to Chapter 4: Orthobiologics)
4. Injectate:
   a. For corticosteroids: Use a 22-gauge 3.5-in needle to inject the solution into the deep peritendinous space or bursa.
   b. For dextrose prolotherapy or PRP (refer to Chapter 4: Orthobiologics): Use a 22-gauge 3.5-in needle to inject the solution into the tendon itself. Administer a total volume (1-2 mL) of 15% dextrose prolotherapy or PRP in small aliquots (0.5 mL or less).
5. Utilize real-time ultrasound guidance throughout to ensure accurate needle placement and minimize the risk of complications (Fig. 11.23).
6. Upon completion of the procedure, carefully withdraw the needle. Adhere to established postprocedure care protocols and ensure appropriate follow-up as recommended.

PEARLS

- Needle visualization is generally better in the first half of the curvilinear transducer, closer to the needle insertion site.
- "Toe" the transducer to improve visualization. If an air gap forms, use a sterile gel standoff.
- Greater trochanteric pain syndrome is most commonly caused by gluteus medius and minimus tendinopathy. Gluteus medius inserts on the posterior and lateral facets of

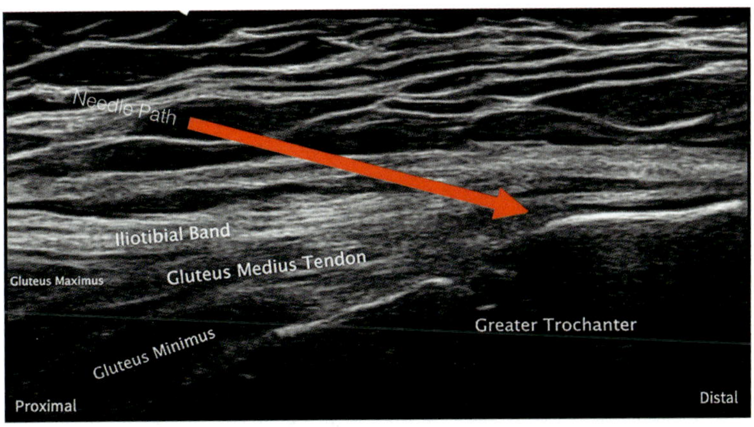

FIGURE 11.23 ● Greater trochanter coronal ultrasound image.

the greater trochanter. Gluteus minimus inserts on the anterior facet of the greater trochanter. Ultrasound imaging can aid in diagnosing tendinopathy and/or bursitis.

Videos showing landmark-guided and ultrasound-guided greater trochanteric pain syndrome injections can be found in the companion eBook.

REFERENCES

1. Williams BS, Cohen SP. Greater trochanteric pain syndrome: a review of anatomy, diagnosis and treatment. *Anesth Analg.* 2009;108(5):1662-1670.
2. Torres A, Fernández-Fairen M, Sueiro-Fernández J. Greater trochanteric pain syndrome and gluteus medius and minimus tendinosis: nonsurgical treatment. *Pain Manag.* 2018;8(1):45-55.
3. Brinks A, van Rijn RM, Willemsen SP, et al. Corticosteroid injections for greater trochanteric pain syndrome: a randomized controlled trial in primary care. *Ann Fam Med.* 2011;9(3):226-234.
4. McEvoy JR, Lee KS, Blankenbaker DG, del Rio AM, Keene JS. Ultrasound-guided corticosteroid injections for treatment of greater trochanteric pain syndrome: greater trochanter bursa versus subgluteus medius bursa. *AJR Am J Roentgenol.* 2013;201(2):W313-W317.
5. Fitzpatrick J, Bulsara MK, O'Donnell J, McCrory PR, Zheng MH. The effectiveness of platelet-rich plasma injections in gluteal tendinopathy: a randomized, double-blind controlled trial comparing a single platelet-rich plasma injection with a single corticosteroid injection. *Am J Sports Med.* 2018;46(4):933-939.
6. Jacobson JA, Yablon CM, Henning PT, et al. Greater trochanteric pain syndrome: percutaneous tendon fenestration versus platelet-rich plasma injection for treatment of gluteal tendinosis. *J Ultrasound Med.* 2016;35(11):2413-2420.
7. Brennan KL, Allen BC, Maldonado YM. Dry needling versus cortisone injection in the treatment of greater trochanteric pain syndrome: a noninferiority randomized clinical trial. *J Orthop Sports Phys Ther.* 2017;47(4):232-239.
8. Mitchell WG, Kettwich SC, Sibbitt WL, et al. Outcomes and cost-effectiveness of ultrasound-guided injection of the trochanteric bursa. *Rheumatol Int.* 2018;38(3):393-401.
9. Gazendam A, Ekhtiari S, Axelrod D, et al. Comparative efficacy of nonoperative treatments for greater trochanteric pain syndrome: a systematic review and network meta-analysis of randomized controlled trials. *Clin J Sport Med.* 2022;32(4):427-432.

Gluteal Pain Syndrome

The gluteus medius and minimus muscles function as primary hip abductors. They originate at the external surface of the ilium and insert onto the superior, posterior lateral surface of the greater trochanter. Gluteal pain syndrome, a term used to describe pain involving tendinopathy and gluteus bursitis, is now recognized as a primary local source of lateral hip pain.[1] It is more common than most practitioners realize. This disorder may occur secondary to acute direct trauma, changes in activity with a repetitive motion injury, chronic excessive hip adduction, or abnormal biomechanics due to conditions involving distal structures. It is frequently seen in middle-aged women who start a vigorous exercise program. Pain typically occurs with hip flexion such as walking, climbing stairs, or getting out of a car or a chair. Night pain while lying on the affected side is classic. Occasionally, snapping may be present over the lateral hip with hip flexion or extension. On examination, pain is palpated over the superior, posterior lateral aspect of the femoral trochanter and increases with resisted hip abduction. Diagnostic ultrasound may be performed to determine the presence of gluteal bursa fluid, echogenic features of tendinopathy, or tears of the gluteus medius tendon.

Management includes education, activity modification, ice, heat, therapeutic ultrasound, physical therapy, and NSAIDs.[2] Corticosteroid injections given with or without ultrasound guidance have been traditionally employed, but effectiveness past the short to medium term has not been demonstrated.[3] Ultrasound-guided PRP injections have shown greater clinical improvement at 12 weeks than corticosteroid injections.[4] A recent well-designed study revealed 2-year sustained improvement in pain following ultrasound-guided leukocyte-rich PRP.[5] Ultrasound-guided gluteal tendon fenestration compared to injections of PRP showed no statistically significant difference in pain scores at 90 days.[6] Patients who do not respond to these measures may be candidates for open or arthroscopic repair of gluteus medius tears.[7]

Relevant Anatomy: (Fig. 11.24)

PATIENT POSITION

- Lying on the examination table in the lateral decubitus position on the unaffected hip.

LANDMARKS

1. With the patient lying on the examination table in the lateral decubitus position on the unaffected hip, the clinician stands behind the patient.
2. Identify and mark the area(s) of maximal tenderness over the superior, posterior, lateral aspect of the greater trochanter.

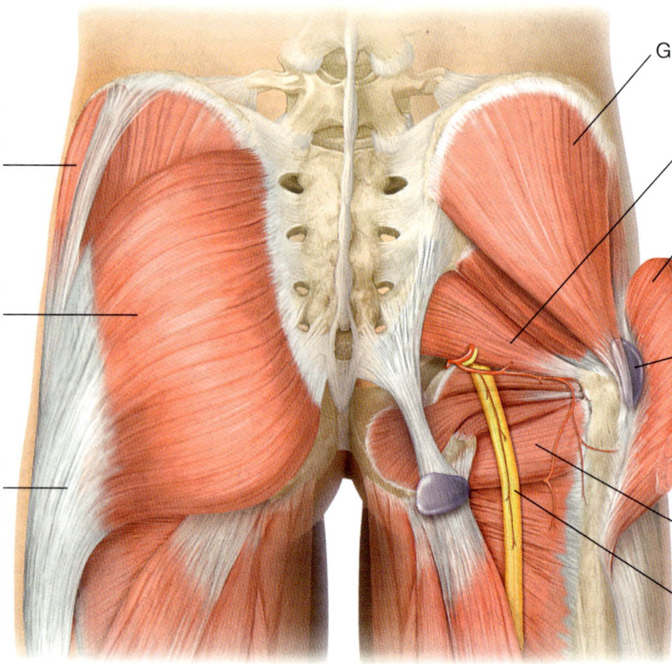

FIGURE 11.24 ● Muscles of gluteal region.

3. At that area, press firmly on the skin with the retracted tip of a ballpoint pen. This indentation represents the entry point(s) for the needle.
4. After the landmarks are identified, the patient should not move the hip.

ANESTHESIA

- Local anesthesia of the skin with topical vapocoolant spray may be used.

EQUIPMENT

- Topical vapocoolant spray
- 5-mL syringe
- 25-gauge 2-in needle
- 3 mL of 1% lidocaine without epinephrine
- 1 mL of the steroid solution (40 mg of triamcinolone acetonide)
- One alcohol prep pad
- Two povidone-iodine or chlorhexidine prep pads
- Sterile gauze pads
- Sterile adhesive bandage

TECHNIQUE

1. Prep the insertion site(s) with alcohol followed by the povidone-iodine or chlorhexidine pads.
2. Achieve good local anesthesia by using topical vapocoolant spray.

3. Position the needle and syringe perpendicular to the skin with the tip of the needle directed medially.
4. Using the no-touch technique, quickly introduce the needle at the insertion site(s) (Fig. 11.25).
5. Advance the needle toward the femoral trochanter until the needle tip touches the bone. Back up the needle 1 to 2 mm.
6. Withdraw the plunger of the syringe to ensure that there is no blood return.
7. Inject the lidocaine/corticosteroid solution as a bolus steadily in the area of the gluteus medius and minimus tendons. The injected solution should flow smoothly into the space. If increased resistance is encountered, advance or withdraw the needle slightly before attempting further injection.
8. Repeat the injection at other adjacent painful areas if needed.
9. Following injection(s), withdraw the needle.
10. Apply a sterile adhesive bandage(s).
11. Instruct the patient to massage the area and move their hip through its full range of motion. This movement distributes the lidocaine/corticosteroid solution throughout the gluteal tendons and bursa.
12. Reexamine the area of the gluteal tendons/bursa in 5 minutes to assess pain relief.

AFTERCARE

- Avoid excessive hip movement over the next 2 weeks.
- NSAIDs, ice, heat, and/or physical therapy as indicated.
- Consider follow-up examination in 2 weeks.

PEARLS

- Consider "fanning" this injection to disperse the corticosteroid solution along the course of the gluteus medius and minimus tendons.

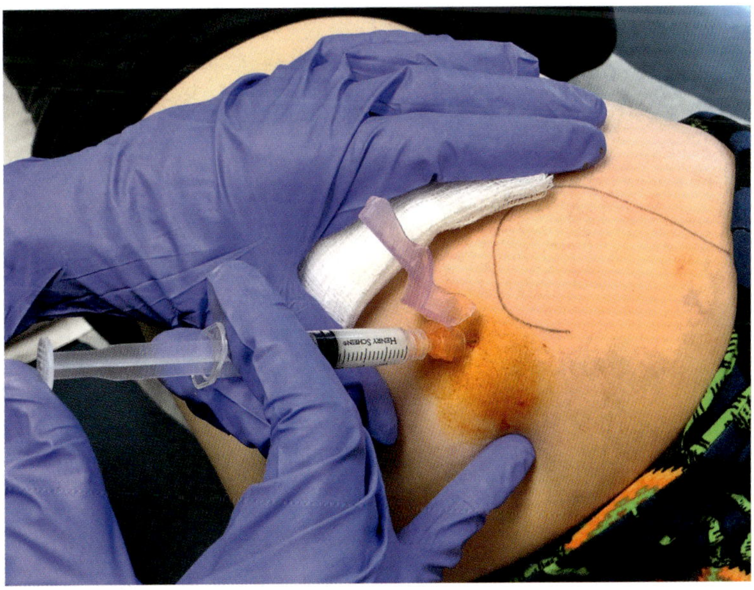

FIGURE 11.25 ● Injection for gluteal pain syndrome—superior and posterior to the right femoral trochanter.

A video showing a landmark-guided gluteal pain syndrome injection can be found in the companion eBook.

REFERENCES

1. Grimaldi A, Mellor R, Hodges P, et al. Gluteal tendinopathy: a review of mechanisms, assessment and management. *Sports Med.* 2015;45(8):1107-1119.
2. Ladurner A, Fitzpatrick J, O'Donnell JM. Treatment of gluteal tendinopathy: a systematic review and stage-adjusted treatment recommendation. *Orthop J Sports Med.* 2021;9(7):23259671211016850.
3. Bolton WS, Kidanu D, Dube B, Grainger AJ, Rowbotham E, Robinson P. Do ultrasound guided trochanteric bursa injections of corticosteroid for greater trochanteric pain syndrome provide sustained benefit and are imaging features associated with treatment response? *Clin Radiol.* 2018;73(5):505.e9-505.e15.
4. Fitzpatrick J, Bulsara MK, O'Donnell J, McCrory PR. The effectiveness of platelet-rich plasma injections in gluteal tendinopathy: a randomized, double-blind controlled trial comparing a single platelet-rich plasma injection with a single corticosteroid injection. *Am J Sports Med.* 2018;46(4):933-939.
5. Fitzpatrick J, Bulsara MK, O'Donnell J, Zheng MH. Leucocyte-rich platelet-rich plasma treatment of gluteus medius and minimus tendinopathy: a double-blind randomized controlled trial with 2-year follow-up. *Am J Sports Med.* 2019;47(5):1130-1137.
6. Jacobson JA, Yablon CM, Henning PT, et al. Greater trochanteric pain syndrome: percutaneous tendon fenestration versus platelet-rich plasma injection for treatment of gluteal tendinosis. *J Ultrasound Med.* 2016;35(11):2413-2420.
7. LaPorte C, Vasaris M, Gossett L, Boykin R, Menge T. Gluteus medius tears of the hip: a comprehensive approach. *Phys Sportsmed.* 2019;47(1):15-20.

Hip Adductor Tendon

Patients uncommonly present to the primary care office for the evaluation and treatment of pain upon adduction of the hip. The pectineus, adductor longus, magnus, and medius muscles connect the medial aspect of the femur to the pubic bone. Acute injury or chronic overuse may cause tendonitis or tendinopathy of the hip adductors. The adductor longus is most commonly injured, and patients classically present with pain upon palpation of the muscle belly and insertion, passive stretching, and resistance to contraction. In chronic tendinopathy, treatment is often lengthy and difficult. Physical therapy is the cornerstone of treatment. It may be facilitated by the judicious use of corticosteroid injections given around the affected tendon(s).

Relevant Anatomy: (Fig. 11.26)

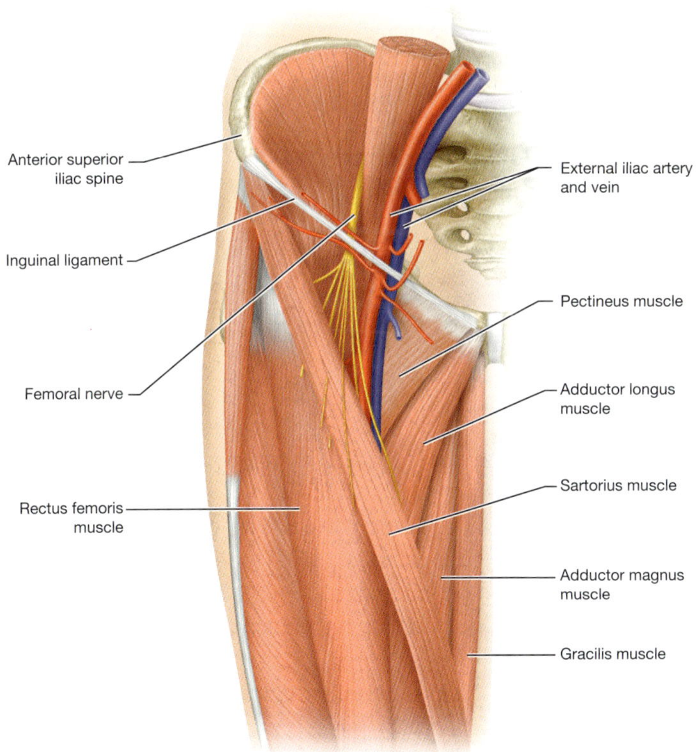

FIGURE 11.26 ● Right thigh and femoral triangle structures. (Modified with permission from Gest TR. *Lippincott® Atlas of Anatomy*. 2nd ed. Wolters Kluwer; 2020.)

PATIENT POSITION

- Lying supine on the examination table.
- Place the hip in a position of combined flexion, abduction, and external rotation.
- Rotate the patient's head away from the side that is being injected. This minimizes anxiety and pain perception.

LANDMARKS

1. With the patient lying supine on the examination table, the clinician stands lateral and posterior to the affected hip.
2. Locate the symphysis pubis and firmly palpate the pubic bone laterally until meeting the origin of the hip adductor muscles.
3. Determine the site of maximal tenderness over the tendons, and mark it with an ink pen.
4. At that site, press firmly on the skin with the retracted tip of a ballpoint pen. This indentation represents the entry point for the needle.
5. After the landmarks are identified, the patient should not move the hip.

ANESTHESIA

- Local anesthesia of the skin using a topical vapocoolant spray.

EQUIPMENT

- Topical vapocoolant spray
- 3-mL syringe
- 25-gauge 2-in needle
- 1 mL of 1% lidocaine without epinephrine
- 1 mL of the steroid solution (40 mg of triamcinolone acetonide)
- One alcohol prep pad
- Two povidone-iodine or chlorhexidine prep pads
- Sterile gauze pads
- Sterile adhesive bandage

TECHNIQUE

1. Prep the insertion site with alcohol followed by the povidone-iodine or chlorhexidine pads.
2. Achieve good local anesthesia by using a topical vapocoolant spray.
3. Position the needle and syringe at an angle of 30° to the skin with the tip of the needle directed proximally toward the pubic bone.
4. Using the no-touch technique, quickly introduce the needle at the insertion site (Fig. 11.27).
5. Advance the needle so that it is positioned around the affected tendon but not in the substance of the tendon.
6. Withdraw the plunger of the syringe to ensure that there is no blood return.
7. Inject the lidocaine/corticosteroid solution as a bolus around the adductor tendon(s). The injected solution should flow smoothly into the space. If increased resistance

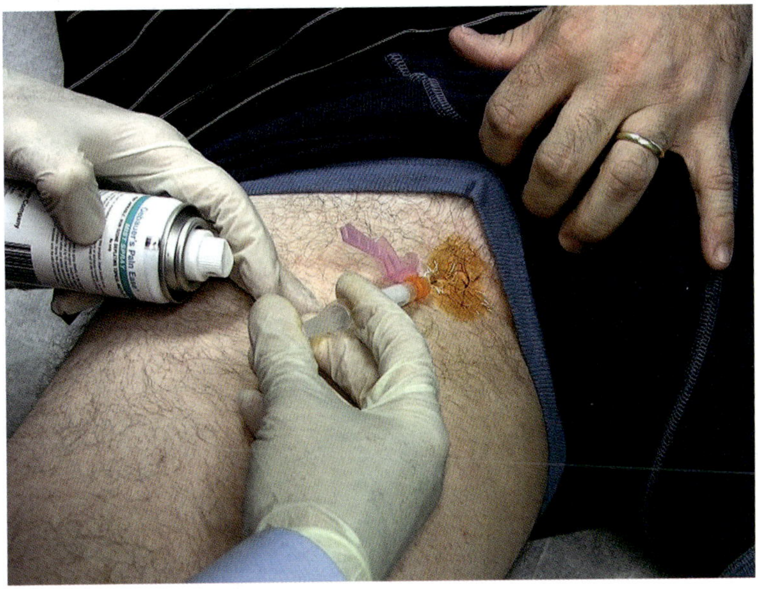

FIGURE 11.27 • Hip adductor tendonitis injection.

is encountered, advance or withdraw the needle slightly before attempting further injection.

8. Following injection, withdraw the needle.
9. Apply a sterile adhesive bandage.
10. Instruct the patient to massage the area and move their hip through its full range of motion. This movement distributes the lidocaine/corticosteroid solution along the adductor tendon(s).
11. Reexamine the medial aspect of the hip in 5 minutes to assess pain relief.

AFTERCARE

- Avoid excessive use of the hip—especially hip abduction and adduction over the next 2 weeks.
- Begin a program of physical therapy.
- NSAIDs, ice, and heat as indicated.
- Consider follow-up examination in 2 weeks.

PEARLS

- This injection can be superficial—especially in thin persons. Depositing corticosteroid in the subcutaneous tissues can result in the complication of skin atrophy and hypopigmentation. Avoid the development of a subdermal wheal while performing all injections of corticosteroid solutions.

ULTRASOUND-GUIDED PROCEDURE

Please refer to the introductory ultrasound chapter for preprocedure, sterile prep, post-procedure, and documentation information and recommendations.

PATIENT POSITION

- Supine on the examination table.
- On the affected side, place the hip in a flexed, abducted, and externally rotated position resting on the examination table. The flexed, abducted, and externally rotated position can be adjusted to improve visualization.
- Place a pillow under their head for comfort.
- Adjust the patient's position as needed to ensure comfort.

PROVIDER/ULTRASOUND POSITION

- The provider stands on the same side of the table as the affected adductor tendon.
- Adjust the examination table to position the injection site between the provider's umbilicus and axillary level, ensuring optimal ergonomics and visualization of the ultrasound screen, transducer, and needle's approach (Fig. 11.28).
- Place the ultrasound machine on the opposite side of the table at the level of the patient's head with the screen facing the provider.

ANESTHESIA

- Local anesthesia of the skin using topical vapocoolant spray.

EQUIPMENT

- 3-mL syringe
- 22-gauge 2-in needle (adjust needle length as needed)

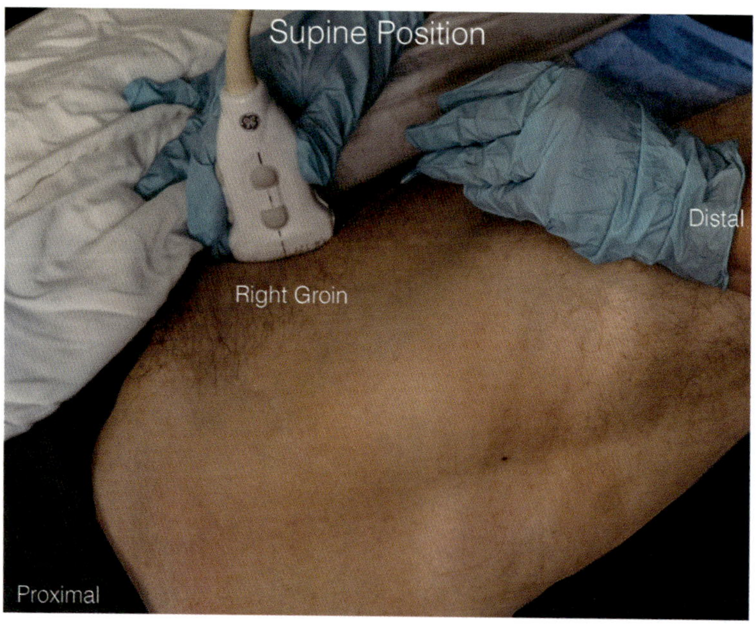

FIGURE 11.28 Ultrasound-guided right adductor–related tendon injection. Supine position with the affected hip resting on examination table. Feet positioned at the right of the image. Provider positioned ipsilaterally distal to the injection site.

- 1 mL of 1% lidocaine without epinephrine
- 1 mL of 40 mg/mL of triamcinolone acetonide
- Three chlorhexidine swabs
- 12-4 MHz linear ultrasound transducer and machine
- Sterile ultrasound transducer cover
- Sterile ultrasound gel
- Nonlatex sterile or nonsterile gloves
- Two 4 × 4 sterile gauze pads
- One sterile adhesive bandage
- Topical vapocoolant spray

TECHNIQUE

1. Position a high-frequency linear 12-4 MHz ultrasound transducer in the coronal oblique plane over the adductor longus tendon in long axis with the pubic symphysis beneath the proximal end.
2. Advance a 22-gauge 2-in needle using an in-plane approach, directing it from distal to proximal, with an initial needle angle of approximately 10° to 15° relative to the skin surface where the transducer is positioned.
3. Target area:
   a. For corticosteroids: The deep peritendinous space
   b. For dextrose prolotherapy or PRP: The tendon itself (refer to Chapter 4: Orthobiologics)
4. Injectate:
   a. For corticosteroids: Use a 22-gauge 2-in needle to inject the solution into the deep peritendinous space.
   b. For dextrose prolotherapy or PRP (refer to Chapter 4: Orthobiologics): Use a 22-gauge 2-in needle to inject the solution into the area of tendinopathy in the tendon. Administer a total volume (1-2 mL) of 15% dextrose prolotherapy or PRP in small aliquots (0.5 mL or less).
5. Utilize real-time ultrasound guidance throughout to ensure accurate needle placement and minimize the risk of complications (Fig. 11.29).
6. Upon completion of the procedure, carefully withdraw the needle. Adhere to established postprocedure care protocols and ensure appropriate follow-up as recommended.

PEARLS

- Adductor-related groin pain is most commonly caused by adductor longus tendinopathy, which originates from the anterolateral surface of the pubic symphysis. Corticosteroid injections around the adductor tendons warrant careful consideration and patient counseling, especially in the cases of tendinosis.
- Exercise caution to avoid inadvertent penetration of the spermatic cord, round ligament, and surrounding neurovascular structures during needle advancement.

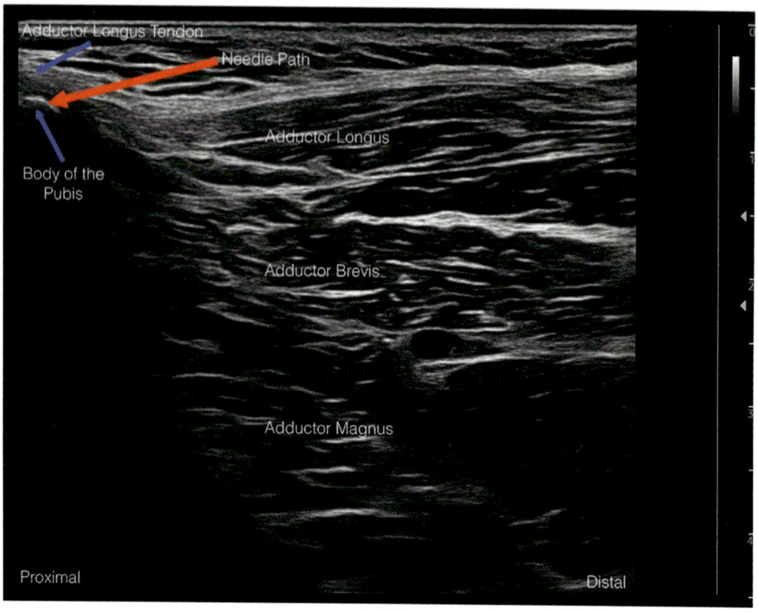

FIGURE 11.29 ● Hip adductor coronal oblique ultrasound image.

Videos showing landmark-guided and ultrasound-guided hip adductor tendon injections can be found in the companion eBook.

Knee Joint Injections

The need for aspiration and injection of the knee joint is commonly encountered by primary care providers. The most common indications for this procedure include evaluation and treatment of monoarthritis, osteoarthritis, and inflammatory arthritis; to rule out septic arthritis; and removal of blood following acute trauma or reactive fluid from overuse. Arthrocentesis (aspiration) is employed to remove fluid from a joint for diagnostic synovial fluid analysis, to enhance comfort, to improve proprioception,[1] and to minimize dilution of injected substances. Injections of various products are also employed including corticosteroids,[2] HA viscosupplements,[3-5] PRP,[6] dextrose (prolotherapy),[7] etanercept,[8,9] botulinum toxin,[10,11] and others.

Most practitioners use one of four palpation-based, anatomic landmark-guided approaches to perform aspirations and injections of the knee joint. Figure 11.30A and B shows the most common knee joint approaches—the extended-knee lateral suprapatellar, extended-knee lateral midpatellar, flexed-knee anteromedial, and flexed-knee anterolateral portals. The author avoids the medial suprapatellar and medial midpatellar approaches because of the limited operating space on the medial aspect of the knee/leg, to preserve patient modesty, and due to the lack of demonstrated accuracy and effectiveness in the medical literature. There is a general lack of consensus among experts regarding the best technique for knee joint injection and aspiration. An examination of the current medical literature (below), however, gives us some guidance. Although it appears that the lateral suprapatellar and lateral midpatellar approaches have an advantage over the others, the individual provider will ultimately determine the desired portal based on the scientific data, their expertise, history of success, and other patient-specific factors.

A comprehensive review of intra-articular knee joint injection accuracy was published in 2013 by Maricar et al[12] Data from 23 publications were pooled and revealed that injections at the lateral suprapatellar portal were most accurate (87%), while medial midpatellar (64%) and anterolateral joint line sites (70%) were least accurate. Furthermore, lateral suprapatellar, medial midpatellar, and medial suprapatellar sites were more accurate when using image guidance than when using anatomic landmarks. Another systematic review of nine studies by Hermans et al[13] found the extended-leg lateral suprapatellar approach (91%) to be the most accurate, as compared with the lateral midpatellar (85%), anteromedial (72%), and anterolateral (67%) approaches. This success makes sense when the location of synovial fluid in the knee joint is considered. Hirsch et al[14] demonstrated that small effusions were more commonly detected in the lateral suprapatellar pouch than elsewhere. In patients with painful knee arthritis, fluid distributes maximally to the lateral suprapatellar pouch in the extended knee. Furthermore, Zhang et al[15] found a "dry tap" rate of 10% in the extended-leg supine position and 25% in the sitting position.

In an individual study by Jackson et al[16] using a 1½-in 21-gauge needle, the landmark-based, lateral midpatellar approach was significantly more accurate (93%) than were the anteromedial (75%) and anterolateral (71%) approaches. Toda and

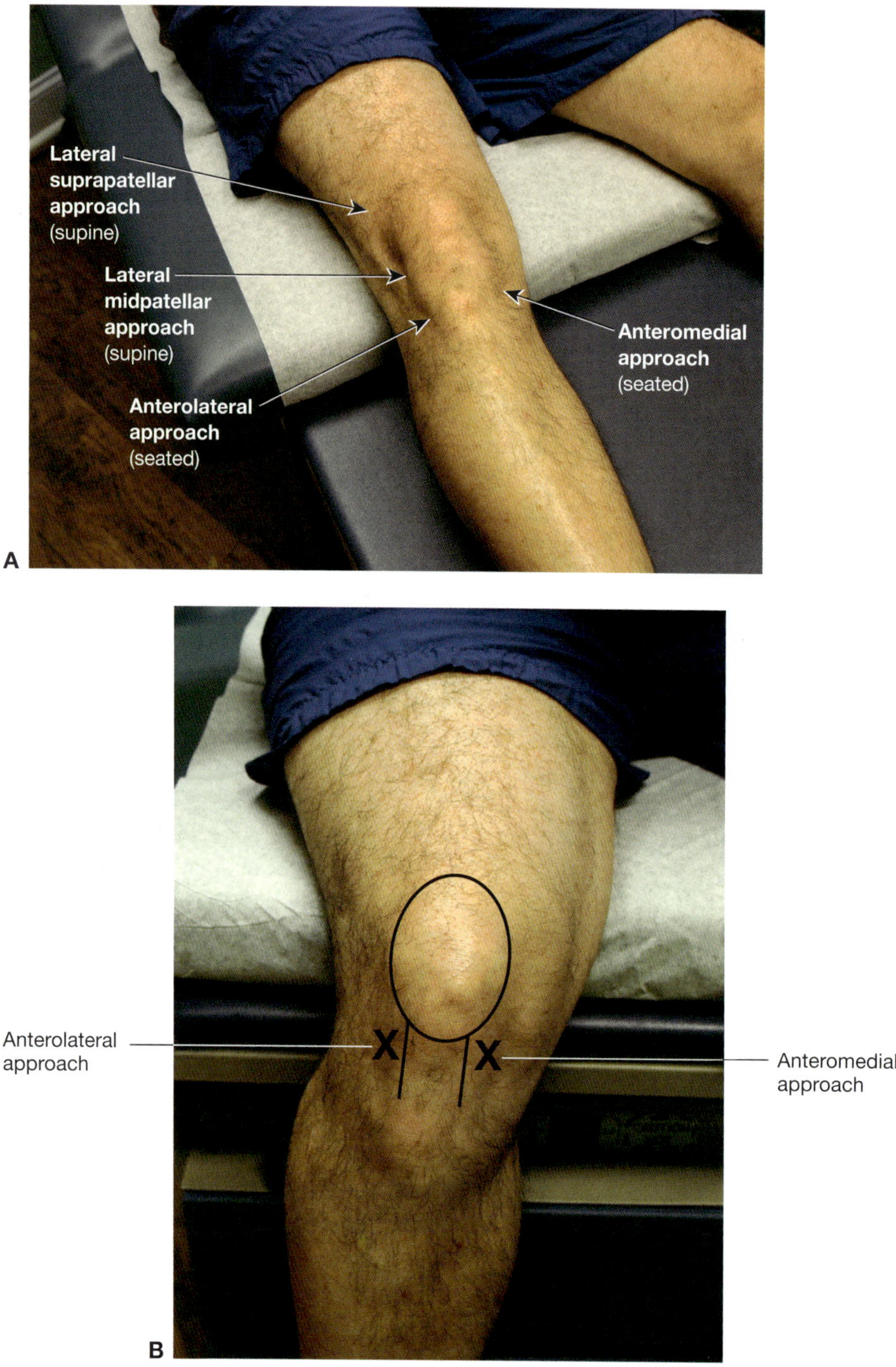

FIGURE 11.30 ● **A.** Right knee—the most common knee joint approaches. **B.** Flexed knee showing landmarks.

Tsukimura[17] reported that a modified 30° flexed-knee approach incorporating distal knee traction was significantly more accurate (86%) than were seated anteromedial (62%) and extended-leg lateral suprapatellar (70%) approaches using a 1½-in 25-gauge needle. Accuracy rates increased with the presence of severe osteoarthritis. In another investigation by Chavez-Chiang et al,[18] an anterolateral knee portal with 90° flexion targeting the synovial membrane of the medial femoral condyle with a 2-in 21-gauge needle yielded an accuracy rate of 97%. This approach might be useful for patients who cannot lie down, transfer to an examination table, extend the knee, or those with flexion contractures.

The use of musculoskeletal ultrasound dramatically increases the accuracy of knee injections. A number of studies now demonstrate significantly increased accuracy rates of injections when using ultrasound-guided techniques. The use of ultrasound increases the success rate to nearly 100%, even when performed by less experienced practitioners.[19] A study of ultrasound-guided injections in patients with moderate osteoarthritis using a 1½-in 25-gauge needle showed success rates of 100% for the lateral suprapatellar, 95% for the lateral midpatellar, and 75% for the anteromedial approaches.[20] A review of 13 studies of the knee showed that imaging guidance with ultrasound improved the accuracy of intra-articular injections of the knee to 95.8% versus 77.8%, $P < .001$.[21] Employing a joint cupping maneuver from an inferior approach also improves the detection and removal of knee joint effusion by improving ultrasound visualization of the effusion.[22] The use of image-guided techniques is particularly important in patients without joint effusion and especially when injecting intra-articular viscosupplements to treat osteoarthritis of the knee.[23,24] Most importantly, there is statistically significant improvement in short-term (2 weeks) patient outcomes of pain and function with a reduction in adverse events when ultrasound-guided injections are compared to those guided by palpation of landmarks. These image-guided techniques also cause significantly less procedural pain, take no additional time to perform, lead to greater provider confidence with the procedure, and improve cost-effectiveness.[18,25,26]

The extended knee, lateral suprapatellar approach, for a knee joint intra-articular injection is relatively easy to perform, easily lends itself to ultrasound guidance without bony obstruction, and is well accepted by patients. Additionally, because of supine positioning, patients may not see the approaching needle and anxiety is diminished. For these reasons and based on the published studies, this approach is the author's preferred technique and is highly recommended to others.

REFERENCES

1. Cho YR, Hong BY, Lim SH, et al. Effects of joint effusion on proprioception in patients with knee osteoarthritis: a single-blind, randomized controlled clinical trial. *Osteoarthritis Cartilage.* 2011;19(1):22-28.
2. Leung A, Liew D, Lim J, et al. The effect of joint aspiration and corticosteroid injections in osteoarthritis of the knee. *Int J Rheum Dis.* 2011;14(4):384-389.
3. Saito S, Kotake S. Is there evidence in support of the use of intra-articular hyaluronate in treating rheumatoid arthritis of the knee? A meta-analysis of the published literature. *Mod Rheumatol.* 2009;19(5):493-501.
4. Foti C, Cisari C, Carda S, et al. A prospective observational study of the clinical efficacy and safety of intra-articular sodium hyaluronate in synovial joints with osteoarthritis. *Eur J Phys Rehabil Med.* 2011;47(3):407-415.
5. Tarantino D, Forte AM, Picone A, Sirico F, Ruosi C. The effectiveness of a single hyaluronic acid injection in improving symptoms and muscular strength in patients with knee osteoarthritis: a multicenter, retrospective study. *J Pers Med.* 2024;14(8):784.
6. Spaková T, Rosocha J, Lacko M, Harvanová D, Gharaibeh A. Treatment of knee joint osteoarthritis with autologous platelet-rich plasma in comparison with hyaluronic acid. *Am J Phys Med Rehabil.* 2012;91(5):411-417.
7. Sit RWS, Wu RWK, Rabago D, et al. Efficacy of intra-articular hypertonic dextrose (prolotherapy) for knee osteoarthritis: a randomized controlled trial. *Ann Fam Med.* 2020;18(3):235-242.
8. Liang DF, Huang F, Zhang JL, et al. A randomized, single-blind, parallel, controlled clinical study on single intra-articular injection of etanercept in treatment of inflammatory knee arthritis. *Zhonghua Nei Ke Za Zhi* 2010;49(11):930-934.
9. Zhang F, Ma C. Comparison of the effectiveness on intra-articular and subcutaneous TNF inhibitor in rheumatoid arthritis patients. *Clin Rheumatol.* 2018;37(1):199-204.

10. Chou CL, Lee SH, Lu SY, Tsai K-L, Ho C-Y, Lai H-C. Therapeutic effects of intra-articular botulinum neurotoxin in advanced knee osteoarthritis. *J Chin Med Assoc.* 2010;73(11):573-580.
11. Wu T, Song HX, Dong Y, Ye Y, Li J-H. Intra-articular injections of botulinum toxin a for refractory joint pain: a systematic review and meta-analysis. *Clin Rehabil.* 2017;31(4):435-443.
12. Maricar N, Parkes MJ, Callaghan MJ, Felson DT, O'Neill TW. Where and how to inject the knee—a systematic review. *Semin Arthritis Rheum.* 2013;43(2):195-203.
13. Hermans J, Bierma-Zeinstra SM, Bos PK, Verhaar JAN, Reijman M. The most accurate approach for intra-articular needle placement in the knee joint: a systematic review. *Semin Arthritis Rheum.* 2011;41(2):106-115.
14. Hirsch G, O'Neill T, Kitas G, Klocke R. Distribution of effusion in knee arthritis as measured by high-resolution ultrasound. *Clin Rheumatol.* 2012;31(8):1243-1246.
15. Zhang Q, Zhang T, Lv H, et al. Comparison of two positions of knee arthrocentesis: how to obtain complete drainage. *Am J Phys Med Rehabil.* 2012;91(7):611-615.
16. Jackson DW, Evans NA, Thomas BM. Accuracy of needle placement into the intra-articular space of the knee. *J Bone Joint Surg Am.* 2002;84-A(9):1522-1527.
17. Toda Y, Tsukimura N. A comparison of intra-articular hyaluronan injection accuracy rates between three approaches based on radiographic severity of knee osteoarthritis. *Osteoarthritis Cartilage.* 2008;16(9):980-985.
18. Chavez-Chiang CE, Sibbitt WL Jr, Band PA, Chavez-Chiang NR, DeLea SL, Bankhurst AD. The highly accurate anteriolateral portal for injecting the knee. *Sports Med Arthrosc Rehabil Ther Technol.* 2011;3(1):6.
19. Curtiss HM, Finnoff JT, Peck E, Hollman J, Smith J. Accuracy of ultrasound-guided and palpation-guided knee injections by an experienced and less-experienced injector using a superolateral approach: a cadaveric study. *PM R.* 2011;3(6):507-515.
20. Park Y, Lee SC, Nam HS, Lee J, Nam SH. Comparison of sonographically guided intra-articular injections at 3 different sites of the knee. *J Ultrasound Med.* 2011;30(12):1669-1676.
21. Berkoff DJ, Miller LE, Block JE. Clinical utility of ultrasound guidance for intra-articular knee injections: a review. *Clin Interv Aging.* 2012;7:89-95.
22. Uryasev O, Joseph OC, McNamara JP, Dallas AP. Novel joint cupping clinical maneuver for ultrasonographic detection of knee joint effusions. *Am J Emerg Med.* 2013;31(11):1598-1600.
23. Punzi L, Oliviero F. Arthrocentesis and synovial fluid analysis in clinical practice: value of sonography in difficult cases. *Ann N Y Acad Sci.* 2009;1154:152-158.
24. Elsawy NA, Ibrahiem AH, Younis GA, Meheissen MA, Abdel-Fattah YH. Clinical examination, ultrasound assessment and aspiration of knee effusion in primary knee osteoarthritis patients. *J Orthop Surg Res.* 2023;18(1):422.
25. Wiler JL, Costantino TG, Satz W. Comparison of ultrasound-guided and standard landmark techniques for knee arthrocentesis. *J Emerg Med.* 2010;39(1):76-82.
26. Sibbitt WL Jr, Kettwich LG, Band PA, et al. Does ultrasound guidance improve the outcomes of arthrocentesis and corticosteroid injection of the knee? *Scand J Rheumatol.* 2012;41(1):66-72.

Knee Joint—Preferred Lateral Suprapatellar Approach

The supine, extended-leg, lateral suprapatellar approach to the knee joint is relatively easy to perform and is well accepted by patients. Because of supine positioning, patients may not see the approaching needle and anxiety is diminished. This approach is considered a safe procedure since there are no major arteries or nerves in the immediate path of the needle. Also, since the injection is done using the suprapatellar approach, it is extraarticular, but still within the joint capsule. As a result, joint fluid can be removed and injections performed without direct, large-needle injury to articular cartilage. With the use of local anesthetic, this injection can help the clinician differentiate the etiology of knee pain. After pain has been eliminated as a confounding factor, the knee can be reexamined to assess structural integrity of the ligaments and menisci. For the reasons previously noted, the extended-leg, lateral suprapatellar approach is the preferred technique to perform landmark-guided knee joint aspirations and injections.

Relevant Anatomy: (Fig. 11.31)

PATIENT POSITION

- Lying supine on the examination table with the knee extended, or slightly flexed and supported with a pillow or folded chucks pads as needed for patient comfort.
- Rotate the patient's head away from the side that is being injected. This minimizes anxiety and pain perception.

LANDMARKS

1. With the patient lying supine on the examination table, the clinician stands lateral to the affected knee.
2. Locate the superior aspect of the patella.
3. Draw a line vertically 1 cm superior to the proximal margin of the patella (Fig. 11.32).
4. Next, draw a line horizontally along the posterior edge of the patella.
5. Identify the point where these two lines intersect. Make sure that this intersection lies underneath the quadriceps tendon.
6. At that site, press firmly on the skin with the retracted tip of a ballpoint pen. This indentation represents the entry point for the needle.
7. After the landmarks are identified, the patient should not move the knee.

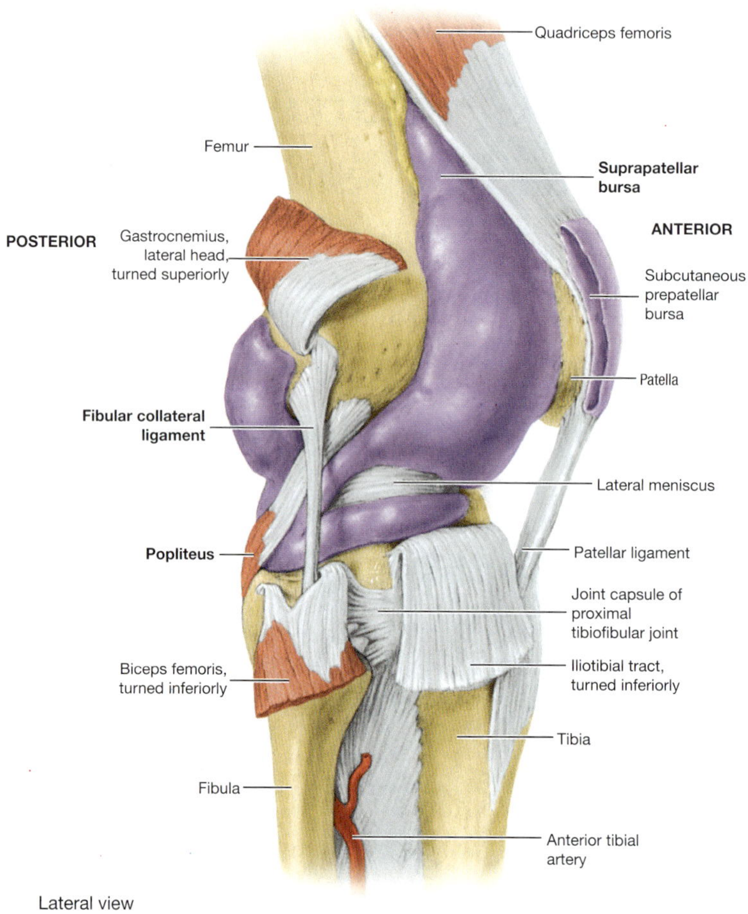

FIGURE 11.31 ● Lateral aspect of the right knee showing the extent of the knee joint capsule. (Reprinted with permission from Agur AMR, Dalley AF II. *Grant's Atlas of Anatomy*. 16th ed. Wolters Kluwer; 2025.)

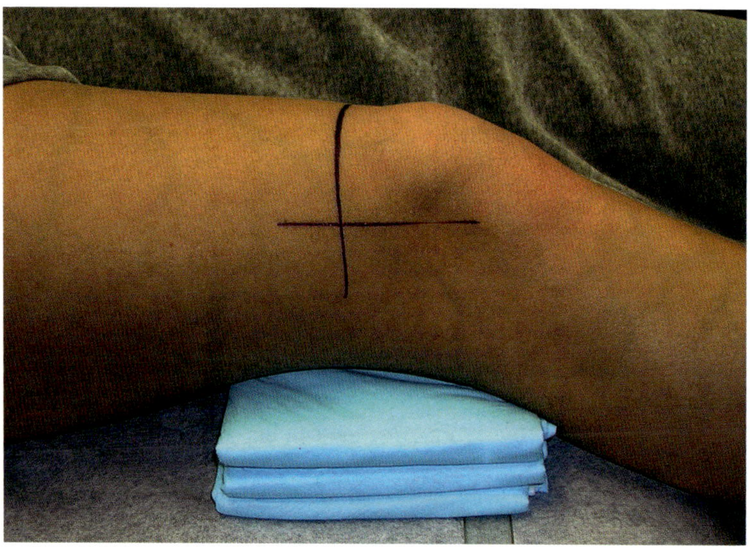

FIGURE 11.32 ● Lateral aspect of the right knee with lines drawn.

ANESTHESIA

- Local anesthesia of the skin using topical vapocoolant spray.
- (Optional) Local anesthesia and vasoconstriction of the skin and soft tissues may be augmented using an injection of 2 to 4 mL of 1% lidocaine with epinephrine (see "Pearls").

EQUIPMENT

- Topical vapocoolant spray
- 3-mL syringe—for injection of the mepivacaine/corticosteroid mixture
- 25-gauge 2-in needle—for direct injection of the mepivacaine/corticosteroid mixture
- (Optional) 10- to 60-mL syringe(s)—for aspiration
- (Optional) 5-mL syringe—for injection of 1% lidocaine with epinephrine to provide augmented local tissue anesthesia
- (Optional) 25-gauge 1½-in needle—for injection of 1% lidocaine with epinephrine to provide local tissue anesthesia—in preparation for an 18-gauge needle
- (Optional) 18-gauge 1½-in needle—for aspiration
- (Optional) 2 to 4 mL of 1% lidocaine with epinephrine—for local tissue anesthesia of skin and knee joint capsule—in preparation for an 18-gauge needle
- 1 mL of 1% mepivacaine without epinephrine—to dilute the corticosteroid
- 1 mL of the corticosteroid solution (40 mg of triamcinolone acetonide)
- (Optional) Viscosupplementation agent of choice—if indicated
- One alcohol prep pad
- Two povidone-iodine or chlorhexidine prep pads
- Sterile gauze pads
- Sterile adhesive bandage
- Nonsterile, clean chucks pad

TECHNIQUE

1. (Optional) Use ultrasound to image the knee joint structures using an adjacent, but separate, acoustic window. This allows separate imaging from the injection site so that there is no contamination from the ultrasound gel. Alternatively, the entire site may be prepped in an aseptic manner and sterile ultrasound gel utilized (Fig. 11.33).
2. Create an aseptic insertion site by wiping with a single alcohol prep pad followed by two 10% povidone-iodine or chlorhexidine prep pads. Allow this site to completely dry by evaporation.
3. If significant intra-articular fluid accumulation is not suspected, or not seen on ultrasound examination, then proceed with direct injection of the mepivacaine/corticosteroid solution (step 4). If fluid is suspected or confirmed on ultrasound, proceed to step 10.
4. Achieve good local anesthesia by using topical vapocoolant spray.
5. Position the 25-gauge 2-in needle and syringe perpendicularly to the skin, parallel to the floor, at a right angle to the other two previously drawn skin lines and with the tip of the needle directed medially.
6. Using the aseptic, no-touch technique, quickly introduce that needle at the insertion site.

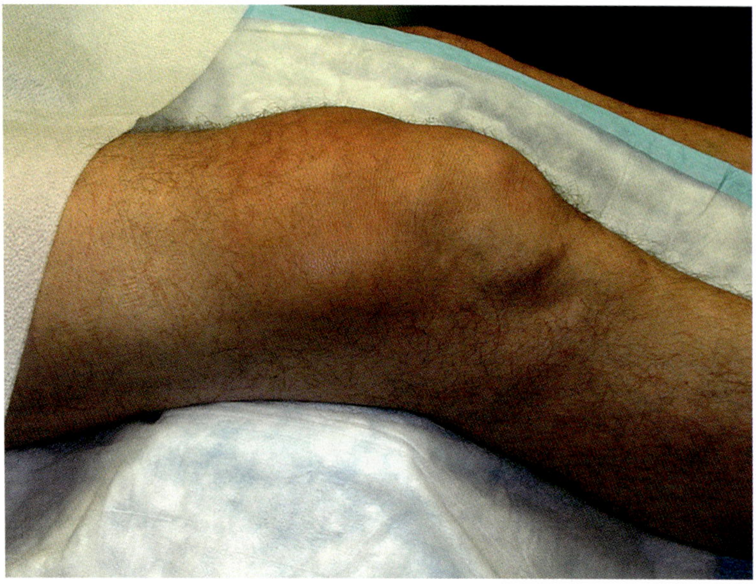

FIGURE 11.33 ● Right knee joint—distended with a large amount of intra-articular fluid. Note bulging of the joint capsule (suprapatellar bursa) proximal to the patella.

7. Advance the 25-gauge 2-in needle under the quadriceps tendon and toward the anterior surface of the distal femur until the needle tip is located within the joint capsule. The needle may contact the distal femur itself. Should that happen, withdraw the needle a few centimeters and advance the needle as needed to "walk" it over the anterior aspect of the femur.
8. Withdraw the plunger of the syringe to ensure that there is no blood return.
9. Inject the mepivacaine/corticosteroid solution as a bolus into the knee joint. The injected solution should flow smoothly into the joint space. If increased resistance is encountered, advance or withdraw the needle slightly before attempting further injection (Fig. 11.34). (Proceed to step 18.)
10. (Optional) Achieve good local anesthesia by using topical vapocoolant spray.
11. Using the no-touch technique, introduce the 25-gauge 1½-in needle for local anesthesia at the insertion site. Inject 2 to 4 mL of 1% lidocaine with epinephrine to provide adequate local anesthesia. Infuse the anesthetic under the skin and at the joint capsule.
12. Position the 18-gauge 1½-in needle and syringe perpendicularly to the skin, parallel to the floor, at a right angle to the other two previously drawn skin lines and with the tip of the needle directed medially.
13. Using the aseptic, no-touch technique, quickly introduce that needle at the insertion site.
14. Advance the 18-gauge 1½- in needle under the quadriceps tendon and toward the anterior surface of the distal femur until the needle tip is located in the joint capsule. (This may occur after advancing only 1 to 2 cm if the lateral pocket of a distended knee joint capsule is present.) Apply suction to the syringe while advancing the needle. The appearance of fluid in the syringe confirms that the joint capsule has been entered (Fig. 11.35). If fluid is aspirated, stop advancing the needle. The needle may contact the distal femur itself. Should that happen, withdraw the needle a few centimeters and advance the needle as needed to "walk" it over the femur and into the joint capsule.

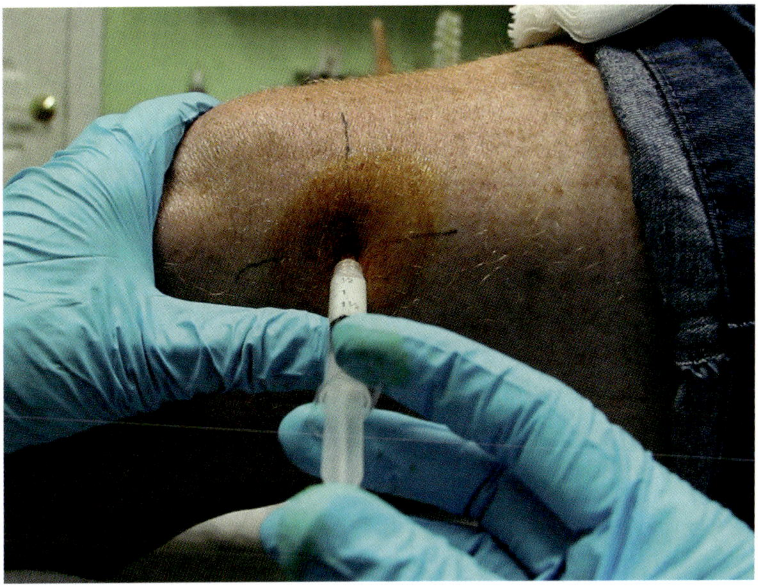

FIGURE 11.34 • Landmark-guided left knee corticosteroid injection.

15. Multiple syringes may be required in order to drain all of the synovial fluid if a large effusion is present.
16. If injection following aspiration is elected, remove the large syringe from the 18-gauge needle and then attach the 3-mL syringe filled with the mepivacaine/corticosteroid solution (Fig. 11.34) or a proprietary glass syringe prefilled with viscosupplement.
17. Inject the mepivacaine/corticosteroid solution or viscosupplement as a bolus into the knee joint. The injected solution should flow smoothly into the joint space. If increased resistance is encountered, advance or withdraw the needle slightly, and confirm aspiration of a small amount of joint fluid before attempting further injection.
18. Following injection, withdraw the needle.
19. Apply a sterile adhesive bandage.
20. Instruct the patient to move their knee through its full range of motion. This movement distributes the mepivacaine/corticosteroid solution or viscosupplement throughout the knee joint.
21. Reexamine the knee in 5 minutes to assess pain relief.

AFTERCARE

- Avoid more than light use of the affected knee over the next 2 weeks.
- Use other complementary treatment modalities including physical therapy as indicated.
- Consider follow-up examination in 2 weeks.

PEARLS

- Although both the lateral and medial suprapatellar approaches may be used, the preferred landmark-guided injection approach is from the lateral aspect. This approach affords the operator more room, avoids inadvertent kicking of the clinician by the patient with the uninvolved leg, and preserves patient modesty.

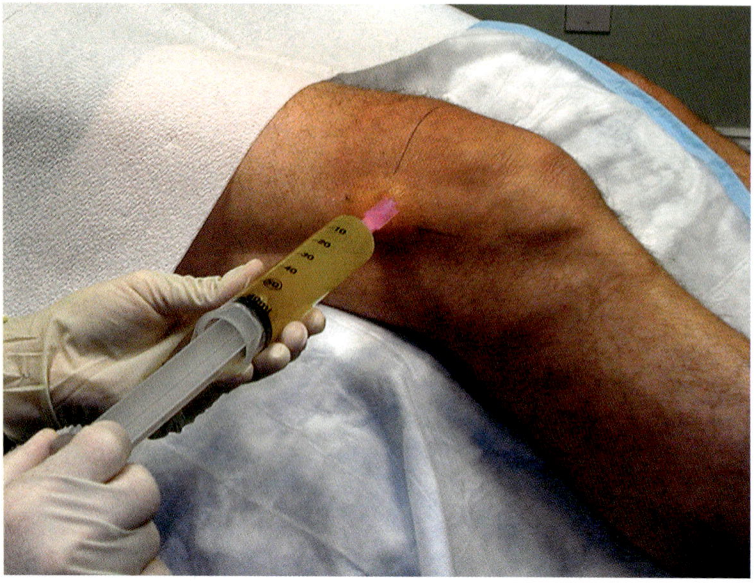

FIGURE 11.35 ● Right knee large volume aspiration of distended joint using the preferred lateral suprapatellar approach.

- Usually, this procedure can be conducted in a pain-free manner with the use of topical vapocoolant spray. However, an occasional patient may complain of pain when the 18-gauge needle is advanced into contact with the joint capsule. In this case, that needle should be withdrawn and a 1½-in 25-gauge needle advanced in the same direction. A total of 2 to 4 mL of 1% lidocaine with epinephrine is deposited under the skin and at the margin of the joint capsule. In almost all such cases where pain is reported, it is the author's experience that an ultrasound examination often shows that the synovial capsule is thickened and presumably inflamed.
- If the clinician encounters the unusual situation of experiencing difficulty finding the joint capsule, then either of the following maneuvers can be attempted:
  - Ask the patient to activate (tighten) their quadriceps muscles. This concentrates the volume of intra-articular fluid into the suprapatellar pouch.
  - Firmly squeeze the anterodistal aspect of the patella and displace it posteriorly and proximally (the "cupping" maneuver) thereby shifting the joint fluid and filling the suprapatellar pouch.[1]
  - Redirect the needle in a distal direction to target the undersurface of the patella. However, this technique may potentially result in injury to the patellar cartilage.
- Ultrasound-guided aspiration and injection are indicated when an effusion is not detected, or in a very obese patient. Ultrasound is also very useful in locating fluid in the knee joint to ensure absolute placement accuracy when injecting expensive viscosupplement products.

ULTRASOUND-GUIDED PROCEDURE

Please refer to the introductory ultrasound chapter for preprocedure, sterile prep, post-procedure, and documentation information and recommendations.

PATIENT POSITION

- Supine on the examination table.
- On the affected side, place the knee in 30° of flexion with a bump.
- Place a rolled-up towel or small bolster under the knee to achieve approximately 30° of flexion.
- Place a pillow under their head for comfort.
- Adjust the patient's position as needed to ensure comfort.

PROVIDER/ULTRASOUND POSITION

- The provider sits on the same side of the table as the affected knee.
- Adjust the examination table to position the injection site between the provider's umbilicus and axillary level, ensuring optimal ergonomics and visualization of the ultrasound screen, transducer, and needle's approach (Figs. 11.36 and 11.37).
- Place the ultrasound machine on the opposite side of the table at the level of the patient's knee with the screen facing the provider.

LANDMARKS

- See the landmarks for the landmark-guided injection procedure.

ANESTHESIA

- Local anesthesia of the skin using topical vapocoolant spray.

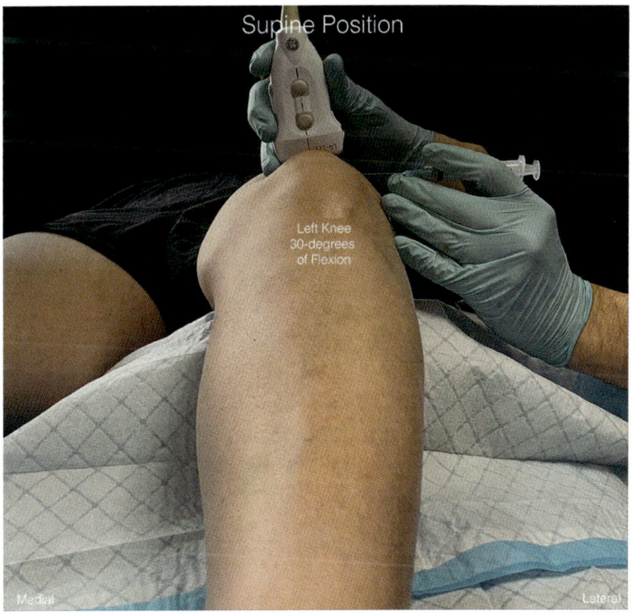

FIGURE 11.36 • Ultrasound-guided left knee injection. Supine position with the affected knee resting at 30° on the examination table. Feet positioned at the bottom of the image. Provider positioned ipsilaterally at the injection site.

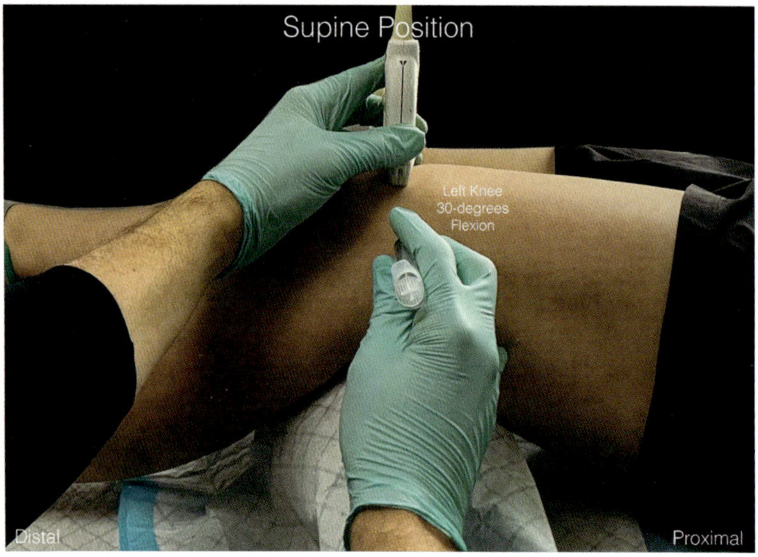

FIGURE 11.37 ● Ultrasound-guided left knee injection. Supine position with the affected knee resting at 30° on the examination table. Feet positioned at the left of the image. Provider positioned ipsilaterally at the injection site.

EQUIPMENT

- 3-mL syringe
- 25-gauge 1.5-in needle (adjust needle length as needed)
- 1 mL of 1% mepivacaine without epinephrine
- 1 mL of 40 mg/mL triamcinolone acetonide
- Alternative setup for aspiration
  - 5-mL syringe (anesthesia)
    - 25-gauge 1.5-in needle (adjust needle length as needed)
    - 5 mL of 1% lidocaine without epinephrine
  - 50-mL syringe (aspiration)
    - 18-gauge 1.5-in needle (adjust needle length as needed)
- Three chlorhexidine swabs
- 12-4 MHz linear ultrasound transducer and machine
- Sterile ultrasound transducer cover
- Sterile ultrasound gel
- Nonlatex sterile or nonsterile gloves
- Two 4 × 4 sterile gauze pads
- One sterile adhesive bandage
- Topical vapocoolant spray

TECHNIQUE

1. Position a high-frequency linear 12-4 MHz ultrasound transducer in an axial plane 1 cm proximal to the superior pole of the patella with the suprapatellar recess centered beneath it.
2. Advance a 25-gauge 1.5-in needle using an in-plane approach, directing it from lateral to medial, with an initial needle angle of approximately 0° to 15° relative to the skin surface where the transducer is positioned.

3. The target area is the suprapatellar recess.
4. Utilize real-time ultrasound guidance throughout the procedure to precisely place the needle within the desired target area and minimize the risk of inadvertently injuring surrounding structures (Figs. 11.38 and 11.39).
5. For intra-articular steroid injection:
   a. Slowly inject the desired volume of mepivacaine and corticosteroid solution directly into the joint.
6. For situations requiring anesthesia, aspiration, or both:
   a. Utilize a separate 25-gauge 1.5-in needle with a 5-mL syringe to inject 5 mL of 1% lidocaine without epinephrine into the soft tissues overlying the joint.
   b. For aspiration, use an 18-gauge 1.5-in needle with a 50-mL syringe to withdraw the effusion.
   c. If a steroid injection is indicated following aspiration, replace the aspiration syringe with the mepivacaine and corticosteroid solution syringe and reconfirm accurate needle placement using real-time ultrasound guidance before injection.

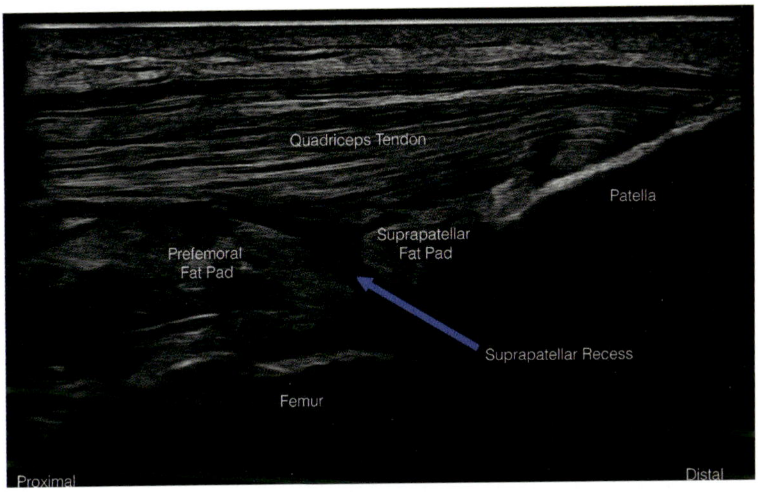

FIGURE 11.38 • Knee ultrasound image—sagittal.

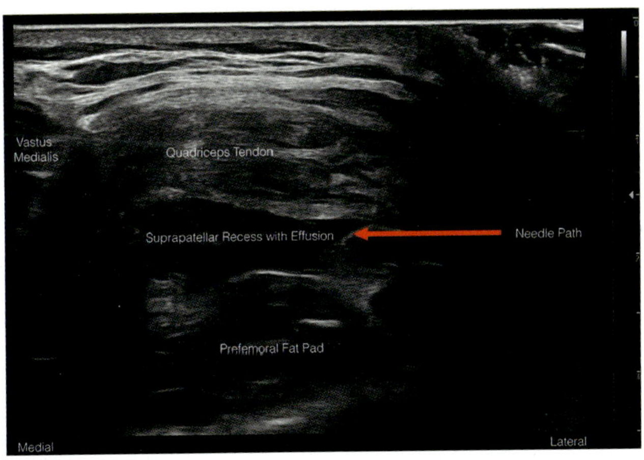

FIGURE 11.39 • Knee ultrasound image—axial.

7. Upon completion of the procedure, carefully withdraw the needle. Adhere to established postprocedure care protocols and ensure appropriate follow-up as recommended.

PEARLS

- Consider a longer needle (eg, 2 in, 25 gauge).
- To improve suprapatellar recess visualization, position the transducer in long axis to the quadriceps tendon (sagittal plane) and instruct the patient to actively extend the knee. Alternatively, push on the quadriceps tendon and suprapatellar fat pad from the medial aspect of the knee while the ultrasound is in short axis (axial plane) to the quadriceps tendon. Both maneuvers may improve visualization by demonstrating the sliding motion between the prefemoral and suprapatellar fat pads. The layer between these two fat pads is the suprapatellar recess.
- Observe for distention of the joint capsule during injection to confirm intra-articular placement.
- Exercise caution to avoid inadvertent penetration of the quadriceps tendon during needle advancement.

Videos showing landmark-guided and ultrasound-guided knee joint aspirations and injections utilizing the preferred lateral suprapatellar approach can be found in the companion eBook.

REFERENCE

1. Uryasev O, Joseph OC, McNamara JP, Dallas AP. Novel joint cupping clinical maneuver for ultrasonographic detection of knee joint effusions. *Am J Emerg Med.* 2013;31(11):1598-1600.

Knee Joint—Lateral Midpatellar Approach

The supine, landmark-guided, extended-leg, lateral midpatellar approach to the knee joint is relatively easy to perform and is well accepted by patients. As noted previously, a landmark-guided injection through this portal has a high likelihood of success. Because of supine positioning, patients may not see the approaching needle and anxiety is diminished. This approach is considered a safe procedure since there are no major arteries or nerves in the immediate path of the needle. Since the needle tip may come into contact with the lateral aspect of the patellar cartilage, direct articular trauma may result, but this is usually lateral to the appositional joint surface and should not be clinically significant. With the use of local anesthetic, this injection can help the clinician differentiate the etiology of knee pain. After pain has been eliminated as a confounding factor, the knee can be reexamined to assess structural integrity of the ligaments and menisci.

Relevant Anatomy: (see Fig. 11.40)

PATIENT POSITION

- Lying supine on the examination table with the knee extended, or slightly flexed and supported with a pillow or folded chucks pads as needed for patient comfort.
- Rotate the patient's head away from the side that is being injected. This minimizes anxiety and pain perception.

LANDMARKS

1. With the patient lying supine on the examination table, the clinician stands lateral to the affected knee.
2. Locate the lateral aspect of the patella.
3. Have the patient relax the quadriceps muscles; then, apply pressure to the medial aspect of the patella in order to displace it laterally.
4. Identify the sulcus at the midpatella that develops between the lateral undersurface of the patella and the lateral femoral condyle (Fig. 11.41).
5. At that site, press firmly on the skin with the retracted tip of a ballpoint pen. This indentation represents the entry point for the needle.
6. After this landmark is identified, the patient should not move the knee.

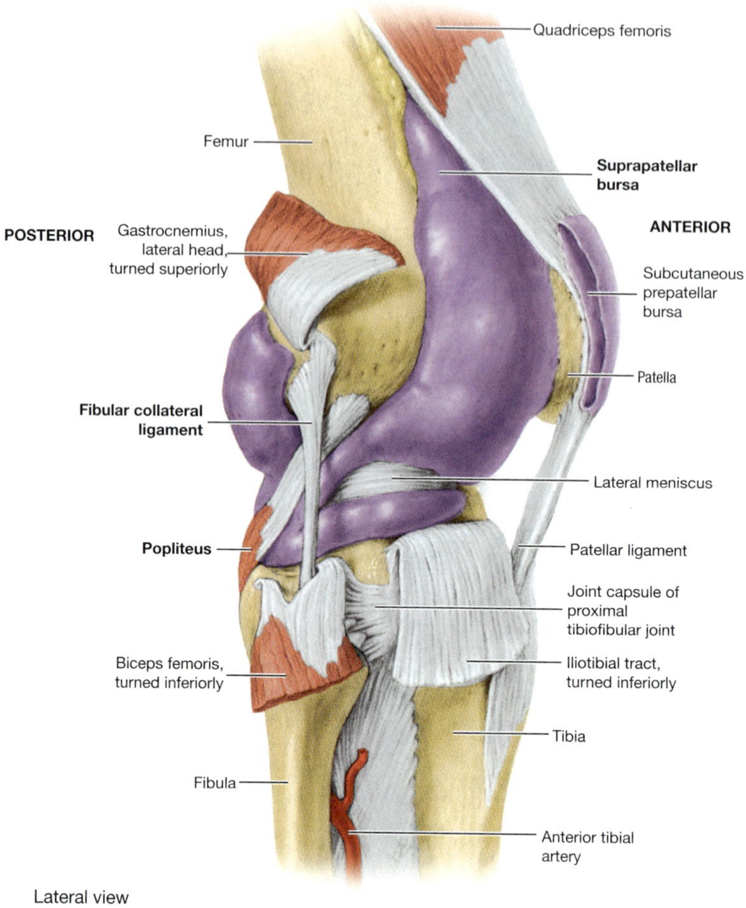

FIGURE 11.40 ● Lateral aspect of the right knee showing the extent of the knee joint capsule. (Reprinted with permission from Agur AMR, Dalley AF II. *Grant's Atlas of Anatomy*. 16th ed. Wolters Kluwer; 2025.)

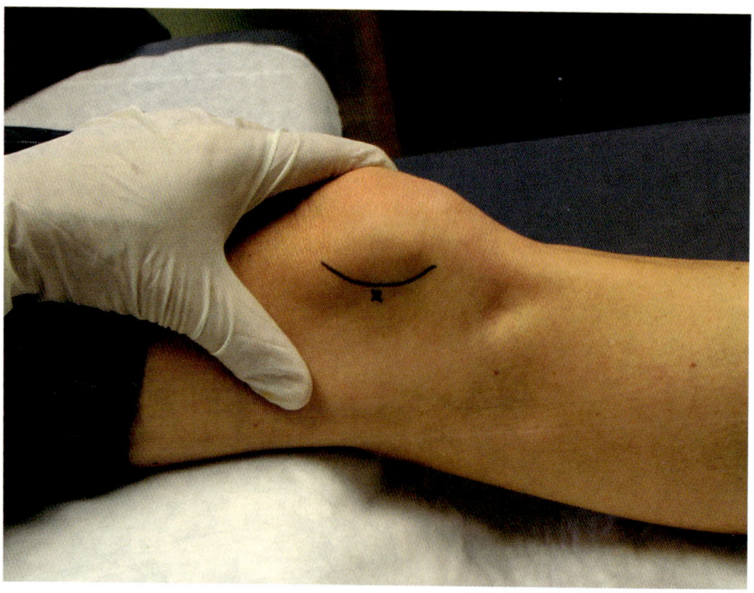

FIGURE 11.41 ● Lateral aspect of the right knee with patella outlined and injection site drawn.

ANESTHESIA

- Local anesthesia of the skin using topical vapocoolant spray.
- (Optional) Local anesthesia and vasoconstriction of the skin and soft tissues may be augmented using an injection of 2 to 4 mL of 1% lidocaine with epinephrine (see Pearls).

EQUIPMENT

- Topical vapocoolant spray
- 3-mL syringe—for injection of the mepivacaine/corticosteroid mixture
- 25-gauge 1½ in needle—for direct injection of the mepivacaine/corticosteroid mixture
- (Optional) 10- to 60-mL syringe(s)—for aspiration
- (Optional) 5-mL syringe—for injection of 1% lidocaine with epinephrine to provide augmented local tissue anesthesia
- (Optional) 25-gauge 1-in needle—for injection of 1% lidocaine with epinephrine to provide local tissue anesthesia—in preparation for an 18-gauge needle
- (Optional) 18-gauge 1½-in needle—for aspiration
- (Optional) 2 to 4 mL of 1% lidocaine with epinephrine—for local tissue anesthesia of skin and knee joint capsule—in preparation for an 18-gauge needle
- 1 mL of 1% mepivacaine without epinephrine—to dilute the corticosteroid
- 1 mL of the corticosteroid solution (40 mg of triamcinolone acetonide)
- (Optional) Viscosupplementation agent of choice—if indicated
- One alcohol prep pad
- Two povidone-iodine or chlorhexidine prep pads
- Sterile gauze pads
- Sterile adhesive bandage
- Nonsterile, clean chucks pad

TECHNIQUE

1. (Optional) Use ultrasound to image the knee joint structures using an adjacent, but separate, acoustic window. This allows separate imaging from the injection site so that there is no contamination from the ultrasound gel. Alternatively, the entire site may be prepped in an aseptic manner and sterile ultrasound gel utilized.
2. Create an aseptic insertion site by wiping with a single alcohol prep pad followed by two 10% povidone-iodine or chlorhexidine prep pads. Allow this site to completely dry by evaporation.
3. Have the patient relax the quadriceps muscles; then, have an assistant apply pressure to the medial aspect of the patella in order to displace it laterally.
4. If significant intra-articular fluid accumulation is not suspected, or not seen on ultrasound examination, then proceed with direct injection of the mepivacaine/corticosteroid solution (step 5). If fluid is suspected or confirmed on ultrasound, proceed to step 11.
5. Achieve good local anesthesia by using topical vapocoolant spray.
6. Position the 25-gauge 1½-in needle and syringe perpendicularly to the skin, parallel to the floor, at a right angle to the other two previously drawn skin lines, and with the tip of the needle directed medially.
7. Using the aseptic, no-touch technique, quickly introduce that needle at the insertion site (Fig. 11.42).

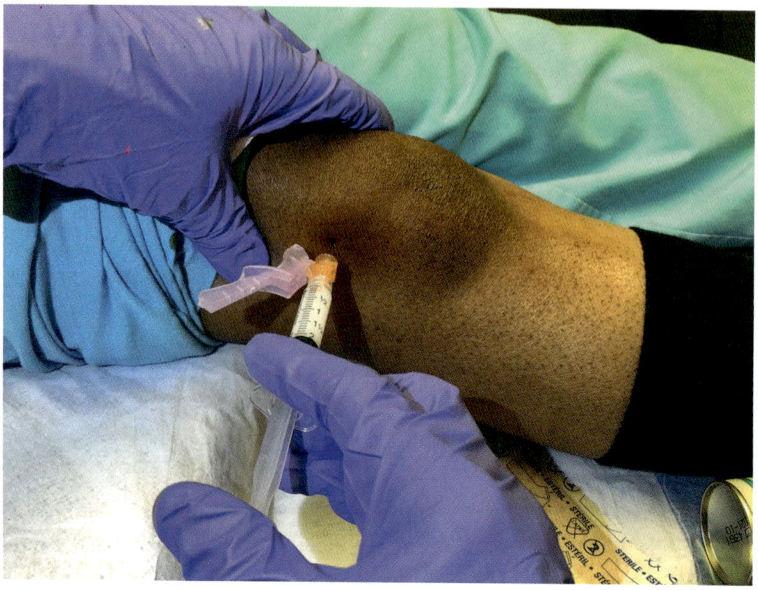

FIGURE 11.42 ● Right knee injection using the lateral midpatellar approach.

8. Advance the 25-gauge 1½-in needle medially underneath the patella and over the lateral femoral condyle until the needle tip is located within the joint capsule in the patellofemoral articulation.
9. Withdraw the plunger of the syringe to ensure that there is no blood return.
10. Inject the mepivacaine/corticosteroid solution as a bolus into the knee joint. The injected solution should flow smoothly into the joint space. If increased resistance is encountered, advance or withdraw the needle slightly before attempting further injection. Proceed to step 19.
11. (Optional) Achieve good local anesthesia by using topical vapocoolant spray.
12. Using the no-touch technique, introduce the 25-gauge 1-in needle for local anesthesia at the insertion site. Inject 2 to 4 mL of 1% lidocaine with epinephrine to provide adequate local anesthesia. Infuse the anesthetic under the skin and at the joint capsule.
13. Position the 18-gauge 1½-in needle and syringe perpendicularly to the skin, parallel to the floor, at a right angle to the other two previously drawn skin lines and with the tip of the needle directed medially.
14. Using the aseptic, no-touch technique, quickly introduce that needle at the insertion site (Fig. 11.42).
15. Advance the 18-gauge 1½-in needle medially underneath the patella and over the lateral femoral condyle until the needle tip is located within the joint capsule in the patellofemoral articulation. Apply suction to the syringe while advancing the needle. The appearance of fluid in the syringe confirms that the joint capsule has been entered. If fluid is aspirated, stop advancing the needle.
16. Multiple syringes may be required in order to drain all of the synovial fluid if a large effusion is present.
17. If injection following aspiration is elected, remove the large syringe from the 18-gauge needle and then attach the 3-mL syringe filled with the mepivacaine/corticosteroid solution or a proprietary glass syringe prefilled with viscosupplement.
18. Inject the mepivacaine/corticosteroid solution or viscosupplement as a bolus into the knee joint. The injected solution should flow smoothly into the joint space.

If increased resistance is encountered, advance or withdraw the needle slightly, and confirm aspiration of a small amount of joint fluid before attempting further injection.

19. Following injection, withdraw the needle.
20. Apply a sterile adhesive bandage.
21. Instruct the patient to move their knee through its full range of motion. This movement distributes the mepivacaine/corticosteroid solution or viscosupplement throughout the knee joint.
22. Reexamine the knee in 5 minutes to assess pain relief.

AFTERCARE

- Avoid more than light use of the affected knee over the next 2 weeks.
- Use other complementary treatment modalities including physical therapy as indicated.
- Consider follow-up examination in 2 weeks.

PEARLS

- Although both the lateral and medial midpatellar approaches may be used, the preferred approach is from the lateral aspect. This approach affords the operator more room, avoids inadvertent kicking of the clinician by the patient with the uninvolved leg, and preserves patient modesty.
- Usually, this procedure can be conducted in a pain-free manner with the use of topical vapocoolant spray. However, an occasional patient may complain of pain when the 18-gauge needle is advanced into contact with the joint capsule. In this case, that needle should be withdrawn and a 1-in 25-gauge needle advanced in the same direction. A total of 2 to 4 mL of 1% lidocaine with epinephrine is deposited under the skin and in the soft tissue at the joint capsule.
- If the clinician encounters the unusual situation of experiencing difficulty finding the joint capsule, then either of the following maneuvers can be attempted:
  - Firmly squeeze the anterodistal aspect of the patella and displace it posteriorly and proximally (the "cupping" maneuver) thereby shifting the joint fluid and filling the suprapatellar pouch.[1]
  - Abandon this approach and use the lateral suprapatellar portal.
  - Utilize ultrasound guidance for the aspiration/injection procedure—also using the lateral suprapatellar approach.
- Ultrasound-guided aspiration and injection are indicated when an effusion is not detected or in a very obese patient. Ultrasound is also very useful in locating fluid in the knee joint to ensure placement accuracy when injecting expensive viscosupplement products (Fig. 11.43).
- Ultrasound-guided aspiration and injection are technically quite difficult for this approach. Thus, if ultrasound guidance is desired, then utilize the lateral suprapatellar approach.

ULTRASOUND-GUIDED PROCEDURE

Please refer to the introductory ultrasound chapter for preprocedure, sterile prep, post-procedure, and documentation information and recommendations.

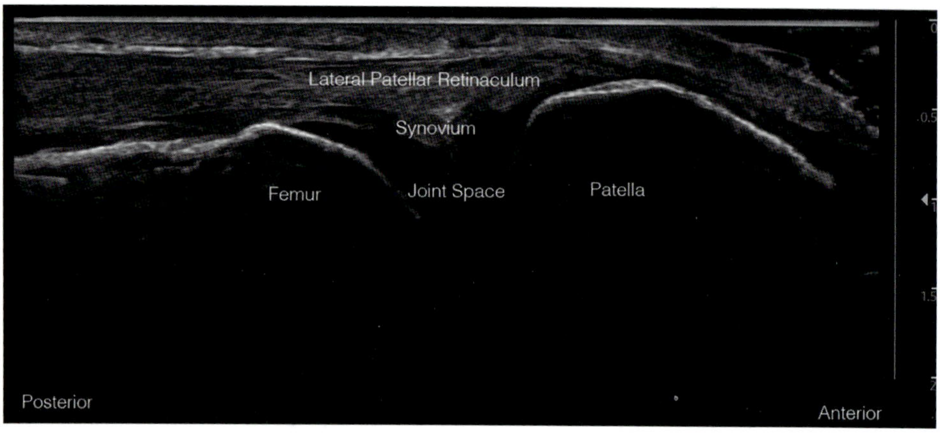

FIGURE 11.43 ● Knee—lateral midpatellar ultrasound image.

A video showing a landmark-guided knee joint aspiration and injection utilizing the lateral midpatellar approach can be found in the companion eBook.

REFERENCE

1. Uryasev O, Joseph OC, McNamara JP, Dallas AP. Novel joint cupping clinical maneuver for ultrasonographic detection of knee joint effusions. *Am J Emerg Med.* 2013;31(11):1598-1600.

Knee Joint—Anteromedial and Anterolateral Approaches

The infrapatellar anteromedial and anterolateral approaches to the knee joint are more difficult to successfully perform than the extended-leg lateral approaches using landmark-guided injection technique. They are also less well accepted by patients since they are usually performed with patients sitting where they can see the approaching needle. There may be increased anxiety with these procedures, and the patients are at increased risk of injury if they develop a vasovagal reaction and fall from the examination table. Alternatively, the patient may be placed supine with hip and knee flexion so the plantar aspect of the foot contacts the examination tabletop. Since these injections are intra-articular, the knee cartilage over the distal femur may suffer direct damage from gouging by an aggressively placed 18-gauge needle. For these reasons, and documented lower success rates as compared to the extended-leg approaches, the anteromedial and anterolateral techniques are considered secondary options. However, they represent a valuable alternative technique in patients who are confined to a wheelchair and in those who cannot be easily moved up onto an examination table.

Unfortunately, direct visualization by ultrasound is not possible with this injection approach.

Relevant Anatomy: (see Fig. 11.40)

- See previous chapter.

PATIENT POSITION

- Sitting on the examination table with the affected knee flexed at an angle of 90°.
- Alternatively, the patient may be sitting in a wheelchair or side chair or even lying supine on the examination table with both knees flexed at 90°.
- Rotate the patient's head away from the side that is being injected. This may minimize anxiety and pain perception.

LANDMARKS

1. With the patient sitting up on the examination table or in a chair, the clinician sits on an examination stool in front of the affected knee.
2. With the patient lying supine on the examination table, the clinician stands medial or lateral to the affected knee.
3. Palpate the anterior aspect of the knee to locate the patellar tendon.
4. At the midpoint of the tendon, move about 2 cm medially or laterally. There is usually a soft depression at that spot. Mark it with ink.

5. At that site, press firmly on the skin with the retracted tip of a ballpoint pen. This indentation represents the entry point for the needle.
6. After the landmarks are identified, the patient should not move the knee (Fig. 11.44A and B).

ANESTHESIA

- Local anesthesia of the skin using topical vapocoolant spray.
- (Optional) Local anesthesia and vasoconstriction of the skin and soft tissues may be augmented using an injection of 2 to 4 mL of 1% lidocaine with epinephrine (see "Pearls").

A

B

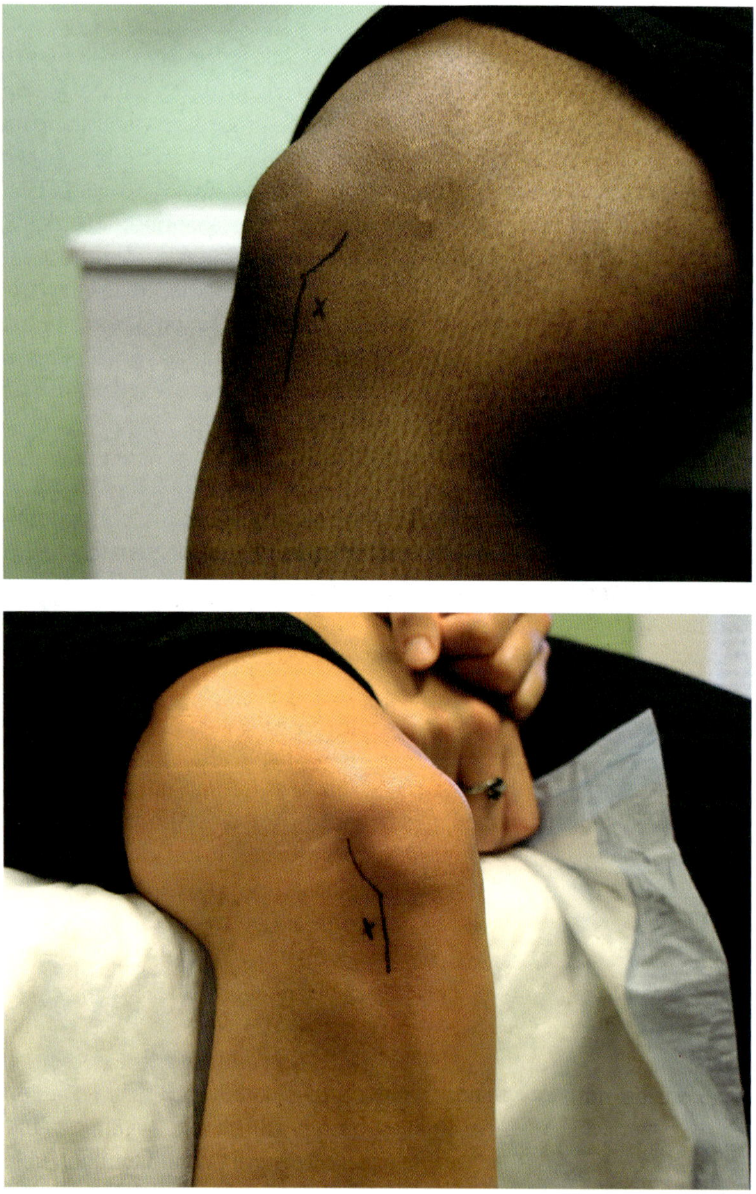

FIGURE 11.44 ● **A.** Anteromedial aspect of the right knee with injection sites drawn. **B.** Anterolateral aspect of the right knee with injection sites drawn.

EQUIPMENT

- Topical vapocoolant spray
- 3-mL syringe—for injection of the mepivacaine/corticosteroid mixture
- 25-gauge 2-in needle—for direct injection of the mepivacaine/corticosteroid mixture
- (Optional) 10- to 60-mL syringe(s)—for aspiration
- (Optional) 5-mL syringe—for injection of 1% lidocaine with epinephrine to provide augmented local tissue anesthesia
- (Optional) 25-gauge 1½-in needle—for injection of 1% lidocaine with epinephrine to provide local tissue anesthesia—in preparation for an 18-gauge needle
- (Optional) 18-gauge 1½-in needle—for aspiration
- (Optional) 2 to 4 mL of 1% lidocaine with epinephrine—for local tissue anesthesia of skin and knee joint capsule—in preparation for an 18-gauge needle
- 1 mL of 1% mepivacaine without epinephrine—to dilute the corticosteroid
- 1 mL of the corticosteroid solution (40 mg of triamcinolone acetonide)
- (Optional) Viscosupplementation agent of choice—if indicated
- One alcohol prep pad
- Two povidone-iodine or chlorhexidine prep pads
- Sterile gauze pads
- Sterile adhesive bandage
- Nonsterile, clean chucks pad

TECHNIQUE

1. (Optional) Use ultrasound to image the knee joint structures using an adjacent, but separate, acoustic window. This allows separate imaging from the injection site so that there is no contamination from the ultrasound gel. Alternatively, the entire site may be prepped in an aseptic manner and sterile ultrasound gel utilized.
2. Create an aseptic insertion site by wiping with a single alcohol prep pad followed by two 10% povidone-iodine or chlorhexidine prep pads. Allow this site to completely dry by evaporation.
3. If significant intra-articular fluid accumulation is not suspected, or not seen on ultrasound examination, then proceed with direct injection of the mepivacaine/corticosteroid solution (step 4). If fluid is suspected or confirmed on ultrasound, proceed to step 10.
4. Achieve good local anesthesia by using topical vapocoolant spray.
5. Position the 25-gauge 2-in needle and syringe perpendicularly to the skin, parallel to the floor, with the tip of the needle directed at a 45° angle into the center of the knee (Fig. 11.45A and B).
6. Using the aseptic, no-touch technique, quickly introduce that needle at the insertion site.
7. Advance the 25-gauge 2-in needle toward the center of the knee until the needle tip is located in the joint capsule or contacts the cartilage over the distal femur deep in center of the knee joint.
8. Withdraw the plunger of the syringe to ensure that there is no blood return.
9. Inject the mepivacaine/corticosteroid solution as a bolus into the knee joint. The injected solution should flow smoothly into the joint space. If increased resistance is encountered, advance or withdraw the needle slightly before attempting further injection (proceed to step 18).

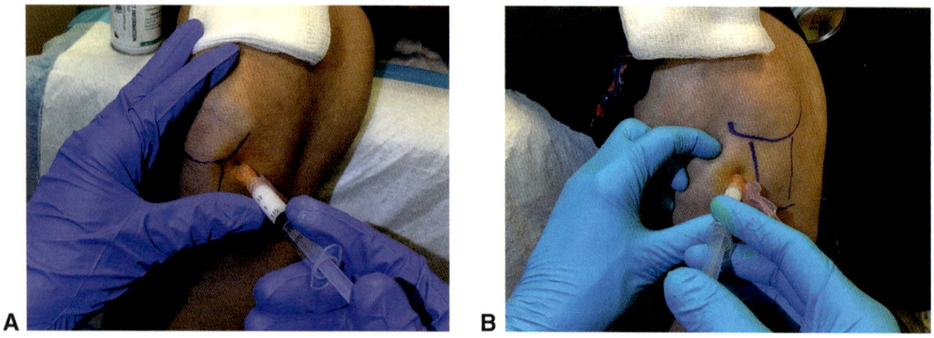

FIGURE 11.45 ● **A.** Right knee injection using the anteromedial approach. **B.** Right knee injection using the anterolateral approach.

10. (Optional) Achieve good local anesthesia by using topical vapocoolant spray.
11. Using the no-touch technique, introduce the 25-gauge, 1½-in needle for local anesthesia at the insertion site. Inject 2 to 4 mL of 1% lidocaine with epinephrine to provide adequate local anesthesia. Infuse the anesthetic under the skin and at the joint capsule.
12. Position the 18-gauge 1½-in needle and syringe perpendicularly to the skin, parallel to the floor, with the tip of the needle directed at a 45° angle into the center of the knee.
13. Using the aseptic, no-touch technique, quickly introduce that needle at the insertion site.
14. Advance the 18-gauge 1½-in needle toward the center of the knee until the needle tip is located in the joint capsule or contacts the cartilage over the distal femur deep in center of the knee joint. Apply suction to the syringe while advancing the needle. The appearance of fluid in the syringe confirms that the joint capsule has been entered. If fluid is aspirated, stop advancing the needle.
15. Multiple syringes may be required to drain all of the synovial fluid if a large effusion is present.
16. If injection following aspiration is elected, remove the large syringe from the 18-gauge needle and then attach the 3-mL syringe filled with the mepivacaine/corticosteroid solution or a proprietary glass syringe prefilled with viscosupplement.
17. Inject the mepivacaine/corticosteroid solution or viscosupplement as a bolus into the knee joint. The injected solution should flow smoothly into the joint space. If increased resistance is encountered, advance or withdraw the needle slightly, and confirm aspiration of a small amount of joint fluid before attempting further injection.
18. Following injection, withdraw the needle.
19. Apply a sterile adhesive bandage.
20. Instruct the patient to move their knee through its full range of motion. This movement distributes the mepivacaine/corticosteroid solution throughout the knee joint.
21. Reexamine the knee in 5 minutes to assess pain relief.

AFTERCARE

- Avoid more than light use of the affected knee over the next 2 weeks.
- Use other complementary treatment modalities including physical therapy as indicated.
- Consider follow-up examination in 2 weeks.

PEARLS

- Because of potential direct needle injury to articular cartilage and documented decreased success rates, the landmark-guided medial and lateral infrapatellar approaches should only be used in special circumstances where the lateral suprapatellar and midpatellar approaches cannot be performed. This may occur in patients with local cellulitis or soft tissue injury, or in a patient confined to a wheelchair who cannot be easily moved onto an examination table.
- Ultrasound-guided aspiration and injection are not possible unless using an indirect technique. Thus, ultrasound guidance for these approaches is not recommended.

Videos showing landmark-guided anteromedial and anterolateral knee joint injections can be found in the companion eBook.

Knee Joint—Popliteal Synovial (Baker) Cyst

A popliteal synovial (Baker) cyst is a fluid- and fibrin-filled structure over the posterior aspect of the knee. It is an uncommon presentation in a primary care medical office. This structure forms when an excessive amount of synovial fluid is produced in the knee joint, usually as a result of osteoarthritis. Other associated conditions include inflammatory synovitis and meniscal tears. Fluid pressure causes the gradual formation of a synovial outpouching in the medial inferior aspect of the popliteal fossa in an area of relative weakness located in the gastrocnemio-semimembranosus bursa.[1] The cyst communicates with the knee joint via a slender neck that functions as a one-way check valve. Baker cysts typically present as an enlarging cystic structure over the posterior aspect of the knee that may be tender, cause lower leg swelling, or limit full flexion of the knee.

Popliteal synovial cysts may be effectively treated with aspiration and corticosteroid injection. Caution is advised when performing large-diameter needle-based procedures in the popliteal area due to the presence of the popliteal artery, popliteal vein, and the tibial nerve running longitudinally in the center of this area. Care must be taken to direct the needle anterior-medially and away from these critical structures. For this reason, ultrasound guidance is recommended.

Treatment of symptomatic cysts can be done by direct aspiration of the fluid contents combined with corticosteroid injection either into the cyst[2-4] or separately into the knee joint.[5] Needle fenestration has also shown benefit.[6] The aspiration and injection procedures are augmented when combined with physical therapy.[7] Ultrasound guidance enhances safety, accuracy, and favorably affects the treatment outcomes of pain and disability.[8,9] Patients who fail conservative management (usually because of the presence of a complex vs simple cyst) may be referred for surgical excision.

Relevant Anatomy: (Fig. 11.46)

PATIENT POSITION

- Lying prone on the examination table with the knee extended.

LANDMARKS

1. With the patient lying prone on the examination table, the clinician stands lateral to the affected knee.
2. Locate the most prominent aspect of the popliteal cyst that is located over the medial inferior aspect of the popliteal space.
3. At that site, press firmly on the skin with the retracted tip of a ballpoint pen. This indentation represents the entry point for the needle.
4. After the landmarks are identified, the patient should not move the knee.

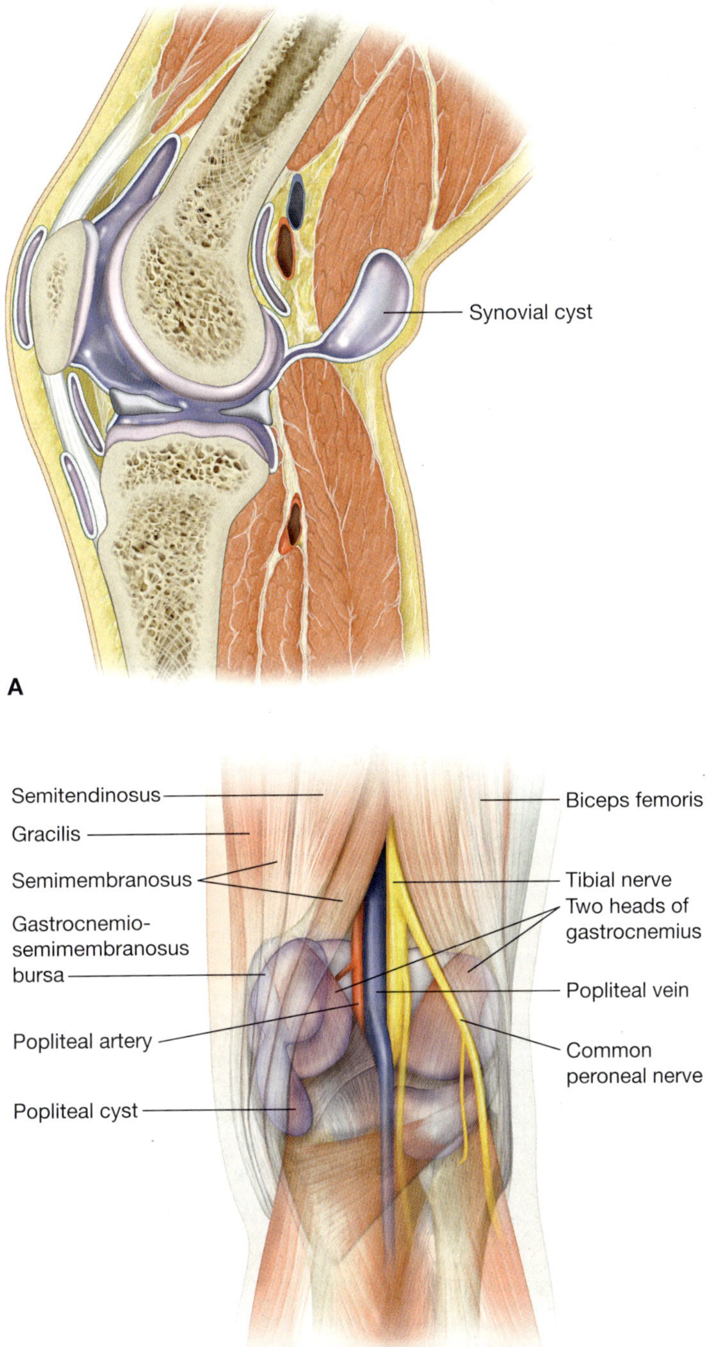

FIGURE 11.46 ● **A.** Popliteal anatomy—sagittal. **B.** Popliteal anatomy—coronal—with location of the gastrocnemio-semimembranosus bursa marked.

ANESTHESIA

- Local anesthesia of the skin using topical vapocoolant spray.

EQUIPMENT

- Topical vapocoolant spray
- 10- to 20-mL syringe—for aspiration
- 18-gauge 1½-in needle—for aspiration of the Baker cyst
- 3-mL syringe—for injection of the mepivacaine/corticosteroid mixture
- 1 mL of 1% mepivacaine without epinephrine—to dilute the corticosteroid
- 1 mL of the corticosteroid solution (40 mg of triamcinolone acetonide)
- One alcohol prep pad
- Two povidone-iodine or chlorhexidine prep pads
- Sterile gauze pads
- Sterile adhesive bandage
- Nonsterile, clean chucks pad

TECHNIQUE

1. (Optional) Use ultrasound to image the posterior knee joint structures (see Ultrasound-Guided Procedure section).
2. Create an aseptic insertion site by wiping with a single alcohol prep pad followed by two 10% povidone-iodine or chlorhexidine prep pads. Allow this site to completely dry by evaporation.
3. Achieve good local anesthesia by using topical vapocoolant spray.
4. Position the 18-gauge 1½-in needle and syringe perpendicularly to the skin and with the tip of the needle directed anterior-medially.
5. Using the aseptic, no-touch technique, quickly introduce that needle at the insertion site (Fig. 11.47).

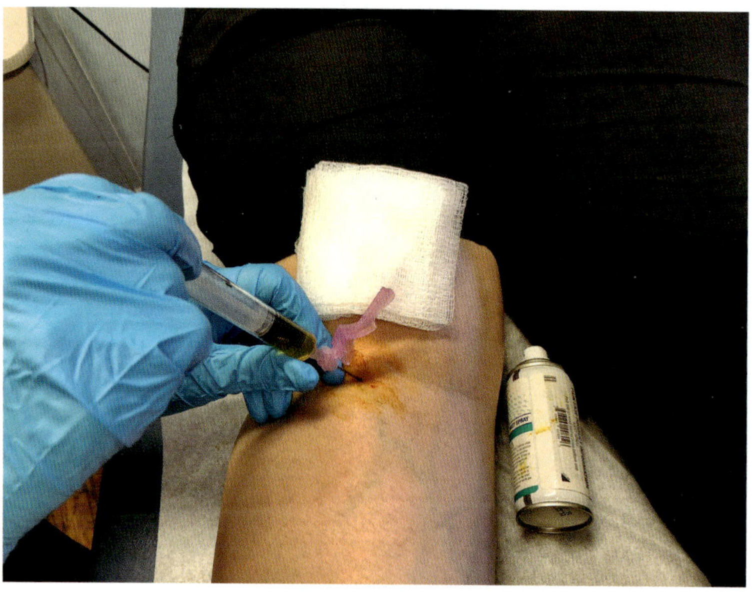

FIGURE 11.47 ● Baker cyst aspiration.

6. While withdrawing the plunger of the syringe, advance the needle into the popliteal synovial cyst.
7. Stop the advancement when clear fluid is aspirated. Then completely aspirate the cyst contents.
8. Next, remove the large syringe from the 18-gauge needle and then attach the 3-mL syringe filled with the mepivacaine/corticosteroid solution.
9. Inject the mepivacaine/corticosteroid solution as a bolus into the cyst. The injected solution should flow smoothly into the joint space. If increased resistance is encountered, advance or withdraw the needle slightly.
10. Following injection, withdraw the needle.
11. Apply a sterile adhesive bandage.
12. Instruct the patient to move their knee through its full range of motion. This movement distributes the mepivacaine/corticosteroid solution throughout the synovial cyst.
13. Reexamine the knee in 5 minutes to assess pain relief.

AFTERCARE

- Avoid more than light use of the affected knee over the next 2 weeks.
- Use other complementary treatment modalities including physical therapy as indicated.
- Consider follow-up examination in 2 weeks.

PEARLS

- Be very careful to avoid inadvertent injury to the popliteal artery, popliteal vein, and the tibial nerve running longitudinally in the center of the popliteal space.
- Direct the needle anterior-medially and away from these critical structures.
- Ultrasound-guided aspiration and injection are recommended to guide needle placement and ensure safety of this procedure.

ULTRASOUND-GUIDED PROCEDURE

Please refer to the introductory ultrasound chapter for preprocedure, sterile prep, post-procedure, and documentation information and recommendations.

PATIENT POSITION

- Prone on the examination table.
- On the affected side, place the hip and knee in a neutral position resting on the examination table with the patient's feet off the end of the table.
- Place a pillow under their head for comfort.
- Adjust the patient's position as needed to ensure comfort.

PROVIDER/ULTRASOUND POSITION

- The provider sits on the same side of the table as the affected knee.
- Adjust the examination table to position the injection site between the provider's umbilicus and axillary level, ensuring optimal ergonomics and visualization of the ultrasound screen, transducer, and needle's approach (Fig. 11.48).
- Place the ultrasound machine on the opposite side of the table from at the level of the patient's head with the screen facing the provider.

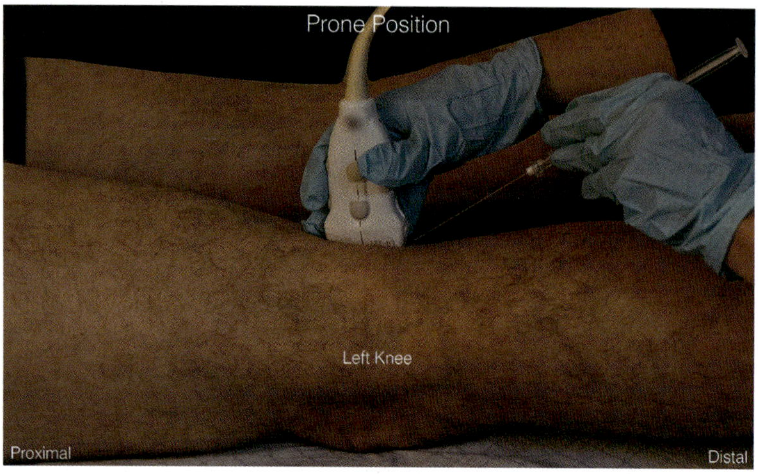

FIGURE 11.48 ● Ultrasound-guided left-sided Baker cyst injection. Prone position with their affected knee resting on the examination table. Feet positioned at the right of the image. Provider positioned ipsilaterally distal to the injection site.

LANDMARKS

- See the landmarks for the landmark-guided injection procedure.

ANESTHESIA

- Local anesthesia of the skin using topical vapocoolant spray.

EQUIPMENT

- 3-mL syringe
- 22-gauge 3.5-in needle (adjust needle length as needed)
- 1 mL of 1% mepivacaine without epinephrine
- 1 mL of 40 mg/mL triamcinolone acetonide
- Alternative setup for aspiration
  - 5-mL syringe (anesthesia)
    - 22-gauge 3.5-in needle (adjust needle length as needed)
    - 5 mL of 1% lidocaine without epinephrine
  - 50-mL syringe
    - 18-gauge 3.5-in needle (adjust needle length as needed)
- Three chlorhexidine swabs
- 12-4 MHz linear ultrasound transducer and machine
- Sterile ultrasound transducer cover
- Nonlatex sterile or nonsterile gloves
- Two 4 × 4 sterile gauze pads
- One sterile adhesive bandage
- Topical vapocoolant spray

TECHNIQUE

1. Position a high-frequency linear 12-4 MHz ultrasound transducer in the sagittal plane with the Baker cyst centered underneath it.

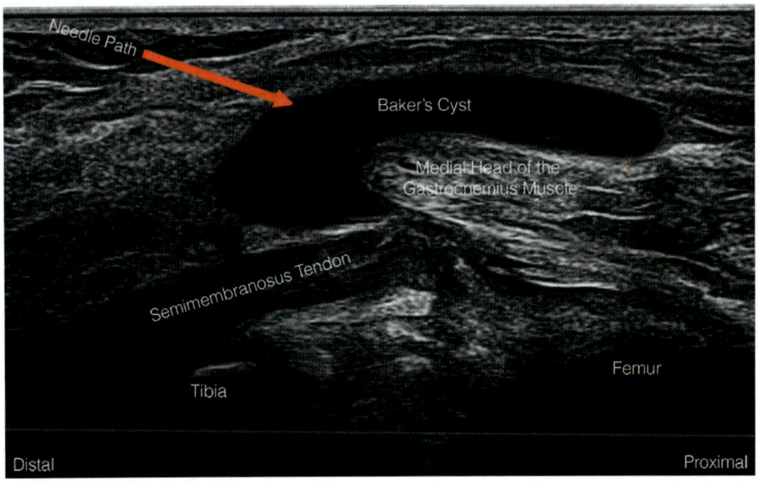

FIGURE 11.49 ● Baker cyst ultrasound image.

2. Using an in-plane approach, insert a 22-gauge 3.5-in needle at the center of the transducer at approximately a 30° to 45° angle, directing it distal to proximal.
3. The target area is the Baker cyst.
4. Utilize real-time ultrasound guidance throughout the procedure to precisely place the needle within the desired target area and minimize the risk of inadvertently injuring surrounding structures (Fig. 11.49).
5. For steroid injection:
   a. Slowly inject the desired volume of mepivacaine and corticosteroid solution directly into the cyst.
6. For situations requiring anesthesia, aspiration, or both:
   a. Utilize a separate 22-gauge 3.5-in needle with a 5-mL syringe to inject 5 mL of 1% lidocaine without epinephrine into the soft tissues overlying the joint.
   b. For aspiration, use an 18-gauge 3.5-in needle with a 5-mL syringe to withdraw the effusion.
   c. If injection is indicated following aspiration, replace the aspiration syringe with the mepivacaine and corticosteroid solution syringe and reconfirm accurate needle placement using real-time ultrasound guidance before injection.

PEARLS

- A Baker cyst is positioned between the medial head of the gastrocnemius muscle and the semimembranosus tendon. If other cystic-like structures are identified in the popliteal fossa outside this area, or the structure does not have the appearance of a cyst, consider consultation with orthopedics or vascular to consider other advanced imaging in this area.

A video showing a landmark-guided aspiration can be found in the companion eBook.

REFERENCES

1. Herman AM, Marzo JM. Popliteal cysts: a current review. *Orthopedics.* 2014;37(8):e678-ee84.
2. Köroğlu M, Callıoğlu M, Eriş HN, et al. Ultrasound guided percutaneous treatment and follow-up of Baker's cyst in knee osteoarthritis. *Eur J Radiol.* 2012;81(11):3466-3471.
3. Bandinelli F, Fedi R, Generini S, et al. Longitudinal ultrasound and clinical follow-up of Baker's cysts injection with steroids in knee osteoarthritis. *Clin Rheumatol.* 2012;31(4):727-731.
4. Fredericksen K, Kiel J. Bedside ultrasound-guided aspiration and corticosteroid injection of a Baker's cyst in a patient with osteoarthritis and recurrent knee pain. *J Am Coll Emerg Physicians Open.* 2021;2(2):e12424.
5. Di Sante L, Paoloni M, Ioppolo F, Dimaggio M, Renzo SD, Santilli V. Ultrasound-guided aspiration and corticosteroid injection of Baker's cysts in knee osteoarthritis: a prospective observational study. *Am J Phys Med Rehabil.* 2010;89(12):970-975.
6. Smith MK, Lesniak B, Baraga MG, Kaplan L, Jose J. Treatment of popliteal (Baker) cysts with ultrasound-guided aspiration, fenestration, and injection: long-term follow-up. *Sports Health.* 2015;7(5):409-414.
7. Di Sante L, Paoloni M, Dimaggio M, et al. Ultrasound-guided aspiration and corticosteroid injection compared to horizontal therapy for treatment of knee osteoarthritis complicated with Baker's cyst: a randomized, controlled trial. *Eur J Phys Rehabil Med.* 2012;48(4):561-567.
8. Çağlayan G, Özçakar L, Kaymak SU, Kaymak B. Effects of Sono-feedback during aspiration of Baker's cysts: a controlled clinical trial. *J Rehabil Med.* 2016;48(4):386-389.
9. Stroiescu AE, Laurinkiene J, Courtney K, Moriarty HK, Kelly IP, Ryan AG. Management of symptomatic Baker's cysts with ultrasound and fluoroscopic-guided aspiration followed by therapeutic injection with Depomedrone and Bupivacaine leads to a durable reduction in pain symptoms in a majority of patients: a case series and literature review. *Ulster Med J.* 2023;92(1):24-28.

Prepatellar Bursa

Prepatellar bursitis is a fairly common condition encountered by primary care practitioners. Approximately one-third of cases are septic and two-thirds of cases are nonseptic. General conservative treatment measures consist of bursal aspiration, NSAIDs, and a combination of protection, rest, ice, compression, and elevation. Analysis of the fluid from the bursa is critical to distinguish septic from noninfectious cases. Successful aspiration is usually easily accomplished because the location of bursa is readily evident. Ultrasound guidance of the procedure is usually not needed.

The subcutaneous prepatellar bursa may become inflamed and accumulate fluid when subjected to repeated excessive pressure or friction. A large-diameter needle is selected since the fluid collection may consist of blood in acute trauma, thick proteinaceous mucoid fluid after repetitive injury, or purulence if infected. For patients with confirmed nonseptic bursitis and high athletic or occupational demands, intrabursal corticosteroid injection may be performed. In the case of septic bursitis, antibiotic therapy should be initiated. Surgical treatment, that is, incision, drainage, endoscopic bursectomy, or open bursectomy, should be restricted to severe, refractory, or chronic/recurrent cases.[1,2] Unfortunately, there are no studies found in the peer-reviewed medical literature that address injection treatment.

Relevant Anatomy: (Fig. 11.50)

PATIENT POSITION

- Lying supine on the examination table with the knee extended, or slightly flexed and supported with a pillow or folded chucks pads as needed for patient comfort.
- Rotate the patient's head away from the side that is being injected. This minimizes anxiety and pain perception.

LANDMARKS

1. With the patient lying supine on the examination table, the clinician stands lateral to the affected knee.
2. The point of maximal fluctuance is identified.
3. At that site, press firmly on the skin with the retracted tip of a ballpoint pen. This indentation represents the entry point for the needle.
4. After the landmarks are identified, the patient should not move the knee.

ANESTHESIA

- Local anesthesia of the skin using topical vapocoolant spray.

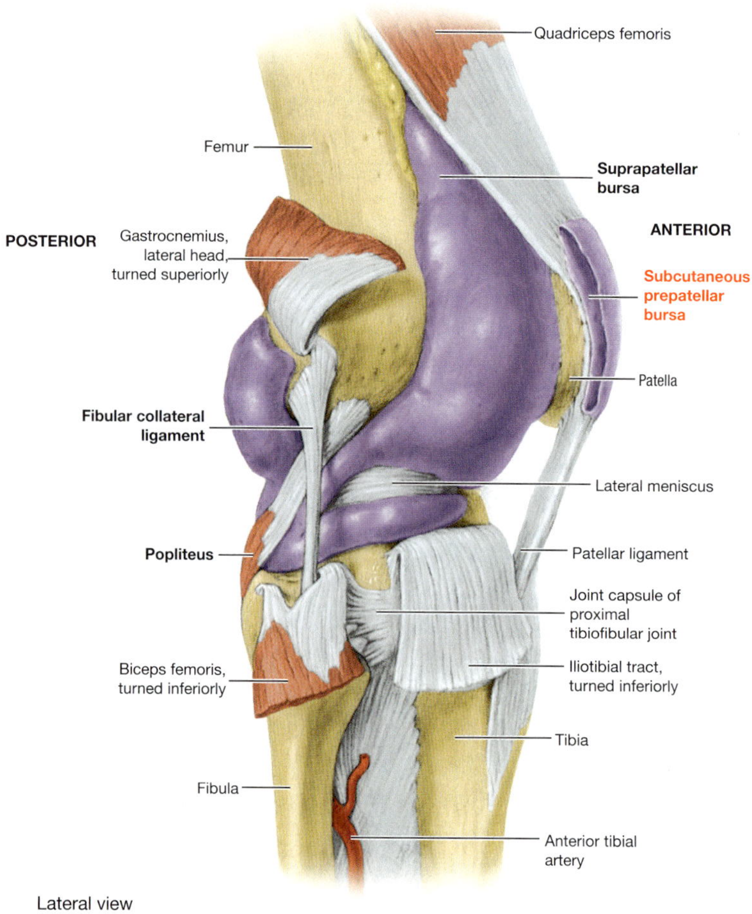

FIGURE 11.50 Lateral aspect of the right knee showing the extent of the knee joint capsule (in *purple*). (Reprinted with permission from Agur AMR, Dalley AF II. *Grant's Atlas of Anatomy*. 16th ed. Wolters Kluwer; 2025.)

EQUIPMENT

- Topical vapocoolant spray
- 20-mL syringe
- 3-mL syringe—for optional injection
- 18-gauge 1½-in needle
- 1 mL of 1% lidocaine without epinephrine—for optional injection
- 1 mL of the steroid solution (40 mg of triamcinolone acetonide)—for optional injection
- One alcohol prep pad
- Two povidone-iodine or chlorhexidine prep pads
- Sterile gauze pads
- Sterile adhesive bandage
- Nonsterile, clean chucks pad

TECHNIQUE

1. Prep the insertion site with alcohol followed by the povidone-iodine or chlorhexidine pads.
2. Achieve good local anesthesia by using topical vapocoolant spray.

3. Stabilize the soft tissues by grasping the bursa firmly with the nondominant hand thumb and index finger. Then, squeeze to compress the fluid accumulation.
4. Position the 18-gauge needle and syringe with the tip of the needle directed toward the center of maximal fluid collection.
5. Using the no-touch technique, quickly introduce the needle at the insertion site (Fig. 11.51).
6. Advance the needle into the center of the bursa.
7. Aspiration should be easily accomplished. Use multiple syringes if the effusion is large.
8. (Optional) If a corticosteroid injection following aspiration is elected, do not remove the needle. Grasp the hub of the 18-gauge needle, remove the large syringe, and then attach the 3-mL syringe filled with the lidocaine/corticosteroid solution.
9. The injected solution should flow smoothly into the space. If increased resistance is encountered, advance or withdraw the needle slightly before attempting further injection.
10. Following completed aspiration, and possible injection, withdraw the needle.
11. Apply a sterile adhesive bandage followed by a compressive elastic bandage.
12. Reexamine the knee in 5 minutes to assess pain relief.

AFTERCARE

- Avoid excessive use of the affected knee over the next 2 weeks.
- Consider the use of a knee compression wrap.
- NSAIDs, and a combination of protection, rest, ice, compression, and elevation as indicated.
- Consider follow-up examination in 2 weeks.

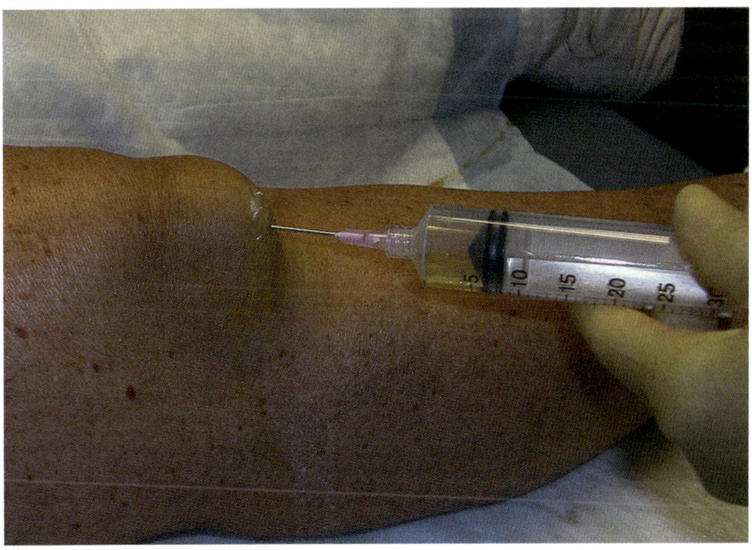

FIGURE 11.51 • Prepatellar bursitis aspiration.

PEARLS

- If the prepatellar bursitis is due to an infection or acute hemorrhagic event, do not follow aspiration with corticosteroid injection.
- Injection of corticosteroid solution is usually reserved for recurrent bursitis.

A video showing a landmark-guided prepatellar bursitis aspiration can be found in the companion eBook.

REFERENCES

1. Baumbach SF, Lobo CM, Badyine I, Mutschler W, Kanz K-G. Prepatellar and olecranon bursitis: literature review and development of a treatment algorithm. *Arch Orthop Trauma Surg.* 2014;134(3):359-370.
2. Brown OS, Smith TO, Parsons T, Benjamin M, Hing CB. Management of septic and aseptic prepatellar bursitis: a systematic review. *Arch Orthop Trauma Surg.* 2022;142(10):2445-2457.

Patellar Tendon

Patients occasionally present to the primary care office for the evaluation and treatment of pain over the patellar tendon. This tendon connects the patella and therefore the quadriceps muscles to the anterior, proximal tibia at the tibial tubercle. The usual inciting factor is chronic overuse (primarily repetitive jumping) that causes tendonitis, tendinopathy, or disruption of the patellar tendon. Predisposing conditions include older age, diabetes, collagen vascular disease, glucocorticoids, and fluoroquinolone use.[1] The primary presenting complaint is the insidious onset of pain located directly over the patellar tendon. The pain increases with direct palpation over the tendon, passive stretching, and active knee extension—particularly with jumping. Patellar tendinopathy and dysfunction are often long-standing and limit athletic and daily activities. The diagnosis is usually easily made on the basis of clinical examination without imaging.

In chronic tendinopathy, treatment is often lengthy and difficult. Physical therapy utilizing eccentric exercise is the primary treatment. Corticosteroid injection therapy is contraindicated due to the increased risk of devastating tendon rupture.[2] Injections of dextrose, polidocanol, PRP, and multiple dry needling have showed potential short-term (1-3 months) or medium-term (6 months) treatment benefits.[3] There is still no evidence for injection interventions with long-term therapeutic benefit. When refractory to conservative management, patellar tendon injuries may be treated with arthroscopic or open surgical techniques.[4-6]

Relevant Anatomy: (Fig. 11.52)

LANDMARKS

1. With the patient lying supine on the examination table with the knee in 30° of flexion, the clinician stands lateral to the affected knee.
2. The point of maximal tenderness over the patellar tendon is identified.
3. At that site, press firmly on the skin with the retracted tip of a ballpoint pen. This indentation represents the entry point for the needle.
4. After the landmarks are identified, the patient should not move the knee.

PEARLS

- Corticosteroid injection therapy is contraindicated due to the risk of devastating tendon rupture.

ULTRASOUND-GUIDED PROCEDURE

Please refer to the introductory ultrasound chapter for preprocedure, sterile prep, postprocedure, and documentation information and recommendations.

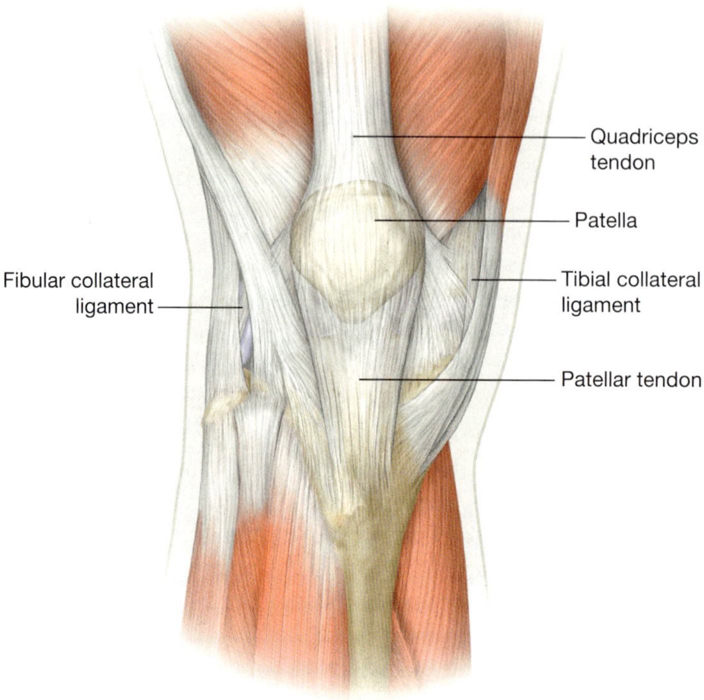

FIGURE 11.52 ● Patellar tendon.

PATIENT POSITION

- Supine on the examination table.
- On the affected side, place the knee in 30° of flexion with a bump.
- Place a rolled-up towel or small bolster under the knee to achieve approximately 30° of flexion.
- Place a pillow under their head for comfort.
- Adjust the patient's position as needed to ensure comfort.

PROVIDER/ULTRASOUND POSITION

- The provider sits on the same side of the table as the affected knee.
- Adjust the examination table to position the injection site between the provider's umbilicus and axillary level, ensuring optimal ergonomics and visualization of the ultrasound screen, transducer, and needle's approach.
- Place the ultrasound machine on the same side of the table at the level of the patient's head with the screen facing the provider (Fig. 11.53).

LANDMARKS

- See the landmarks for the landmark-guided injection procedure.

ANESTHESIA

- Local anesthesia of the skin using topical vapocoolant spray.

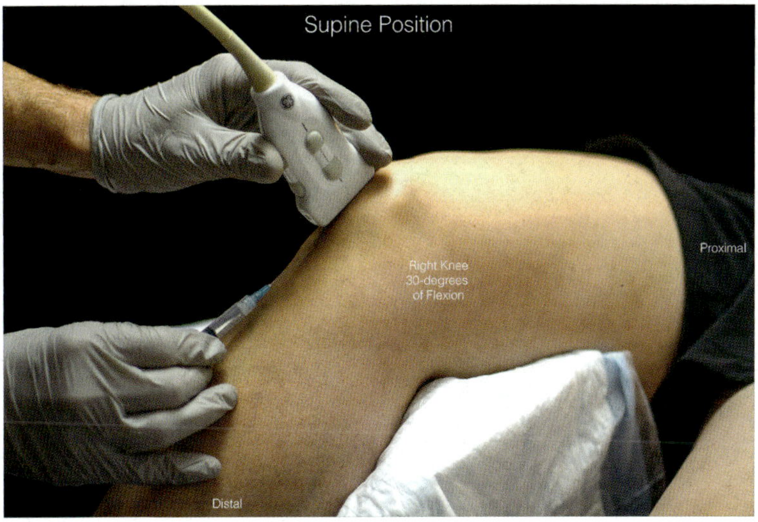

FIGURE 11.53 • Ultrasound-guided right patellar tendon injection. Supine position with the affected knee flexed to 30° resting on the examination table. Feet positioned at the left of the image. Provider positioned ipsilaterally distal to the injection site.

EQUIPMENT

- 3-mL syringe
- 22-gauge 1.5-in needle (adjust needle length as needed)
- 1 to 2 mL of 15% dextrose prolotherapy solution or 1 to 2 mL of PRP
- Three chlorhexidine swabs
- 12-4 MHz linear ultrasound transducer and machine
- Sterile ultrasound transducer cover
- Sterile ultrasound gel
- Nonlatex sterile or nonsterile gloves
- Two 4 × 4 sterile gauze pads
- One sterile adhesive bandage
- Topical vapocoolant spray

TECHNIQUE

1. Position a high-frequency linear 12-4 MHz ultrasound transducer in the sagittal plane over the patellar tendon in long axis centered beneath it.
2. Advance a 22-gauge 1.5-in needle using an in-plane approach, directing it from distal to proximal, with an initial needle angle of approximately 5° to 15° relative to the skin surface where the transducer is positioned.
3. For dextrose prolotherapy or PRP (refer to Chapter 4: Orthobiologics), inject the solution into the area of tendinopathy in the tendon. Administer a total volume (1-2 mL) of 15% dextrose prolotherapy or PRP in small aliquots (0.5 mL or less).
4. Utilize real-time ultrasound guidance throughout to ensure accurate needle placement and minimize the risk of complications (Fig. 11.54).
5. Upon completion of the procedure, carefully withdraw the needle. Adhere to established postprocedure care protocols and ensure appropriate follow-up as recommended.

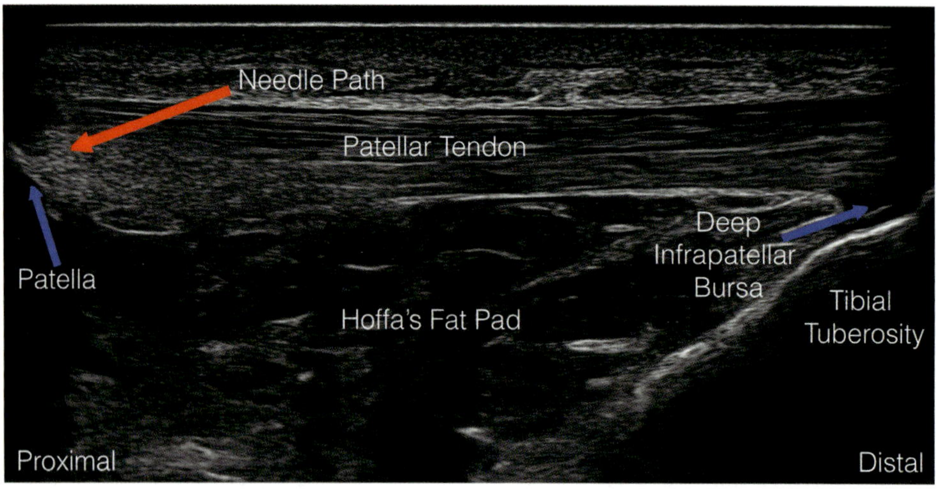

FIGURE 11.54 ● Patellar tendon sagittal ultrasound image.

PEARLS

- Consider a longer needle (eg, 2 in, 22 gauge).
- Exercise caution to avoid inadvertent penetration of the knee joint space during needle advancement.

A video showing ultrasound-guided patellar tendon injection can be found in the companion eBook.

REFERENCES

1. Alves C, Mendes D, Marques FB. Fluoroquinolones and the risk of tendon injury: a systematic review and meta-analysis. *Eur J Clin Pharmacol.* 2019;75(10):1431-1443.
2. Nuhmani S, Ahsan M, Bari MA, et al. Patellar tendinopathy-does injection therapy have a role? A systematic review of randomised control trials. *J Clin Med.* 2022;11(7):2006.
3. Wang S, Lyu B. Effectiveness of injection strategies on patients with patellar tendonitis (jumpers' knee): a network meta-analysis of randomized controlled trials. *Sports Health.* 2025;17(3):556-563.
4. Pestka JM, Lang G, Maier D, Südkamp NP, Ogon P, Izadpanah K. Arthroscopic patellar release allows timely return to performance in professional and amateur athletes with chronic patellar tendinopathy. *Knee Surg Sports Traumatol Arthrosc.* 2018;26(12):3553-3559.
5. Khan WS, Smart A. Outcome of surgery for chronic patellar tendinopathy: asystematic review. *Acta Orthop Belg.* 2016;82(3):610-326.
6. Stuhlman CR, Stowers K, Stowers L, Smith J. Current concepts and the role of surgery in the treatment of jumper's knee. *Orthopedics.* 2016;39(6):e1028-e1035.

Pes Anserine Syndrome

The pes anserinus is the shared insertion for the tendons of the sartorius, gracilis, and semitendinosus muscles. It is located over the medial aspect of the proximal tibia about 2 to 5 cm distal to the anteromedial joint margin of the knee. Pain involving this site, pes anserine syndrome, is a fairly common condition encountered in clinical practice. This pain may originate from bursitis, tendinopathy, or neuritis of the inferior medial genicular nerve.[1] Pain and swelling may occur with overuse or excessive valgus stress on the knee. It is most commonly seen in overweight, middle-aged, and older women, with diabetes as a risk factor. Pes anserine bursitis is commonly associated with knee osteoarthritis and increases in prevalence with its severity.[2,3] A fluid collection is rarely encountered. This syndrome may be treated with injections of corticosteroids or PRP.[4,5]

Relevant Anatomy: (Fig. 11.55)

PATIENT POSITION

- Lying supine on the examination table with the affected knee extended or slightly flexed and supported with folded towels or chucks pads as needed for patient comfort.
- Rotate the patient's head away from the side that is being injected. This minimizes anxiety and pain perception.

LANDMARKS

1. With the patient lying supine on the examination table, the clinician stands lateral to the affected knee.
2. The point of maximal tenderness over the proximal medial anterior tibia is identified.
3. At that site, press firmly on the skin with the retracted tip of a ballpoint pen. This indentation represents the entry point for the needle.
4. After the landmarks are identified, the patient should not move the knee.

ANESTHESIA

- Local anesthesia of the skin using topical vapocoolant spray.

EQUIPMENT

- Topical vapocoolant spray
- 3-mL syringe
- 25-gauge 1-in needle

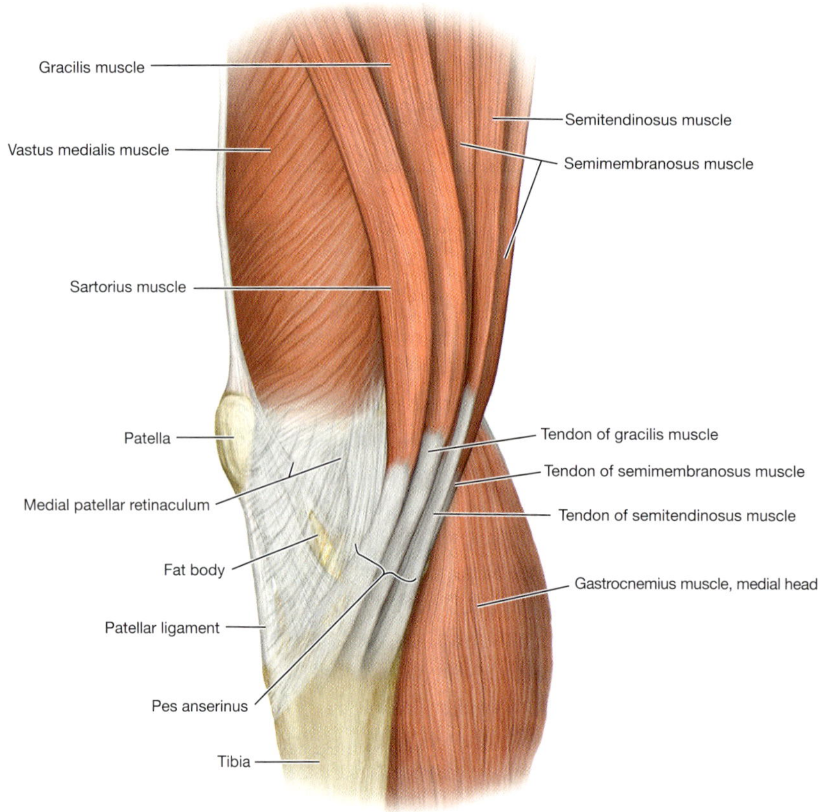

FIGURE 11.55 ● Medial aspect of the right knee/leg.

- 1 mL of 1% lidocaine without epinephrine
- 0.5 to 1 mL of the steroid solution (20-40 mg of triamcinolone acetonide)
- One alcohol prep pad
- Two povidone-iodine or chlorhexidine prep pads
- Sterile gauze pads
- Sterile adhesive bandage
- Nonsterile, clean chucks pad

TECHNIQUE

1. Prep the insertion site with alcohol followed by the povidone-iodine or chlorhexidine pads.
2. Achieve good local anesthesia by using topical vapocoolant spray.
3. Position the needle and syringe perpendicular to the skin with the tip of the needle directed toward the area of maximal tenderness at the insertion of the tendons.
4. Using the no-touch technique, quickly introduce the needle at the insertion site (Fig. 11.56).
5. Advance the needle toward the bone of the proximal medial tibia. Back up the needle 1 to 2 mm.
6. Withdraw the plunger of the syringe to ensure that there is no blood return.

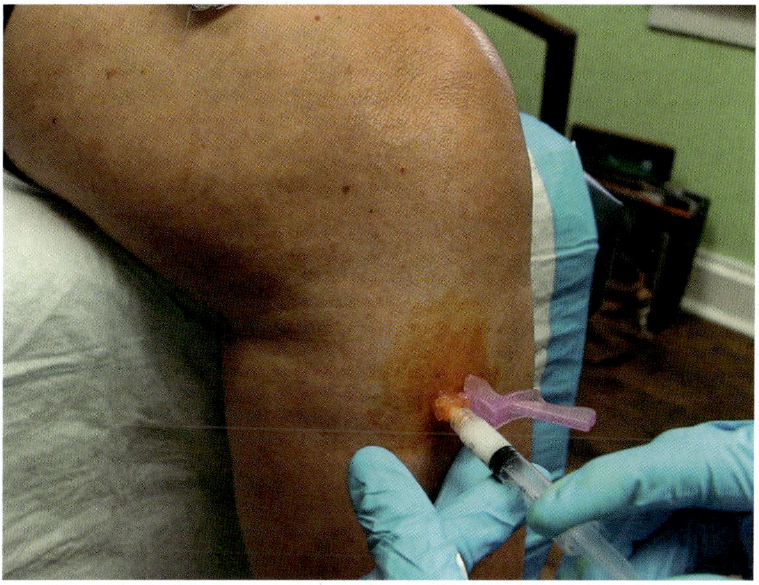

FIGURE 11.56 • Left knee pes anserine bursitis injection.

7. Inject the lidocaine/corticosteroid solution as a bolus into this area. The injected solution should flow smoothly into the space. If increased resistance is encountered, advance or withdraw the needle slightly before attempting further injection.
8. Following injection, withdraw the needle.
9. Apply a sterile adhesive bandage.
10. Instruct the patient to massage this area and move their knee through its full range of motion. This movement distributes the steroid solution throughout the pes anserine bursa and related tendons.
11. Reexamine the pes anserine bursa in 5 minutes to assess pain relief.

AFTERCARE

- Avoid excessive knee extension and adduction over the next 2 weeks.
- Consider the use of a compression wrap.
- NSAIDs, ice, heat, and/or physical therapy as indicated.
- Consider follow-up examination in 2 weeks.

PEARLS

- The pes anserine bursa is superficial. As a result, this injection can be complicated by the development of skin atrophy and hypopigmentation. Avoid the development of a subdermal wheal while injecting the corticosteroid solution.
- Since this is an unusual diagnosis, also consider a medial meniscal tear, chondral fracture, or osteonecrosis of the tibia.

ULTRASOUND-GUIDED PROCEDURE

Please refer to the introductory ultrasound chapter for preprocedure, sterile prep, postprocedure, and documentation information and recommendations.

PATIENT POSITION

- Lateral decubitus with the affected leg positioned down on the examination table.
- Position the affected leg slightly behind the contralateral leg, with the knee flexed to approximately 20° to 30°.
- Place a pillow under their head for comfort.
- Adjust the patient's position as needed to ensure comfort.

PROVIDER/ULTRASOUND POSITION

- The provider stands behind the patient proximal to the level of the affected knee.
- Adjust the examination table to position the injection site between the provider's umbilicus and axillary level, ensuring optimal ergonomics and visualization of the ultrasound screen, transducer, and needle's approach (Fig. 11.57).
- Place the ultrasound machine on the opposite side of the table at the level of the patient's feet with the screen facing the provider.

LANDMARKS

- See the landmarks for the landmark-guided injection procedure.

ANESTHESIA

- Local anesthesia of the skin using topical vapocoolant spray.

EQUIPMENT

- 3-mL syringe
- 25-gauge 1.5-in needle (adjust needle length as needed)

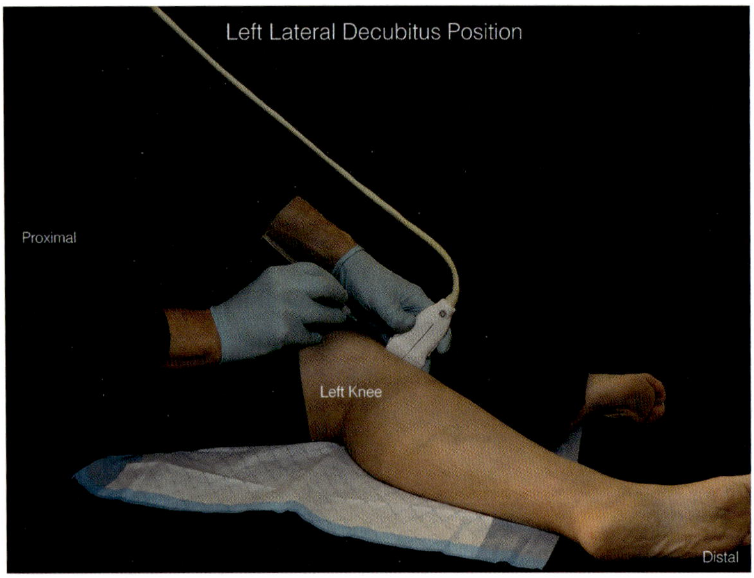

FIGURE 11.57 ● Ultrasound-guided left pes anserine injection. Left lateral decubitus position with the affected leg resting on the examination table. Provider positioned behind the patient proximal to the injection site.

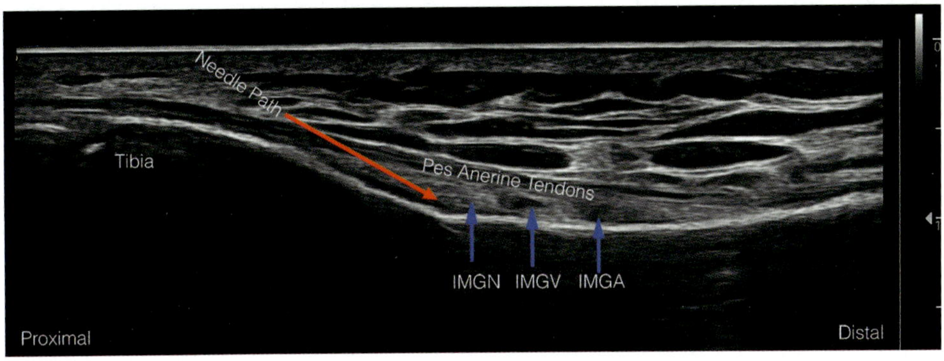

FIGURE 11.58 • Pes anserine tendons coronal oblique ultrasound image with inferior medial genicular nerve (IMGN), inferior medial genicular vein (IMGV), and inferior medial genicular artery (IMGA).

- 1 mL of 1% lidocaine without epinephrine
- 0.5 to 1 mL of 40 mg/mL triamcinolone acetonide
- Three chlorhexidine swabs
- 12-4 MHz linear ultrasound transducer and machine
- Sterile ultrasound transducer cover
- Sterile ultrasound gel
- Nonlatex sterile or nonsterile gloves
- Two 4 × 4 sterile gauze pads
- One sterile adhesive bandage
- Topical vapocoolant spray

TECHNIQUE

1. Position a high-frequency linear 12-4 MHz ultrasound transducer in a coronal oblique plane with the pes anserine tendons as they insert onto the tibia centered beneath it.
2. Advance a 25-gauge 1.5-in needle using an in-plane approach, directing it from posterior to anterior, with an initial needle angle of approximately 5° relative to the skin surface where the transducer is positioned.
3. The target area is deep to the pes tendons or in the pes anserine bursa, if an effusion is present.
4. Utilize real-time ultrasound guidance throughout the procedure to precisely place the needle within the desired target area and minimize the risk of inadvertently injuring surrounding structures (Fig. 11.58).
5. Upon completion of the procedure, carefully withdraw the needle. Adhere to established postprocedure care protocols and ensure appropriate follow-up as recommended.

PEARLS

- Consider a longer needle (eg, 2 in, 25 gauge).
- Carefully identify and avoid the neurovascular structures deep to the pes anserine tendons during needle advancement.

Videos showing landmark-guided and ultrasound-guided pes anserine injections can be found in the companion eBook.

REFERENCES

1. Helfenstein M Jr, Kuromoto J. Anserine syndrome. *Rev Bras Reumatol.* 2010;50(3):313-327.
2. Uysal F, Akbal A, Gökmen F, Adam G. Prevalence of pes anserine bursitis in symptomatic osteoarthritis patients: an ultrasonographic prospective study. *Clin Rheumatol.* 2015;34(3):529-533.
3. Kim IJ, Kim DH, Song YW, et al. The prevalence of periarticular lesions detected on magnetic resonance imaging in middle-aged and elderly persons: a cross-sectional study. *BMC Musculoskelet Disord.* 2016;17:186.
4. Gouda W, Abbas AS, Abdel-Aziz TM, et al. Comparing the efficacy of local corticosteroid injection, platelet-rich plasma, and extracorporeal shockwave therapy in the treatment of pes anserine bursitis: a prospective, randomized, comparative study. *Adv Orthop.* 2023;2023:5545520.
5. Karabaş Ç, Talay Çaliş H, Topaloğlu US, Karakükçü Ç. Effects of ultrasound guided leukocyte-rich platelet-rich plasma (LR-PRP) injection in patients with pes anserinus tendinobursitis. *Transfus Apher Sci.* 2021;60(3):103048.

Iliotibial Band Friction Syndrome

ITB friction syndrome is a common overuse injury typically seen in runners, cyclists, triathletes, and military recruits. Affected patients report lateral knee pain associated with repetitive motion activities. Several etiologies have been proposed for ITB syndrome, including friction of the ITB as it rubs against the lateral femoral epicondyle, compression of the fat and connective tissue deep to the ITB, and chronic inflammation of the ITB bursa.[1] Another factor is a greater strain throughout the support phase of running.[2] In the acute phase of this condition, conservative treatment includes activity modification, ice, and NSAIDs. Corticosteroid injections may be used in cases of severe pain or swelling.[3] However, there is a paucity of research available and only a single, small study to support the use of injected corticosteroids.[4] A small-diameter needle is used since there is no collection of fluid to aspirate. There is a promising study showing that an injection of botulinum toxin into the tensor fasciae latae, combined with physical therapy, rendered significant long-term pain relief.[5]

Relevant Anatomy: (Fig. 11.59)

PATIENT POSITION

- Lying supine on the examination table with the knee extended, or slightly flexed and supported with a pillow or folded chucks pads as needed for patient comfort.
- Rotate the patient's head away from the side that is being injected. This minimizes anxiety and pain perception.

LANDMARKS

1. With the patient lying supine on the examination table, the clinician stands lateral to the affected knee.
2. The point of maximal tenderness over the lateral femoral condyle is identified.
3. At that site, press firmly on the skin with the retracted tip of a ballpoint pen. This indentation represents the entry point for the needle.
4. After the landmarks are identified, the patient should not move the knee.

ANESTHESIA

- Local anesthesia of the skin using topical vapocoolant spray.

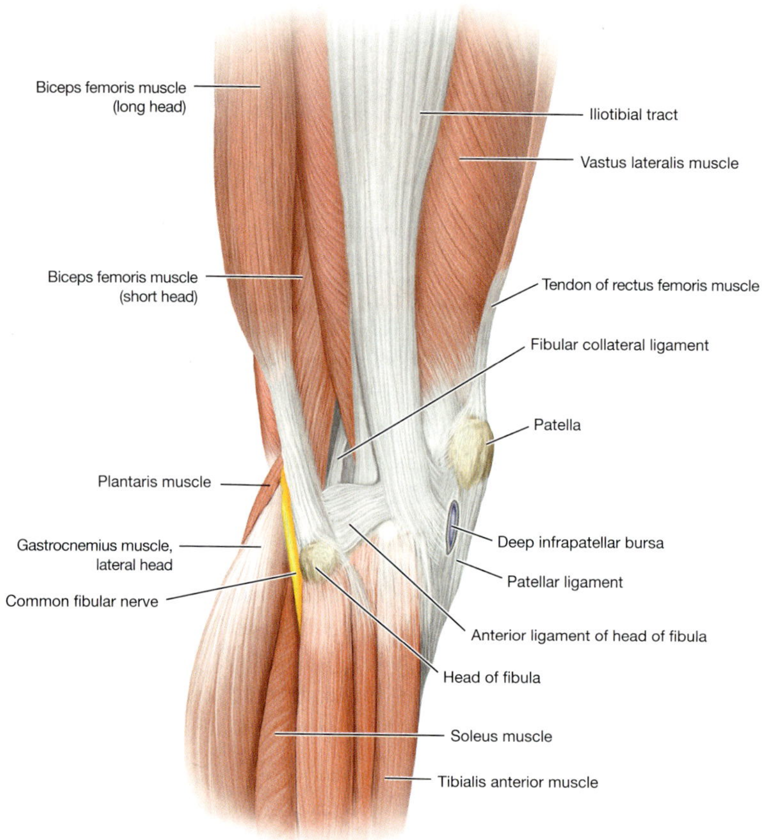

FIGURE 11.59 Lateral aspect of the right knee/leg. (Modified with permission from Gest TR. *Lippincott® Atlas of Anatomy*. 2nd ed. Wolters Kluwer; 2020.)

EQUIPMENT

- Topical vapocoolant spray
- 3-mL syringe
- 25-gauge 1-in needle
- 1 mL of 1% lidocaine without epinephrine
- 1 mL of the steroid solution (40 mg of triamcinolone acetonide)
- One alcohol prep pad
- Two povidone-iodine or chlorhexidine prep pads
- Sterile gauze pads
- Sterile adhesive bandage
- Nonsterile, clean chucks pad

TECHNIQUE

1. Prep the insertion site with alcohol followed by the povidone-iodine or chlorhexidine pads.
2. Achieve good local anesthesia by using topical vapocoolant spray.

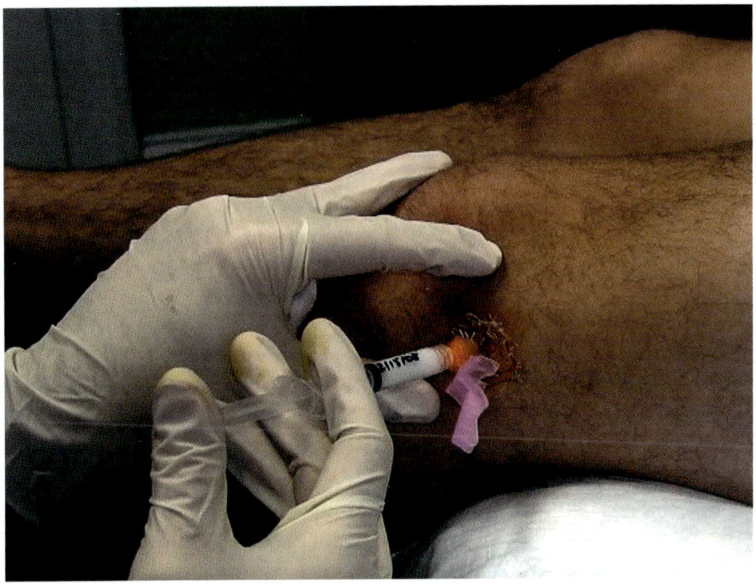

FIGURE 11.60 ● Left leg iliotibial band injection.

3. Position the needle and syringe perpendicular to the skin with the tip of the needle directed toward the area of maximal tenderness over the lateral femoral condyle.
4. Using the no-touch technique, quickly introduce the needle at the insertion site (Fig. 11.60).
5. Advance the needle through the ITB and touch the bone of the lateral femoral condyle. Back up the needle 1 to 2 mm.
6. Withdraw the plunger of the syringe to ensure that there is no blood return.
7. Inject the lidocaine/corticosteroid solution as a bolus into this area. The injected solution should flow smoothly into the tissues. If increased resistance is encountered, advance or withdraw the needle slightly before attempting further injection.
8. Following injection, withdraw the needle.
9. Apply a sterile adhesive bandage.
10. Instruct the patient to massage this area and move their knee through its full range of motion. This movement distributes the lidocaine/corticosteroid solution throughout the iliotibial tract and related structures.
11. Reexamine the lateral aspect of the knee in 5 minutes to assess pain relief.

AFTERCARE

- Relative rest with avoidance of the precipitating activity for at least 2 weeks.
- ITB stretching exercises.
- NSAIDs, ice, heat, and/or physical therapy as indicated.
- Consider follow-up examination in 2 weeks.

PEARLS

- The ITB can be superficial, especially in thin persons. As a result, this injection can be complicated by the development of skin atrophy and hypopigmentation. Avoid the development of a subdermal wheal while injecting the corticosteroid solution.

ULTRASOUND-GUIDED PROCEDURE

Please refer to the introductory ultrasound chapter for preprocedure, sterile prep, post-procedure, and documentation information and recommendations.

PATIENT POSITION

- Lateral decubitus on the examination table with the affected knee upward.
- Position the patient in lateral decubitus with the affected hip and knee flexed to approximately 15° to 20°.
- Place a pillow under their head for comfort.
- Adjust the patient's position as needed to ensure comfort.

PROVIDER/ULTRASOUND POSITION

- The provider stands behind the patient proximal to the level of the affected knee.
- Adjust the examination table to position the injection site between the provider's umbilicus and axillary level, ensuring optimal ergonomics and visualization of the ultrasound screen, transducer, and needle's approach (Fig. 11.61).
- Place the ultrasound machine on the opposite side of the table at the level of the patient's feet with the screen facing the provider.

LANDMARKS

- See the landmarks for the landmark-guided injection procedure.

ANESTHESIA

- Local anesthesia of the skin using topical vapocoolant spray.

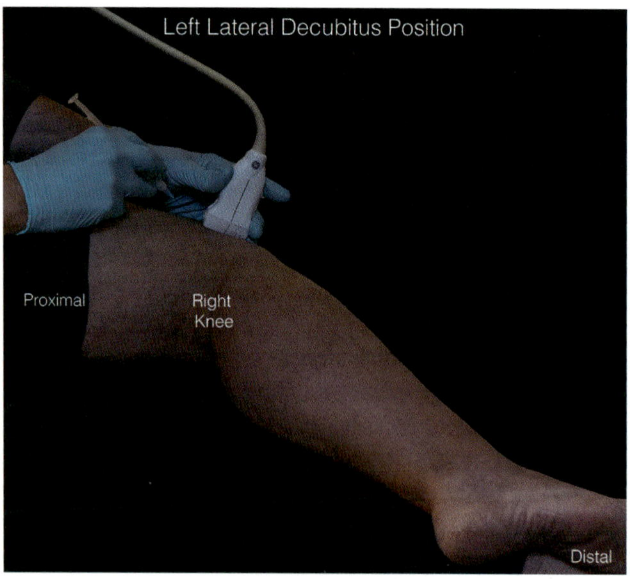

FIGURE 11.61 ● Ultrasound-guided right iliotibial band syndrome injection. Left lateral decubitus position with the affected knee upward. Provider positioned behind the patient proximal to the injection site.

EQUIPMENT

- 3-mL syringe
- 25-gauge 1.5-in needle (adjust needle length as needed)
- 1 mL of 1% lidocaine without epinephrine
- 1 mL of 40 mg/mL triamcinolone acetonide
- Three chlorhexidine swabs
- 12-4 MHz linear ultrasound transducer and machine
- Sterile ultrasound transducer cover
- Sterile ultrasound gel
- Nonlatex sterile or nonsterile gloves
- Two 4 × 4 sterile gauze pads
- One sterile adhesive bandage
- Topical vapocoolant spray

TECHNIQUE

1. Position a high-frequency linear 12-4 MHz ultrasound transducer in the coronal plane with the ITB syndrome in long axis as it crosses the lateral epicondyle of the femur centered beneath it.
2. Advance a 25-gauge 1.5-in needle using an in-plane approach, directing it from proximal to distal, with an initial needle angle of approximately 15° to 30° relative to the skin surface where the transducer is positioned.
3. The target area is deep to the ITB or inside the ITB bursa, if an effusion is present.
4. Utilize real-time ultrasound guidance throughout the procedure to precisely place the needle within the desired target area and minimize the risk of inadvertently injuring surrounding structures (Fig. 11.62).
5. Upon completion of the procedure, carefully withdraw the needle. Adhere to established postprocedure care protocols and ensure appropriate follow-up as recommended.

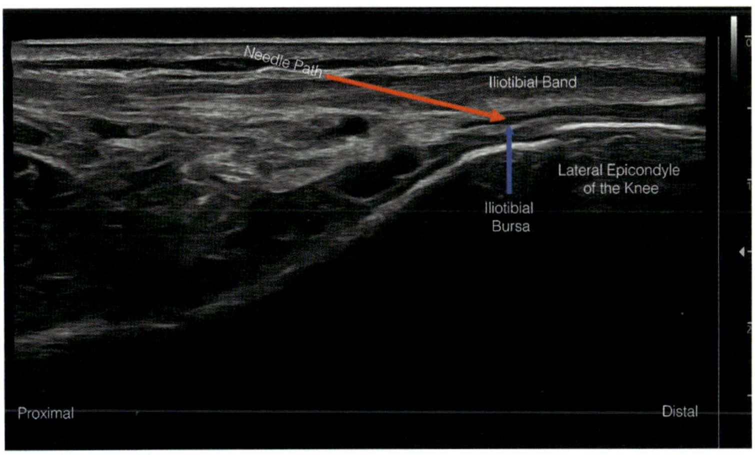

FIGURE 11.62 • Iliotibial band ultrasound coronal image.

PEARLS

- Consider a longer needle (eg, 2 in, 25 gauge).

A video showing ultrasound-guided ITB injection can be found in the companion eBook.

REFERENCES

1. Strauss EJ, Kim S, Calcei JG, Park D. Iliotibial band syndrome: evaluation and management. *J Am Acad Orthop Surg.* 2011;19(12):728-736.
2. Hamill J, Miller R, Noehren B, Davis I. A prospective study of iliotibial band strain in runners. *Clin Biomech (Bristol, Avon).* 2008;23(8):1018-1025.
3. Fredericson M, Weir A. Practical management of iliotibial band friction syndrome in runners. *Clin J Sport Med.* 2006;16(3):261-268.
4. Gunter P, Schwellnus MP. Local corticosteroid injection in iliotibial band friction syndrome in runners: a randomised controlled trial. *Br J Sports Med.* 2004;38(3):269-272.
5. Stephen JM, Urquhart DW, van Arkel RJ, et al. The use of sonographically guided botulinum toxin type a (Dysport) injections into the tensor fasciae latae for the treatment of lateral patellofemoral overload syndrome. *Am J Sports Med.* 2016;44(5):1195-1202.

Achilles Tendon

Patients occasionally present to the primary care office for the evaluation and treatment of pain over the Achilles tendon. The Achilles tendon connects the gastrocnemius and soleus muscles to the posterior calcaneus. Acute injury or chronic overuse may cause tendonitis, tendinopathy, or disruption of the Achilles tendon. Predisposing conditions include older age, pes cavus, foot hyperpronation, diabetes, collagen vascular disease, glucocorticoids, and use of fluoroquinolones.[1] The primary presenting complaint is pain over the posterior lower leg that increases with direct palpation over the tendon, passive stretching, and active plantarflexion. Achilles tendinopathy and dysfunction are often long-standing and limit athletic and daily activities. Physical examination may be aided by either ultrasound or MRI to delineate the anatomic pathology and extent of injury.

Corticosteroid injections' impact on the underlying tendinopathy remains unclear. Multiple studies, including those by Subotnick and Sisney,[2] and Read and Motto,[3,4] consistently reported Achilles tendinopathy rupture rates of 3% to 8% across various treatment modalities, including steroid injections. These rates are influenced by factors such as injury severity, the timing and technique of injection, and postinjection activity levels. The consistent rupture rates across different modalities suggest that the inherent severity of the tendinopathy itself may be a significant risk factor for rupture. Corticosteroid injections around the Achilles tendon warrant careful consideration and patient counseling, especially in the case of tendinosis.

In chronic tendinopathy, treatment is often lengthy and difficult. Physical therapy emphasizing a progressive loading eccentric exercise program is the primary treatment. Although Wetke et al[5] demonstrated decreased pain, increased participation in physical therapy, and improved clinical outcomes following corticosteroid injections, corticosteroid injection therapy is traditionally avoided due to the increased risk of devastating tendon rupture. However, a randomized controlled trial demonstrated that corticosteroid injections combined with exercise therapy were associated with better outcomes in the treatment of Achilles tendinopathy compared with placebo injections and exercise therapy.[6] Morath's[7] systematic review of prolotherapy using injected dextrose showed it to be beneficial. Two meta-analyses came to the conclusion that PRP injections do not reduce pain, tendon thickness, or color Doppler activity.[8,9] A recent literature review revealed conflicting results with PRP injections.[10] When refractory to conservative management, Achilles injuries may be surgically treated with débridement and reattachment.

Relevant Anatomy: (Fig. 11.63)

LANDMARKS

1. With the patient lying prone and the patient's feet off the end of the table.
2. The point of maximal tenderness over the Achilles tendon is identified.

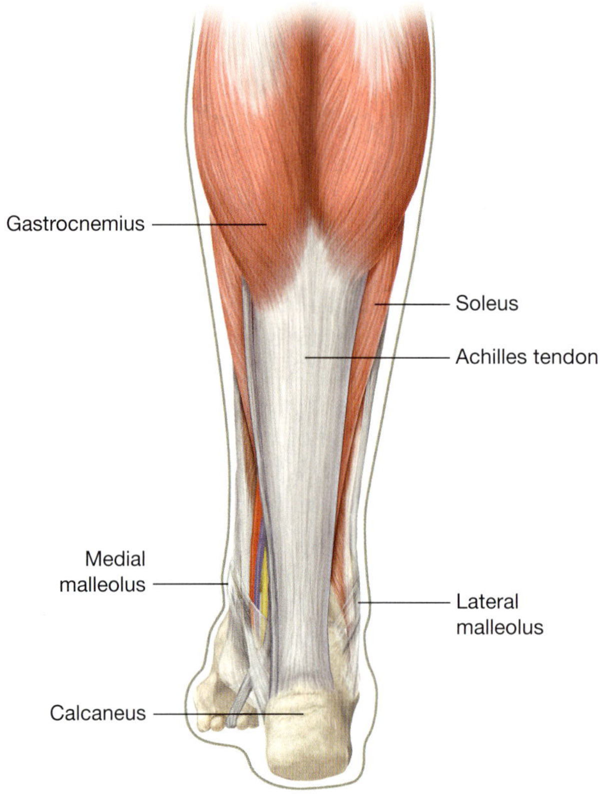

FIGURE 11.63 ● Achilles tendon.

3. At that site, press firmly on the skin with the retracted tip of a ballpoint pen. This indentation represents the entry point for the needle.
4. After the landmarks are identified, the patient should not move the leg or foot.

PEARLS

- Corticosteroid injection therapy is contraindicated due to the risk of devastating Achilles tendon rupture.

ULTRASOUND-GUIDED PROCEDURE

Please refer to the introductory ultrasound chapter for preprocedure, sterile prep, post-procedure, and documentation information and recommendations.

PATIENT POSITION

- Prone on the examination table.
- On the affected side, place the hip in a neutral position resting on the examination table with the patient's feet off the end of the table.
- Slight ankle dorsiflexion can improve visualization.
- Place a pillow under their head for comfort.
- Adjust the patient's position as needed to ensure comfort.

PROVIDER/ULTRASOUND POSITION

- The provider sits on the same side of the table as the affected Achilles tendon.
- Adjust the examination table to position the injection site between the provider's umbilicus and axillary level, ensuring optimal ergonomics and visualization of the ultrasound screen, transducer, and needle's approach (Fig. 11.64).
- Place the ultrasound machine at the end of the table at the level of the patient's feet with the screen facing the provider.

LANDMARKS

- See the landmarks for the landmark-guided injection procedure.

ANESTHESIA

- Local anesthesia of the skin using topical vapocoolant spray.

EQUIPMENT

- 3-mL syringe
- 22-gauge 1.5-in needle (adjust needle length as needed)
- 1 to 2 mL of 15% dextrose prolotherapy solution or 1 to 2 mL of PRP
- Three chlorhexidine swabs
- 12-4 MHz linear ultrasound transducer and machine
- Sterile ultrasound transducer cover
- Sterile ultrasound gel
- Nonlatex sterile or nonsterile gloves
- Two 4 × 4 sterile gauze pads
- One sterile adhesive bandage
- Topical vapocoolant spray

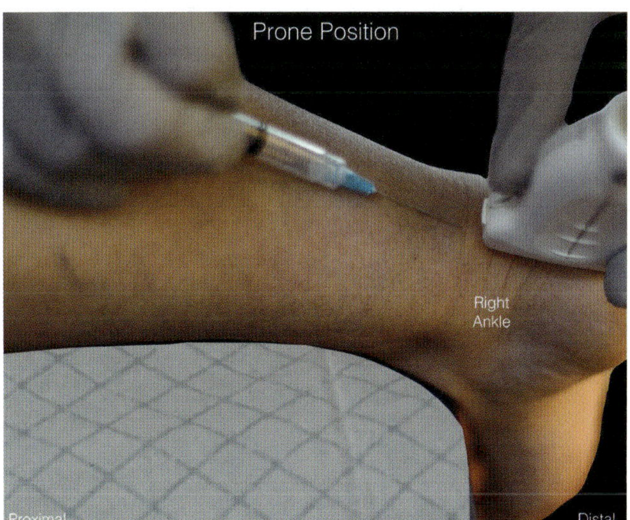

FIGURE 11.64 ● Ultrasound-guided right Achilles tendon injection. Prone position with affected foot off the examination table. Provider positioned ipsilaterally proximal to the injection site.

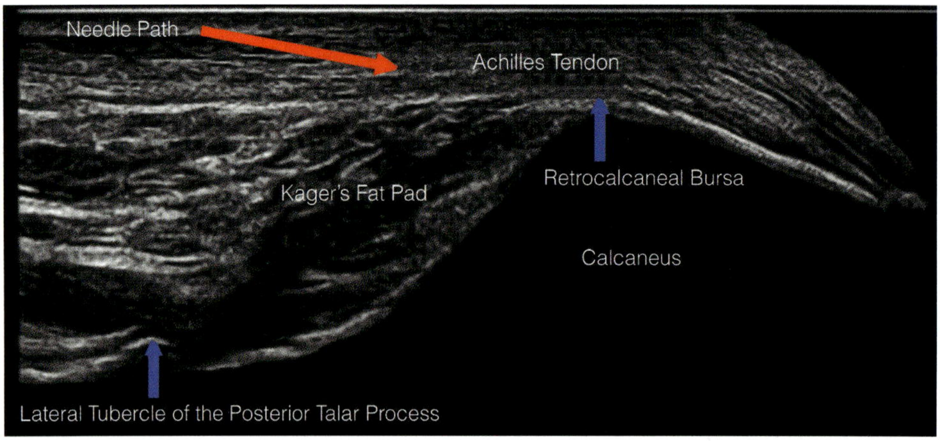

FIGURE 11.65 ● Achilles tendon ultrasound sagittal image.

TECHNIQUE

1. Position a high-frequency linear 12-4 MHz ultrasound transducer in the sagittal plane over the Achilles tendon in long axis centered beneath it.
2. Advance a 22-gauge 1.5-in needle using an in-plane approach, directing it from proximally to distally, with an initial needle angle of approximately 5° to 15° relative to the skin surface where the transducer is positioned.
3. Target area:
   a. Insertional Achilles tendinopathy: Target the area of the tendon where the pathology is located as the tendon inserts onto the calcaneus.
   b. Midsubstance Achilles tendinopathy: Target the area of the tendon where the pathology is located from the myotendinous junction to the insertion.
4. For dextrose prolotherapy or PRP (refer to Chapter 4: Orthobiologics), use a 22-gauge 1.5-in needle to inject the solution into the area of tendinopathy in the tendon. Administer a total volume (1-2 mL) of 15% dextrose prolotherapy or PRP in small aliquots (0.5 mL or less).
5. Utilize real-time ultrasound guidance throughout to ensure accurate needle placement and minimize the risk of complications (Fig. 11.65).
6. Upon completion of the procedure, carefully withdraw the needle. Adhere to established postprocedure care protocols and ensure appropriate follow-up as recommended.

PEARLS

- Consider a longer needle (eg, 2 in, 25 gauge).

Videos showing ultrasound-guided Achilles tendon injections can be found in the companion eBook.

REFERENCES

1. Alves C, Mendes D, Marques FB. Fluoroquinolones and the risk of tendon injury: a systematic review and meta-analysis. *Eur J Clin Pharmacol.* 2019;75(10):1431-1443.
2. Subotnick SI, Sisney P. Treatment of Achilles tendinopathy in the athlete. *J Am Podiatr Med Assoc.* 1986;76(10):552-557.

3. Read MT, Motto SG. Tendo Achillis pain: steroids and outcome. *Br J Sports Med.* 1992;26(1):15-21. doi:10.1136/bjsm.26.1.15
4. Read MT. Safe relief of rest pain that eases with activity in achillodynia by intrabursal or peritendinous steroid injection: the rupture rate was not increased by these steroid injections. *Br J Sports Med.* 1999;33(2):134-135.
5. Wetke E, Johannsen F, Langberg H. Achilles tendinopathy: a prospective study on the effect of active rehabilitation and steroid injections in a clinical setting. *Scand J Med Sci Sports.* 2015;25(4):e392-e399.
6. Johannsen F, Olesen JL, Øhlenschläger TF, et al. Effect of ultrasonography-guided corticosteroid injection vs placebo added to exercise therapy for Achilles tendinopathy: a randomized clinical trial. *JAMA Netw Open.* 2022;5(7):e2219661.
7. Morath O, Kubosch EJ, Taeymans J, et al. The effect of sclerotherapy and prolotherapy on chronic painful Achilles tendinopathy-a systematic review including meta-analysis. *Scand J Med Sci Sports.* 2018;28(1):4-15.
8. Lin MT, Chiang CF, Wu CH, et al. Meta-analysis comparing autologous blood-derived products (including platelet-rich plasma) injection versus placebo in patients with Achilles tendinopathy. *Arthroscopy.* 2018;34(6):1966-1975.e5.
9. Zhang YJ, Xu SZ, Gu PC, et al. Is Platelet-rich plasma injection effective for chronic Achilles tendinopathy? A meta-analysis. *Clin Orthop Relat Res.* 2018;476(8):1633-1641.
10. Desouza C, Dubey R, Shetty V. Platelet-rich plasma in chronic Achilles tendinopathy. *Eur J Orthop Surg Traumatol.* 2023;33(8):3255-3265.

Tibialis Posterior Tendonitis

Tibialis posterior tendonitis is not commonly encountered by primary care clinicians. The tibialis posterior muscle originates from the interosseous membrane and the adjacent posterior surface of the tibia in the proximal third of the leg. It courses behind the medial malleolus, passes under the flexor retinaculum, and inserts into the tuberosity of the navicular bone. The muscle plantar flexes the ankle and inverts the foot. Tibialis posterior tendon dysfunction is an often unrecognized disabling cause of progressive flatfoot deformity and is the most frequently ruptured tendon in the rear foot. Tenosynovitis of the tibialis posterior tendon occurs as a result of acute trauma, altered mechanics of the foot, and chronic overuse or with inflammatory conditions such as rheumatoid arthritis. Patients present with pain, difficulty walking, and swelling along the medial malleolus and the arch of the foot. Conservative management includes the use of orthotics, stretching, as well as eccentric and concentric progressive resistive exercises.[1] Ultrasound-guided corticosteroid injections into the posterior tibialis tendon sheath have been demonstrated as a safe treatment option for posterior tibialis tenosynovitis.[2] Surgery is required in the case of tendon rupture or the failure to respond to conservative therapy.

Relevant Anatomy: (Fig. 11.66)

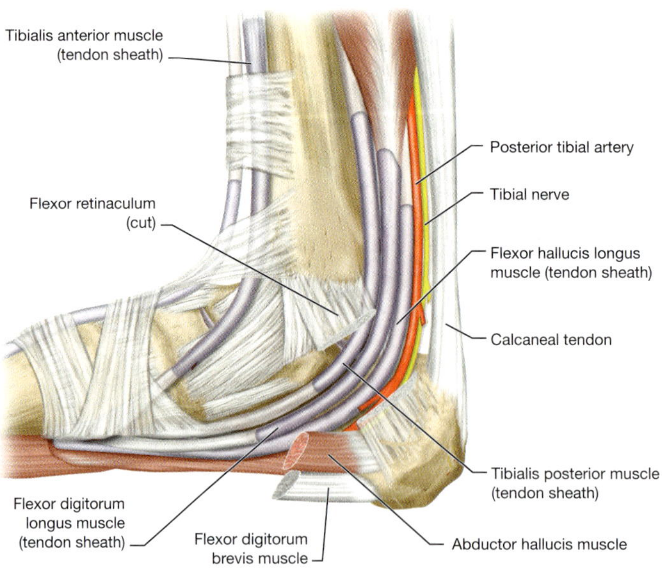

FIGURE 11.66 ● Medial aspect of the right foot.

PATIENT POSITION

- Supine on the examination table with the hip in full external rotation, knee slightly flexed, and the ankle in a neutral position.
- Alternatively, lying on the examination table on the affected side with the knee slightly flexed and the ankle in a neutral position.
- Rotate the patient's head away from the side that is being injected. This minimizes anxiety and pain perception.

LANDMARKS

1. With the patient lying supine on the examination table, the clinician stands or sits medial to the affected ankle.
2. Palpate the medial malleolus of the tibia.
3. Locate the tibialis posterior tendon immediately behind and below the medial malleolus.
4. Determine the location of maximal tenderness along the tendon.
5. Identify a point along the tendon 1 cm distal to the point of maximal tenderness and mark it in ink.
6. At that site, press firmly on the skin with the retracted tip of a ballpoint pen. This indentation represents the entry point for the needle.
7. After the landmarks are identified, the patient should not move the ankle.

ANESTHESIA

- Local anesthesia of the skin with topical vapocoolant spray.

EQUIPMENT

- Topical vapocoolant spray
- 3-mL syringe
- 25-gauge 5/8-in needle
- 0.5 mL of 1% lidocaine without epinephrine
- 0.5 mL of the steroid solution (20 mg of triamcinolone acetonide)
- One alcohol prep pad
- Two povidone-iodine or chlorhexidine prep pads
- Sterile gauze pads
- Sterile adhesive bandage
- Nonsterile, clean chucks pad

TECHNIQUE

1. Prep the insertion site with alcohol followed by the povidone-iodine or chlorhexidine pads.
2. Achieve good local anesthesia by using topical vapocoolant spray.
3. Position the needle and syringe with the needle tip directed proximally at a 30° angle to the surface of the skin.
4. Using the no-touch technique, quickly introduce the needle at the insertion site (Fig. 11.67).

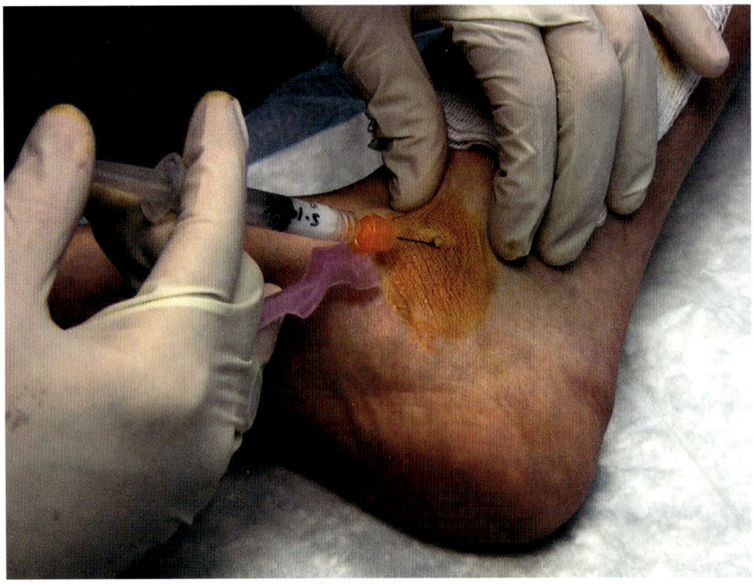

FIGURE 11.67 ● Tibialis posterior tendonitis injection.

5. Advance the needle until it touches the tibialis posterior tendon. Back up the needle 1 to 2 mm.
6. Withdraw the plunger of the syringe to ensure that there is no blood return.
7. Slowly inject the lidocaine/corticosteroid solution around the tendon. The injected solution should flow smoothly into the synovial sheath. If increased resistance is encountered, advance or withdraw the needle slightly before attempting further injection.
8. Following injection, withdraw the needle.
9. Apply a sterile adhesive bandage.
10. Instruct the patient to move their ankle through its full range of motion. This movement distributes the lidocaine/corticosteroid solution throughout the tibialis posterior tendon sheath.
11. Reexamine the tendon in 5 minutes to assess pain relief.

AFTERCARE

- Avoid excessive use of the foot over the next 2 weeks.
- Begin a program of physical therapy.
- Use orthotics or "motion-control" running shoes if there is excessive foot pronation.
- NSAIDs, ice, and heat as indicated.
- Consider follow-up examination in 2 weeks.

PEARLS

- This injection can be superficial. Depositing corticosteroid in the subcutaneous tissues can result in the complication of skin atrophy and hypopigmentation. Avoid the development of a subdermal wheal while performing all injections of corticosteroid solutions.

ULTRASOUND-GUIDED PROCEDURE

Please refer to the introductory ultrasound chapter for preprocedure, sterile prep, postprocedure, and documentation information and recommendations.

PATIENT POSITION

- Lateral decubitus on the examination table with the affected leg downward.
- Position the affected leg slightly behind the contralateral leg, with the ankle in a neutral position.
- Consider placing a small bolster or rolled towel under the calcaneus of the affected side to elevate the heel and improve visualization of the tendon and needle approach.
- Place a pillow under their head for comfort.
- Adjust the patient's position as needed to ensure comfort.

PROVIDER/ULTRASOUND POSITION

- The provider sits behind the patient at the level of the affected tendon.
- Adjust the examination table to position the injection site between the provider's umbilicus and axillary level, ensuring optimal ergonomics and visualization of the ultrasound screen, transducer, and needle's approach (Fig. 11.68).
- Place the ultrasound machine on the opposite side of the table from the provider at the level of the patient's toes with the screen facing the provider.

LANDMARKS

- See the landmarks for the landmark-guided injection procedure.

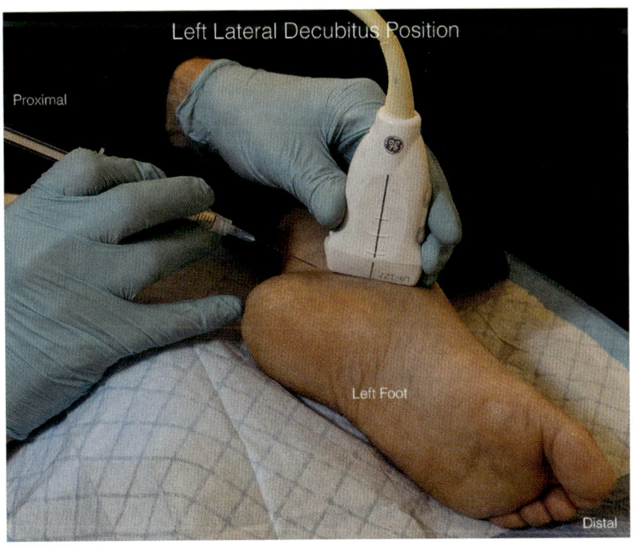

FIGURE 11.68 • Ultrasound-guided left posterior tibialis tendon or tendon sheath injection. Left lateral decubitus position with affected ankle resting on table. Provider positioned behind the patient at the level of the injection.

ANESTHESIA

- Local anesthesia of the skin using topical vapocoolant spray.

EQUIPMENT

- 3-mL syringe
- 25-gauge 1.5-in needle (adjust needle length as needed)
- 0.5 mL of 1% lidocaine without epinephrine
- 0.5 mL of 40 mg/mL of triamcinolone acetonide
- Three chlorhexidine swabs
- 12-4 MHz linear ultrasound transducer and machine
- Sterile ultrasound transducer cover
- Sterile ultrasound gel
- Nonlatex sterile or nonsterile gloves
- Two 4 × 4 sterile gauze pads
- One sterile adhesive bandage
- Topical vapocoolant spray

TECHNIQUE

1. Position a high-frequency linear 12-4 MHz ultrasound transducer in the axial oblique plane posterior to the medial malleolus over the posterior tibialis tendon in short axis centered beneath it.
2. Advance a 25-gauge 1.5-in needle using an in-plane approach, directing it from posterior to anterior, with an initial needle angle of approximately 5° to 15° relative to the skin surface where the transducer is positioned.
3. Target area:
   a. For corticosteroids: Inside the tendon sheath
   b. For dextrose prolotherapy or PRP (refer to Chapter 4: Orthobiologics): The area of tendinopathy in the tendon
4. Injectate:
   a. For corticosteroids: Use a 25-gauge 1.5-in needle to inject the solution into the tendon sheath.
   b. For dextrose prolotherapy or PRP (refer to Chapter 4: Orthobiologics): Use a 22-gauge 1.5-in needle to inject the solution into the area of tendinopathy in the tendon. Administer a total volume (1-2 mL) of 15% dextrose prolotherapy or PRP in small aliquots (0.5 mL or less).
5. Utilize real-time ultrasound guidance throughout to ensure accurate needle placement and minimize the risk of complications (Fig. 11.69).
6. Upon completion of the procedure, carefully withdraw the needle. Adhere to established postprocedure care protocols and ensure appropriate follow-up as recommended.

PEARLS

- To improve needle visualization, if the proximal edge of the transducer lifts off the skin, creating an air gap, place a sterile ultrasound gel standoff between the transducer face and the skin. This will effectively fill the gap and enhance image visualization.

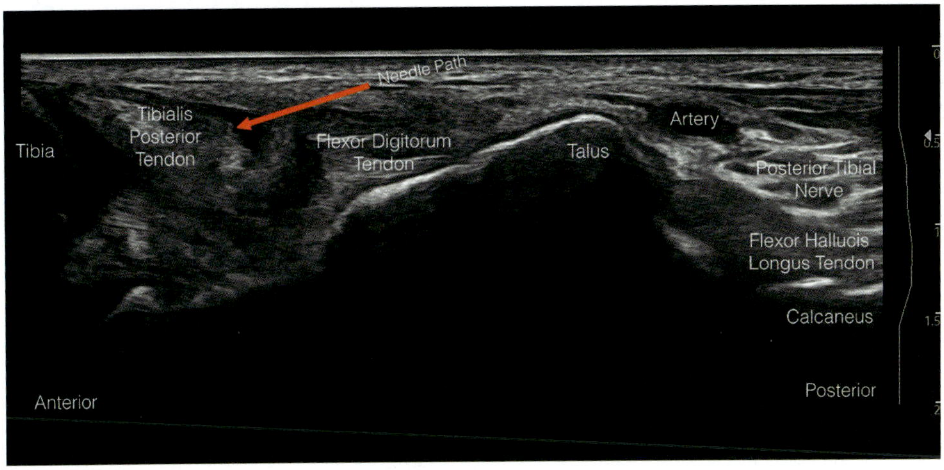

FIGURE 11.69 • Tarsal tunnel ultrasound axial image.

- Posterior tibialis tenosynovitis can present with pain and swelling around the posterior medial malleolus. Prior to injection, it is crucial to differentiate tenosynovitis from a tendon tear, which may exhibit similar symptoms. Diagnostic imaging modalities such as ultrasound or MRI can aid in this differential diagnosis.
- Exercise caution to avoid inadvertent penetration of the posterior tibial artery and nerve during needle advancement.

Videos showing landmark-guided and ultrasound-guided tibialis posterior tendon injections can be found in the companion eBook.

REFERENCES

1. Kulig K, Reischl SF, Pomrantz AB, et al. Nonsurgical management of posterior tibial tendon dysfunction with orthoses and resistive exercise: a randomized controlled trial. *Phys Ther.* 2009;89(1):26-37.
2. Spencer M, Hall M, Schafer A, Geaney LE. Clinical outcomes of posterior tibial tendon sheath ultrasound-guided corticosteroid injections. *Australas J Ultrasound Med.* 2023;26(3):169-174.

Tarsal Tunnel Syndrome

Tarsal tunnel syndrome is a rare condition encountered in primary care. It represents an entrapment neuropathy of the posterior tibial nerve or its branches as it passes underneath the flexor retinaculum at the level of the medial malleolus. It may occur due to trauma from crush injury, stretch injury, fractures, dislocations, severe ankle sprains, radiculopathy, ganglion cysts, lipomas, accessory muscles, tenosynovitis, and venous engorgement. Other causes include overuse in athletes, valgus foot deformity, compression from bony prominences, and systemic conditions, such as diabetes, hypothyroidism, rheumatoid arthritis, or amyloidosis. Typical symptoms include pain and paresthesias that radiate from the medial ankle. A positive Tinel sign may be elicited posterior to the medial malleolus. Electrodiagnostic tests frequently yield false-negative results.[1] Diagnostic imaging such as ultrasound or MRI can help differentiate the cause of the nerve entrapment. Once an accurate diagnosis is obtained, treatment is aimed at reducing external pressure, minimizing inflammation, correcting any causative foot and ankle deformities, and ultimately releasing any constrictive tissues.[2] Conservative treatment modalities include relative rest, physical therapy, orthotics, splints, and, perhaps, the injection of corticosteroids. However, uncertainties still exist about the best conservative treatment including the use of injections.[3] Complete surgical decompression of the tarsal tunnel is required for patients with persistent symptoms.[4]

Relevant Anatomy: (Fig. 11.70)

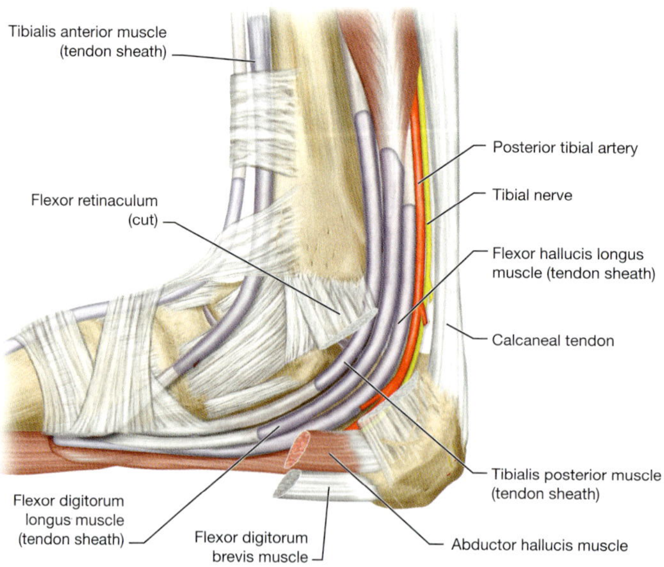

FIGURE 11.70 ● Medial aspect of the right foot.

PATIENT POSITION

- Supine on the examination table with the hip in full external rotation, the knee slightly flexed, and the ankle in a neutral position.
- Alternatively, lying on the examination table on the affected side with the knee slightly flexed and the ankle in a neutral position.
- Rotate the patient's head away from the side that is being injected. This minimizes anxiety and pain perception.

LANDMARKS

1. With the patient lying supine on the examination table, the clinician stands or sits medial to the affected ankle.
2. Locate the medial malleolus of the tibia and then the insertion of the Achilles tendon into the calcaneus.
3. Midway between these two structures, palpate the posterior tibial artery.
4. The posterior tibial nerve is located about 0.5 cm posterior to the posterior tibial artery. Mark the nerve with ink.
5. At that site, press firmly on the skin with the retracted tip of a ballpoint pen. This indentation represents the entry point for the needle.
6. After the landmarks are identified, the patient should not move the ankle.

ANESTHESIA

- Local anesthesia of the skin using a topical vapocoolant spray.

EQUIPMENT

- Topical vapocoolant spray
- 3-mL syringe
- 25-gauge 5/8-in needle
- 1 mL of 1% lidocaine without epinephrine
- 1 mL of the steroid solution (40 mg of triamcinolone acetonide)
- One alcohol prep pad
- Two povidone-iodine or chlorhexidine prep pads
- Sterile gauze pads
- Sterile adhesive bandage
- Nonsterile, clean chucks pad

TECHNIQUE

1. Prep the insertion site with alcohol followed by the povidone-iodine or chlorhexidine pads.
2. Achieve good local anesthesia by using a topical vapocoolant spray.
3. Position the needle and syringe with the needle tip directed perpendicularly to the surface of the skin with the tip of the needle directed laterally toward the nerve.
4. Using the no-touch technique, quickly introduce the needle at the insertion site (Fig. 11.71).

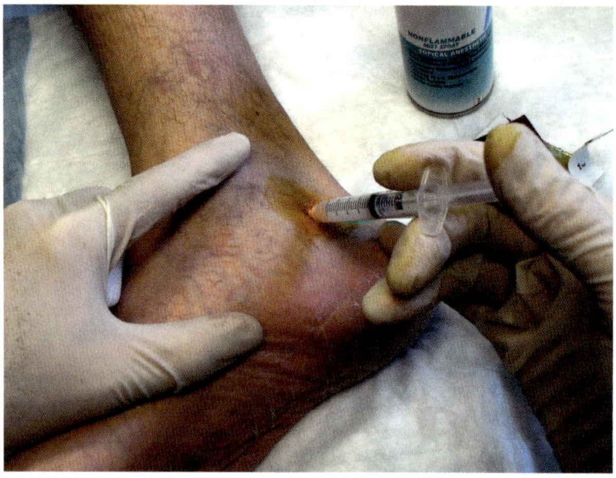

FIGURE 11.71 ● Tarsal tunnel injection.

5. Advance the needle about 1 cm deep. If any pain, paresthesia, or numbness is encountered, back up the needle 1 to 2 mm.
6. Withdraw the plunger of the syringe to ensure that there is no blood return.
7. Slowly inject the lidocaine/corticosteroid as a bolus around the posterior tibial nerve and into the tarsal tunnel. If increased resistance is encountered, advance or withdraw the needle slightly before attempting further injection.
8. Following injection, withdraw the needle.
9. Apply a sterile adhesive bandage.
10. Instruct the patient to move their ankle through its full range of motion. This movement distributes the lidocaine/corticosteroid solution along the nerve and throughout the tarsal tunnel.
11. Reexamine the foot in 5 minutes to assess pain relief and/or the development of numbness from the local anesthetic in the distribution of the posterior tibial nerve.

AFTERCARE

- Avoid excessive use of the foot over the next 2 weeks.
- Begin a program of physical therapy.
- Use orthotics or "motion-control" running shoes if there is excessive foot pronation.
- Consider splinting—especially at night.
- NSAIDs, ice, and heat as indicated.
- Consider follow-up examination in 2 weeks.

PEARLS

- Warn the patient that the posterior tibial nerve may be contacted when using this approach. Ask them to calmly report any pain or electrical shock sensation without jerking their foot away.
- This injection can be superficial. Depositing corticosteroid in the subcutaneous tissues can result in the complication of skin atrophy and hypopigmentation. Avoid the development of a subdermal wheal while performing all injections of the corticosteroid solutions.

ULTRASOUND-GUIDED PROCEDURE

Please refer to the introductory ultrasound chapter for preprocedure, sterile prep, post-procedure, and documentation information and recommendations.

PATIENT POSITION

- Lateral decubitus on the examination table with the affected leg downward.
- Position the affected leg slightly behind the contralateral leg, with the ankle in a neutral position.
- Consider placing a small bolster or rolled towel under the calcaneus of the affected side to elevate the heel and improve visualization of the tendon and needle approach.
- Place a pillow under their head for comfort.
- Adjust the patient's position as needed to ensure comfort.

PROVIDER/ULTRASOUND POSITION

- The provider sits behind the patient at the level of the affected tarsal tunnel.
- Adjust the examination table to position the injection site between the provider's umbilicus and axillary level, ensuring optimal ergonomics and visualization of the ultrasound screen, transducer, and needle's approach (Fig. 11.72).
- Place the ultrasound machine on the opposite side of the table from the provider at the level of the patient's toes with the screen facing the provider.

LANDMARKS

- See the landmarks for the landmark-guided injection procedure.

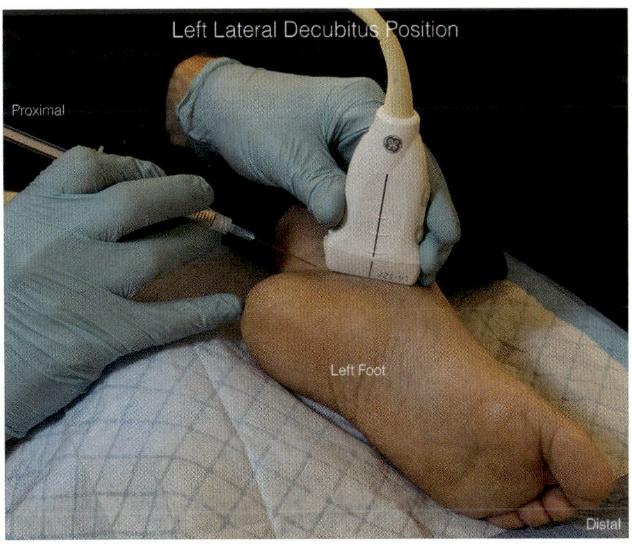

FIGURE 11.72 ● Ultrasound-guided right perineural tibial nerve injection. Left lateral decubitus position with affected ankle resting on examination table. Provider behind the patient at the level of the injection.

ANESTHESIA

- Local anesthesia of the skin using topical vapocoolant spray.

EQUIPMENT

- 3-mL syringe
- 25-gauge 1.5-in needle (adjust needle length as needed)
- 1 mL of 1% lidocaine without epinephrine
- 1 mL of 40 mg/mL triamcinolone acetonide
- Three chlorhexidine swabs
- 12-4 MHz linear ultrasound transducer and machine
- Sterile ultrasound transducer cover
- Sterile ultrasound gel
- Nonlatex sterile or nonsterile gloves
- Two 4 × 4 sterile gauze pads
- One sterile adhesive bandage
- Topical vapocoolant spray

TECHNIQUE

1. Position a high-frequency linear 12-4 MHz ultrasound transducer in the axial oblique plane posterior to the medial malleolus over the tibial nerve in short axis, centered beneath it, located between the posterior tibial vein and flexor hallucis longus tendon.
2. Prior to the procedure, activate power Doppler imaging to precisely localize the neurovascular structures. This visualization is essential for preventing inadvertent injury to the neurovascular bundle.
3. Advance a 25-gauge 1.5-in needle using an in-plane approach, directing it from posterior to anterior, with an initial needle angle of approximately 5° to 15° relative to the skin surface where the transducer is positioned.
4. The target area is the perineural space surrounding the tibial nerve.
5. Utilizing real-time ultrasound guidance throughout the procedure to precisely place the needle within the desired target area and minimize the risk of inadvertently injuring surrounding structures (Fig. 11.73).

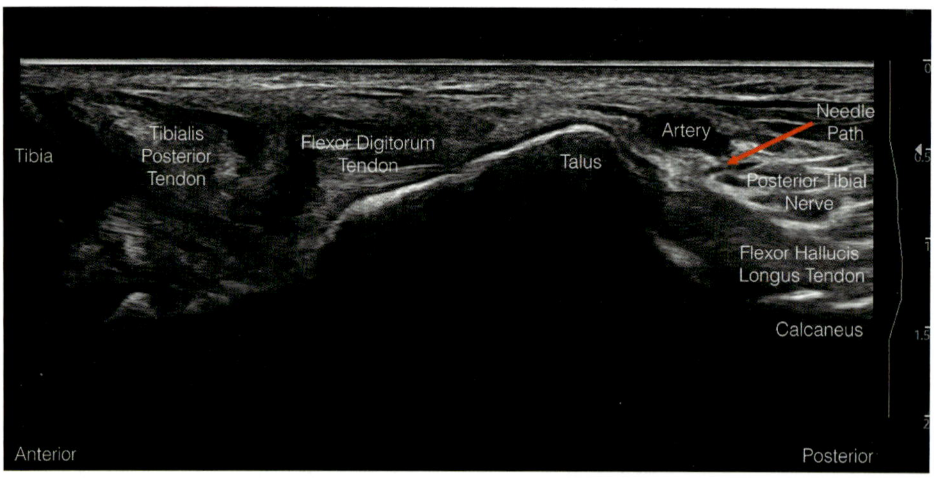

FIGURE 11.73 ● Tarsal tunnel axial oblique image.

6. Upon completion of the procedure, carefully withdraw the needle. Adhere to established postprocedure care protocols and ensure appropriate follow-up as recommended.

PEARLS

- If an air gap forms between the transducer and the skin during the ultrasound-guided procedure, use a sterile ultrasound gel standoff to improve needle visualization.
- Be aware of the anatomical variability of the tibial nerve and its branches within the tarsal tunnel.
- Advance the needle slowly and with controlled movements, continuously monitoring its position under ultrasound, to avoid intraneural injection.

A video showing an ultrasound-guided tarsal tunnel injection can be found in the companion eBook.

REFERENCES

1. Ahmad M, Tsang K, Mackenney PJ, Adedapo AO. Tarsal tunnel syndrome: a literature review. *Foot Ankle Surg*. 2012;18(3):149-152.
2. Pomeroy G, Wilton J, Anthony S. Entrapment neuropathy about the foot and ankle: an update. *J Am Acad Orthop Surg*. 2015;23(1):58-66.
3. Doneddu PE, Coraci D, Loreti C, Piccinini G, Padua L. Tarsal tunnel syndrome: still more opinions than evidence. Status of the art. *Neurol Sci*. 2017;38(10):1735-1739.
4. Franson J, Baravarian B. Tarsal tunnel syndrome: a compression neuropathy involving four distinct tunnels. *Clin Podiatr Med Surg*. 2006;23(3):597-609.

Ankle Joint—Anterolateral Approach

Ankle pain is a common presenting complaint in primary care. However, injection of the joint is rarely done due to provider unfamiliarity and reluctance to perform this procedure. Ankle joint pain may occur following acute trauma or with osteoarthritis, posttraumatic arthritis, gout, rheumatoid arthritis, or other inflammatory conditions. Conservative treatment of osteoarthritis includes weight loss, physical therapy, bracing, orthoses, and the use of NSAIDs.[1] The effectiveness of the anterolateral approach to the ankle, especially when combined with imaging guidance, has been verified.[2] A small-diameter needle is usually selected as this technique is primarily used to inject steroid solution into a painful ankle joint. Uncommonly, joint fluid may need to be aspirated.

There is a growing collection of studies that demonstrate short- to medium-term benefit from corticosteroid injections.[3-5] However, corticosteroids should not be administered immediately following ankle arthroscopy[6] and not within 3 months prior to total ankle arthroplasty.[7] There is increasing favorable data on improvement in pain and function in patients treated with HA viscosupplements.[8,9] However, this treatment is still not approved by the U.S. Food and Drug Administration at the time of publication. The combination of exogenous HA and corticosteroid showed greater and longer analgesic effects and function improvement in comparison with isolated intra-articular corticosteroids.[10] Other treatment modalities that appear promising include injections of PRP[11] and mesenchymal stem cells.[12] Those patients who fail conservative interventions may eventually require surgery. Total ankle arthroplasty has supplanted ankle arthrodesis as the most functional and safest treatment option in the management of end-stage degenerative arthritis.[13]

Relevant Anatomy: (Fig. 11.74)

PATIENT POSITION

- Supine on the examination table.
- The knee on the affected side is placed in 90° of flexion.
- The ankle is slightly plantarflexed so that the plantar surface is in full contact with the chucks pad covering the examination table.
- Rotate the patient's head away from the side that is being injected. This minimizes anxiety and pain perception.

LANDMARKS

1. With the patient lying supine on the examination table, the clinician stands or sits lateral to the affected ankle.

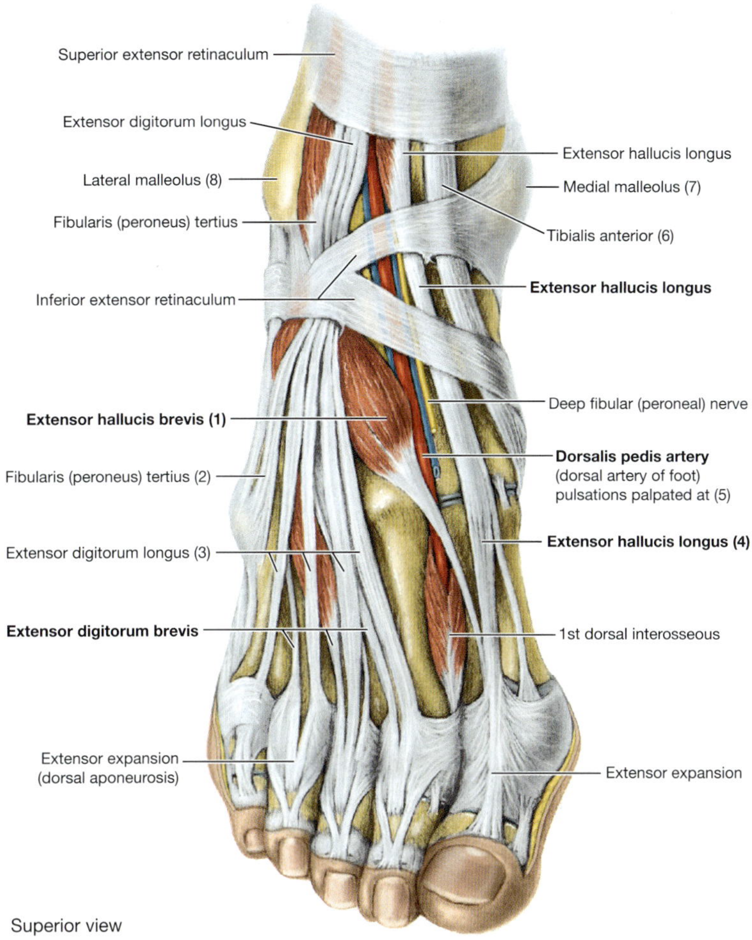

FIGURE 11.74 • Anterior aspect of the right ankle.

2. Identify the junction over the anterolateral aspect of the ankle that is located between the anterior medial aspect of the distal fibula, anterior lateral aspect of the distal tibia, and superior lateral aspect of the talus.
3. Mark a point over this articulation. There is normally a soft depression in that area.
4. At that site, press firmly on the skin with the retracted tip of a ballpoint pen. This indentation represents the entry point for the needle.
5. After the landmarks are identified, the patient should not move the ankle.

ANESTHESIA

- Local anesthesia of the skin using topical vapocoolant spray.

EQUIPMENT

- Topical vapocoolant spray
- 3-mL syringe—for injection
- 10- or 20-mL syringe—for optional aspiration
- 25-gauge 1½-in needle—if not aspirating fluid
- 20-gauge 1-in needle—for optional aspiration

- 1 mL of 1% mepivacaine without epinephrine
- 1 mL of the steroid solution (40 mg of triamcinolone acetonide)
- One alcohol prep pad
- Two povidone-iodine or chlorhexidine prep pads
- Sterile gauze pads
- Sterile adhesive bandage
- Nonsterile, clean chucks pad

TECHNIQUE

1. Prep the insertion site with alcohol followed by the povidone-iodine or chlorhexidine pads.
2. Achieve good local anesthesia by using topical vapocoolant spray.
3. Position the needle and syringe perpendicular to the skin with the tip of the needle directed posteriorly.
4. Using the no-touch technique, quickly introduce the needle at the insertion site (Fig. 11.75).
5. Advance the needle into the ankle joint. This places the needle tip between the distal tibia and fibula within the ankle joint.
6. If only injecting mepivacaine/corticosteroid solution, use a 25-gauge 1½-in needle with the 3-mL syringe.
7. If aspirating, withdraw the fluid using a 20-gauge 1½-in needle with a 10- or 20-mL syringe.
8. If injection following aspiration is elected, remove the large syringe from the 20-gauge needle and then attach the 3-mL syringe filled with the mepivacaine/corticosteroid solution.
9. Inject the mepivacaine/corticosteroid solution as a bolus into the ankle joint. The injected solution should flow smoothly into the space. If increased resistance is encountered, advance or withdraw the needle slightly before attempting further injection.

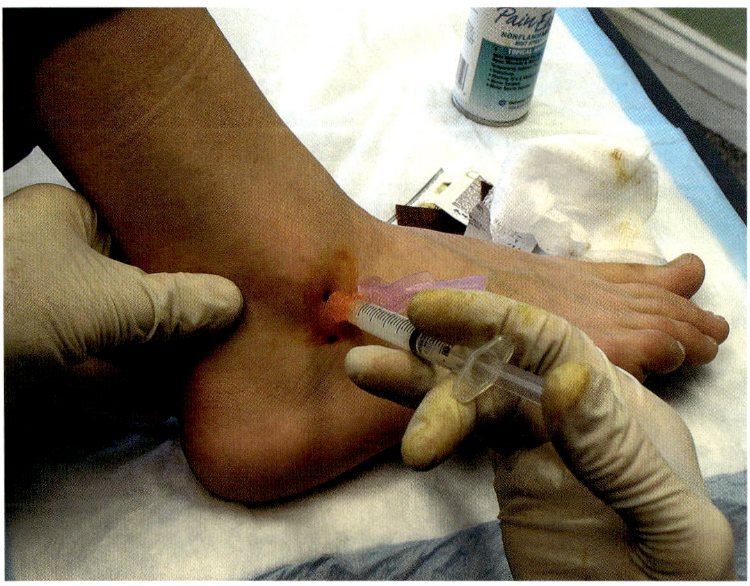

FIGURE 11.75 ● Right anterolateral ankle joint injection.

10. Following injection, withdraw the needle.
11. Apply a sterile adhesive bandage.
12. Instruct the patient to move their ankle through its full range of motion. This movement distributes the mepivacaine/corticosteroid solution throughout the ankle joint.
13. Reexamine the ankle in 5 minutes to assess pain relief.

AFTERCARE

- Consider the use of an ankle brace.
- Avoid vigorous use of the ankle over the next 2 weeks.
- NSAIDs, ice, and/or physical therapy as indicated.
- Consider follow-up examination in 2 weeks.

ULTRASOUND-GUIDED PROCEDURE

See the next chapter: Ankle Joint—Anteromedial Approach.

A video showing a landmark-guided ankle joint injection can be found in the companion eBook.

REFERENCES

1. Khlopas H, Khlopas A, Samuel LT, et al. Current concepts in osteoarthritis of the ankle: review. *Surg Technol Int.* 2019;35:280-294.
2. Fox MG, Wright PR, Alford B, Patrie JT, Anderson MW. Lateral mortise approach for therapeutic ankle injection: an alternative to the anteromedial approach. *AJR Am J Roentgenol.* 2013;200(5):1096-1100.
3. Furtado RNV, Machado FS, Luz KRD, et al. Intra-articular injection with triamcinolone hexacetonide in patients with rheumatoid arthritis: prospective assessment of goniometry and joint inflammation parameters. *Rev Bras Reumatol Engl Ed.* 2017;57(2):115-121.
4. Ward ST, Williams PL, Purkayastha S. Intra-articular corticosteroid injections in the foot and ankle: a prospective 1-year follow-up investigation. *J Foot Ankle Surg.* 2008;47(2):138-144.
5. Vannabouathong C, Del Fabbro G, Sales B, et al. Intra-articular injections in the treatment of symptoms from ankle arthritis: a systematic review. *Foot Ankle Int.* 2018;39(10):1141-1150.
6. Brand JC. Editorial commentary: big data suggest that because of a significant increased risk of postoperative infection, steroid injection is not recommended after ankle arthroscopy. *Arthroscopy.* 2016;32(2):355.
7. Uçkay I, Hirose CB, Assal M. Does intra-articular injection of the ankle with corticosteroids increase the risk of subsequent periprosthetic joint infection (PJI) following total ankle arthroplasty (TAA)? If so, how long after a prior intra-articular injection can TAA be safely performed? *Foot Ankle Int.* 2019; 40(1 Suppl):3S-4S.
8. Papalia R, Albo E, Russo F, et al. The use of hyaluronic acid in the treatment of ankle osteoarthritis: a review of the evidence. *J Biol Regul Homeost Agents.* 2017;31(4 Suppl 2):91-102.
9. Boffa A, Previtali D, Di Laura FG, Vannini F, Candrian C, Filardo G. Evidence on ankle injections for osteochondral lesions and osteoarthritis: a systematic review and meta-analysis. *Int Orthop.* 2021;45(2):509-523.
10. Gomes FF, Maranho DA, Gomes MS, de Castro Jr, Mansur H. Effects of hyaluronic acid with intra-articular corticosteroid injections in the management of subtalar post-traumatic osteoarthritis—randomized comparative trial. *J Foot Ankle Surg.* 2023;62(1):14-20.
11. Sun SF, Hsu CW, Lin GC, et al. Efficacy and safety of a single intra-articular injection of platelet-rich plasma on pain and physical function in patients with ankle osteoarthritis—a prospective study. *J Foot Ankle Surg.* 2021;60(4):676-682.
12. McIntyre JA, Jones IA, Han B, Vangsness CT. Intra-articular mesenchymal stem cell therapy for the human joint: a systematic review. *Am J Sports Med.* 2018;46(14):3550-3563.
13. Almutairi TA, Ragab KM, Elsayed SM, et al. Safety and efficacy of total ankle arthroplasty versus ankle arthrodesis for ankle osteoarthritis: a systematic review and meta-analysis. *Foot (Edinb).* 2023;55:101980.

Ankle Joint—Anteromedial Approach

Ankle pain is a common presenting complaint in primary care. However, injection of the joint is rarely done due to provider unfamiliarity and reluctance to perform this procedure. Ankle joint pain may occur following acute trauma or with osteoarthritis, posttraumatic arthritis, gout, rheumatoid arthritis, or other inflammatory conditions. Conservative treatment of osteoarthritis includes weight loss, physical therapy, bracing, orthoses, and the use of NSAIDs.[1] A small-diameter needle is usually selected as this technique is primarily used to inject steroid solution into a painful ankle joint. Uncommonly, joint fluid may need to be aspirated.

There is a growing collection of studies that demonstrate short- to medium-term benefit from corticosteroid injections.[2-4] However, corticosteroids should not be administered immediately following ankle arthroscopy[5] and not within 3 months prior to total ankle arthroplasty.[6] There is increasing favorable data on improvement in pain and function in patients treated with HA viscosupplements.[7,8] However, this treatment is still not approved by the U.S. Food and Drug Administration at the time of publication. The combination of exogenous HA and corticosteroid showed greater and longer analgesic effects and function improvement in comparison with isolated intra-articular corticosteroids.[9] Other treatment modalities that appear promising include injections of PRP[10] and mesenchymal stem cells.[11] Those patients who fail conservative interventions may eventually require surgery. Total ankle arthroplasty has supplanted ankle arthrodesis as the most functional and safest treatment option in the management of end-stage degenerative arthritis.[12]

Relevant Anatomy: (Fig. 11.76)

PATIENT POSITION

- Supine on the examination table.
- The knee on the affected side is placed in 90° of flexion.
- The ankle is slightly plantarflexed so that the plantar surface is in full contact with the chucks pad covering the examination table.
- Rotate the patient's head away from the side that is being injected. This minimizes anxiety and pain perception.

LANDMARKS

1. With the patient lying supine on the examination table, the clinician stands or sits medial to the affected ankle.
2. Locate the junction between the distal tibia and talus over the anteromedial aspect of the ankle.

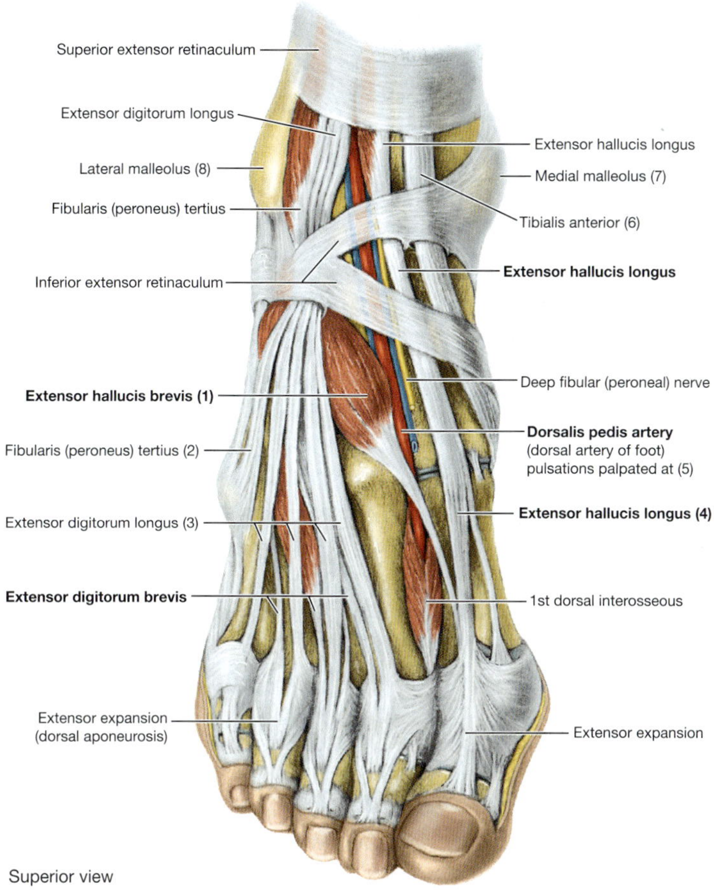

FIGURE 11.76 • Right anterior ankle.

3. Identify the anterior tibialis tendon by asking the patient to extend their great toe.
4. Mark a point over the ankle joint line that is 1 cm medial to the anterior tibialis tendon. There is normally a soft depression in that area.
5. At that site, press firmly on the skin with the retracted tip of a ballpoint pen. This indentation represents the entry point for the needle.
6. After the landmarks are identified, the patient should not move the ankle.

ANESTHESIA

- Local anesthesia of the skin using topical vapocoolant spray.

EQUIPMENT

- Topical vapocoolant spray
- 10- or 20-mL syringe—for optional aspiration
- 3-mL syringe—for injection
- 20-gauge 1-in needle—for optional aspiration
- 25-gauge 1½-in needle—if not aspirating fluid
- 1 mL of 1% mepivacaine without epinephrine

- 1 mL of the steroid solution (40 mg of triamcinolone acetonide)
- One alcohol prep pad
- Two povidone-iodine or chlorhexidine prep pads
- Sterile gauze pads
- Sterile adhesive bandage
- Nonsterile, clean chucks pad

TECHNIQUE

1. Prep the insertion site with alcohol followed by the povidone-iodine or chlorhexidine pads.
2. Achieve good local anesthesia by using topical vapocoolant spray.
3. Position the needle and syringe perpendicular to the skin with the tip of the needle directed posteriorly.
4. Using the no-touch technique, quickly introduce the needle at the insertion site (Fig. 11.77).
5. Advance the needle into the ankle joint. This places the needle tip between the distal tibia and talus in the ankle joint.
6. If aspirating, withdraw the fluid using a 20-gauge 1½-in needle with the 10- or 20-mL syringe.
7. If only injecting mepivacaine/corticosteroid solution, use a 25-gauge 1½-in needle with the 3-mL syringe.
8. If injection following aspiration is elected, remove the large syringe from the 20-gauge needle and then attach the 3-mL syringe filled with the mepivacaine/corticosteroid solution.
9. Inject the mepivacaine/corticosteroid solution as a bolus into the ankle joint. The injected solution should flow smoothly into the space. If increased resistance is encountered, advance or withdraw the needle slightly before attempting further injection.

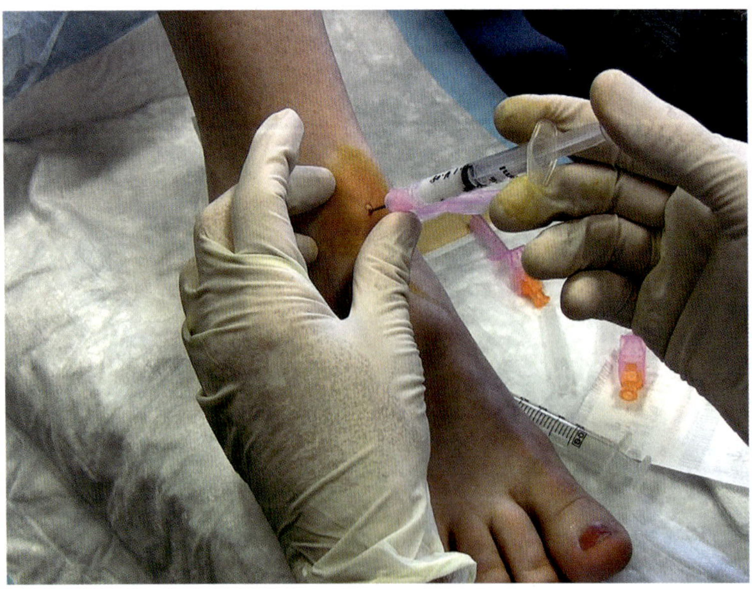

FIGURE 11.77 ● Right anteromedial ankle joint injection.

10. Following injection, withdraw the needle.
11. Apply a sterile adhesive bandage.
12. Instruct the patient to move their ankle through its full range of motion. This movement distributes the mepivacaine/corticosteroid solution throughout the ankle joint.
13. Reexamine the ankle in 5 minutes to assess pain relief.

AFTERCARE

- Consider the use of an ankle brace.
- Avoid vigorous use of the affected ankle over the next 2 weeks.
- NSAIDs, ice, and/or physical therapy as indicated.
- Consider follow-up examination in 2 weeks.

PEARLS

- Insert the needle medially to the anterior tibialis tendon in order to avoid injury to the anterior tibial artery, anterior tibial vein, and deep fibular nerve.

ULTRASOUND-GUIDED PROCEDURE

Please refer to the introductory ultrasound chapter for preprocedure, sterile prep, postprocedure, and documentation information and recommendations.

PATIENT POSITION

- Supine on the examination table with the affected foot plantarflexed on a chux pad.
- Place the unaffected extremity tucked underneath the affected extremity for patient comfort.
- Place a pillow under their head for comfort.
- Adjust the patient's position as needed to ensure comfort.

PROVIDER/ULTRASOUND POSITION

- The provider sits on the opposite side at the level of the affected tibiotalar joint.
- Adjust the examination table to position the injection site between the provider's umbilicus and axillary level, ensuring optimal ergonomics and visualization of the ultrasound screen, transducer, and needle's approach (Fig. 11.78).
- Place the ultrasound machine on the opposite side of the table from the provider at the level of the patient's ankle with the screen facing the provider.

LANDMARKS

- See the landmarks for the landmark-guided injection procedure.

ANESTHESIA

- Local anesthesia of the skin using topical vapocoolant spray.

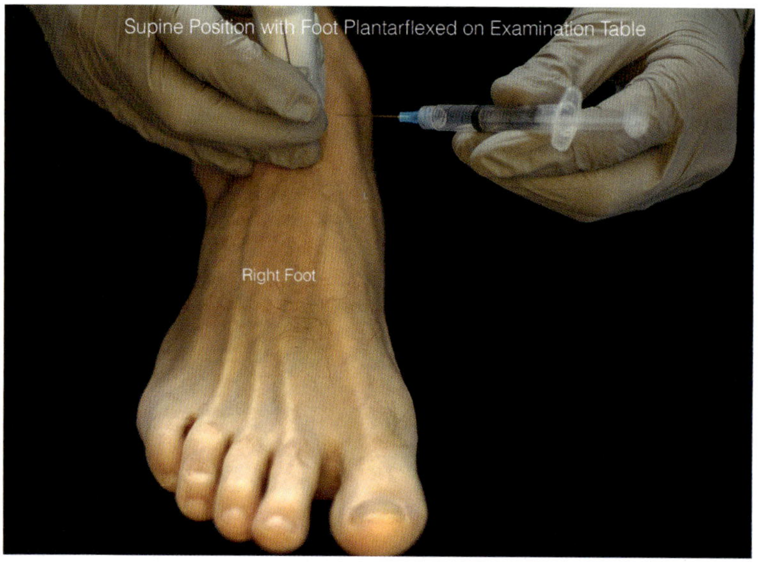

FIGURE 11.78 ● Ultrasound-guided right tibiotalar joint injection. Supine position with affected foot plantarflexed onto the examination table. Provider positioned contralaterally at the level of the injection site.

EQUIPMENT

- 3-mL syringe
- 25-gauge 1.5-in needle (adjust needle length as needed)
- 1 mL of 1% mepivacaine without epinephrine
- 1 mL of 40 mg/mL of triamcinolone acetonide
- Alternative setup for aspiration
  - 5-mL syringe (anesthesia)
    - 25-gauge 1.5-in needle (adjust needle length as needed)
    - 5 mL of 1% lidocaine without epinephrine
  - 5-mL syringe
    - 18-gauge 1.5-in needle (adjust needle length as needed)
- Three chlorhexidine swabs
- 12-4 MHz linear ultrasound transducer and machine
- Sterile ultrasound transducer cover
- Sterile ultrasound gel
- Nonlatex sterile or nonsterile gloves
- Two 4 × 4 sterile gauze pads
- One sterile adhesive bandage
- Topical vapocoolant spray

TECHNIQUE

1. Position a high-frequency linear 12-4 MHz ultrasound transducer in the sagittal plane over the tibialis anterior tendon in long axis with the tibiotalar joint centered beneath it.
2. Advance a 25-gauge 1.5-in needle using an out-of-plane approach, directing it from anteromedial to posterolateral, with an initial needle angle of approximately 45° to 60° distally and 45° to 60° laterally relative to the skin surface where the transducer is positioned.

3. The target area is the affected tibiotalar joint.
4. Utilize real-time ultrasound guidance throughout the procedure to precisely place the needle within the desired target area and minimize the risk of inadvertently injuring surrounding structures (Fig. 11.79).
5. For intra-articular steroid injection:
   a. Slowly inject the desired volume of mepivacaine and corticosteroid solution directly into the joint.
6. For situations requiring anesthesia, aspiration, or both:
   a. Utilize a separate 25-gauge 1.5-in needle with a 5-mL syringe to inject 5 mL of 1% lidocaine without epinephrine into the soft tissues overlying the joint.
   b. For aspiration, use an 18-gauge 1.5-in needle with a 5-mL syringe to withdraw the effusion.
   c. If a corticosteroid injection is indicated following aspiration, replace the aspiration syringe with the mepivacaine and corticosteroid solution syringe and reconfirm accurate needle placement using real-time ultrasound guidance before injection.
7. Upon completion of the procedure, carefully withdraw the needle. Adhere to established postprocedure care protocols and ensure appropriate follow-up as recommended.

PEARLS

- Observe for distention of the joint capsule during injection to confirm intra-articular placement.
- Exercise caution to avoid inadvertent penetration of the neurovascular bundle during needle advancement.

Videos showing landmark-guided and ultrasound-guided anteromedial ankle joint injections can be found in the companion eBook.

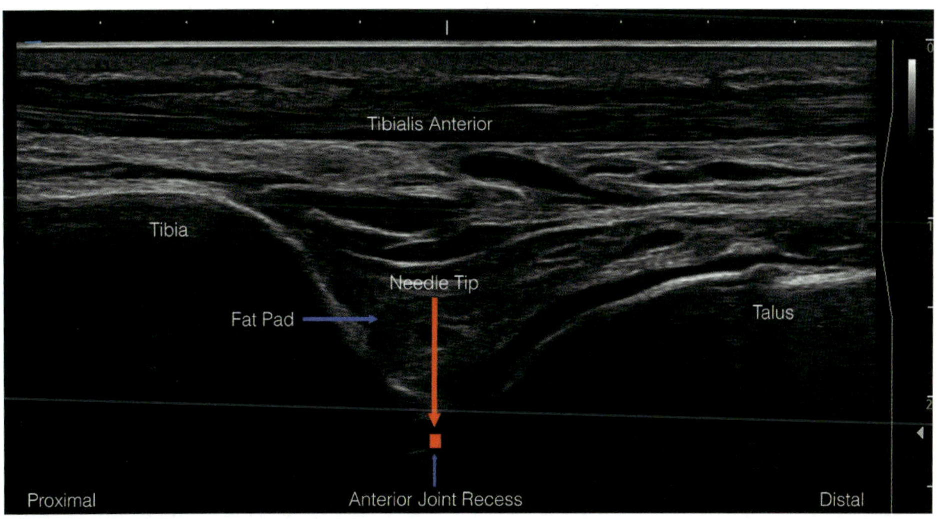

FIGURE 11.79 • Tibiotalar joint ultrasound sagittal image.

REFERENCES

1. Khlopas H, Khlopas A, Samuel LT, et al. Current concepts in osteoarthritis of the ankle: review. *Surg Technol Int.* 2019;35:280-294.
2. Furtado RNV, Machado FS, Luz KRD, et al. Intra-articular injection with triamcinolone hexacetonide in patients with rheumatoid arthritis: prospective assessment of goniometry and joint inflammation parameters. *Rev Bras Reumatol Engl Ed.* 2017;57(2):115-121.
3. Ward ST, Williams PL, Purkayastha S. Intra-articular corticosteroid injections in the foot and ankle: a prospective 1-year follow-up investigation. *J Foot Ankle Surg.* 2008;47(2):138-144.
4. Vannabouathong C, Del Fabbro G, Sales B, et al. Intra-articular injections in the treatment of symptoms from ankle arthritis: a systematic review. *Foot Ankle Int.* 2018;39(10):1141-1150.
5. Brand JC. Editorial commentary: big data suggest that because of a significant increased risk of postoperative infection, steroid injection is not recommended after ankle arthroscopy. *Arthroscopy.* 2016;32(2):355.
6. Uçkay I, Hirose CB, Assal M. Does Intra-articular Injection of the ankle with corticosteroids increase the risk of subsequent periprosthetic joint infection (PJI) following total ankle arthroplasty (TAA)? If so, how long after a prior intra-articular injection can TAA be safely performed? *Foot Ankle Int.* 2019; 40(1 Suppl):3S-4S.
7. Papalia R, Albo E, Russo F, et al. The use of hyaluronic acid in the treatment of ankle osteoarthritis: a review of the evidence. *J Biol Regul Homeost Agents.* 2017;31(4 Suppl 2):91-102.
8. Boffa A, Previtali D, Di Laura FG, Vannini F, Candrian C, Filardo G. Evidence on ankle injections for osteochondral lesions and osteoarthritis: a systematic review and meta-analysis. *Int Orthop.* 2021;45(2):509-523.
9. Gomes FF, Maranho DA, Gomes MS, de Castro IM Jr, Mansur H. Effects of hyaluronic acid with intra-articular corticosteroid injections in the management of subtalar post-traumatic osteoarthritis—randomized comparative trial. *J Foot Ankle Surg.* 2023;62(1):14-20.
10. Sun SF, Hsu CW, Lin GC, et al. Efficacy and safety of a single intra-articular injection of platelet-rich plasma on pain and physical function in patients with ankle osteoarthritis—a prospective study. *J Foot Ankle Surg.* 2021;60(4):676-682.
11. McIntyre JA, Jones IA, Han B, Vangsness CT. Intra-articular mesenchymal stem cell therapy for the human joint: a systematic review. *Am J Sports Med.* 2018;46(14):3550-3563.
12. Almutairi TA, Ragab KM, Elsayed SM, et al. Safety and efficacy of total ankle arthroplasty versus ankle arthrodesis for ankle osteoarthritis: a systematic review and meta-analysis. *Foot (Edinb).* 2023;55:101980.

Fibularis Brevis Tendonitis

Injection of corticosteroids for the treatment of tendonitis of the fibularis brevis (formerly known as the peroneus brevis) tendon is a fairly uncommon procedure for primary care physicians. The fibularis longus and brevis tendons are often injured with inversion ankle sprains. This can cause tendinopathy and chronic subluxation of the tendons. Overuse from repeated forceful plantarflexion and resisted foot eversion may also occur. Corticosteroids injections are commonly provided. Ultrasound-guided corticosteroid injections into the tendon sheath of the fibularis brevis and longus tendons have been shown to be a safe and effective treatment option for tenosynovitis.[1] The most common sonographic finding is peritendinous fluid and sheath thickening. Alternatively, a single case report shows treatment success with application of ultrasound-guided needle tenotomy.[2]

Relevant Anatomy: (Fig. 11.80)

PATIENT POSITION

- Supine on the examination table.
- The ankle and the knee on the affected side are supported by placing rolled towels underneath them.
- The ankle is in a neutral position.
- Rotate the patient's head away from the side that is being injected. This minimizes anxiety and pain perception.

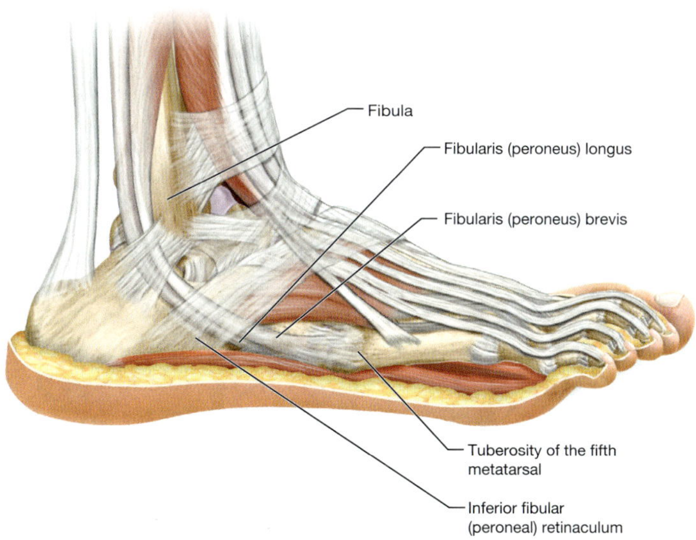

FIGURE 11.80 ● Lateral aspect of the right foot.

LANDMARKS

1. With the patient lying supine on the examination table, the clinician stands or sits lateral to the affected foot.
2. While the foot is held in a position of active eversion, identify tenderness at and immediately proximal to the head of the fifth metatarsal bone.
3. Palpate the fibularis brevis tendon along its course from posterior and distal to the lateral malleolus to its insertion into the head of the fifth metatarsal bone.
4. Locate the area of maximal tenderness.
5. At that site, press firmly with the retracted tip of a ballpoint pen. This indentation represents the entry point for the needle.
6. After the landmarks are identified, the patient should not move the ankle.

ANESTHESIA

- Local anesthesia of the skin using a topical vapocoolant spray.

EQUIPMENT

- Topical vapocoolant spray
- 3-mL syringe
- 25-gauge 5/8-in needle
- 0.5 mL of 1% lidocaine without epinephrine
- 0.5 mL of the steroid solution (20 mg of triamcinolone acetonide)
- One alcohol prep pad
- Two povidone-iodine or chlorhexidine prep pads
- Sterile gauze pads
- Sterile adhesive bandage
- Nonsterile, clean chucks pad

TECHNIQUE

1. Prep the insertion site with alcohol followed by the povidone-iodine or chlorhexidine pads.
2. Achieve good local anesthesia by using a topical vapocoolant spray.
3. If treating tendonitis at the insertion of the fibularis brevis on the fifth metacarpal:
   a. Position the needle and syringe perpendicularly to the skin with the needle tip directed medially.
   b. Using the no-touch technique, introduce the needle at the insertion site.
   c. Advance the needle slowly until the needle tip touches the tendon/bone junction. Back up the needle 1 to 2 mm.
   d. Withdraw the plunger of the syringe to ensure that there is no blood return.
   e. Inject the lidocaine/corticosteroid solution slowly as a bolus around the insertion of the fibularis brevis tendon into the head of the fifth metatarsal. The injected solution should flow smoothly into the space. If increased resistance is encountered, advance or withdraw the needle slightly before attempting further injection.
4. If treating tendonitis along the course of the fibularis brevis tendon proximal to its insertion:
   a. Position the needle and syringe at an angle of 45° to the skin with the needle tip directed proximally.

   b. Using the no-touch technique, quickly introduce the needle at the insertion site (Fig. 11.81).
   c. Advance the needle slowly until the needle tip touches the tendon. Back up the needle 1 to 2 mm.
   d. Withdraw the plunger of the syringe to ensure that there is no blood return.
   e. Inject the lidocaine/corticosteroid solution slowly as a bolus around the fibularis brevis tendon. A small bulge in the shape of a sausage may develop in the tendon sheath. The injected solution should flow smoothly into the tenosynovial space. If increased resistance is encountered, advance or withdraw the needle slightly before attempting further injection.
5. Following injection, withdraw the needle.
6. Apply a sterile adhesive bandage.
7. Instruct the patient to move their ankle through its full range of inversion and eversion. This movement distributes the lidocaine/corticosteroid solution throughout the fibularis brevis tenosynovial sheath.
8. Reexamine the foot in 5 minutes to assess pain relief.

AFTERCARE

- Ensure no excessive plantarflexion over the next 2 weeks by the use of an ankle-foot orthosis or a walking cast boot.
- NSAIDs, ice, heat, and/or physical therapy as indicated.
- Consider follow-up examination in 2 weeks.

PEARLS

- The fibularis brevis tendon is superficial. As a result, this injection can be complicated by the development of skin atrophy and hypopigmentation. Avoid the development of a subdermal wheal while injecting the corticosteroid solution.

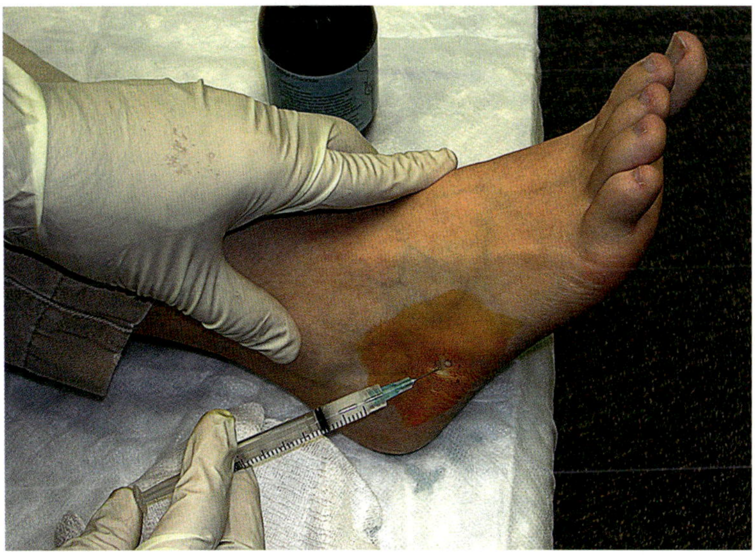

FIGURE 11.81 ● Injection of the right fibularis brevis tendon insertion.

ULTRASOUND-GUIDED PROCEDURE

Please refer to the introductory ultrasound chapter for preprocedure, sterile prep, postprocedure, and documentation information and recommendations.

PATIENT POSITION

- Lateral decubitus position on the examination table with the affected leg upward.
- Position the affected leg slightly behind the contralateral leg, with the ankle in a neutral, or slightly dorsiflexed, position.
- Consider placing a small bolster or rolled towel under the calcaneus of the affected side to elevate the heel and improve visualization of the tendon and needle approach.
- Place a pillow under their head for comfort.
- Adjust the patient's position as needed to ensure comfort.

PROVIDER/ULTRASOUND POSITION

- The provider sits behind the patient at the level of the affected tendon.
- Adjust the examination table to position the injection site between the provider's umbilicus and axillary level, ensuring optimal ergonomics and visualization of the ultrasound screen, transducer, and needle's approach (Fig. 11.82).
- Place the ultrasound machine on the opposite side of the table from the provider at the level of the patient's toes with the screen facing the provider.

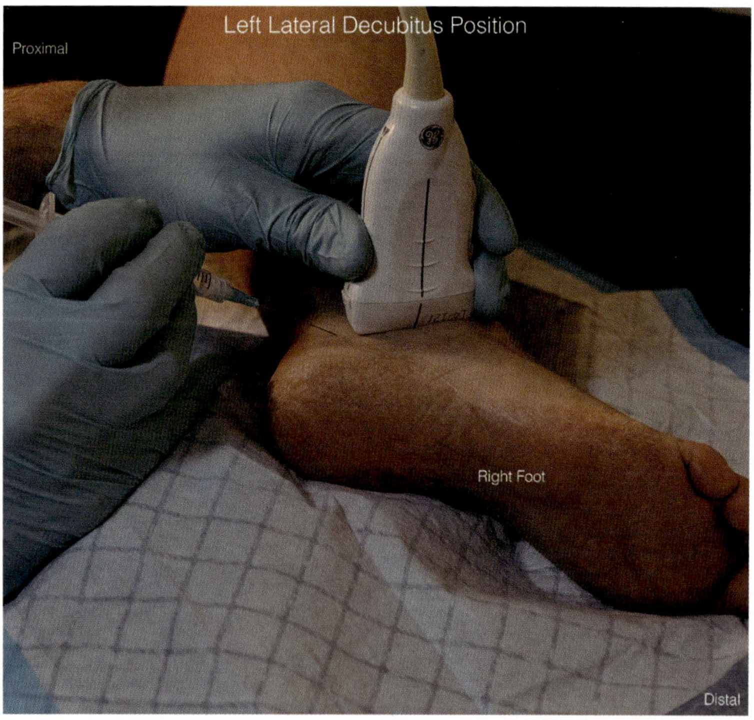

FIGURE 11.82 ● Ultrasound-guided right fibularis longus or brevis tendon sheath injection. Left lateral decubitus position with the affected foot resting on the examination table. Provider positioned behind the patient at the level of the injection.

LANDMARKS

- See the landmarks for the landmark-guided injection procedure.

ANESTHESIA

- Local anesthesia of the skin using topical vapocoolant spray.

EQUIPMENT

- 3-mL syringe
- 25-gauge 1.5-in needle (adjust needle length as needed)
- 0.5 mL of 1% lidocaine without epinephrine
- 0.5 mL of 40 mg/mL triamcinolone acetonide
- Three chlorhexidine swabs
- 12-4 MHz linear ultrasound transducer and machine
- Sterile ultrasound transducer cover
- Sterile ultrasound gel
- Nonlatex sterile or nonsterile gloves
- Two 4 × 4 sterile gauze pads
- One sterile adhesive bandage
- Topical vapocoolant spray

TECHNIQUE

1. Position a high-frequency linear 12-4 MHz ultrasound transducer in the axial oblique plane posterior to the lateral malleolus over the fibularis tendons in short axis centered beneath them.
2. Advance a 25-gauge 1.5-in needle using an in-plane approach, directing it from anterior to posterior, with an initial needle angle of approximately 15° to 30° relative to the skin surface where the transducer is positioned.
3. The target area is in the tendon sheath of the fibularis brevis and longus tendon.
4. Utilize real-time ultrasound guidance throughout the procedure to precisely place the needle within the desired target area and minimize the risk of inadvertently injuring surrounding structures (Fig. 11.83).
5. Upon completion of the procedure, carefully withdraw the needle. Adhere to established postprocedure care protocols and ensure appropriate follow-up as recommended.

PEARLS

- If an air gap forms between the transducer and the skin, place a sterile ultrasound gel standoff between them to improve needle visualization.
- Fibularis brevis and longus tendon tenosynovitis can present with pain and swelling around the posterior lateral malleolus. Before considering an injection, it is crucial to distinguish tenosynovitis from a tendon tear, which may have similar symptoms. Diagnostic imaging such as ultrasound or MRI can help differentiate these conditions.
- Exercise caution to avoid inadvertent needle penetration of the sural nerve and saphenous vein, which are typically superficial to the fibularis tendon sheath.

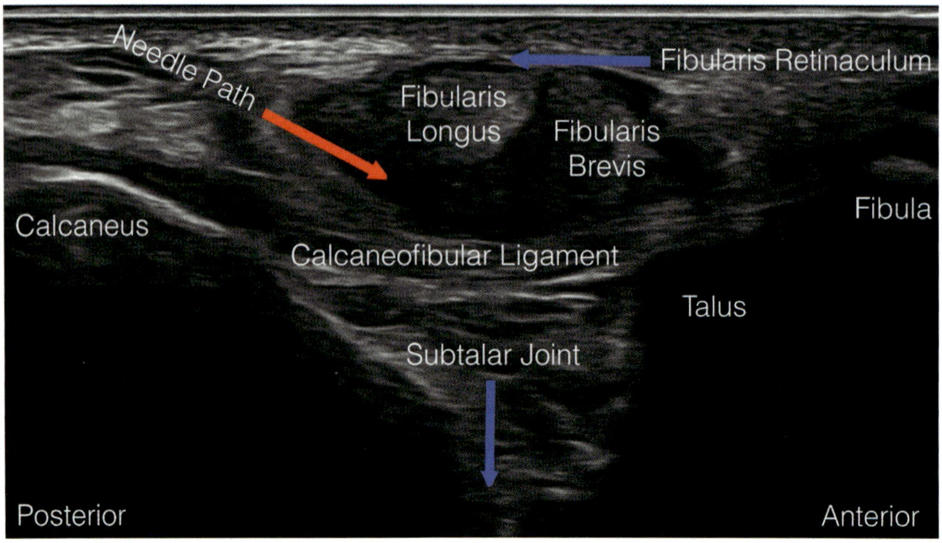

FIGURE 11.83 ● Ultrasound axial image of the fibularis longus and brevis tendons.

Videos showing landmark-guided and ultrasound-guided fibularis brevis tendon injections can be found in the companion eBook.

REFERENCES

1. Fram BR, Rogero R, Fuchs D, Shakked RJ, Raikin SM, Pedowitz DI. Clinical outcomes and complications of peroneal tendon sheath ultrasound-guided corticosteroid injection. *Foot Ankle Int.* 2019;40(8):888-894.
2. Sussman WI, Hofmann K. Treatment of insertional peroneus brevis tendinopathy by ultrasound-guided percutaneous ultrasonic needle tenotomy: a case report. *J Foot Ankle Surg.* 2019;58(6):1285-1287.

Plantar Fascia

Foot pain due to plantar fasciopathy is the most common cause of heel pain in adults. This repetitive motion injury typically involves microtrauma leading to chronic degeneration and tendinosis involving the origin of the plantar aponeurosis at the medial tubercle of the calcaneus. It is usually caused by excessive repetitive pronation of the foot—especially in persons with pes planus. The pain with this condition is greatest when bearing weight after a period of rest. Conservative treatment modalities include relative rest, stretching of the heel cords/plantar fascia, ice massage, and NSAIDs. Many standard treatments such as night splints and orthoses have actually not shown benefit over placebo.[1]

Corticosteroid injections have been a mainstay of treatment and demonstrate at least short-term symptomatic improvement.[2,3] Efficacy increases with ultrasound guidance.[4,5] Ultrasound-guided corticosteroid injections performed deep to the plantar fascia have been shown to provide safe and effective short-term therapeutic benefits in terms of pain relief, disability, and quality of life.[6] In a recent systematic review, corticosteroid injections were shown to be more effective for pain reduction than noninvasive treatments (physical therapy and shock wave therapy) within 3 months.[7] Furthermore, a combination of both corticosteroid injections and physical therapy provides improved short- and long-term pain and functional outcomes compared to each treatment individually.[8]

Other injection treatment options that demonstrate improvements in both pain and function compared to corticosteroid injections include prolotherapy,[9] PRP,[10,11] and botulinum toxin.[12,13] Surgical procedures should be considered if conservative management fails.

Relevant Anatomy: (Fig. 11.84)

PATIENT POSITION

- Supine on the examination table with the hip in full external rotation, the knee slightly flexed, and the ankle in a neutral position.
- Alternatively, lying on the examination table on the affected side with the knee slightly flexed and the ankle in a neutral position.
- Rotate the patient's head away from the side that is being injected. This minimizes anxiety and pain perception.

LANDMARKS

1. With the patient lying supine on the examination table, the clinician stands or sits in front of the affected foot.
2. Identify the point of maximal tenderness over the plantar aspect of the foot. This is usually just medial of midline over the medial tubercle of the calcaneus.

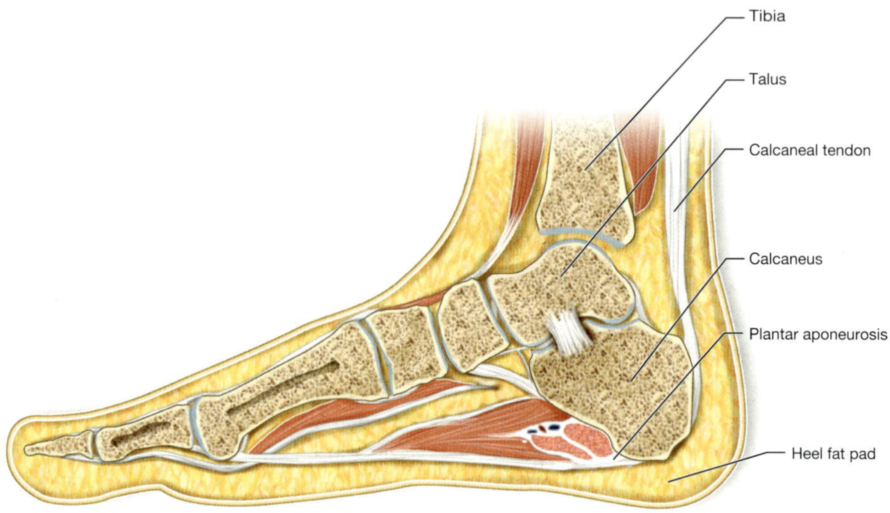

FIGURE 11.84 ● Medial right foot—sagittal section.

3. Draw a vertical line down the posterior border of the tibia.
4. Draw a horizontal line one fingerbreadth above the plantar surface.
5. Mark the point where these two lines intersect over the medial aspect of the foot.
6. At that site, press firmly on the skin with the retracted tip of a ballpoint pen. This indentation represents the entry point for the needle.
7. After the landmarks are identified, the patient should not move the foot or ankle.

ANESTHESIA

- Local anesthesia of the skin using a topical vapocoolant spray.

EQUIPMENT

- Topical vapocoolant spray
- 3-mL syringe
- 25-gauge 1½-in needle
- 1 mL of 1% lidocaine without epinephrine
- 1 mL of the steroid solution (40 mg of triamcinolone acetonide)
- One alcohol prep pad
- Two povidone-iodine or chlorhexidine prep pads
- Sterile gauze pads
- Sterile adhesive bandage
- Nonsterile, clean chucks pad

TECHNIQUE

1. Prep the insertion site with alcohol followed by the povidone-iodine or chlorhexidine pads.
2. Achieve good local anesthesia by using topical vapocoolant spray.
3. Position the needle and syringe perpendicular to the skin and the intersection of the two landmark lines with the tip of the needle directed laterally.

4. Using the no-touch technique, quickly introduce the needle at the insertion site (Fig. 11.85).
5. Advance the needle toward the medial tubercle of the calcaneus until the needle tip is located at the origin of the plantar fascia.
6. Withdraw the plunger of the syringe to ensure that there is no blood return.
7. Inject the lidocaine/corticosteroid solution as a bolus at the origin of the plantar fascia. The injected solution should flow smoothly into the space. If increased resistance is encountered, advance or withdraw the needle slightly before attempting further injection.
8. Following injection, withdraw the needle.
9. Apply a sterile adhesive bandage.
10. Instruct the patient to massage the area and then take several steps. This movement distributes the lidocaine/corticosteroid solution along the plantar fascia.
11. Reexamine the foot in 5 minutes to assess pain relief.

AFTERCARE

- NSAIDs, ice, heat, and/or physical therapy as indicated.
- Instruct the patient to perform heel cord static stretching exercises of the gastrocnemius and soleus muscles four times a day.
- Wear proper shoes or orthotics as indicated.
- Consider the use of a tension night splint.
- Consider follow-up examination in 2 weeks.

PEARLS

- The plantar fascia injection may occasionally be quite painful. This is especially true if the injection is performed through the plantar surface of the foot. The medial

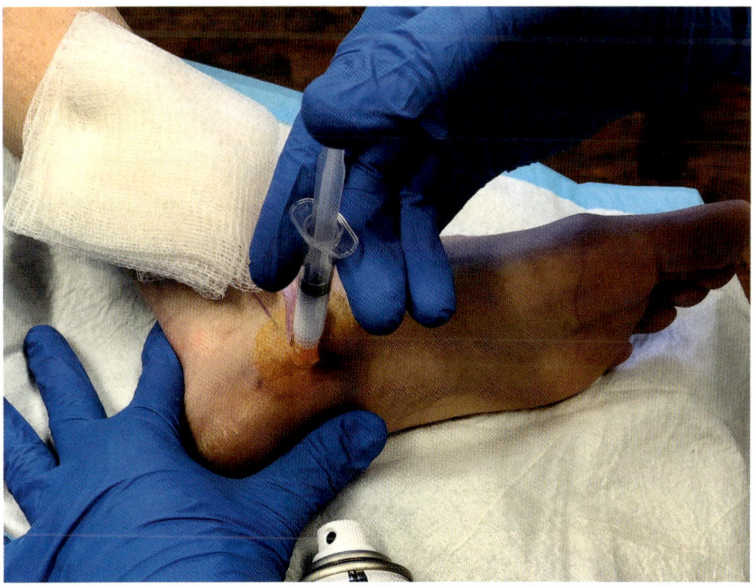

FIGURE 11.85 • Left foot plantar fasciitis injection.

approach described above minimizes the pain of this procedure. Vapocoolant spray should always be used.
- Notice the thickness of the plantar fat pad in the anatomic drawing. The injection should be placed superior to the fat pad in order to prevent fat atrophy in this critical area.

ULTRASOUND-GUIDED PROCEDURE

Please refer to the introductory ultrasound chapter for preprocedure, sterile prep, post-procedure, and documentation information and recommendations.

PATIENT POSITION

- Prone on the examination table with the affected foot resting over the end of the table.
- Place a pillow under their head for comfort.
- Adjust the patient's position as needed to ensure comfort.

PROVIDER/ULTRASOUND POSITION

- The provider sits on the opposite side at the level of the affected foot.
- Adjust the examination table to position the injection site between the provider's umbilicus and axillary level, ensuring optimal ergonomics and visualization of the ultrasound screen, transducer, and needle's approach (Fig. 11.86).
- Place the ultrasound machine on the opposite side of the table from the provider at the level of the patient's foot with the screen facing the provider.

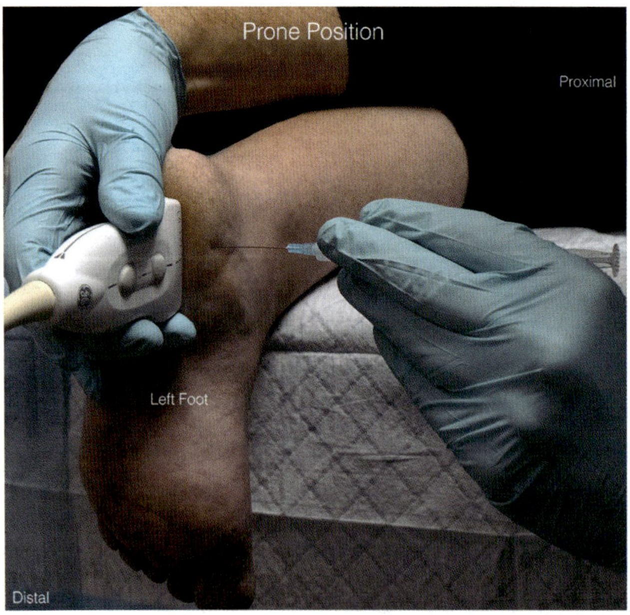

FIGURE 11.86 ● Ultrasound-guided left plantar fascia injection. Prone position with affected foot extended over the end of the examination table. Provider positioned on the contralateral side at the level of the affected foot.

LANDMARKS

- See the landmarks for the landmark-guided injection procedure.

ANESTHESIA

- Local anesthesia of the skin using topical vapocoolant spray.

EQUIPMENT

- 3-mL syringe
- 25-gauge 1.5-in needle (adjust needle length as needed)
- 1 mL of 1% lidocaine without epinephrine
- 1 mL of 40 mg/mL triamcinolone acetonide
- Three chlorhexidine swabs
- 12-4 MHz linear ultrasound transducer and machine
- Sterile ultrasound transducer cover
- Sterile ultrasound gel
- Nonlatex sterile or nonsterile gloves
- Two 4 × 4 sterile gauze pads
- One sterile adhesive bandage
- Topical vapocoolant spray

TECHNIQUE

1. Position a high-frequency linear 12-4 MHz ultrasound transducer in the sagittal plane over the plantar fascia in long axis with the medial calcaneal tubercle centered beneath it.
2. Advance a 25-gauge 1.5-in needle using an in-plane approach, directing it from medial to lateral, with an initial needle entry site about 2 cm deep from the transduce face with an angle of approximately 0° to 5° relative to the skin surface where the transducer is positioned.
3. The target area is deep to the plantar fascia at the medial calcaneal tubercle.
4. Utilize real-time ultrasound guidance throughout the procedure to precisely place the needle within the desired target area and minimize the risk of inadvertently injuring surrounding structures (Fig. 11.87).
5. Upon completion of the procedure, carefully withdraw the needle. Adhere to established postprocedure care protocols and ensure appropriate follow-up as recommended.

PEARLS

- To improve needle visualization, if an air gap forms between the transducer and the skin, place a sterile ultrasound gel standoff between them.
- Exercise caution during needle advancement to prevent inadvertent penetration of the medial calcaneal nerve and Baxter nerve. Avoid injecting corticosteroid into the plantar fascia or calcaneal fat pad.

Videos showing landmark-guided and ultrasound-guided plantar fascia injections can be found in the companion eBook.

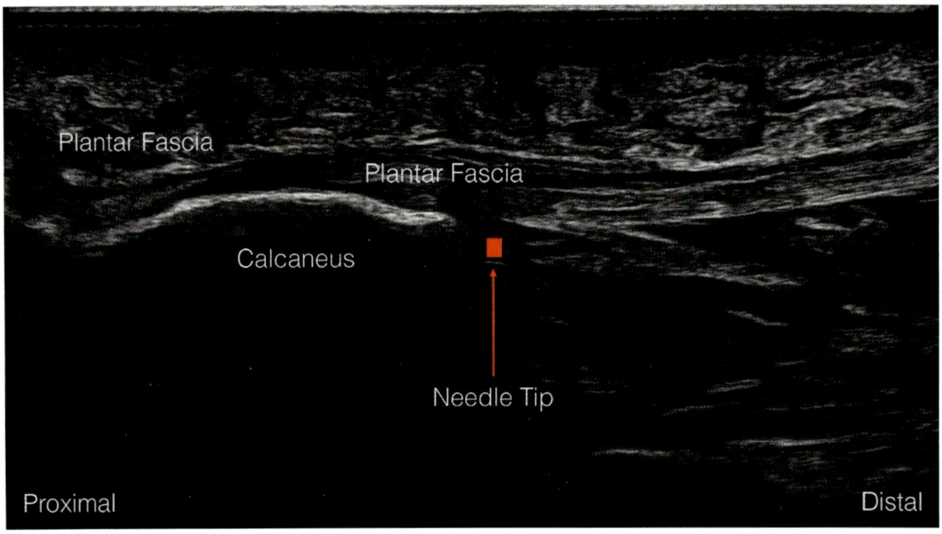

FIGURE 11.87 Plantar fascia ultrasound sagittal image.

REFERENCES

1. Trojian T, Tucker AK. Plantar fasciitis. *Am Fam Physician.* 2019;99(12):744-750.
2. Ball EM, McKeeman HM, Patterson C, et al. Steroid injection for inferior heel pain: a randomised controlled trial. *Ann Rheum Dis.* 2013;72(6):996-1002.
3. Whittaker GA, Munteanu SE, Menz HB, Bonanno DR, Gerrard JM, Landorf KB. Corticosteroid injection for plantar heel pain: a systematic review and meta-analysis. *BMC Musculoskelet Disord.* 2019;20(1):378.
4. Chen CM, Chen JS, Tsai WC, Hsu H-C, Chen K-H, Lin C-H. Effectiveness of device-assisted ultrasound-guided steroid injection for treating plantar fasciitis. *Am J Phys Med Rehabil.* 2013;92(7):597-605.
5. McMillan AM, Landorf KB, Gilheany MF, Bird AR, Morrow AD, Menz HB. Ultrasound guided corticosteroid injection for plantar fasciitis: randomised controlled trial. *BMJ.* 2012;344:e3260.
6. Gurcay E, Kara M, Karaahmet OZ, Ata AM, Onat SS, Özçakar L. Shall we inject superficial or deep to the plantar fascia? an ultrasound study of the treatment of chronic plantar fasciitis. *J Foot Ankle Surg.* 2017;56(4):783-787.
7. Chen CM, Lee M, Lin CH, Chang C-H, Lin C-H. Comparative efficacy of corticosteroid injection and non-invasive treatments for plantar fasciitis: a systematic review and meta-analysis. *Sci Rep.* 2018;8(1):4033.
8. Johannsen FE, Herzog RB, Malmgaard-Clausen NM, Hoegberget-Kalisz M, Magnusson SP, Kjaer M. Corticosteroid injection is the best treatment in plantar fasciitis if combined with controlled training. *Knee Surg Sports Traumatol Arthrosc.* 2019;27(1):5-12.
9. Mansiz-Kaplan B, Nacir B, Pervane-Vural S, Duyur-Cakit B, Genc H. Effect of dextrose prolotherapy on pain intensity, disability, and plantar fascia thickness in unilateral plantar fasciitis: a randomized, controlled, double-blind study. *Am J Phys Med Rehabil.* 2020;99(4):318-324.
10. Kothari U, Shah S, Pancholi D, Chaudhary C. Efficacy and safety of platelet-rich plasma injection for chronic plantar fasciitis: a prospective study on functional restoration and pain relief. *Cureus.* 2024;16(1):e52414.
11. Shetty SH, Dhond A, Arora M, Deore S. Platelet-rich plasma has better long-term results than corticosteroids or placebo for chronic plantar fasciitis: randomized control trial. *J Foot Ankle Surg.* 2019;58(1):42-46.
12. Acosta-Olivo C, Simental-Mendía LE, Vilchez-Cavazos F, Peña-Martínez VM, Elizondo-Rodíguez J, Simental-Mendía M. Clinical efficacy of botulinum toxin in the treatment of plantar fasciitis: a systematic review and meta-analysis of randomized controlled trials. *Arch Phys Med Rehabil.* 2022;103(2):364-371.e2.
13. Elizondo-Rodriguez J, Araujo-Lopez Y, Moreno-Gonzalez JA, Cardenas-Estrada E, Mendoza-Lemus O, Acosta-Olivo C. A comparison of botulinum toxin a and intralesional steroids for the treatment of plantar fasciitis: a randomized, double-blinded study. *Foot Ankle Int.* 2013;34(1):8-14.

Midfoot Joints

Midfoot joint pain is an unusual presenting complaint in primary care. This may occur following acute trauma or with osteoarthritis, gout, rheumatoid arthritis, or other inflammatory conditions. Conservative treatment of osteoarthritis includes weight loss, physical therapy, bracing, orthoses, and the use of acetaminophen or NSAIDs. A small-diameter needle is employed as this technique is used to inject steroid solution into painful midfoot joints. A recent study shows that corticosteroid injections are a viable diagnostic and short- to mid-term therapeutic option. The results at 4 months were statistically significant for decreased pain and with the additional finding of a difference observed between obese and nonobese patients.[1]

Relevant Anatomy: (Fig. 11.88)

PATIENT POSITION

- Supine on the examination table.
- The knee on the affected side is placed in 90° of flexion.
- The ankle is slightly plantarflexed so that the plantar surface is in full contact with the chucks pad covering the examination table.
- Rotate the patient's head away from the side that is being injected. This minimizes anxiety and pain perception.

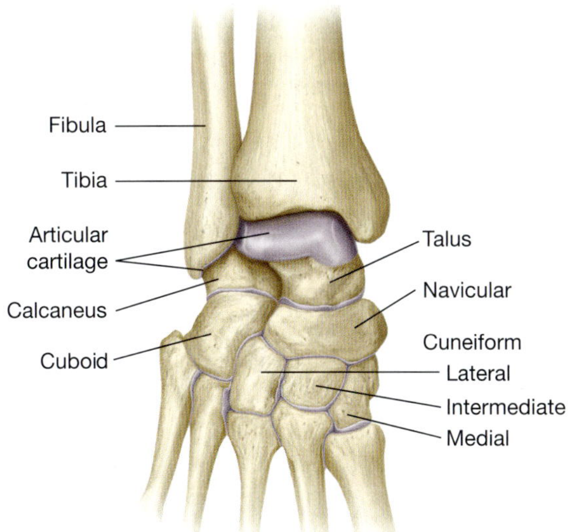

FIGURE 11.88 ● Midfoot joints.

LANDMARKS

1. With the patient lying supine on the examination table, the clinician stands or sits directly in front of the affected foot.
2. Identify the painful articulation over the dorsal aspect of the midfoot.
3. Mark a point over this articulation. There is normally a soft depression in that area.
4. At that site, press firmly on the skin with the retracted tip of a ballpoint pen. This indentation represents the entry point for the needle.
5. After the landmarks are identified, the patient should not move the foot.

ANESTHESIA

- Local anesthesia of the skin using topical vapocoolant spray.

EQUIPMENT

- Topical vapocoolant spray
- 3-mL syringe—for injection
- 25-gauge 5/8-in needle
- 0.5 mL of 1% mepivacaine without epinephrine
- 0.5 mL of the steroid solution (20 mg of triamcinolone acetonide)
- One alcohol prep pad
- Two povidone-iodine or chlorhexidine prep pads
- Sterile gauze pads
- Sterile adhesive bandage
- Nonsterile, clean chucks pad

TECHNIQUE

1. Prep the insertion site with alcohol followed by the povidone-iodine or chlorhexidine pads.
2. Achieve good local anesthesia by using topical vapocoolant spray.
3. Position the needle and syringe perpendicular to the skin with the tip of the needle directed inferiorly into the midfoot joint.
4. Using the no-touch technique, quickly introduce the needle at the insertion site (Fig. 11.89).
5. Advance the needle into the midfoot joint.
6. Withdraw the plunger of the syringe to ensure that there is no blood return.
7. Inject the mepivacaine/corticosteroid solution as a bolus into the midfoot joint. The injected solution should flow smoothly into the space. If increased resistance is encountered, advance or withdraw the needle slightly before attempting further injection.
8. Following injection, withdraw the needle.
9. Apply a sterile adhesive bandage.
10. Instruct the patient to move their foot through its full range of motion. This movement distributes the mepivacaine/corticosteroid solution throughout the midfoot joint.
11. Reexamine the foot in 5 minutes to assess pain relief.

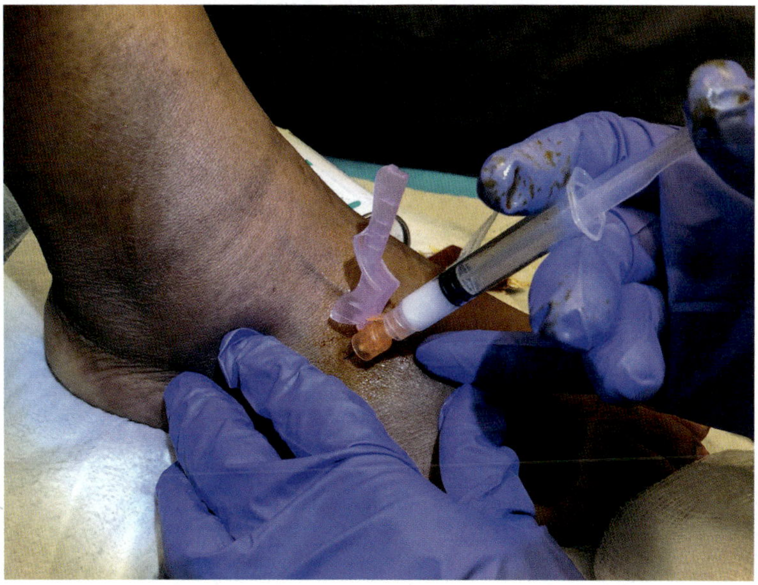

FIGURE 11.89 • Midfoot joint injection.

AFTERCARE

- Consider the use of an ankle foot orthosis.
- Avoid vigorous use of the foot over the next 2 weeks.
- NSAIDs, ice, and/or physical therapy as indicated.
- Consider follow-up examination in 2 weeks.

ULTRASOUND-GUIDED PROCEDURE

Please refer to the introductory ultrasound chapter for preprocedure, sterile prep, post-procedure, and documentation information and recommendations.

PATIENT POSITION

- Supine on the examination table with the affected foot plantarflexed on a chux pad.
- Place a pillow under their head for comfort.
- Adjust the patient's position as needed to ensure comfort.

PROVIDER/ULTRASOUND POSITION

- The provider sits on the same side at the level of the affected midfoot joint.
- Adjust the examination table to position the injection site between the provider's umbilicus and axillary level, ensuring optimal ergonomics and visualization of the ultrasound screen, transducer, and needle's approach (Fig. 11.90).
- Place the ultrasound machine on the opposite side of the table from the provider at the level of the patient's ankle with the screen facing the provider.

LANDMARKS

- See the landmarks for the landmark-guided injection procedure.

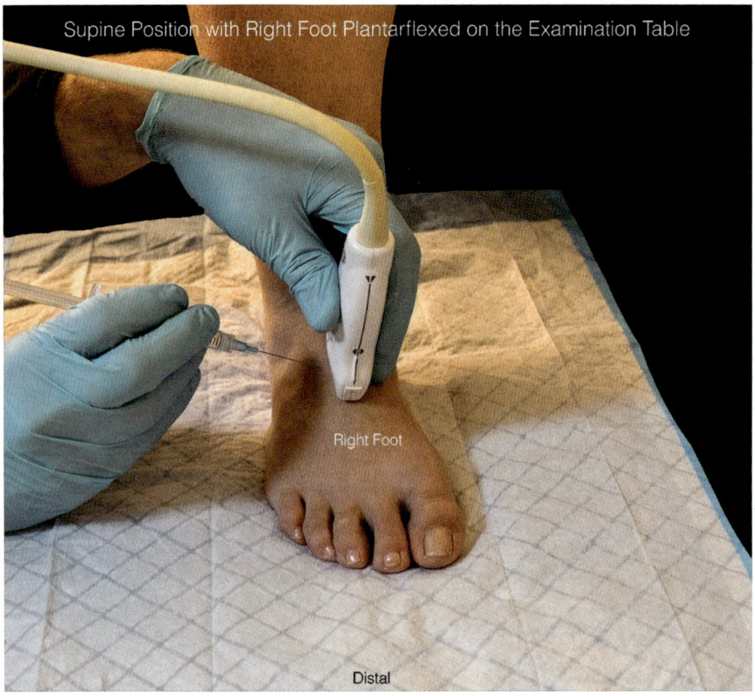

FIGURE 11.90 Ultrasound-guided right midfoot joint injection. Supine position with affected foot plantarflexed resting on the examination table. Provider positioned ipsilaterally at the level of the injection.

ANESTHESIA

- Local anesthesia of the skin using topical vapocoolant spray.

EQUIPMENT

- 3-mL syringe
- 25-gauge 1.5-in needle (adjust needle length as needed)
- 0.5 mL of 1% mepivacaine without epinephrine
- 0.5 mL of 40 mg/mL triamcinolone acetonide
- Three chlorhexidine swabs
- 12-4 MHz linear ultrasound transducer and machine
- Sterile ultrasound transducer cover
- Sterile ultrasound gel
- Nonlatex sterile or nonsterile gloves
- Two 4 × 4 sterile gauze pads
- One sterile adhesive bandage
- Topical vapocoolant spray

TECHNIQUE

1. Position a high-frequency linear 12-4 MHz ultrasound transducer in the sagittal plane with the affected midfoot joint centered beneath it.
2. Advance a 25-gauge 1.5-in needle using an out-of-plane approach, directing it from anterolateral to posteromedial, with an initial needle angle of approximately 15° to 30° relative to the skin surface where the transducer is positioned.

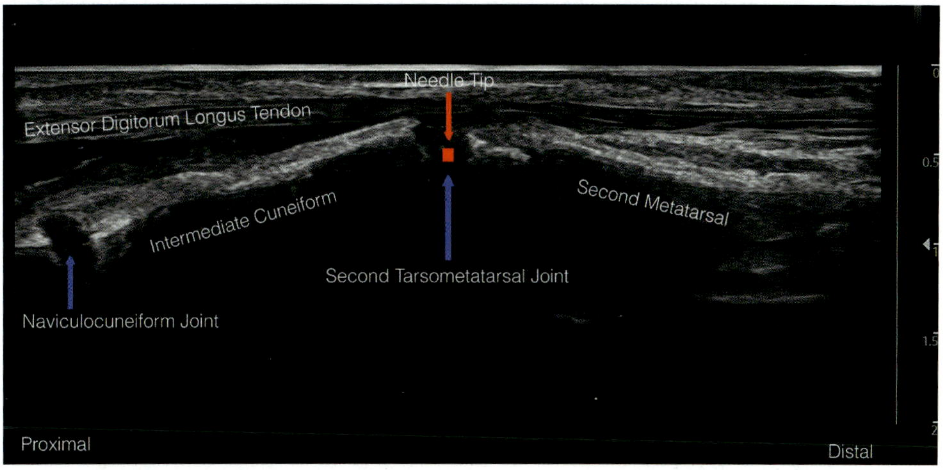

FIGURE 11.91 • Second tarsometatarsal joint ultrasound sagittal image.

3. The target area is the joint space of the affected midfoot joint (eg, second tarsometatarsal joint).
4. Utilize real-time ultrasound guidance throughout the procedure to precisely place the needle within the desired target area and minimize the risk of inadvertently injuring surrounding structures (Fig. 11.91).
5. Upon completion of the procedure, carefully withdraw the needle. Adhere to established postprocedure care protocols and ensure appropriate follow-up as recommended.

PEARLS

- While ultrasound-guided injections can be performed in any midfoot joint with appropriate indications, the cuneiform-second metatarsal joint is a frequent target due to its high prevalence of osteoarthritis.[2]
- Observe for distention of the joint capsule during injection to confirm intra-articular placement.
- Due to the small size of the midfoot joints, precise needle placement is crucial for successful intra-articular injection.

Videos showing landmark-guided and ultrasound-guided midfoot injections can be found in the companion eBook.

REFERENCES

1. Protheroe D, Gadgil A. Guided intra-articular corticosteroid injections in the midfoot. *Foot Ankle Int.* 2018;39(8):1001-1004.
2. Roddy E, Menz HB. Foot osteoarthritis: latest evidence and developments. *Ther Adv Musculoskelet Dis.* 2018;10(4):91-103.

First Metatarsophalangeal Joint

Pain involving the first metatarsophalangeal (MTP) joint of the foot is frequently encountered by primary medical providers. It is a common aspiration and injection site for diagnostic and therapeutic purposes. This great toe MTP is the most frequently involved joint by gout and is the most common site of osteoarthritis in the foot. Conservative treatment of osteoarthritis includes weight loss, physical therapy, bracing, orthoses, and the use of acetaminophen or NSAIDs. Sivera et al[1] described the use of a 29-gauge needle to successfully aspirate this joint. Corticosteroids are effective in the treatment of arthritis of the MTP joint.[2] Ultrasound may be used as a tool to select joints that will benefit from intra-articular injections.[3] Injected corticosteroids are also useful in patients with mild but not severe grades of hallux rigidus.[4]

Relevant Anatomy: (Fig. 11.92)

PATIENT POSITION

- Supine on the examination table.
- The knee on the affected side is placed in 90° of flexion.
- The ankle is slightly plantarflexed so that the plantar surface is in full contact with the chucks pad covering the examination table.
- Rotate the patient's head away from the side that is being injected. This minimizes anxiety and pain perception.

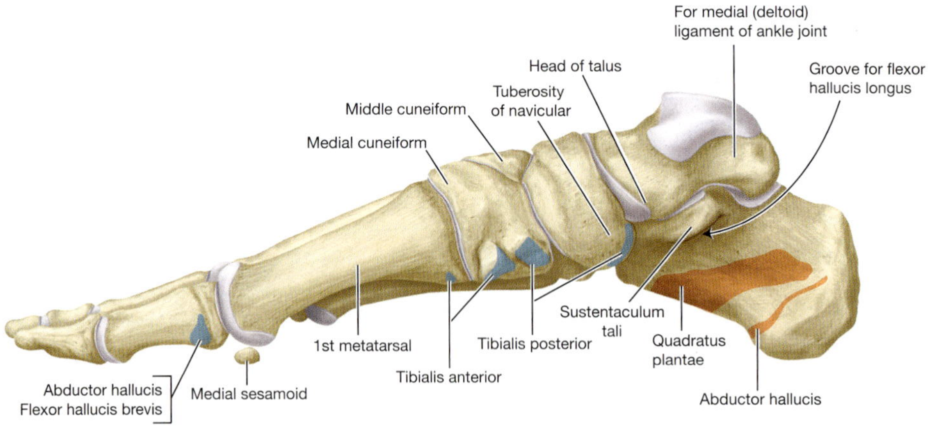

FIGURE 11.92 ● Medial aspect of the right foot—bony anatomy. (Reprinted with permission from Agur AMR, Dalley AF II. *Grant's Atlas of Anatomy*. 16th ed. Wolters Kluwer; 2025.)

LANDMARKS

1. With the patient lying supine on the examination table, the clinician stands or sits medial to the affected foot.
2. Locate the first MTP joint with simultaneous palpation and flexion/extension of the great toe proximal phalanx. The patient will report tenderness in this joint, and there may be associated erythema and swelling.
3. The injection point is directly over the first MTP joint.
4. At that site, press firmly on the skin with the retracted tip of a ballpoint pen. This indentation represents the entry point for the needle.
5. After the landmarks are identified, the patient should not move the foot or toe.

ANESTHESIA

- Local anesthesia of the skin using topical vapocoolant spray.

EQUIPMENT

- Topical vapocoolant spray
- 3-mL syringe
- 3-mL syringe—for optional aspiration
- 25-gauge 5/8-in needle for injection
- 25-gauge 5/8-in needle for optional aspiration
- 0.25 to 0.5 mL of 1% mepivacaine without epinephrine
- 0.25 to 0.5 mL of the steroid solution (10-20 mg of triamcinolone acetonide)
- One alcohol prep pad
- Two povidone-iodine or chlorhexidine prep pads
- Sterile gauze pads
- Sterile adhesive bandage
- Nonsterile, clean chucks pad

TECHNIQUE

1. Prep the insertion site with alcohol followed by the povidone-iodine or chlorhexidine pads.
2. Achieve good local anesthesia by using topical vapocoolant spray.
3. Position the needle and syringe perpendicular to the skin with the tip of the needle directed into the center of the joint.
4. Using the no-touch technique, quickly introduce the needle at the insertion site (Fig. 11.93).
5. Advance the needle until the tip is located in the joint capsule. If the needle contacts bone or cartilage, back up the needle 1 to 2 mm.
6. If aspirating, withdraw fluid using the 25-gauge 5/8-in needle with a 3-mL syringe.
7. If injection following aspiration is elected, remove the 3-mL syringe from the 25-gauge needle and then attach the 3-mL syringe filled with the mepivacaine/corticosteroid solution.
8. If only injecting mepivacaine/corticosteroid solution, use a 25-gauge 5/8-in needle with the 3-mL syringe.

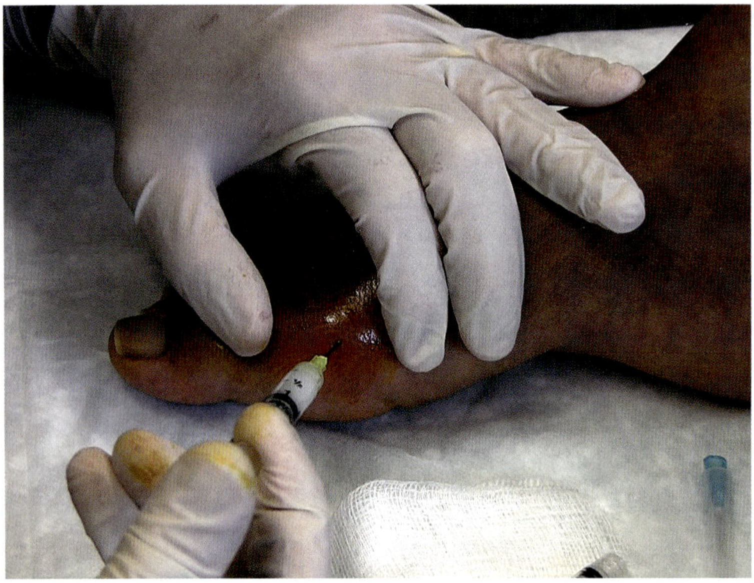

FIGURE 11.93 ● Right first metatarsophalangeal joint injection.

9. Inject the mepivacaine/corticosteroid solution as a bolus into the joint capsule. The injected solution should flow smoothly into the space. If increased resistance is encountered, advance or withdraw the needle slightly before attempting further injection.
10. Following injection, withdraw the needle.
11. Apply a sterile adhesive bandage.
12. Instruct the patient to move their toe through its full range of motion. This movement distributes the mepivacaine/corticosteroid solution throughout the joint capsule.
13. Reexamine the first MTP joint in 5 minutes to assess pain relief.

AFTERCARE

- Avoid excessive movement of the first MTP joint over the next 2 weeks.
- NSAIDs, ice, and/or physical therapy as indicated.
- Consider the use of an ankle-foot orthotic or wooden-soled shoe.
- Consider follow-up examination in 2 weeks.

PEARLS

- Applying traction to the great toe in a distal direction may help open up the joint to accommodate the needle.

ULTRASOUND-GUIDED PROCEDURE

Please refer to the introductory ultrasound chapter for preprocedure, sterile prep, postprocedure, and documentation information and recommendations.

PATIENT POSITION

- Supine on the examination table with the affected foot plantarflexed on a chux pad.
- Place the unaffected extremity tucked underneath the affected extremity for patient comfort.
- Place a pillow under their head for comfort.
- Adjust the patient's position as needed to ensure comfort.

PROVIDER/ULTRASOUND POSITION

- The provider sits on the opposite side at the level of the affected MTP joint.
- Adjust the examination table to position the injection site between the provider's umbilicus and axillary level, ensuring optimal ergonomics and visualization of the ultrasound screen, transducer, and needle's approach (Fig. 11.94).
- Place the ultrasound machine on the opposite side of the table from the provider at the level of the patient's foot with the screen facing the provider.

LANDMARKS

- See the landmarks for the landmark-guided injection procedure.

ANESTHESIA

- Local anesthesia of the skin using topical vapocoolant spray.

EQUIPMENT

- 3-mL syringe
- 25-gauge 1.5-in needle (adjust needle length as needed)

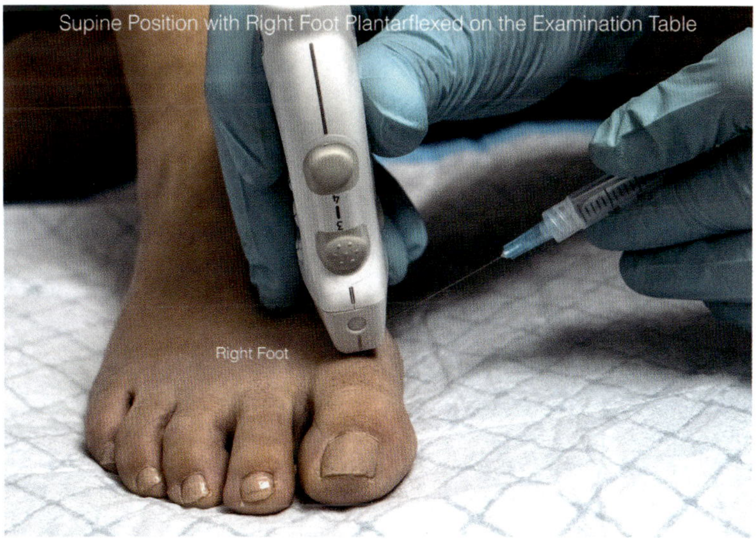

FIGURE 11.94 ● Ultrasound-guided right first metatarsophalangeal joint injection. Supine position with affected foot plantarflexed resting on the examination table. Provider positioned contralaterally at the injection site.

- 0.5 mL of 1% mepivacaine without epinephrine
- 0.5 mL of 40 mg/mL triamcinolone acetonide
- Alternative setup for aspiration
  - 3-mL syringe (anesthesia)
    - 22-gauge 1.5-in needle (adjust needle length as needed)
    - 3 mL of 1% lidocaine without epinephrine
  - 3-mL syringe
    - 18-gauge 1.5-in needle (adjust needle length as needed)
- Three chlorhexidine swabs
- 12-4 MHz linear ultrasound transducer and machine
- Sterile ultrasound transducer cover
- Sterile ultrasound gel
- Nonlatex sterile or nonsterile gloves
- Two 4 × 4 sterile gauze pads
- One sterile adhesive bandage
- Topical vapocoolant spray

TECHNIQUE

1. Position a high-frequency linear 12-4 MHz ultrasound transducer in the sagittal plane over the first MTP joint with the joint space centered beneath it.
2. Advance a 25-gauge 1.5-in needle using an out-of-plane approach, directing it from anteromedial to posterolateral, with an initial needle angle of approximately 15° to 30° relative to the skin surface where the transducer is positioned.
3. The target area is the affected first MTP joint.
4. Utilize real-time ultrasound guidance throughout the procedure to precisely place the needle within the desired target area and minimize the risk of inadvertently injuring surrounding structures (Fig. 11.95).
5. For intra-articular steroid injection:
   a. Slowly inject the desired volume of mepivacaine and corticosteroid solution directly into the joint.
6. For situations requiring anesthesia, aspiration, or both:
   a. Utilize a separate 25-gauge 1.5-in needle with a 3-mL syringe to inject 3 mL of 1% lidocaine without epinephrine into the soft tissues overlying the joint.
   b. For aspiration, use an 18-gauge 1.5-in needle with a 3-mL syringe to withdraw the effusion.

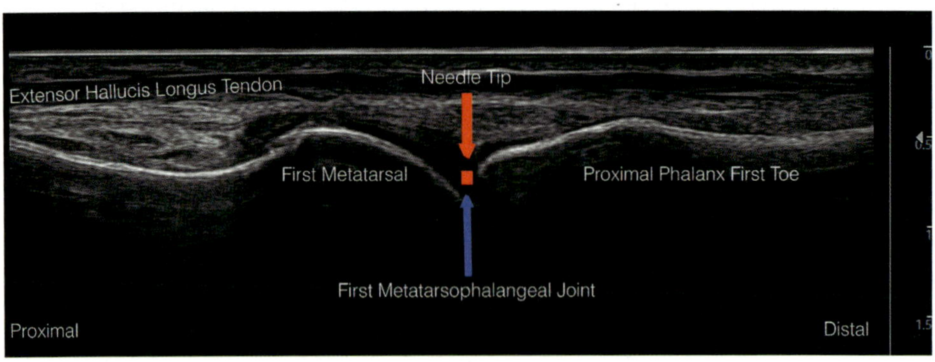

FIGURE 11.95 ● First metatarsophalangeal joint ultrasound sagittal image.

   c. If a corticosteroid injection is indicated following aspiration, replace the aspiration syringe with the mepivacaine and corticosteroid solution syringe and reconfirm accurate needle placement using real-time ultrasound guidance before injection.
7. Upon completion of the procedure, carefully withdraw the needle. Adhere to established postprocedure care protocols and ensure appropriate follow-up as recommended.

PEARLS

- Observe for distention of the joint capsule during injection to confirm intra-articular placement.
- Due to the small size of the first MTP joint, precise needle placement is crucial for successful intra-articular injection.

Videos showing landmark-guided and ultrasound-guided first MTP joint injections can be found in the companion eBook.

REFERENCES

1. Sivera F, Aragon R, Pascual E. First metatarsophalangeal joint aspiration using a 29-gauge needle. *Ann Rheum Dis.* 2008;67(2):273-275.
2. Emami Razavi SZ, Azadvari M, Fateh HR, Akbari MG, Kazemi S, Rezaee E. Short-term efficacy of ultrasonographic guidance for intra-articular corticosteroid injection in hallux rigidus: a single-blind randomized controlled trial. *Foot Ankle Int.* 2021;42(11):1410-1418.
3. Nordberg LB, Lillegraven S, Aga AB, et al. The impact of ultrasound on the use and efficacy of intraarticular glucocorticoid injections in early rheumatoid arthritis: secondary analyses from a randomized trial examining the benefit of ultrasound in a clinical tight control regimen. *Arthritis Rheumatol.* 2018;70(8):1192-1199.
4. Solan MC, Calder JD, Bendall SP. Manipulation and injection for hallux rigidus: is it worthwhile? *J Bone Joint Surg Br.* 2001;83:706-708.

Intermetatarsal (Morton) Neuroma

Compression of the interdigital nerves as they course between the metatarsal bones in the foot can result in a painful condition referred to as a Morton neuroma. This is a fairly common condition seen by primary care clinicians. The disorder is a compressive neuropathy often causing inflammation, perineural fibrosis, and enlargement of the interdigital nerve(s). It presents symptoms of significant lancinating pain and dysesthesias with weight bearing—especially when wearing shoes with a narrow toe box. Usually, the neuroma lies between the second and third or the third and fourth metatarsal heads. Conservative treatment strategies include shoe-wear modifications, custom-made orthotics, and corticosteroid injections.

Corticosteroid injections to treat Morton neuromas have been demonstrated to be safe and effective for both short- to medium-term pain relief.[1,2] Corticosteroid injections and manipulation/mobilization are the two interventions with the strongest evidence for pain reduction.[3] Ultrasound-guided steroid injections in Morton neuroma leads to a higher percentage of short-term pain relief and fewer skin side effects than landmark-based injections.[4] However, treatment failures are encountered. The size of the neuroma on ultrasonography is the sole predictor of corticosteroid injection failure.[5] With a cut-off value of 6.3 mm, larger Morton neuromas are associated with failure of corticosteroid injection.[6]

Sclerosant treatment with ultrasound-guided alcohol injections into the substance of the neuroma is a promising intervention as summarized in a recent systematic review.[7] Perini et al[8] also demonstrated significant relief of neuropathic symptoms and a good safety profile using this technique in a relatively large study. Patients who do not respond to conservative management and injections may require operative intervention with nerve decompression or neurectomy.

Relevant Anatomy: (Fig. 11.96)

PATIENT POSITION

- Supine on the examination table.
- The knee on the affected side is placed in 90° of flexion.
- The ankle is slightly plantarflexed so that the plantar surface is in full contact with the chucks pad covering the examination table.
- Rotate the patient's head away from the side that is being injected. This minimizes anxiety and pain perception.

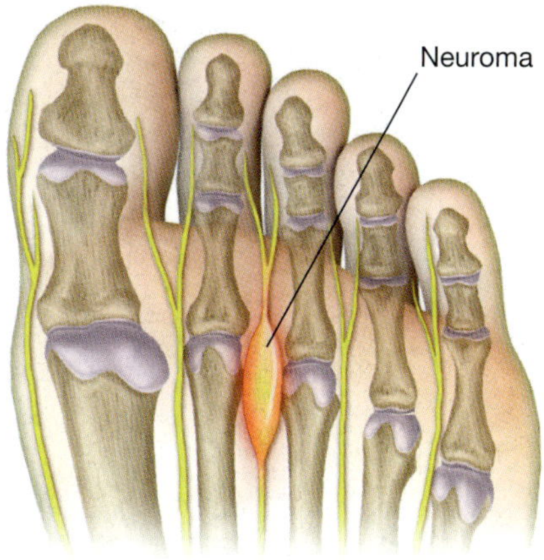

FIGURE 11.96 • Dorsal aspect of the right foot.

LANDMARKS

1. With the patient lying supine on the examination table, the clinician stands or sits in front of the affected foot.
2. Locate the site of maximal tenderness. This is found between the heads of the metatarsals. The most common sites are located between the second and third, or the third and fourth metatarsal heads.
3. The injection point is on the dorsal aspect of the distal foot directly over the area of maximal tenderness. A tender nodule may be palpated occasionally at this site.
4. At that site, press firmly on the skin with the retracted tip of a ballpoint pen. This indentation represents the entry point for the needle.
5. After the landmarks are identified, the patient should not move the foot.

ANESTHESIA

- Local anesthesia of the skin using topical vapocoolant spray.

EQUIPMENT

- Topical vapocoolant spray
- 3-mL syringe
- 25-gauge 1-in needle
- 0.5 mL of 1% lidocaine without epinephrine
- 0.5 mL of the steroid solution (20 mg of triamcinolone acetonide)
- One alcohol prep pad
- Two povidone-iodine or chlorhexidine prep pads
- Sterile gauze pads
- Sterile adhesive bandage
- Nonsterile, clean chucks pad

TECHNIQUE

1. Prep the insertion site with alcohol followed by the povidone-iodine or chlorhexidine pads.
2. Achieve good local anesthesia by using topical vapocoolant spray.

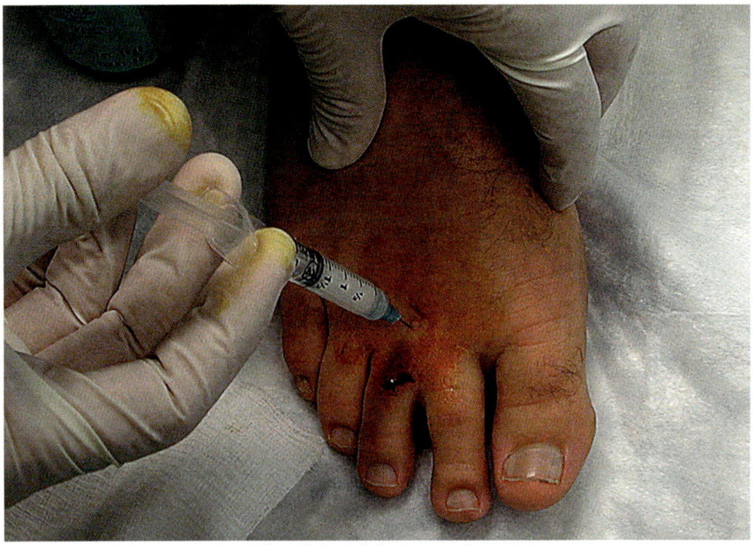

FIGURE 11.97 ● Morton neuroma injection.

3. Position the needle and syringe perpendicular to the skin with the tip of the needle directed inferiorly between the affected metatarsal heads.
4. Using the no-touch technique, quickly introduce the needle at the insertion site (Fig. 11.97).
5. Advance the needle until the needle tip is located in the neuroma between the metatarsal heads.
6. Withdraw the plunger of the syringe to ensure that there is no blood return.
7. Inject the lidocaine/corticosteroid solution as a bolus into or around the neuroma. The injected solution should flow smoothly. If increased resistance is encountered, advance or withdraw the needle slightly before attempting further injection.
8. Following injection, withdraw the needle.
9. Apply a sterile adhesive bandage.
10. Instruct the patient to massage the area of injection. This movement distributes the lidocaine/corticosteroid solution around the neuroma.
11. Reexamine the foot in 5 minutes to assess pain relief.

AFTERCARE

- Avoid wearing shoes with a narrow toe box.
- NSAIDs, ice, and/or physical therapy as indicated.
- Consider metatarsal pads or custom orthotics.
- Consider follow-up examination in 2 weeks.

ULTRASOUND-GUIDED PROCEDURE

Please refer to the introductory ultrasound chapter for preprocedure, sterile prep, post-procedure, and documentation information and recommendations.

PATIENT POSITION

- Supine on the examination table with the affected foot plantarflexed on a chux pad.
- Place a pillow under their head for comfort.
- Adjust the patient's position as needed to ensure comfort.

PROVIDER/ULTRASOUND POSITION

- The provider sits at the affected webspace.
- Adjust the examination table to position the injection site between the provider's umbilicus and axillary level, ensuring optimal ergonomics and visualization of the ultrasound screen, transducer, and needle's approach (Fig. 11.98).
- Place the ultrasound machine on the same side of the table from at the level of the patient's hip with the screen facing the provider.

LANDMARKS

- See the landmarks for the landmark-guided injection procedure.

ANESTHESIA

- Local anesthesia of the skin using topical vapocoolant spray.

EQUIPMENT

- 3-mL syringe
- 25-gauge 1.5-in needle (adjust needle length as needed)
- 0.5 mL of 1% lidocaine without epinephrine
- 0.5 mL of 40 mg/mL triamcinolone acetonide
- Three chlorhexidine swabs

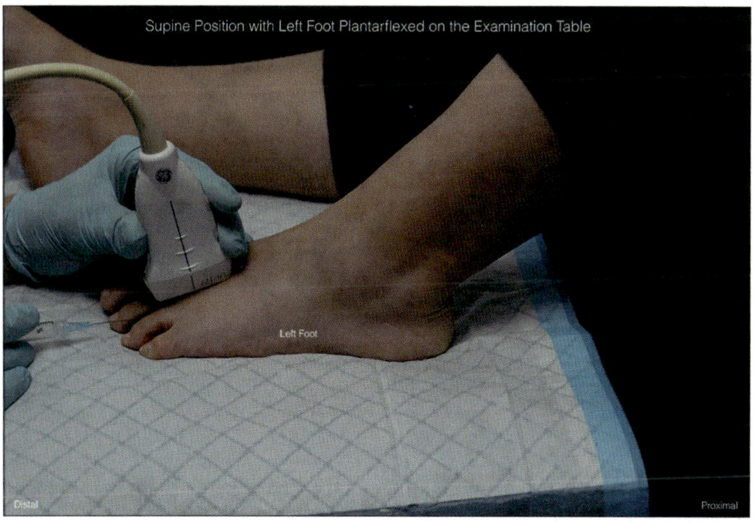

FIGURE 11.98 • Ultrasound-guided left Morton neuroma injection. Supine position with affected foot plantarflexed resting on the examination table. Provider positioned distally to the injection site.

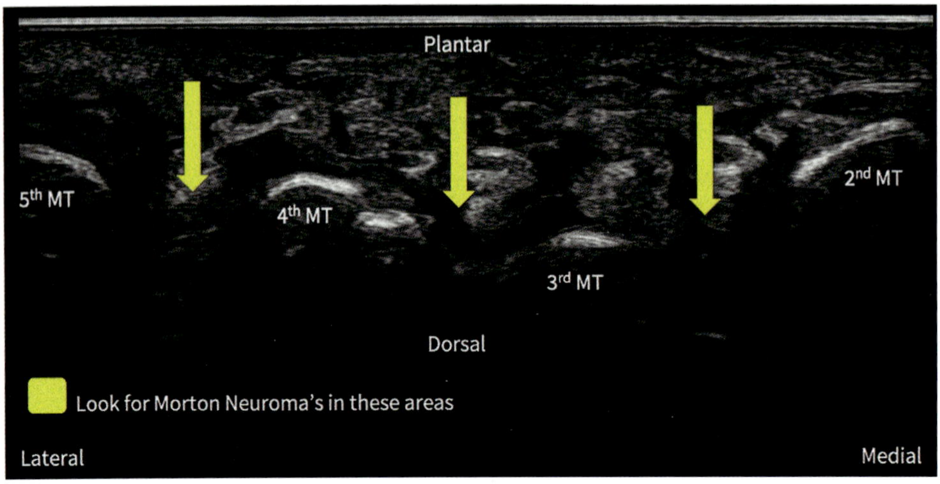

FIGURE 11.99 ● Metatarsal webspace ultrasound axial image.

- 12-4 MHz linear ultrasound transducer and machine
- Sterile ultrasound transducer cover
- Sterile ultrasound gel
- Nonlatex sterile or nonsterile gloves
- Two 4 × 4 sterile gauze pads
- One sterile adhesive bandage
- Topical vapocoolant spray

TECHNIQUE

1. Position a high-frequency linear 12-4 MHz ultrasound transducer in the sagittal plane over the affected metatarsal webspace, centering the Morton neuroma within the image.
2. Advance a 25-gauge 1.5-in needle using an in-plane approach, directing it from distal to proximal, with an initial entry site in the webspace about 1 cm deep to the transducer face and a needle angle of approximately 0° to 5° relative to the skin surface where the transducer is positioned.
3. The target area is the perineural space of the neuroma.
4. Utilize real-time ultrasound guidance throughout the procedure to precisely place the needle within the desired target area and minimize the risk of inadvertently injuring surrounding structures (Fig. 11.99).
5. Upon completion of the procedure, carefully withdraw the needle. Adhere to established postprocedure care protocols and ensure appropriate follow-up as recommended.

PEARLS

- If an air gap forms between the transducer and the skin, use a sterile ultrasound gel standoff to improve image contact and visualization.
- Exercise caution to avoid an intraneural injection or inadvertent penetration of the plantar vessels during needle advancement.

A video showing a landmark-guided intermetatarsal (Morton) neuroma injection can be found in the companion eBook.

REFERENCES

1. Markovic M, Crichton K, Read JW, et al. Effectiveness of ultrasound-guided corticosteroid injection in the treatment of Morton's neuroma. *Foot Ankle Int.* 2008;29(5):483-487.
2. Edwards SR, Fleming S, Landorf KB. Efficacy of a single corticosteroid injection for Morton's neuroma in adults: a systematic review. *J Am Podiatr Med Assoc.* 2021;111(4):Article_13.
3. Matthews BG, Hurn SE, Harding MP, Henry RA, Ware RS. The effectiveness of non-surgical interventions for common plantar digital compressive neuropathy (Morton's neuroma): a systematic review and meta-analysis. *J Foot Ankle Res.* 2019;12:12.
4. Santiago FR, Muñoz PT, Ramos-Bossini AJL, Martínez AM, Olleta NP. Long-term comparison between blind and ultrasound-guided corticoid injections in Morton neuroma. *Eur Radiol.* 2022;32(12):8414-8422.
5. Park YH, Kim TJ, Choi GW, Kim HJ. Prediction of clinical prognosis according to intermetatarsal distance and neuroma size on ultrasonography in Morton neuroma: a prospective observational study. *J Ultrasound Med.* 2019;38(4):1009-1014.
6. Park YH, Lee JW, Choi GW, Kim HJ. Risk factors and the associated cutoff values for failure of corticosteroid injection in treatment of Morton's neuroma. *Int Orthop.* 2018;42(2):323-329.
7. Santos D, Morrison G, Coda A. Sclerosing alcohol injections for the management of intermetatarsal neuromas: a systematic review. *Foot (Edinb).* 2018;35:36-47.
8. Perini L, Perini C, Tagliapietra M, et al. Percutaneous alcohol injection under sonographic guidance in Morton's neuroma: follow-up in 220 treated lesions. *Radiol Med.* 2016;121(7):597-604.

APPENDIX 1

Consent for Needle Aspiration and/or Injection

Date: ________________

I hereby authorize ____

(Provider's name)

to perform upon

____

(Patient's name)

the following procedure(s): ____________________________________

____

____

The procedure(s) consists of: ___________________________________

____

____

____

(Describe in lay language)

Possible risks associated with the performance of a needle injection/aspiration may include but are not limited to:
Bleeding, Infection, Local pain, Fainting, Allergic reaction, or

____

Possible risks with the use of injected corticosteroids may include but are not limited to:

Feeling flushed
Tendon rupture
Abnormal skin color
Impaired immune response
Irregular menstrual periods
Flare-up of joint inflammation
Abnormal thinning of the skin
Worsening blood sugars in diabetes
Disturbance of hormone balance

The nature of this procedure, methods of diagnosis/treatment, and possible alternatives have been explained to me by __________________ or his/her associate. I am aware that there are certain risks associated with this procedure and that the practice of medicine and surgery is not an exact science. I acknowledge that no guarantees have been made to me concerning the results of the procedure or its interpretation.

I certify that I understand the contents of this form:

____

Signature of patient or authorized representative

____

Witness

IF THE PATIENT IS UNABLE TO CONSENT OR IS A MINOR, COMPLETE THE FOLLOWING:

The patient is a minor, ____ years of age, or is unable to consent because ____________

____(strike or define).

The undersigned hereby consents to the performance of the above described diagnostic/therapeutic procedure on the above patient as well as any tests, which are deemed necessary.

____

Signature of authorized representative

APPENDIX 2

Medical Record Documentation

The following is an example of documentation that may be used for a knee aspiration and injection procedure with ultrasound guidance. Creating a text template, either this version or a customized variation, in an electronic medical record provides the practitioner with flexibility to document the diverse scenarios that may be encountered during the procedure.

Patient name: ____ Date: __________

Procedure—Knee Aspiration and Injection with Ultrasound Guidance:
Prior to performance of the knee aspiration and injection, a discussion of the nature of this procedure, proposed benefits, material risks, and alternative treatments was conducted with the patient. All questions were answered.

After written informed consent was obtained, the patient was placed in the supine position on the examination table. The musculoskeletal probe with the [Brand/Model] ultrasound machine was used. An ultrasound survey of the knee joint structures was performed in the sagittal and transverse planes.

Lateral Suprapatellar Approach:
A point at the intersection of a line in the axial plane 2 cm above the patella and a line, perpendicular to the first, in the coronal plane at the undersurface of the patella was identified and marked with the retracted tip of a ball point pen. The superior-lateral aspect of the knee was prepped in a sterile fashion by wiping with a single alcohol prep pad followed by two 10% povidone–iodine (or two 2% chlorhexidine) prep pads. Topical [Brand] vapocoolant spray was used to achieve good transient local anesthesia.

Following the no-touch technique:
For injection only:
❑ a 2″ 25-gauge needle was inserted and directed medially into the knee joint capsule under direct ultrasound guidance with the needle in the long axis and in-plane. The image was documented.

For aspiration and injection:
❑ a 2″ 25-gauge needle was inserted and directed medially into the knee joint capsule under direct ultrasound guidance with the needle in the long axis and in-plane. A total of 4 mL of 1% lidocaine without epinephrine was injected immediately under the skin and also adjacent to the joint capsule over the anterior aspect of the distal femur—to achieve adequate local anesthesia of these structures.

❑ Next, a 1 1/2″ 18-gauge needle was directed medially into the knee joint capsule under direct ultrasound guidance. The image was documented.
❑ No; ❑ A small amount; ❑ A moderate amount; ❑ A large amount; of fluid was observed.
❑ No; ❑ ____ mL of ____________(describe appearance)____________ fluid was removed.

Finally, a mixture of 1 mL of 1% mepivacaine without epinephrine and 1 mL of Kenalog (40 mg) was injected easily into the knee joint through the ❑ 25-gauge needle, ❑ 18-gauge needle

The needle was withdrawn. No bleeding was encountered. The injection site was covered with a sterile adhesive bandage.
The patient tolerated the procedure well without complications.
The patient reported complete relief of pain and demonstrated full range of motion within 5 minutes.
The aftercare handout was provided and instructions discussed. The patient indicated understanding about recurring pain, resting the affected area, watching for and immediately reporting any signs of possible infection.

Other:

____

____

____

____

____
Signature of medical provider

APPENDIX 3

Aspiration and Injection Aftercare Handout

You have just had a procedure done by: ______________________________

Your diagnosis is: ______________________________

The procedure involved placing a needle into the tissues to:

____ withdraw fluid from the ______________________________

____ inject "cortisone" into the ______________________________

____ other ______________________________

Please Follow These Instructions:

Recurring Pain:
Injections are usually done using a local anesthetic such as lidocaine or mepivacaine mixed with cortisone. The anesthetic effect of the lidocaine or mepivacaine usually lasts for 30 to 60 minutes and then wears off. At that time, your pain will return. Improvement in pain from the cortisone injection usually takes 24 to 48 hours. So, expect the pain to return after an hour and hopefully go away in 1 to 2 days.

Rest the Area:
Be careful with the affected area/joint. Usually, the injected medication causes the area to feel numb. Because you may not feel pain, it is easy to suffer further injury to the area. Do not use the area for anything more than mild essential movements for the next 2 weeks.

Watch for Infection:
Although every precaution has been taken to prevent infection, be alert for the following signs—fever above 100 °F, increased warmth in the area, redness at the injection site, redness moving up the arm or leg, and swelling of the area.

If *any* of these symptoms develop, call this office immediately at any time of day or night (INSERT PHONE NUMBER).

Follow the Directions of Any Checked Boxes:
❑ Apply ice to the area every 4 hours for 20 minutes at a time for ____ day(s).
❑ Apply a heating pad to the area every 4 hours for 20 minutes at a time for ____ day(s).
❑ Apply an elastic compression wrap to the area for ____ day(s).
❑ Perform stretching exercises as instructed.

❑ Wear a splint to the area for ____ day(s).
❑ Referral for Physical Therapy.
❑ Take the following medicines in addition to your usual medications:

____

____

____

Return to this office in ____ day(s)/week(s) for further evaluation and management of your condition.

Index

Note: Page numbers followed by '*f*' indicate figures; those followed by '*t*' indicate tables.

D

E

F

G

J

K

L

M

N

V

W